CLINICAL FOCUS SERIES

Tuberculosis
Selected Problems

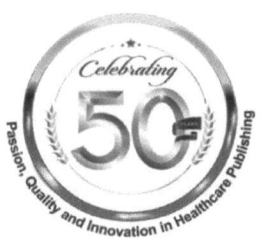

CLINICAL FOCUS SERIES

Tuberculosis
Selected Problems

Editors

Violeta V Mihailovic Vucinic MD
Professor of Internal Medicine and Pulmonology
Vth Clinical Department for Sarcoidosis and
other Granulomatous Diseases
University Hospital of Pulmonology
Clinical Centre of Serbia
Belgrade, Serbia

Dragana M Jovanovic MD PhD
Professor of Internal Medicine
VIth Clinical Department
University Hospital of Pulmonology
Clinical Centre of Serbia
Belgrade, Serbia

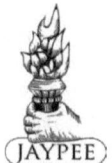

JAYPEE BROTHERS MEDICAL PUBLISHERS
The Health Sciences Publisher
New Delhi | London | Panama

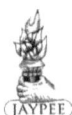

Jaypee Brothers Medical Publishers (P) Ltd

Headquarters

Jaypee Brothers Medical Publishers (P) Ltd
4838/24, Ansari Road, Daryaganj
New Delhi 110 002, India
Phone: +91-11-43574357
Fax: +91-11-43574314
Email: jaypee@jaypeebrothers.com

Overseas Offices

J.P. Medical Ltd
83 Victoria Street, London
SW1H 0HW (UK)
Phone: +44 20 3170 8910
Fax: +44 (0)20 3008 6180
Email: info@jpmedpub.com

Jaypee-Highlights Medical Publishers Inc
City of Knowledge, Bld. 235, 2nd Floor, Clayton
Panama City, Panama
Phone: +1 507-301-0496
Fax: +1 507-301-0499
Email: cservice@jphmedical.com

Jaypee Brothers Medical Publishers (P) Ltd
Bhotahity, Kathmandu, Nepal
Phone: +977-9741283608
Email: kathmandu@jaypeebrothers.com

Website: www.jaypeebrothers.com
Website: www.jaypeedigital.com

© 2019, Jaypee Brothers Medical Publishers

The views and opinions expressed in this book are solely those of the original contributor(s)/author(s) and do not necessarily represent those of editor(s) of the book.

All rights reserved. No part of this publication may be reproduced, stored or transmitted in any form or by any means, electronic, mechanical, photocopying, recording or otherwise, without the prior permission in writing of the publishers.

All brand names and product names used in this book are trade names, service marks, trademarks or registered trademarks of their respective owners. The publisher is not associated with any product or vendor mentioned in this book.

Medical knowledge and practice change constantly. This book is designed to provide accurate, authoritative information about the subject matter in question. However, readers are advised to check the most current information available on procedures included and check information from the manufacturer of each product to be administered, to verify the recommended dose, formula, method and duration of administration, adverse effects and contraindications. It is the responsibility of the practitioner to take all appropriate safety precautions. Neither the publisher nor the author(s)/editor(s) assume any liability for any injury and/or damage to persons or property arising from or related to use of material in this book.

This book is sold on the understanding that the publisher is not engaged in providing professional medical services. If such advice or services are required, the services of a competent medical professional should be sought.

Every effort has been made where necessary to contact holders of copyright to obtain permission to reproduce copyright material. If any have been inadvertently overlooked, the publisher will be pleased to make the necessary arrangements at the first opportunity. The **CD/DVD-ROM** (if any) provided in the sealed envelope with this book is complimentary and free of cost. **Not meant for sale.**

Inquiries for bulk sales may be solicited at: jaypee@jaypeebrothers.com

Clinical Focus Series

Tuberculosis: Selected Problems / Violeta V Mihailovic Vucinic, Dragana M Jovanovic

First Edition: **2019**

ISBN: 978-93-86261-35-9

CONTRIBUTORS

EDITORS

Violeta V Mihailovic Vucinic MD
Professor of Internal Medicine and Pulmonology
Vth Clinical Department for
Sarcoidosis and
other Granulomatous Diseases
University Hospital of Pulmonology
Clinical Centre of Serbia
Belgrade, Serbia

Dragana M Jovanovic MD PhD
Professor of Internal Medicine
VIth Clinical Department
University Hospital of Pulmonology
Clinical Centre of Serbia
Belgrade, Serbia

CONTRIBUTING AUTHORS

Anand Jaiswal MD
Director
Department of Respiratoy Diseases and Sleep Medicine
Medanta-The Medicity
Gurugram, Haryana, India

Anna L Rich FRCP MD
Respiratory Consultant and
Honorary Lecturer
Department of Respiratory Medicine
Nottingham University Hospitals
Nottingham, UK

Ashok Shah DTCD MD Fellow National Academy of Medical Sciences (India)
Director Professor (Retd)
Department of Pulmonary Medicine
Vallabhbhai Patel Chest Institute
University of Delhi
Delhi, India

Atul C Mehta MD FACP FCCP
Professor of Medicine
Lerner College of Medicine
Buoncore Family Endowed Chair in
Lung Transplantation
Staff
Department of Pulmonary Medicine
Respiratory Institute
Cleveland Clinic
Cleveland, Ohio, USA

Bojana Luković MD
Head of the National Reference Laboratory for Tuberculosis
Department of Microbiology
Clinical Center of Serbia
Belgrade, Serbia

Dipti Gothi MD
Professor, Department of Respiratory Diseases
ESI-PGIMSR Hospital
New Delhi, India

Dragica P Pesut MSc PhD
Professor, Internal Medicine Department
University of Belgrade School of Medicine
Head of Department
IVth Clinical Department
Clinical Center of Serbia, Teaching Hospital of
Pulmonology
Belgrade, Republic of Serbia

Hannah Jarvis MBBS BSc MRCP
Specialist Registrar in Respiratory Medicine
Chest and Allergy Department
St Mary's Hospital
Imperial College NHS Trust
London, UK

Kamal Gera MD
Junior Resident
Department of Pulmonary Medicine
Vallabhbhai Patel Chest Institute
University of Delhi
Delhi, India

Kamal K Singhal MD DCH
Associate Professor, Department of Pediatrics
Lady Hardinge Medical College and Kalawati
Saran Children's Hospital
New Delhi, India

Müge Aydoğdu MD
Associate Professor
Department of Pulmonary Diseases
Department and Critical Care Unit
Gazi University
Ankara, Turkey

Onn M Kon MD FRCP
Consultant Respiratory Physician
Chest and Allergy Clinic,
St Mary's Hospital
Imperial College Healthcare NHS Trust
London, UK

Ravindra K Dewan MS MCh
Head, Department of Thoracic Surgery
National Institute of Tuberculosis and
Respiratory Diseases
New Delhi, India

Semra Bilaçeroğlu MD FCCP
Director
Vth Pulmonary Department
Izmir Dr Suat Seren Training and Research
Hospital for Thoracic Medicine
and Surgery
Izmir, Turkey

Shekhar Kunal MBBS
Junior Resident
Department of Pulmonary Medicine
Vallabhbhai Patel Chest Institute
University of Delhi
Delhi, India

Snežana Jovičić PhD
Teaching Assistant
Faculty of Pharmacy
Department of Medical Biochemistry
University of Belgrade
Head of Department at Clinic for Cardiac
Surgery, Center for Medical Biochemistry
Clinical Center of Serbia
Belgrade, Serbia

Varinder Singh MD FRCPCH (Hony)
Director Professor
Department of Pediatrics
Lady Hardinge Medical College and
Kalawati Saran Children's Hospital
New Delhi, India

Vesna Škodrić Trifunović MD PhD
Professor
Department for Tuberculosis and
Nonspecific Pleuropulmonary Diseases
Clinic of Pulmonology
Clinical Center of Serbia
Medical School University of Belgrade
Belgrade, Serbia

Zorica Šumarac PhD
Assistant professor
Faculty of Pharmacy Novi Sad
University Business Academy in Novi Sad
Center for Medical Biochemistry
Clinical Center of Serbia
Belgrade, Serbia

Preface

The global tuberculosis (TB) burden is higher than expected and estimated previously.

Two years ago, when the idea about this book rose, TB still remained one of the top 10 causes of death worldwide.

In the year 2015, the World Health Organization (WHO) reported 10.4 million new TB cases worldwide, 10% among children. There were an estimated 1.4 million TB deaths.

The book on selected problems in TB tends to elucidate special clinical approach to this global health problem. Dealing from the epidemiology of TB infection to non-*Mycobacterium* infection manifestations, authors illuminate different clinical manifestations of TB, which might help doctors in recognizing the disease appearance.

The main purpose of this book is to provide medical fraternity broad review of possible clinical manifestations of TB. It is written for general practitioners, internists and pulmonologists. The book may provide also medical students with much useful information.

Authors of the book "*Tuberculosis: Selected Problems*" wish to contribute to one of the main targets of the WHO "End TB Strategy" that calls for a 90% reduction in TB deaths and an 80% reduction in the TB incidence rate by 2030, compared with 2015.

This is a group effort of the authors of this book to contribute to "Stop TB Millennium Goals".

Violeta V Mihailovic Vucinic
Dragana M Jovanovic

Acknowledgment

Editors appreciate all the authors for their serious work on the chapters of this book. Their contribution is equal to the lifesaving manner they are acting every single day during the work with tuberculosis patients.

The final look of this book was made by careful efforts of Jaypee Brothers Medical Publishers (P) Ltd. and our most sincere appreciations belong to them.

Contents

1. **Microbiology of *Mycobacterium tuberculosis* and Laboratory Diagnosis of Tuberculosis** — 1
   Bojana Luković

2. **Epidemiology of Tuberculosis** — 22
   Anna L Rich

3. **Latent Tuberculosis** — 33
   Hannah Jarvis, Onn M Kon

4. **Diagnosis of Tuberculosis** — 50
   Violeta V Mihailovic Vucinic, Dragana M Jovanovic

5. **Lymph Node Tuberculosis** — 61
   Anand Jaiswal, Dipti Gothi

6. **Conventional and Interventional Bronchoscopy in Tuberculosis** — 77
   Semra Bilaçeroğlu, Atul C Mehta

7. **Bronchogenic Tuberculosis** — 96
   Dragana M Jovanovic, Atul C Mehta

8. **Miliary Tuberculosis** — 128
   Ashok Shah, Shekhar Kunal

9. **Tuberculosis Effusion and the Role of Closed Pleural Biopsy and Pleuroscopy** — 155
   Dragana M Jovanovic, Violeta V Mihailovic Vucinic

10. **Clinically Unrecognized Tuberculosis: Multidisciplinary Approach** — 170
    Vesna Škodrić Trifunović

11. **Challenges in the Diagnosis and Treatment of MDR and XDR Tuberculosis** — 185
    Müge Aydoğdu

12. **Childhood Tuberculosis** — 205
    Varinder Singh, Kamal K Singhal

13. **Tuberculosis in Immunocompromised** — 225
    Vesna Škodrić Trifunović

14. **Smoking and Tuberculosis: A Pernicious Association** 243
    Ashok Shah, Shekhar Kunal, Kamal Gera

15. **Pulmonary Diseases Caused by Nontuberculous Mycobacterium** 257
    Violeta V Mihailovic Vucinic

16. **Treatment of Tuberculosis** 266
    Dragica P Pesut

17. **Management of the Adverse Effects of Antituberculosis Drugs** 281
    Dragica P Pesut

18. **Vitamin D and Tuberculosis** 291
    Snežana Jovičić, Zorica Šumarac

19. **Surgery for Pulmonary Tuberculosis** 298
    Ravindra K Dewan

20. **Prevention of Tuberculosis in Areas with High Tuberculosis Incidence** 306
    Dragana M Jovanovic, Violeta V Mihailovic Vucinic

Index 323

PLATE 1

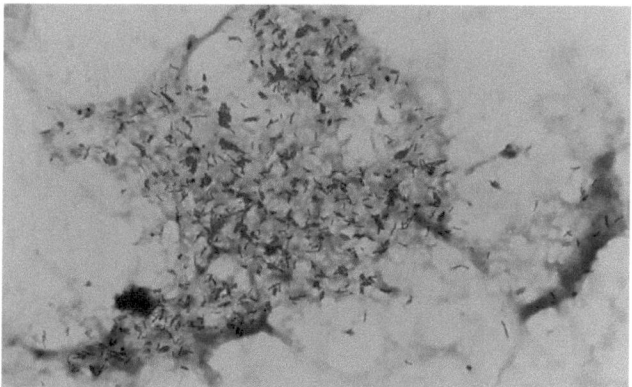

FIG. 1: Acid-fast bacillus in processed sputum smear stained with Ziehl–Neelsen method. *(Chapter 1)*

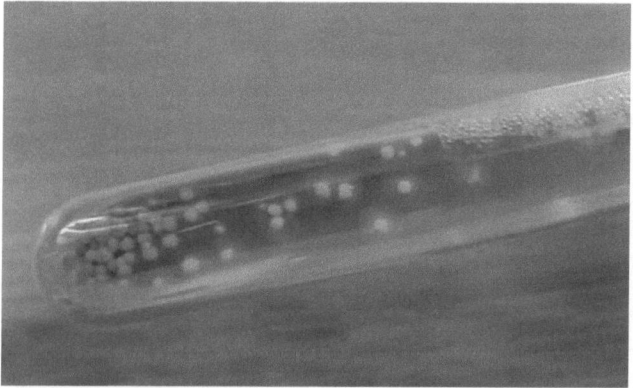

FIG. 2: *Mycobacterium tuberculosis* colonies on Löwenstein–Jensen medium. *(Chapter 1)*

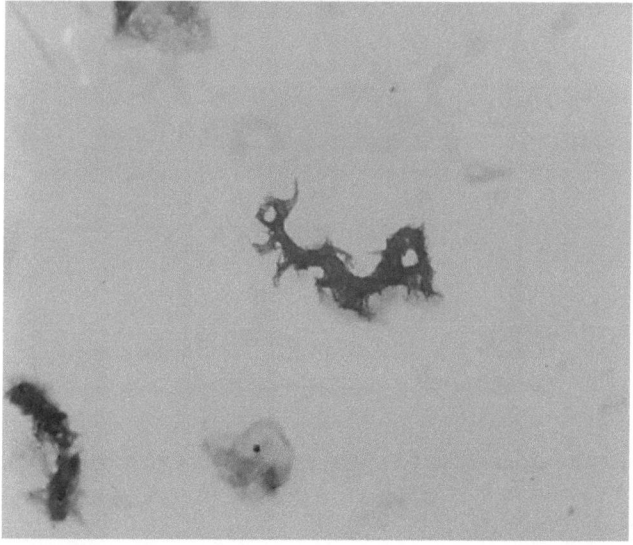

FIG. 3: *Mycobacterium tuberculosis* "serpentine cord". *(Chapter 1)*

PLATE 2

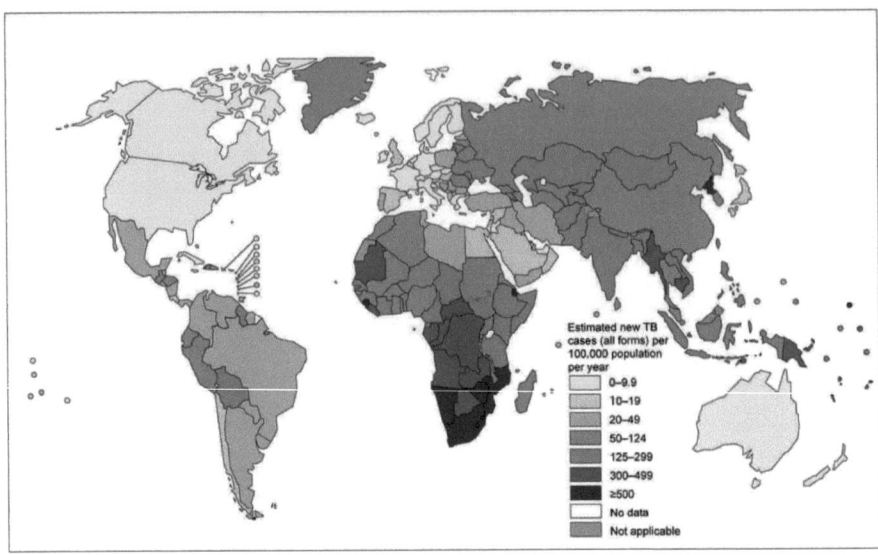

TB, tuberculosis.

FIG. 1: Estimated tuberculosis incidence rates worldwide in 2012. *(Chapter 2)*

Source: World Health Organization.

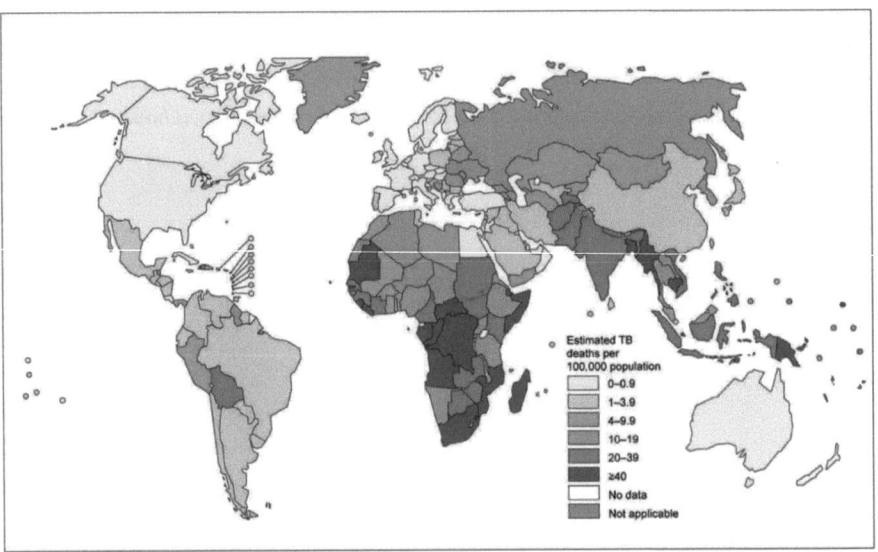

TB, tuberculosis.

FIG. 2: Estimated tuberculosis mortality rates excluding tuberculosis deaths among human immunodeficiency virus-positive people, 2012. *(Chapter 2)*

Source: World Health Organization.

PLATE 3

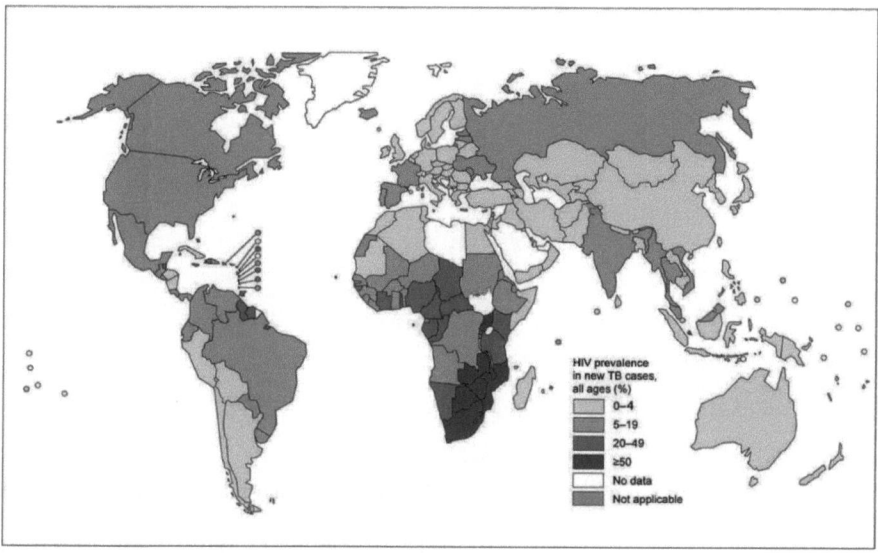

HIV, human immunodeficiency virus; TB, tuberculosis.

FIG. 3: Human immunodeficiency virus prevalence in new cases of tuberculosis in 2012. *(Chapter 2)*

Source: World Health Organization.

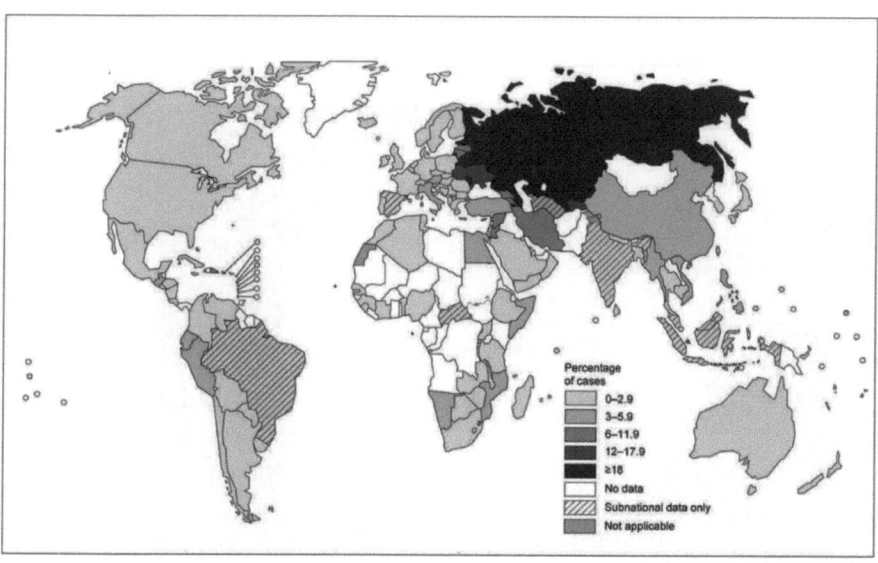

Note: Figures are based on the most recent year for which data has been reported, which varies among countries.

FIG. 4: Percentage of new cases of tuberculosis with multidrug-resistant tuberculosis. *(Chapter 2)*

Source: World Health Organization.

PLATE 4

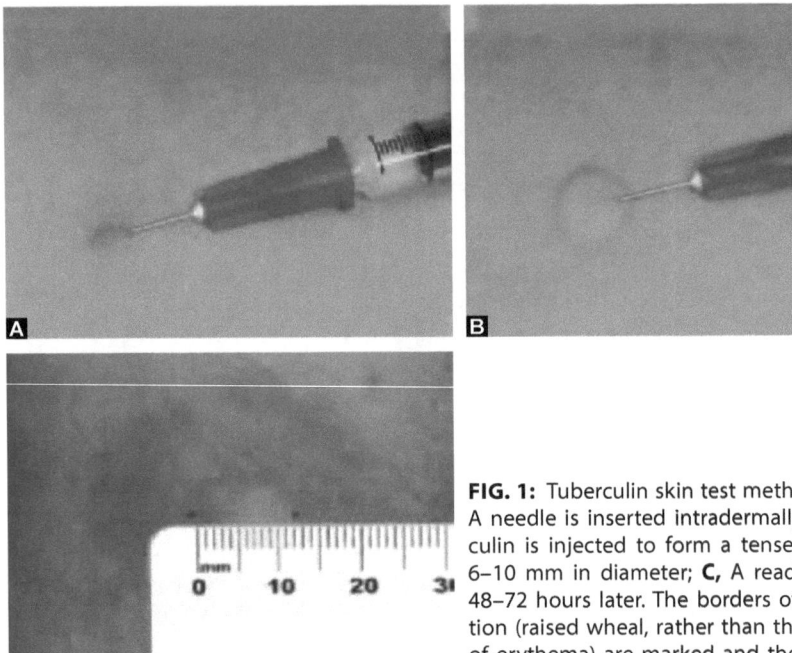

FIG. 1: Tuberculin skin test method. **A** and **B**, A needle is inserted intradermally and tuberculin is injected to form a tense, pale wheal 6–10 mm in diameter; **C,** A reading is made 48–72 hours later. The borders of the induration (raised wheal, rather than the larger area of erythema) are marked and the diameter is measured. *(Chapter 3)*

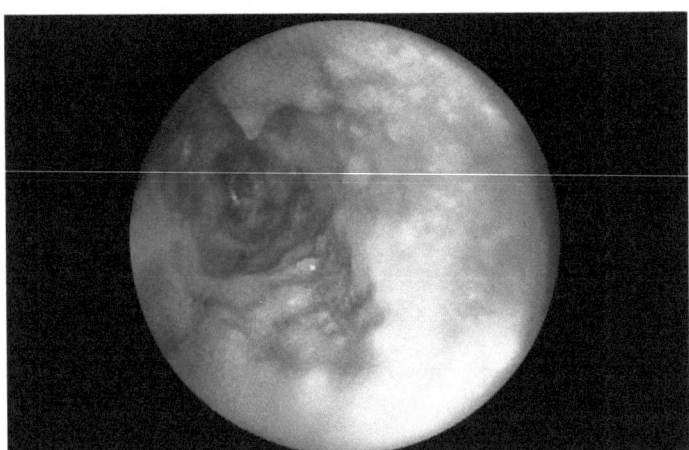

FIG. 8: Extensive pulmonary distraction (bronchopulmonary communication) due to progressive tuberculosis. *(Chapter 4)*
Courtesy: Dr Spasoje Popevic, Bronchologist, University Clinic of Pulmonology, Clinical Center of Serbia, Belgrade.

PLATE 5

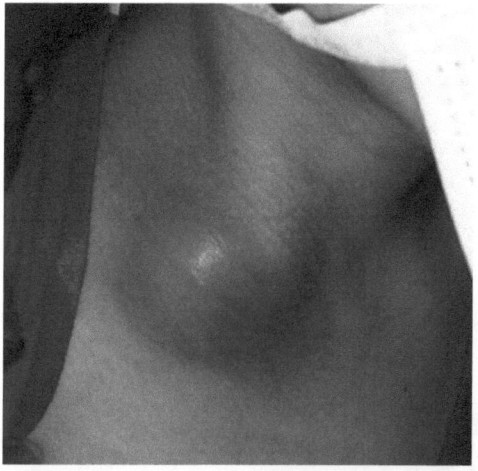

FIG. 1: Cervical lymph node with abscess formation. *(Chapter 5)*

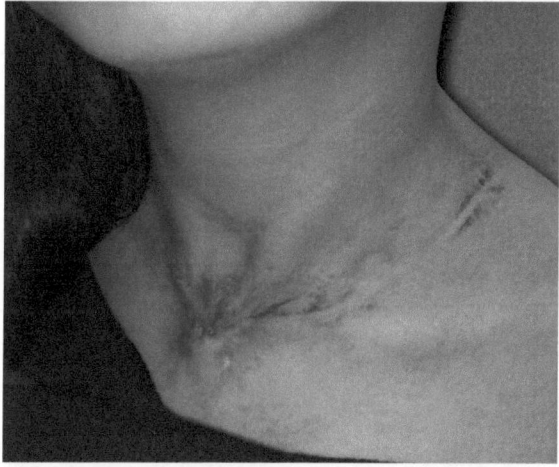

FIG. 2: Multiple scar formation, a complication of cervical lymph node tuberculosis. *(Chapter 5)*

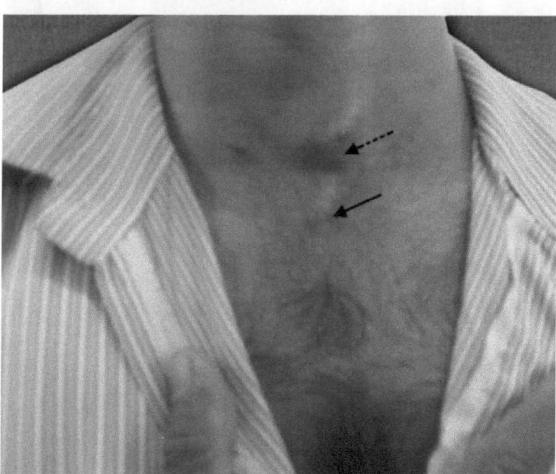

FIG. 5: A 36-year-old man with paradoxical reaction. The solid arrow shows suprasternal lymph node for which he was started on antituberculosis treatment based on cytology showing acid-fast bacilli (AFB). Two months later another lymph node shown by dotted arrow appeared. The culture for AFB was negative confirming paradoxical reaction. *(Chapter 5)*

PLATE 6

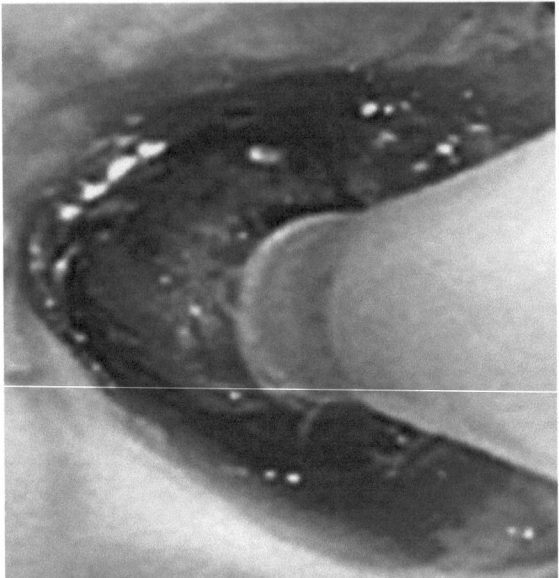

FIG. 1: Balloon dilatation of a bronchial stenosis due to endobronchial tuberculosis. *(Chapter 6)*

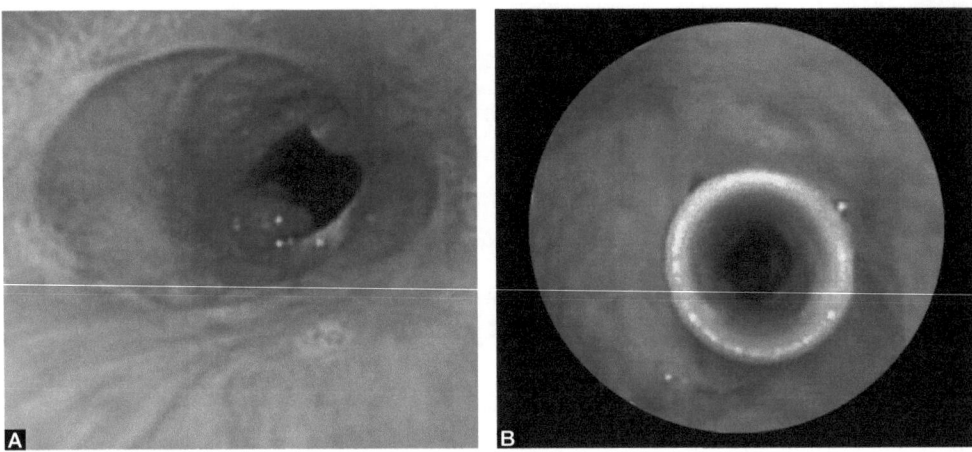

FIG. 2: A, Tracheal stenosis due to tuberculosis; **B,** A Dumon stent is placed and patency of trachea is reestablished. *(Chapter 6)*

PLATE 7

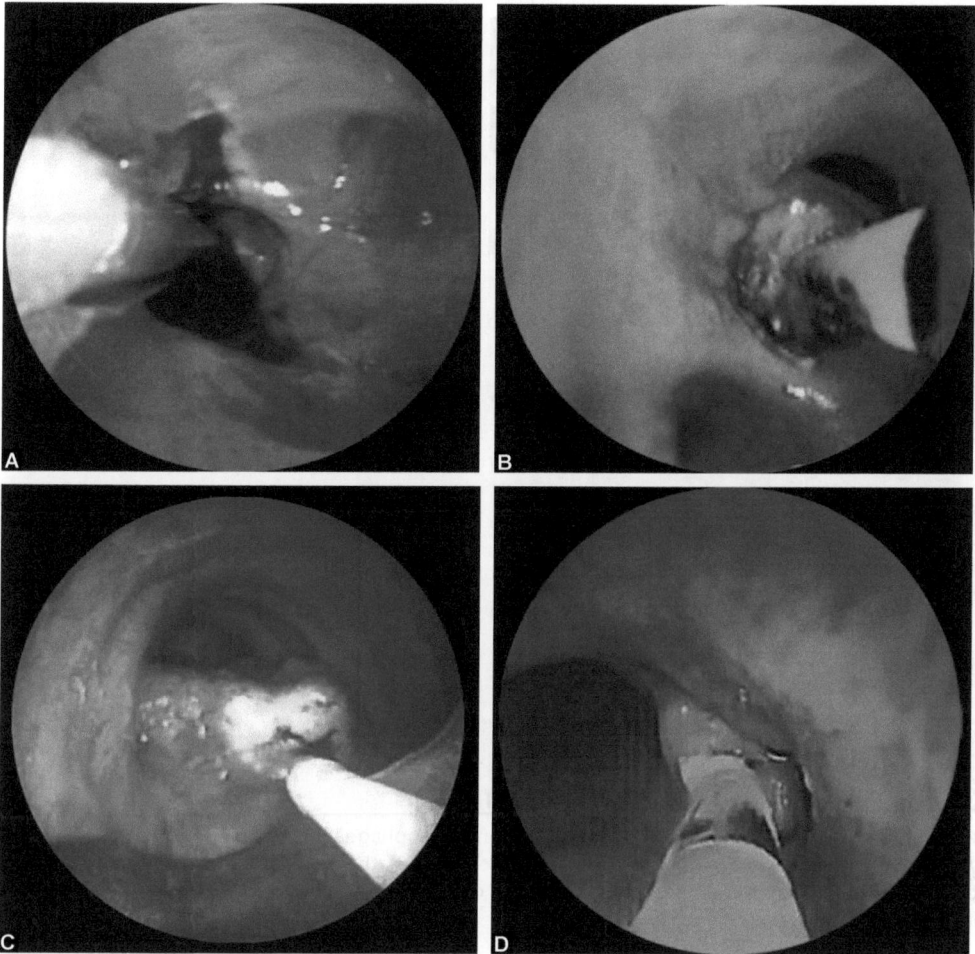

FIG. 3: Ablation of obstructing TB-related web-like and granulomatous tissues in the airways by **A,** electrocautery; **B,** argon plasma coagulation; **C,** laser; and **D,** cryotherapy. *(Chapter 6)*

PLATE 8

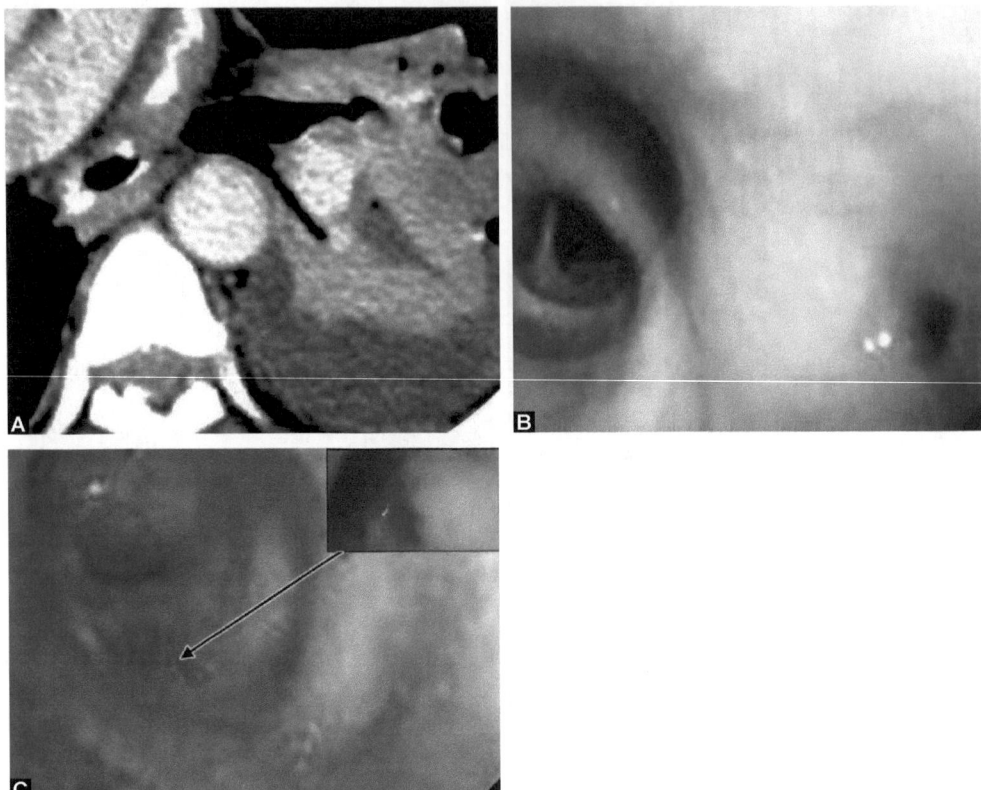

FIG. 4: A, Computed tomography image of a bronchoesophageal fistula (BEF) on the distal medial wall of left main bronchus; **B,** initial bronchoscopic image of the BEF; **C,** bronchoscopic image after closure of the BEF by bronchoscopic injection of cyanoacrylate glue (right upper corner: close-up image of BEF sealed with glue) *(Chapter 6)*

PLATE 9

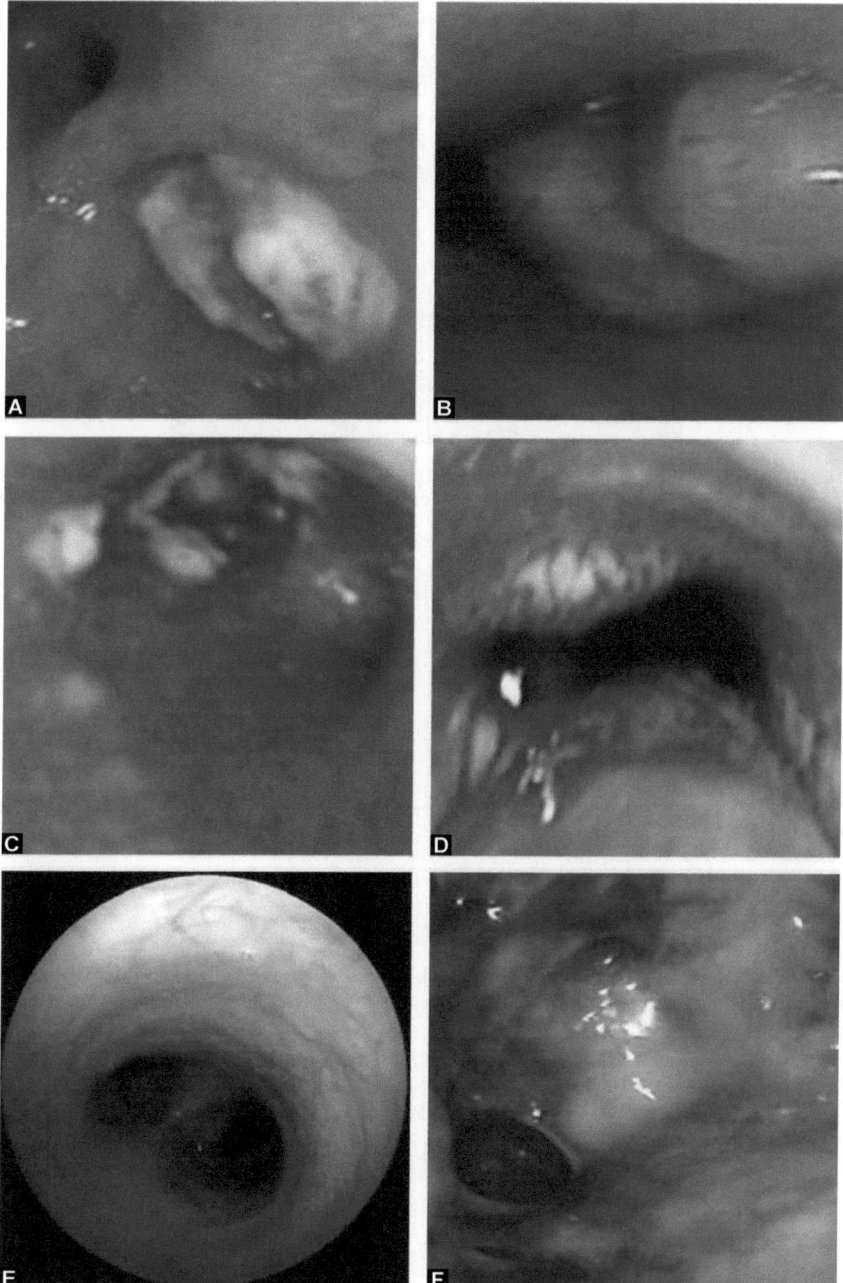

FIG. 5: Bronchoscopic images of different subtypes of endobronchial tuberculosis: **A,** actively caseating (with hyperhemia); **B,** tumorous; **C,** granular and edematous-hyperemic; **D,** ulcerating (with some stenosis); **E,** nonspecific bronchitic; **F,** fibrostenotic (with caseation and antracosis). *(Chapter 6)*

PLATE 10

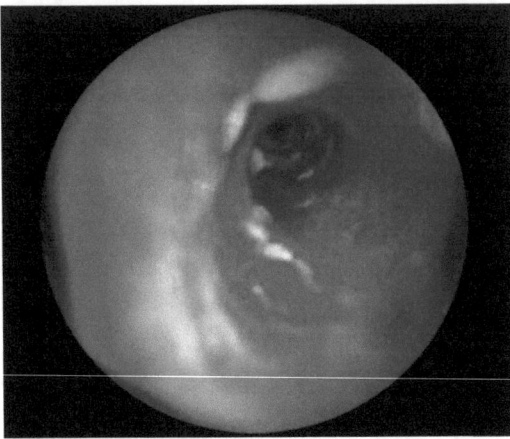

FIG. 12: Hyperemic, edematous mucosa of the trachea, covered with whitish (caseous) debris. Bronchoscopic biopsy revealed tuberculosis. A case of active-caseating form of endobronchial/tracheobronchial tuberculosis. *(Chapter 7)*

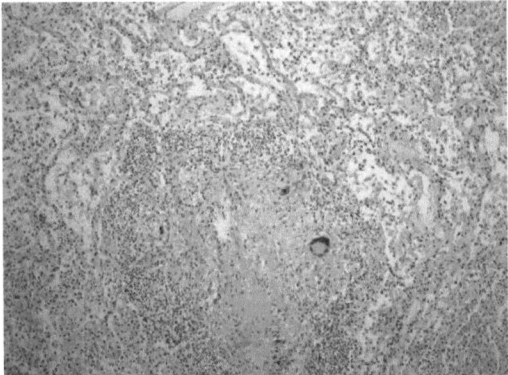

FIG. 2: Histopathology finding—lungs (HE, ×100): Areas of caseous necrosis, which are surrounded by rare epithelioid cells, giant multinucleated cells (Langhans cells), lymphocytes, and fibroblasts. *(Chapter 10)*

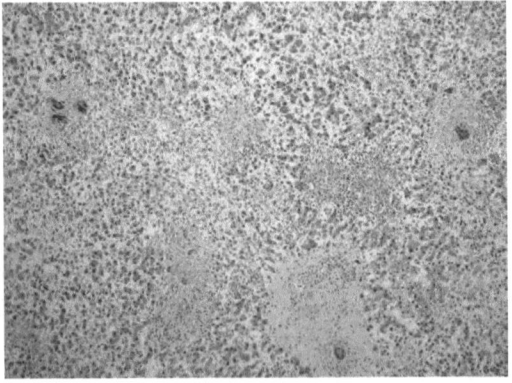

FIG. 3: Histopathology finding—liver (HE, ×100): Areas of caseous necrosis, which are surrounded by rare epithelioid cells, giant multinucleated cells (Langhans cells), and lymphocytes. *(Chapter 10)*

PLATE 11

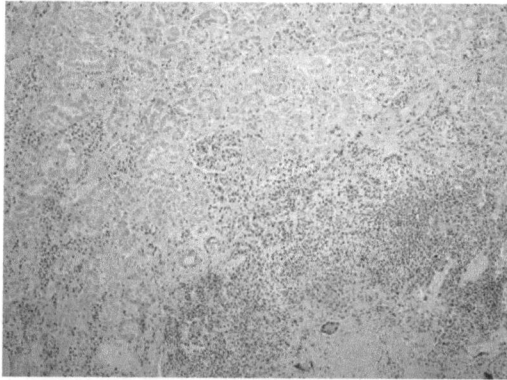

FIG. 4: Histopathology finding—kidney (HE, ×100): Small areas of caseous necrosis, which are surrounded by rare epithelioid cells, giant multinucleated cells (Langhans cells), and lymphocytes. *(Chapter 10)*

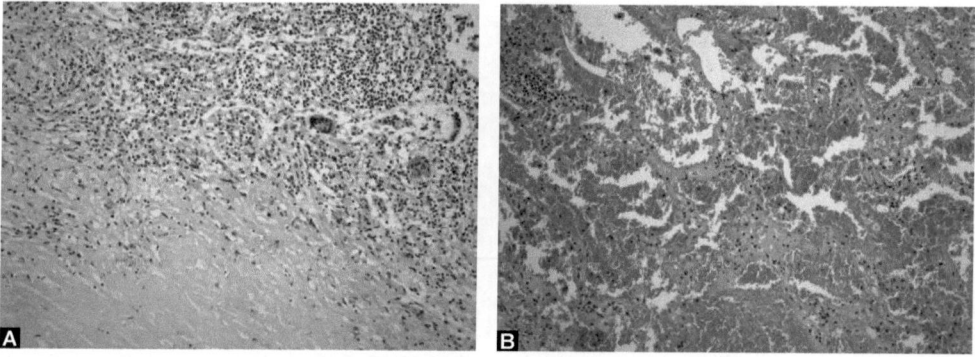

FIG. 7: Histopathology findings—lungs: **A,** Miliary tuberculous granulomas in both lungs are of different ages, primarily organized and calcified; **B,** Alveoli filled with erythrocytes. *(Chapter 10)*

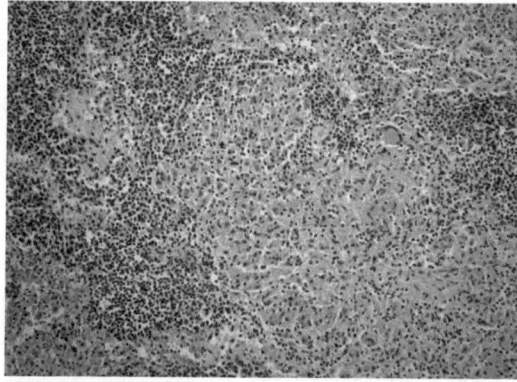

FIG. 8: Pulmonary hilar lymph nodes showed tuberculous granuloma with a field of caseous necrosis. *(Chapter 10)*

Courtesy: Pathologists, Institute of Pathology, Faculty of Medicine, University of Belgrade, Serbia.

PLATE 12

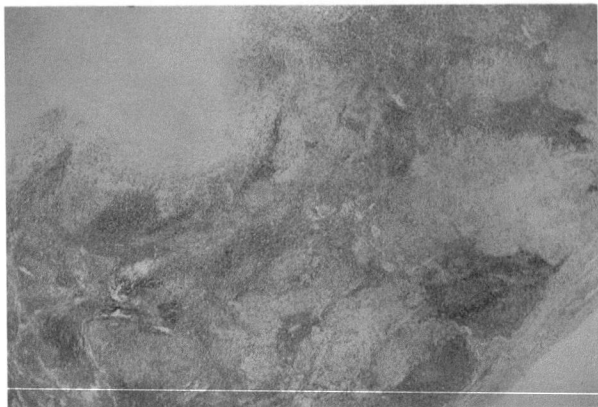

FIG. 13: Histopathology findings: Granulomatous lymphadenitis (HE, ×13). *(Chapter 10)*

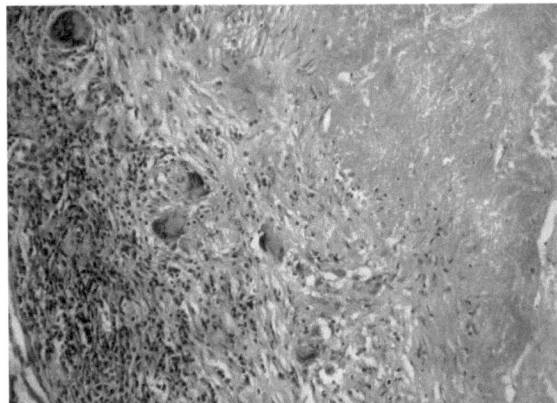

FIG. 9: Histopathology findings: Lung parenchyma (H ×20): Specific granuloma with predominant caseous necrosis surrounded by giant cells of Langhans type. *(Chapter 13)*

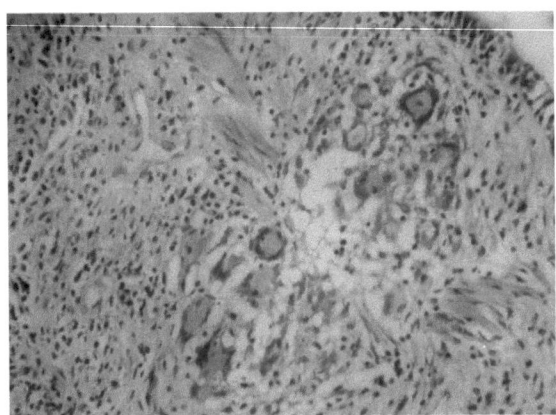

FIG. 10: Histopathology findings (H ×20): Specific bronchiectasis: In bronchial wall are present numerous productive granulomas consisted of epitheloid hystiocytes and giant cells of Langhans type. *(Chapter 13)*
Courtesy: Pathologist Jelena Stojsic Service of pathology, Clinical Center of Serbia, Belgrade, Serbia.

Microbiology of *Mycobacterium tuberculosis* and Laboratory Diagnosis of Tuberculosis

Bojana Luković

INTRODUCTION

Laboratory diagnosis of tuberculosis (TB) is practically a diagnosis of tubercle bacilli, the members of the *Mycobacterium tuberculosis* complex (MTBC).

One of the oldest and most devastating of human afflictions, TB remains a leading cause of infectious death worldwide today, and a serious public health threat. More than 9 million new cases are reported annually, and about 2 million people die.[1]

Mycobacterium tuberculosis complex is in the genus *Mycobacterium*, the only genus of the family *Mycobacteriaceae*. The name *Mycobacterium* (fungus-bacterium) is an allusion to the mold-like pellicles formed when members of this genus are grown in liquid media.[2] Bacteria are classified in the genus *Mycobacterium* on the basis of their strong acid-fastness, the presence of mycolic acids containing 70–90 carbons, and high (61–71 mol%) guanine-cytosine content in their deoxyribonucleic acid (DNA).[3] Mycobacteria possess a complex, lipid rich cell wall, responsible for many of the characteristic properties of the bacteria (acid-fastness, slow growth, resistance to detergents, resistance to common antibacterial antibiotics, antigenicity, and clumping). Porins and other proteins that are found throughout the cell wall are biologically important antigens, stimulating the patient's cellular immune response to infection. Extracted and partially purified preparations of these proteins derivatives [purified protein derivatives (PPDs)] are used as skin test reagents to measure exposure to *M. tuberculosis*.[4,5]

Among more than 150 named species of mycobacteria, obligate pathogens are the leprosy bacillus *Mycobacterium leprae*, and members of the slow growing MTBC. The other species are nontuberculous mycobacteria (NTM), environmental saprophytes, some of which can cause opportunistic disease.

Mycobacterium tuberculosis complex refers to a closely related group of variants of a single species. Several parameters, including analysis of antigenic extracts, target epitopes for monoclonal antibodies, antigenic and DNA-relatedness studies, suggest that they represent a single species.[6] Members of the complex all-cause TB, a chronic granulomatous disease affecting man and many other mammals. The complex includes *M. tuberculosis, M. bovis, M. bovis* Bacillus Calmette–Guérin (BCG strain), *M. africanum, M. caprae, M. canetti, M. microti,* and *M. pinnipedii*.[7]

EPIDEMIOLOGY AND TRANSMISSION

Humans are the only reservoir for the *M. tuberculosis*. *Mycobacterium bovis* is the principal cause of TB in cattle (known as bovine TB), and many other mammals, rare in man because of the widespread pasteurization of milk, the institution of public health measures, and attenuation of a laboratory strain of *M. bovis* and development of the BCG vaccine in

1921. However, *M. bovis* can still jump the species barrier and cause TB in humans. The European badger (*Meles meles*) has been identified as a wildlife reservoir of bovine TB and source of transmission to cattle in Britain and Ireland.[8]

The use of attenuated laboratory strain of *M. bovis* in BCG vaccine for therapy of bladder tumors has resulted in a number of cases of local and disseminated infections with *M. bovis*.[9]

Mycobacterium africanum, intermediate in form between the human and bovin types, causes human TB in equatorial Africa. It can be subdivided into type I (*M. bovis*-like) and type II (*M. tuberculosis*-like). Type I is more common in West Africa and type II is mainly of East African origin. Patients infected with *M. africanum* type II are more likely to present with major lung complications.[10,11]

Mycobacterium caprae, isolated from goats, can be the cause of human TB as well.[12]

Mycobacterium canetti is the emerging disease affecting man in the Horn of Africa.[13]

Mycobacterium pinnipedii primarily infects seals and transmission to humans happens in a zoo with marine mammals.[14]

Mycobacterium microti can be transferred to humans from voles and other small mammals.[15]

Mycobacterium tuberculosis complex replication occurs in the tissues of warm-blooded hosts. Tubercle bacilli are aerobes, nonmotile, nonsporing, noncapsulate, intracellular pathogens, incapable of replicating in or on inanimate objects. However, they can survive in milk and other organic materials and on pastureland so long as they are not exposed to ultraviolet (UV) light, to which they are very sensitive. They are also heat sensitive and are destroyed by pasteurization.[16]

BIOSAFETY IN TUBERCULOSIS LABORATORY

Mycobacterium tuberculosis complex is transmitted primarily through the inhalation of airborne droplet nuclei, approximately 1–5 μm in size, from an active pulmonary TB patient by coughing or from the positive specimens or cultures in the laboratory. Nosocomial transmission of this organism is of major concern to healthcare workers.[17]

Droplet nuclei "meander" in the air and are transmitted to susceptible individuals by inhalation. The risk of the infection is dependent to the load of the bacillus that has been inhaled, level of infectiousness, and the immune competency of the potential host. For personnel in TB laboratory, risk of infection is three to five times greater than it is in other professions. As a result, laboratory safety procedures are aimed at preventing the spread of potentially infective aerosols. The Centers for Disease Control and Prevention (CDC) has recommended that work involving manipulation of TB cultures be done in biosafety level-3 (BSL-3) laboratory.[18] The BSL-3 space which includes the biologic safety cabinet and aerosol-tight centrifuge should have nonpermeable walls and work surfaces, directional airflow (with the lowest air pressure in the laboratory), and double door air lock to prevent the back flow of air. Air from the BSL-3 space should be vented through high efficiency particulate air filters directly to the outside.

All manipulations of infected materials or viable cultures (processing of specimens, smear preparations, inoculum preparation, pipetting, vortexing, mixing, making dilutions, and inoculation of media) must be handled in certified biologic safety cabinet. Gloves, caps, protective disposable gowns, shoe protection, and respirator masks, should be worn at all times when specimens or viable cultures are being handled. Protective clothing should be removed and placed in a bag for autoclaving when work in BSL-3 is completed.

Effective germicides include 3–8% formaldehyde, 0.05–0.5% sodium hypochlorite, 70% ethanol, and 5% phenol. Ultraviolet light is a useful adjunct for surface decontamination.

DIFFERENT TUBERCULOSIS LABORATORY SERVICE LEVELS

Experience with the College of American Pathologists Special Mycobacterial Interlaboratory Survey, over the many years, has shown that increasing numbers of laboratories are restricting their services for mycobacterial infections to the preparation and interpretation of acid-fast stained smears, setting up primary cultures, and referring positive cultures to reference laboratories for identification and susceptibility testing.[19]

Specimen Collection

All specimens for mycobacterial culture must be collected in sterile, disposable containers before the initiation of therapy and promptly transported to the laboratory. If delay is unavoidable, specimen must be refrigerated to prevent the overgrowth of contaminants.

Tubercle bacilli can be recovered from respiratory specimens (sputum, bronchial washes, bronchoalveolar lavage, or bronchial biopsies), gastric lavage, urine, feces, blood, cerebrospinal fluid, tissue biopsies, and deep needle aspirations of virtually any tissue or organ.[20]

Respiratory Specimens

The most frequent type of respiratory sample is sputum. It is important that the patient be instructed to cough deeply to produce the desirable thick exudate. However, any isolate of *M. tuberculosis*, even that in saliva, is considered significant.[21] Conventionally, three early sputum samples (5-10 mL), collected on three consecutive days from persistent coughing patients, are usually sufficient.[22,23] If patients are unable to produce suitable specimens, sputa may be induced with nebulization techniques, specifically inhalation of warm (45°C), aerosolized, sterile 10% sodium chloride (NaCl), or the use of ultrasonic nebulizers, or different bronchoscopy techniques are use.

Gastric Lavage

Gastric lavage may be necessary for infants or very young children and for patients who are comatose or have mental disorders.[24] It is strongly recommended that gastric lavage specimens be collected in containers without preservatives and processed immediately or at least within 4 hours of collection.

Urine

A minimum of five clean catch, first morning urine should be collected on successive 24-hour periods to maximize the chance of recovery of MTBC. Pooled urine is not satisfactory.[25]

Specimen Preparation

Miscellaneous Sterile Specimens

Cerebrospinal fluid, synovial, and other body fluids that are normally sterile, usually need not be decontaminated before culture. Processing can commence with centrifugation.[25]

Tissues and needle biopsy material should be placed in a small quantity of liquid broth (Middlebrook 7H9 or 7H11) as a holding medium, or in the absence of broth, in sterile 0.85% saline or 0.2% bovine albumin, and then inoculated directly onto both solid and liquid media.

Body fluids can contain small numbers of organisms and they should be concentrated before inoculation. These fluids are centrifuged at 3,000–3,800 × g, in aerosol-tight centrifuges with cooling, and the sediment is inoculated to liquid and solid media.

Digestion and Decontamination of Contaminated Specimens

Specimens that contain large amounts of organic debris or are contaminated with a variety of organisms that rapidly outgrow the MTBC, mandate the use of digestion decontamination procedures to liquefy the debris and kill the undesirable contaminants. These specimens are sputum, gastric lavage, urine, feces, and other potentially contaminated body fluids.

Strict adherence to the processing procedures is mandatory because overexposure to these agents also kills the MTBC. The most widely used digestion decontamination procedure is the N-acetyl-L-cysteine (NALC) plus 2% sodium hydroxide (NaOH) method, mild decontamination solution with mucolytic agent NALC to free mycobacteria entrapped in mucus. Exposure to NaOH should be limited to 15 minutes.[26]

Trisodium phosphate (13% solution) plus benzalkonium chloride (Zephiran) is preferred by laboratories that cannot carefully control time of exposure to decontamination solution. Zephiran should be neutralized with lecithin and not inoculated onto egg-based culture medium.[25,27]

Dithiothreitol plus 2% NaOH is very effective mucolytic agent. Exposure to NaOH should be limited to 15 minutes.[28]

NaOH (4% solution) is traditional decontamination solution. Often used for urine samples. Time of exposure must be carefully controlled to no more than 15 minutes.

Cetylpyridinium chloride (1% solution) plus 2% NaCl is effective for sputum specimens mailed from outpatient clinics. Tubercle bacilli have survived 8-day transit without significant loss.[29]

Oxalic acid (5% solution) method is recommended for treating sputum specimens that are consistently contaminated with *Pseudomonas* species.[30]

Centrifugation

After the digestion and decontamination, next important step in TB laboratory is concentration of the specimen by centrifugation in aerosol tight centrifuge with cooling. The high lipid content in the mycobacteria cell wall makes the specific gravity of the organism very low. If the organism is to be maximally sedimented during the centrifugation of the specimen, relative centrifugal force (RCF) should be 3,000 × g or even 3,800 × g. With higher RCF, there is an increase in the correlation of positive smears to positive cultures.[31] Also, considerable heat is generated at high speeds, and refrigerated centrifuges may be required when RCFs exceed 3,000 × g.

MICROSCOPIC EXAMINATION

In spite of modern advances, microscopy remains a cornerstone of TB control because it identifies sputum smear positive cases, infectious reservoirs, and those most likely to spread TB, and is rapid and cheap, although has a limited specificity.

Smears are usually prepared after concentration of the specimen. In situations when rapid evaluation of clinical specimen is needed, a direct smear may be prepared from the specimen. For smear to be positive, it requires approximately 10^4 bacilli/mL of sputum. Patients with extensive disease shed large number of bacilli, with a good correlation between a positive smear and a positive culture. Many patients have minimal or less advanced disease, and the correlation of positive smears to positive cultures in this group may be only 25–40%.

The CDC recommends that positive results from acid-fast bacillus (AFB) smears must be reported after 24 hours of receipt of the specimen.[23,32] It is also important to perform AFB microscopy analysis, following confirmation of TB, to ensure the prescribed treatment is completely successful.[23,33]

After TB drug therapy is started, cultures become negative before the smears do, suggesting that the organisms are not capable of replicating but are capable of binding the stain.

Prolongation of decontamination and concentrating processes from sputum samples, as well as shortening culture incubation time, may result in smear-positive but culture-negative results.[6]

The large amount of lipids in the cell wall of mycobacteria makes them impermeable to the dyes used in Gram stain. When stained with the Gram stain, they vary from Gram-positive to "Gram-ghost" or "Gram-neutral" bacilli.[34] Mycobacteria are able to form stable complexes with certain arylmethane dyes such as fuchsin (stains the cell membrane) and auramine O (binds to deoxyribonucleic or ribonucleic acid). Once these complexes are formed, they are very resistant to decolorization with acid alcohols or strong mineral acids, and are thus, termed acid-fast. The Ziehl–Neelsen (ZN) (heat-fixed smears), Kinyoun (cold stain), and fluorochrome acid-fast staining techniques are used in mycobacteriology. The ZN and Kinyoun methods employ a carbol fuchsin stain and a methylene blue counterstain.[27,30] With a carbol fuchsin stain, AFB stains red and background material stains blue.[35] Tubercle bacilli are straight or slightly curved rods about 3×0.3 µm in size, may occur singly or in small clumps, and many contain heavily red stained areas called beads and often have alternating stained and clear sections, making them appear banded (Fig. 1). Smears stained with these methods are examined with the oil immersion objective of a bright field microscope.

Fluorochrome stained smears (auramine O or the combination of auramine-rhodamine) should be scanned with a fluorescence microscope at lower magnifications, which permits the examination of large area of the smear per unit of time.[23,27] The AFB appear bright yellow to orange in fluorochrome stained smears. If a potassium permanganate counterstain is used, the background appears dark.

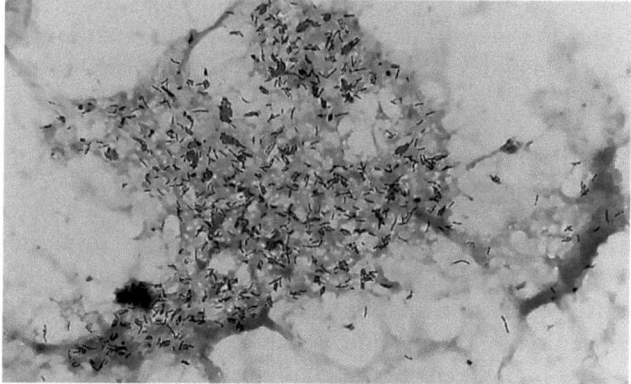

FIG. 1: Acid-fast bacillus in processed sputum smear stained with Ziehl–Neelsen method. *(For color version, see Plate 1)*

TABLE 1	Quantitatively reporting procedure for microscopy of acid-fast bacillus smears
Number of AFB seen	**Report**
0	Negative
1–2 AFB/whole smear	Doubtful positive. Confirm by observing another smear from the same specimen or from another specimen from the same patient
1–9 AFB/100 fields	1+
1–9 AFB/10 fields	2+
1–9 AFB/fields	3+
>9 AFB/field	4+

AFB, acid-fast bacillus.

Microscopist should examine a minimum of 100 fields from each smear before reporting as negative. There are different criteria for degree of positivity, which may be followed to quantitatively report the number of AFB seen on a smear. One of the quantitatively reporting procedures recommended by the CDC is given in table 1.[27]

Despite quick results, microscopy analysis using either ZN or fluorochrome staining dyes may potentially give false-positive results due to cross contamination from many sources, such as the presence of partially acid-fast like *Corynebacterium, Nocardia,* and *Rhodococcus* species.[36,37] False-positive results may also be due to the handling process, suitability of stain, the transfer of AFB from slides to slides, contamination of tap water or distilled water with saprophytic AFB, or contaminated oil. Too thin smears may give false-negative results and debris in smears that are too thick may mask presence of AFB. Factors that may interfere with staining or reduce fluorescence include excessive exposure of the stained smear to potassium permanganate, exposure to solutions of heavy metal ions, high chlorine content of rinse water, and use of absorbent paper during staining procedure.[35]

Furthermore, light and fluorescent microscopy cannot differentiate between MTBC and NTM. A peptide nucleic acids (PNAs) fluorescent technique is another alternative in microscopy, which can be used to distinguish between MTBC and NTM directly in respiratory specimens. This technique uses a peptide-like structure to replace the sugar-phosphate backbone and binds at specific sequences such as 16S ribosomal ribonucleic acid (16S rRNA). Due to the hydrophobicity of PNA, it can enter the mycobacterial cell wall and bind to intracellular nucleic acid sequences and visualized using fluorescent microscopy.[23,38]

CULTURE TECHNIQUES

Because of the insensitivity of AFB microscopic staining for TB detection, culturing concentrated respiratory specimens together with clinical indicators remains the most reliable method of mycobacterial identification. Culture on solid or broth media, selective and nonselective, remains the gold standard method for detection of the phenotypic mycobacteria.[39,40] The option of using solid or liquid media depends on the routine practices and preferences of the laboratory. In 1993, the CDC recommended that every clinical laboratory must use a liquid medium to isolate mycobacteria in conjunction with solid media.[41]

Solid Culture Media

Nonselective solid culture media may be egg-based [Löwenstein-Jensen (LJ), Petragnani, American Thoracic Society medium] or agar-based (Middlebrook 7H10, Middlebrook 7H11 medium). All nonselective media include malachite green, which suppresses the growth of contaminating bacteria. Among the egg-based media, LJ is the most commonly used. The increased content of the malachite green in Petragnani agar makes this medium more suitable for highly contaminated specimens. Conversely, American Thoracic Society medium is more acceptable for specimens less likely to be contaminated (spinal fluids, pleural fluids).[6]

Casein hydrolysate (0.1%) in Middlebrook 7H11 agar-based medium stimulates the growth of difficult to grow drug resistant strains of M. tuberculosis.[42]

The agar media are transparent and are especially useful because they allow easier and more rapid microscopic detection of colonies. Colonies may be observed in 12–14 days, in contrast to 18–24 days with the egg-based media. Microcolony detection with simple light microscopy on plates with thin layer of Middlebrook 7H11 agar medium allows detection of M. tuberculosis in less than 7 days.[43]

Selective solid culture media are the same formulations of LJ, 7H10, or 7H11, with added antimicrobial agents to suppress bacterial and fungal contamination (Gruft's modification of LJ, Mitchison's modification of 7H11).[44,45] Although the selective 7H10 and 7H11 media are very effective, they should be used only in conjunction with the nonselective media, and not as the sole media for the isolation of mycobacteria.[40,46,47]

Broth Culture Media in Automated, Semiautomated, and Manual Systems

Use of broth culture media for the early recovery of mycobacteria is highly recommended. Comparing to solid culture media there is a greater rate of recovery of M. tuberculosis for a shorter period of time, 1–2 weeks earlier. Broth culture media are Middlebrook 7H9, 7H12, 7H13, modified 7H11 broth base, and other Middlebrooks formulations. Different semiautomated and automated mycobacteria detection systems are currently available.

BACTEC 460 TB, a semiautomated liquid culture system, has been long considered the best method for rapid detection of M. tuberculosis. This radiometric technique uses palmitic acid labeled with radioactive carbons (^{14}C palmitic acid), in 7H12 medium to detect the metabolism rather than the visible growth of mycobacteria. If mycobacterium is present in the inoculum, it metabolizes the ^{14}C substrate, leading to the production of radiolabeled carbon dioxide ($^{14}CO_2$) which is measured and reported in terms of growth index. Disadvantages of the system include the inability to observe colony morphology and detect mixed cultures, overgrowth of contaminants, need for disposal of radioactive materials, and extensive use of needles. An Indian study showed that the BACTEC 460 TB radiometric method obtained 87% of positive results within 7 days and 96% within 14 days.[48] The widespread adoption of semiautomated rapid liquid culture systems was frustrated by the demands on staff time and the difficulties associated with the disposal of radioisotopes.

The BACTEC instrument can also be used to differentiate M. tuberculosis and M. bovis from NTM using blood culture vials containing p-nitro-α-acetylamino-β-hydroxy-propiophenone (NAP). Mycobacterium tuberculosis and M. bovis cannot grow in NAP containing culture media, and therefore, will not produce a positive growth index.[6]

BACTEC MGIT 960 TB is a nonradiometric fully automated system that uses the modified 7H9 broth base with special supplement and antibiotic mixture for isolation of mycobacteria from clinical specimens other than blood and urine. A fluorescent compound sensitive to dissolved oxygen in the broth is embedded in silicone on the bottom of the tube. As the actively growing bacteria consume the dissolved oxygen, the fluorescence is unmasked and the sensors can detect it. If the tubes stay negative, instrument incubates them for 42 days.[49] Tortoli and associates found that the MGIT 960 had the shortest mean time to positivity at 13.3 days, compared with 14.8 days for the BACTEC 960 system and 25.6 days for the LJ medium. In this comparison, the MGIT 960 also had the highest contamination rate (10.0%), compared with the radiometric system (3.7%) and the LJ medium (17.0%).[50]

If there is no automated MGIT 960 system in the laboratory, Manual MGIT can be used. The difference is that instead the fluorescence is detected automatically by the instrument, laboratory personnel detect it by observing the mycobacteria growth indicator tube under long wave UV light (Wood's lamp). Growth may also be detected by observing a nonhomogeneous turbidity or small grains or lakes in the culture medium. Positive tubes are stained for AFB, preferably using the ZN technique. Negative tubes are incubated up to 6 weeks.[49]

The MB/BacT is a nonradiometric automated monitoring system designed for the isolation of mycobacteria from clinical specimens other than blood. MB/BacT bottles contain enhanced Middlebrook 7H9 broth. The bottom of each bottle is fitted with a gas permeable sensor that changes from dark green to bright yellow when CO_2 is produced in the broth by metabolizing mycobacteria. It utilizes a colorimetric sensor and reflected light to continuously monitor the CO_2 concentration in the culture medium.[51] A Swiss study showed that the mean time for the detection of *M. tuberculosis* from sputum, cerebrospinal fluid, and urine samples was 17.5 (±6.4) days for MB/BacT, 14.3 (±8.2) days for BACTEC, and 24.2 (±7.5) days for egg-based media cultures.[52]

The ESP Culture System II is an adaptation of the ESP blood culture system. The bottles contain modified Middlebrook 7H9 medium. It is a nonradiometric continuous monitoring system designed for the isolation of mycobacteria from clinical specimens. It utilizes a colorimetric sensor and reflected light to continuously monitor CO_2 concentration in the culture medium. In a study that compared the ESP Culture System II with the BACTEC MGIT 960, examining a total of 3,151 specimens, the mean times to detection members of MTBC were 17.4 days for ESP II and 11.9 days for BACTEC MGIT 960.[53]

BACTEC MYCO/F Lytic culture bottle contains a lytic agent to release the mycobacteria that have been phagocytosed by white blood cells. It is incubated and monitored automatically in a manner similar to the other BACTEC blood culture bottles. In addition to growing mycobacteria, the BACTEC MYCO/F Lytic is a good culture system for bacteria and fungi that may be present in the bloodstream.[54]

Septi-Chek AFB is a manual mycobacterial culture system. It allows simultaneous detection of MTBC and NTM, other respiratory pathogens and even contaminants, from respiratory specimens, urine, stool, body fluids, biopsy tissues, wounds, and skin lesions.[55] Capped bottle contains Middlebrook 7H9 broth and a paddle with agar media. The paddle is covered on one side with nonselective Middlebrook 7H11 agar and on the other side it is divided into two sections, one which allows the differentiation of MTBC from other mycobacteria (7H11 agar with NAP), and the other which ensures detection of contaminants (chocolate agar). This method requires about 3 weeks of incubation.[56] Isenberg et al. found that the Septi-Chek system was more sensitive than LJ, 7H11, and BACTEC broth in the percentage of mycobacterial isolates recovered.[57]

IDENTIFICATION OF MTBC USING CONVENTIONAL METHODS

Environmental Requirements

Tubercle bacilli are slow growing mycobacteria. Generation time is 20–22 hours for *M. tuberculosis* and 16–20 hours for *M. bovis*. They show optimal growth at 35–37°C in 5–10% CO_2. All cultures should be incubated under that conditions and examined after 5–7 days of incubation and weekly thereafter for 8 weeks before being discarded as negative.

Cultural Characteristics

Colony morphology should be observed on individual colonies with a hand lens. An acid-fast smear should be made to ensure that the colony being examined is indeed a MTBC and that no contaminating organisms are present. The texture of *M. tuberculosis* colonies on LJ medium has a characteristic roughness, they are dry, with nodular surface, and irregular thin periphery, and colonies are nonpigmented (Fig. 2). *Mycobacterium tuberculosis* fails to produce pigment beyond a light buff color, even after exposure to light.[6]

An acid-fast smear made from the *M. tuberculosis* colonies, from solid or liquid Middlebrook media, shows long stacked chains of bacilli, twisted rope-like, described as serpentine cords (Fig. 3), owing to the production of "cording factor" a cell surface glycolipid (trehalose 6,6'-dimycolate).[58]

A few relatively simple phenotypic tests are needed to identify most isolates of the MTBC. Phenotypic characteristics for identification of *M. tuberculosis* are formation of nonpigmented, rough, buff colonies after 14–28 days of incubation at 37°C on LJ or Middlebrook media; appearance of microcolonies after 5–7 days incubation on Middlebrook 7H10 or 7H11 agars, with formation of serpentine cords; accumulation of niacin; reduction of nitrates to nitrites; ability to grow in the presence of thiophene-2-carboxylic acid hydrazide (T2H); lack of catalase activity at 68°C; and selective inhibition of growth in broth culture media containing NAP.[6]

Phenotypic characteristics which can differentiate *M. bovis* from classic strains of *M. tuberculosis* are: most strains are niacin-negative, nitrates are not reduced to nitrites, pyrazinamidase is not produced and growth is selectively inhibited by T2H. The classic

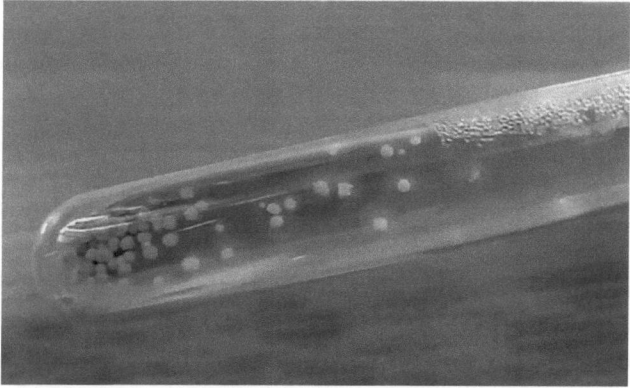

FIG. 2: *Mycobacterium tuberculosis* colonies on Löwenstein–Jensen medium. *(For color version, see Plate 1)*

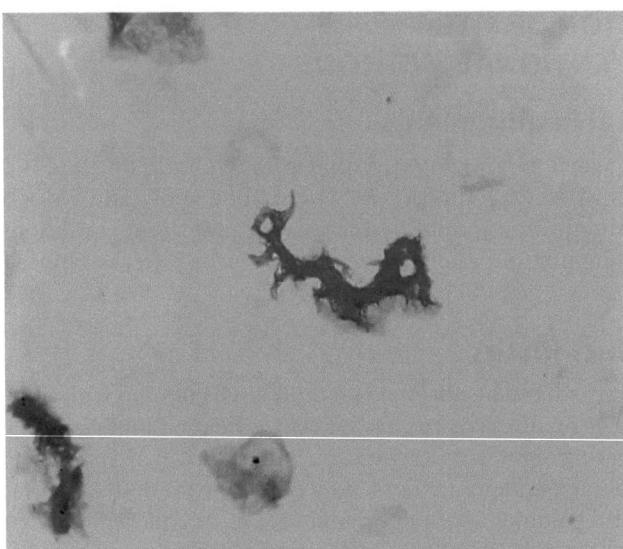

FIG. 3: *Mycobacterium tuberculosis* "serpentine cord". *(For color version, see Plate 1)*

human strains of *M. bovis* have a very slow growth rate, producing dysgonic-appearing colonies on LJ medium after 6–8 weeks. The medium most favorable for *M. bovis* contains 0.4% pyruvate without glycerol. Typical colonies are buff, low, and small and may appear either smooth or rough on egg-based medium. If pyruvate has been added to the medium, colonies may show serpentine cords similar to those of eugonic *M. tuberculosis*. Bacillus Calmette–Guérin strains simulate *M. tuberculosis* by being eugonic or more rapidly growing (3–4 weeks on LJ medium), having a rough, buff appearance and, in some cases, accumulating niacin. However, these strains remain T2H sensitive and can be differentiated on that basis.[59] The microscopic morphology of *M. bovis* cells in acid-fast stained smears is not distinctive.

Laboratories that perform only conventional methods should not use only one biochemical test. *Mycobacterium tuberculosis* accumulates niacin, but *M. simiae*, certain strains of *M. bovis*, and occasional strains of *M. marinum*, *M. africanum*, and *M. chelonae* may also be niacin-positive; therefore, this characteristic must be used in conjunction with other findings. Multiply drug resistant strains of *M. tuberculosis* may be niacin-negative as well.[60] It is essential to have sufficient growth on the primary egg-based media; otherwise, the risk of the obtaining false-negative results is increased.

Most of the mycobacteria produce catalase. However, not all species are capable of producing a positive reaction after heating the culture at 68°C for 20 minutes (heat stable catalase). Most strains of *M. tuberculosis* and other members of the MTBC do not produce heat-stable catalase, except for certain isoniazid (INH) resistant strains.[6]

PERFORMANCE OF RAPID IMMUNOCHROMATOGRAPHIC TESTS FOR IDENTIFICATION OF *MYCOBACTERIUM TUBERCULOSIS* COMPLEX IN LIQUID CULTURE

Rapid and accurate identification of MTBC in positive cultures is essential, particularly as liquid culture is associated with isolation of more NTM.[61] Conventional biochemical identification methods are slow, requiring subculture onto solid media, and cost and limited laboratory capacity preclude nucleic acid amplification tests (NAATs) in low-resource settings. Immunochromatographic tests which detect the MTBC protein fractions (MPT64, MPB64) are cheaper and simpler to use, and thus, may have an important role in these settings.

Immunochromatographic tests (ICTs) are for qualitative detection of these protein fractions that are secreted from MTBC cells during culture. The total assay time is 15 minutes with reactivity determined by visual color development.

Samples are added from positive broth cultures or from resuspended colonies from solid media to the test device, MPT64 antigen binds to anti-MPT64 antibodies conjugated to visualizing particles on the test strip. The antigen-conjugate complex migrates across the test strip to the reaction area and is captured by a second specific MPT64 antibody applied to the membrane. If the MPT64 antigen is present in the sample, a color reaction is produced by the labeled colloidal gold particles and is visualized as a pink to red line.

It is important to make ZN stained smears from tested cultures, and inoculate blood agar (48 h incubation at 37°C) as well, to rule out mixed cultures or potential contamination.

Brent et al. compared one MPT64 ICT, the MGIT TB_C Identification test (TB_C ID; Becton Dickinson, Sparks, MD) with the GenoType MTBC and *Mycobacterium* CM/AS line probe assays (LPAs) (Hain Lifescience GmbH, Nehren, Germany). They processed clinical samples in the MGIT 960 system. The sensitivity and specificity of TBc ID were 97.6 and 100%, respectively. TBc ID and LPA results were concordant for 208 (83 MTBC and 125 non-MTBC isolates: 99%) of 210 AFB-positive cultures. There was no statistical evidence of a difference between the LPA and TBc ID in diagnostic accuracy. A small minority of MTBC isolates are not detected by MPT64 assays due to deletion or mutation of the mpb64 gene, or to low MPT64 concentrations in early cultures or mixed cultures.[62]

Ngamlert et al. in Bangkok study compared ICT Capilia TB Test Kit with biochemical testing (niacin accumulation, nitrate reduction, and paranitrobenzoic acid). Of 247 isolates from broth-based culture (BATEC MGIT 960 system) evaluated, Capilia TB correctly identified 226 isolates as MTBC, and 14 isolates as NTM (97%) using the results of biochemical testing as the gold standard. The median time from specimen receipt in the laboratory and identification of MTBC was 20 days for Capilia TB compared with 45 days for the complete battery of biochemical tests. Six isolates that were Capilia TB negative but positive by biochemical testing were confirmed as MTBC and mutations in the *MPB64* gene, encoding the MPB64 protein, were detected in all.[63]

GAS-LIQUID AND HIGH PERFORMANCE LIQUID CHROMATOGRAPHY FOR IDENTIFICATION OF MYCOBACTERIAL SPECIES

Analysis of cellular long-chain fatty acids by gas-liquid chromatography (GLC) has been used to aid in the characterization of mycobacteria. It is used in reference laboratories for epidemiologic studies, since it can identify different species of mycobacteria after isolation by any type of culture technique, based on the difference between species regarding the length of the colic acid residues in the cell wall, and it can provide results in as little as 2 hours. Chromatography is a highly reproducible technique but the initial cost of the equipment is high.[64] These systems are in direct competition with nucleic acid-based methods for the rapid identification of mycobacteria.

MOLECULAR METHODS FOR DETECTION OF *MYCOBACTERIUM TUBERCULOSIS*

Nucleic Acid Amplification-based Techniques

Nucleic acid amplification tests are the most promising development in TB diagnostics with the purpose of obtaining faster results and early diagnosis of TB from clinical specimens. These tests have high specificity, but limited and variable sensitivity, especially from sputum smear-negative disease. There are different commercially available NAATs.

Amplicor *Mycobacterium tuberculosis* test is a DNA-based test that amplifies a segment of the *16S rRNA* gene using genus-specific primers, which, after hybridization to oligonucleotide probes, is detected in a colorimetric reaction in a microwell plate format.[65] An automated version of the test, the COBAS Amplicor MTB test together with the COBAS Amplicor analyzer allows automation of the amplification and detection steps in one system. More recently, the qualitative COBAS TaqMan MTB test has also been introduced using real-time polymerase chain reaction (PCR) and hybridization and performed in the COBAS TaqMan 48 analyzer running up to 48 samples simultaneously in 2.5 hours. All three tests are meant to be used in decontaminated and concentrated smear-positive respiratory samples from patients without previous treatment. Many studies have evaluated the Amplicor MTB test for the detection of *M. tuberculosis* both in respiratory and extrapulmonary samples.[66,67] Overall sensitivity has ranged from 83 to 92.4% in respiratory samples and from 50 to 95.9% in smear-negative samples. From extrapulmonary samples, the reported sensitivity has been consistently lower. Overall specificity has ranged from 91.3 to 100%.[68]

Amplified *Mycobacterium tuberculosis* Direct Test (MTD) uses isothermal amplification of 16S ribosomal transcripts, which are detected in a hybridization protection assay with an acridinium ester labeled MTBC-specific DNA probe.[69] The test is Food and Drug Administration approved for the direct detection of *M. tuberculosis* in smear-positive and smear-negative respiratory specimens and its interpretation requires the use of a luminometer.[70,71] Piersimoni and Scarparo reported overall sensitivity from 77 to 100%, with values of 90-100% in smear-positive samples and 63-100% in smear-negative samples compared with culture and clinical status of patient.[68]

The BD ProbeTec MTB test was first introduced several years ago as semiautomated system for rapid diagnosis of TB. It is based on the strand displacement amplification technique that uses enzymatic replication of target sequences in IS6110 and the *16S rRNA* gene. The amplified products are then detected with a luminometer. The method was evaluated in studies with respiratory samples with a reported sensitivity of 100% in smear-positive specimens and 92-100% in smear-negative samples. The overall specificity was 96-99% in the same studies.[72,73] The major drawback was that the sample preparation required at least 2 hours. An improved version of this system, the BD ProbeTec ET, which includes an internal amplification control to detect the presence of inhibitors, has been more recently evaluated in respiratory and nonrespiratory specimens in a clinical setting. As with the other NAATs described above, higher sensitivity and specificity have been found in respiratory smear-positive samples.[74]

MOLECULAR METHODS FOR IDENTIFICATION OF *MYCOBACTERIUM TUBERCULOSIS*

The first of such methods commercially available was the AccuProbe based on species-specific DNA probes that hybridize to rRNA for the identification of several important mycobacteria, members of the NTM and MTBC. Results are obtained after about 2 hours from a positive culture. The probes have been extensively evaluated in clinical setting, and have shown sensitivity and specificity greater than 90%. More recently, other molecular commercial systems have also been introduced for the rapid identification of the MTBC: the INNO-LiPA MYCOBACTERIA v2 and GenoType MTBC and GenoType *Mycobacterium* both to be applied on positive cultures.

INNO-LiPA MYCOBACTERIA v2 is a line probe assay that simultaneously detects and identifies the genus *Mycobacterium* and 16 different mycobacterial species, among them MTBC. It is based on nucleotide differences in the *16S-23S rRNA* gene spacers and can be performed on liquid or solid cultures. The test has been evaluated with a large variety of mycobacterial species showing an overall sensitivity of 100% and specificity of 94%.[75]

The GenoType MTBC and the GenoType *Mycobacterium* are also based on the reverse line probe hybridization assay and are intended for the differentiation of members of the MTBC and for the identification of 35 species of mycobacteria including *M. tuberculosis* respectively. The GenoType MTBC is based on 23S rRNA gene fragment specific for the MTBC, together with gyrB sequence polymorphisms, and the RD1 deletion for identification of *M. bovis* BCG.[76] As in other reverse hybridization assays, amplified products from a multiplex PCR assay will hybridize to specific oligonuleotides immobilized on a membrane strip. The GenoType *Mycobacterium* is based on regions of the 23S rRNA gene. After PCR amplification, hybridization is performed on the oligonucleotides immobilized on the membrane strips, and results are interpreted based on the combination of bands that appear. Two kits are offered separately, the GenoType *Mycobacterium* CM (common mycobacteria) allowing identification of 17 species and the GenoType *Mycobacterium* AS (additional species) that identifies 18 less common mycobacterial species.[77] The performance of these three LPAs requires the availability of a thermal cycler and adequate facilities to conduct PCR amplification.

MOLECULAR METHODS FOR DETECTION OF DRUG RESISTANCE OF *MYCOBACTERIUM TUBERCULOSIS*

The continuous emergence of severe forms of drug resistance, such as the extensively drug-resistant tuberculosis (XDR-TB) that has evolved multidrug-resistant tuberculosis (MDR-TB) or resistance to rifampicin (RIF) and isoniazid (INH), as well as to any member of the quinolone family and at least one of the following second line TB treatments: kanamycin, capreomycin, or amikacin, calls for improved and faster methods for its detection. With the purpose of detecting drug resistance in a shorter period of time and for rapid screening of multidrug resistance markers, such as resistance to RIF in certain populations,[78] several molecular approaches have been proposed in the last years. Molecular tests to detect drug resistance in TB look for gene mutations known to be associated with resistance to a particular drug.

Solid Phase Hybridization Assays

This type of assay is based on the reverse hybridization of oligonucleotides on plastic strips to which specific probes have been immobilized. They are also known as line probe assays. Amplified target sequences from the organism under evaluation are then bound to the specific probes, and hybridization is revealed by the development of a colored reaction on the strip.

Commercially available solid phase reverse hybridization assays for the rapid detection of drug resistance in *M. tuberculosis* are: the line probe assay (LiPA; INNO-

LiPA Rif TB assay) for detecting resistance to RIF and the GenoType MTBDRplus for the simultaneous detection of resistance to RIF and INH.

Line probe assay is based on reverse hybridization of amplified DNA from cultured isolates or clinical samples to ten probes covering the core region of the *rpoB* gene of *M. tuberculosis* immobilized on a nitrocellulose strip.[79] The pattern of hybridization obtained indicates the presence or the absence of mutated or wild regions, which is visualized by a colorimetric reaction, and the strain can be considered as resistant or susceptible to RIF.[80] Several studies have been conducted on the application of LiPA for the detection of RIF resistance.

Four studies that performed LiPA on clinical samples showed 100% specificity but the sensitivity ranged from 80 to 100%.[81] Traore et al. performed a larger study, where they assessed the usefulness of LiPA for detecting RIF resistance in 420 sputum samples originated from different countries. A 99.6% agreement was found between results obtained by culture and LiPA. The study showed that with an adequate DNA extraction method, LiPA allows rapid detection of resistance to RIF when performed directly from sputum samples.[82]

The GenoType MTBDRplus, on the other hand, detects resistance to INH and RIF in clinical isolates and sputum samples based on the detection of the most common mutations in *katG*, *inhA*, and *rpoB* genes.[83] It also uses PCR and reverse hybridization to probes immobilized on a plastic strip. In a South African study, Barnard et al. implemented MTBDRplus in a high volume public health laboratory for the rapid screening of MDR-TB. Overall, 97% of results from smear-positive samples were available within 1–2 days. Sensitivity and specificity for detection of RIF resistance were 98.9 and 99.4%, respectively. For INH resistance sensitivity and specificity were 94.2 and 99.7%, respectively, and for detection of MDR-TB, 98.8 and 100%, respectively, as compared with conventional drug susceptibility testing (DST) results.[84]

Real-time Polymerase Chain Reaction Assay

Xpert MTB/RIF assay is fully automated, real-time nucleic acid amplification technology run on the multidisease platform GeneXpert. It was recommended for use by the World Health Organization (WHO) in December 2010. Test simultaneously detects MTBC and RIF resistance conferring mutations, in a closed system, in less than 2 hours, directly from sputum samples.[85] Assay targets a mutation in the RIF resistance determining region of the *rpoB* gene. It is unable to detect INH resistance.[86] Test has high accuracy for pulmonary TB detection (sensitivity 89%, specificity 99%).[87] While Xpert has been approved for TB detection in sputum by regulatory agencies, Xpert for TB detection in nonrespiratory specimens is considered "off-label" use. Denkinger et al. performed a systematic review and meta-analysis to assess the accuracy of Xpert for the detection of extrapulmonary TB. They identified 18 studies involving 4,461 samples. Xpert sensitivity differed substantially between sample types. In lymph node tissues or aspirates, Xpert pooled sensitivity was 83.1% versus culture and 81.2% versus composite reference standards (CRSs). In cerebrospinal fluid, Xpert pooled sensitivity was 80.5% against culture and 62.8% against CRS. In pleural fluid, pooled sensitivity was 46.4% against culture and 21.4% against CRS. Xpert pooled specificity was consistently greater than 98.7% against CRS across different samples types. Based on this systematic review, the WHO now recommends Xpert over conventional tests for diagnosis of TB in lymph nodes and other tissues, and as the preferred initial test for diagnosis of TB meningitis.[88] The poor sensitivity of Xpert in pleural fluid is probably due to the paucibacillary nature of the disease and fact that not pleural fluid but rather pleural biopsy is the sample of choice for the diagnosis of pleural TB (as has been described for culture).[89]

Although not a complete surrogate for MDR-TB, particularly in settings with low resistance levels, RIF resistance is most important indicator of MDR-TB with serious clinical implications for affected patients. Given that most patients enrolled in drug resistance surveys are newly diagnosed with TB and at low risk of RIF resistance, the positive predictive value of any test will not be adequate to identify true positives but the negative predictive value will be sufficiently high to accurately identify true negatives. Xpert MTB/RIF could, therefore, be used as screening tool to identify those with no resistance to RIF, while patients with RIF resistance undergo further confirmatory testing with a second WHO-approved technology.[88]

Any molecular test, including Xpert, is not suitable for patient monitoring as these tests detect DNA from viable and nonviable bacilli. Conventional laboratory diagnostic, is therefore, required to monitor treatment response of patients detected by molecular tests and to conduct additional DST in patients with RIF and/or INH resistance.

DRUG SUSCEPTIBILTY TESTING

Resistance can be associated with the misuse of antimicrobial therapy, or it may occur as process of random evolution, independent of exposure to the agents. The frequency of drug resistant mutants in a culture of tubercle bacilli has been estimated to be about $1:10^5$ bacteria for INH and $1:10^6$ for streptomycin (STR). If two drugs (i.e., INH and STR) are taken together, the incidence of resistance is $1:10^{11}$, which is the sum of the two taken separately. Knowledge of incidence of mutants becomes important because it has been determined that patients with an open pulmonary cavity may have a total bacillary population of 10^7–10^9 bacteria. In as much as 1 of every 10^5–10^6 MTBC may be resistant to a single anti-TB agent, the cavity may contain as many as 10^2–10^4 drug resistant bacilli.[90] Therefore, if these patients are treated with a single anti-TB agent, their cultures may soon show the emergence of the resistant phenotype to that agent, and thus, treatment fails. Consequently, patients with TB must always be treated with at least two, or preferably more drugs.

A second principal of MTBC DST is based on the *in vitro* correlation between the clinical response to an anti-TB agent and the result of *in vitro* susceptibility testing. If more than 1% of the tubercle bacilli present are resistant to a drug *in vitro*, therapy with that drug is not clinically useful. Therefore, most methods for DST must be capable of determining the proportion of bacilli susceptible and resistant to a given drug.

The most commonly used proportion method on LJ medium or Middlebrook agar requires a minimum of 3-4 weeks to produce results.[91] The radiometric BACTEC TB 460 system, on the other hand, using an enriched liquid medium decreased the turnaround time, for both primary and secondary anti-TB agents, and is considered the "gold standard".[41,92] However, due to increasing concern about the use and disposal of radioactive material, there is a rapid trend toward using commercially available nonradiometric broth-based culture and DST methods.

BACTEC MGIT 960 is a new nonradiometric system, which is considered equivalent to the BACTEC 460 in performance. Bemer et al. conducted the multicenter study which evaluated the reproducibility and reliability of the BACTEC MGIT 960 instrument for testing of *M. tuberculosis* susceptibility to the front line drugs: INH, RIF, ethambutol, and STR, and compared the results to those obtained by the radiometric procedure. A total of 110 *M. tuberculosis* strains were evaluated in this study. The proportion method on LJ medium was used to resolve discrepant results by an independent arbiter. After resolution of discrepant results, the sensitivity of BACTEC MGIT 960 system was 100% for all four drugs and specificity ranged from 89.8% for STR to 100% for RIF. Turnaround times were 4.6–11.7 days (median, 6.5 days) for BACTEC MGIT 960 and 4.0–10.0 days (median, 7.0 days) for BACTEC 460 TB.[93]

Another multicenter study for laboratory validation of the BACTEC MGIT 960 technique for testing susceptibilities of *M. tuberculosis* to classical second line drugs and newer antimicrobials was conducted by Rüsch-Gerdes et al.[94] The primary aim of their study was to develop a basic protocol, establish critical test concentrations for seven second line and newer drugs, and test a large number of clinical isolates. For comparison, BACTEC 460 was used as the gold standard, since critical test concentrations of most of the drugs have already been established for this system.[92] The critical concentrations for the seven drugs used in the MGIT 960 system are as follows: amikacin, 1.0 μg/mL; capreomycin, 2.5 μg/mL; ethionamide, 5.0 μg/mL; prothionamide, 2.5 μg/mL; ofloxacin 2.0 μg/mL; rifabutin, 0.5 μg/mL; and linezolid, 1.0 μg/mL.[94] These data demonstrate that the BACTEC MGIT 960 system is an accurate method for rapid susceptibility testing of *M. tuberculosis* to first and second line drugs.

Susceptibility tests should be performed on all initial isolates of *M. tuberculosis* and on isolates from patients who remain culture-positive after 3 months or demonstrate clinical evidence of therapeutic failure.[91]

IMMUNODIAGNOSTIC TESTS FOR TUBERCULOSIS

The ability of TB to infect a patient and remain latent for many years before reactivation is a key obstacle to the control and elimination of TB. Failure to identify and treat latently infected individuals allows the chain of transmission to continue. Testing for latent TB has typically been done by healthcare workers in the form of tuberculin skin testing (TST), using PPD.[95] The widespread use of BCG vaccination, crossreacting environmental antigens, and the presence of anergy in rare cases confounds this test and a more accurate replacement is required.

MPB64 skin patch test provides an approach to distinguish active TB from PPD-positive healthy controls. MPB64 is a mycobacterial antigen specific for MTBC. The test result can be interpreted 3–4 days after patch application. During initial evaluation in Japan, this test showed a sensitivity of 98%, with specificity of 99%.[96]

Interferon-γ Release Assays

Cytokine detection assays measure the cell mediated immune response elicited against *M. tuberculosis*. Interferon-γ release assays (IGRAs) measure the interferon-γ (IFN-γ) released by sensitized white blood cells.

Use of these tests for diagnosis of active disease is based on the presumption that one must have TB infection in order to have TB disease. The greater problem in diagnosis of active TB disease is their poor specificity for disease, because these tests cannot distinguish an immune response to reactivated TB from a response to TB infection that remains latent.

Longitudinal studies have shown that the predictive value of IGRAs for reactivation of TB in immunosuppressed individuals is better than that provided by TST in individuals vaccinated with BCG. High levels of IFN-γ release are detected by these assays in about 70–90% of individuals with active disease and these levels decrease after treatment is completed, although such reductions are not consistently recorded.[97,98]

Different IGRAs are commercially available, using different antigens to stimulate IFN-γ release and different methods of measurement.

QuantiFERON-TB Gold is an enzyme-linked immunosorbent assay test, which detects the release of INF-γ in fresh heparinized whole blood from sensitized persons upon incubation with synthetic peptides simulating early secretory antigenic target-6 (ESAT-6) and culture filtrate protein-10 (CFP-10).[99] The test steps involve blood sample collection, addition of stimulating antigens, incubation for 16-24 hours at 37°C, harvesting of plasma, and addition of conjugate solution. The samples are then incubated for 2 hours at room temperature, the plates are washed at least six times and then the substrate is added. The samples are then incubated for 30 minutes, adding stop solution, reading absorbance at 450 nm, and calculating results using dedicated software. The patient only needs to visit once, for specimen collection, and results can be obtained in 48 hours.

The QuantiFERON-TB Gold In-Tube was developed to overcome the limitation of QuantiFERON-TB Gold, which could only be used in facilities where blood testing could begin within a few hours of its collection. This test uses a mixture of 14 peptides representing ESAT-6, CFP-10, and a part of TB 7.7.[99]

T-SPOT.TB incubates peripheral blood mononuclear cells with mixtures of peptides (ESAT-6, CFP-10) and uses an enzyme-linked immunospot assay to detect increases in the number of cells that secrete INF-γ (spots in each test well).[99]

Although several comparison studies of IGRAs for *M. tuberculosis* have been carried out, their clinical application is still limited, especially among at-risk populations and children.[100,101]

REFERENCES

1. World Health Organization. Global tuberculosis control. WHO report 2011. WHO/HTM/TB/2011.16. Geneva: WHO; 2011.
2. Gangadharam PRJ, Jenkins PA, editors. Mycobacteria: I Basic Aspects. New York: Chapman and Hall; 1997.
3. Lévy-Frébault VV, Portaels F. Proposed minimal standards for the genus *Mycobacterium* and for description of new slowly growing *Mycobacterium* species. Int J Syst Bacteriol. 1992;42:315-23.
4. Karakousis PC, Bishai WR, Dorman SE. *Mycobacterium tuberculosis* cell envelope lipids and the host immune response. Cell Microbiol. 2004;6:105-16.
5. Smith I. *Mycobacterium tuberculosis* pathogenesis and molecular determinants of virulence. Clin Microbiol Rev. 2003;16:463-96.
6. Koneman EW, Allen SD, Janda WM, Schreckenberger PC, Winn WC, editors. Color Atlas and Textbook of Diagnostic Microbiology. 6th ed. Philadelphia: Lippincott Williams & Wilkins. 2006. pp. 1064-124.
7. Homolka S, Post E, Oberhauser B, et al. High genetic diversity among *Mycobacterium tuberculosis* complex strains from Sierra Leone. BMC Microbiol. 2008;8:103.
8. Atkins PJ, Robinson PA. Bovine tuberculosis and badgers in Britain: relevance of the past. Epidemiol Infect. 2013;141:1437-44.
9. Lamm DL, van der Meijden PM, Morales A, et al. Incidence and treatment of complications of bacillus Calmette-Guérin intravesical therapy in superficial bladder cancer. J Urol. 1992;147:596-600.
10. De Jong BC, Antonio M, Gagneux S. *Mycobacterium africanum*—review of an important cause of human tuberculosis in West Africa. PLoS Negl Trop Dis. 2010;4(9):e744.
11. Mostowy S, Onipede A, Gagneux S, et al. Genomic analysis distinguishes *Mycobacterium africanum*. J Clin Microbiol. 2004;42(8):3594-9.
12. Cvetnic Z, Katalinic-Jankovic V, Sostaric B, et al. *Mycobacterium caprae* in cattle and humans in Croatia. Int J Tuberc Lung Dis. 2007;11(6):652-8.
13. Miltgen J, Morillon M, Koeck JL, et al. Two cases of pulmonary tuberculosis caused by *Mycobacterium tuberculosis subsp canetti*. Emerg Infect Dis. 2002;8(11):1350-2.

14. Kiers A, Klarenbeek A, Mendelts B, Van Soolingen D, Koëter G. Transmission of *Mycobacterium pinnipedii* to humans in a zoo with marine mammals. Int J Tuberc Lung Dis. 2008;12(12):1469-73.
15. Frank W, Reisinger EC, Brandt-Hamerla W, Schwede I, Handrick W. *Mycobacterium microti*—pulmonary tuberculosis in an immunocompetent patient. Wien Klin Wochenschr. 2009;121(7-8):282-6.
16. Grange JM. Mycobacterium. In: Greenwood D, Slack R, Peutherer J, Barer M, editors. Medical Microbiology. 17th ed. Philadelphia: Churchill Livingstone Elsevier; 2007. pp. 206-20.
17. Castro KG, Dooley SW. *Mycobacterium tuberculosis* transmission in healthcare settings: is it influenced by coinfection with human immunodeficiency virus? Infect Control Hosp Epidemiol. 1993;14:65-6.
18. Centers for Disease Control and Prevention and National Institutes of Health. Biosafety in microbiological and biomedical laboratories. HHS Publication (CDC) 99-8395. Washington: US Government Printing Office; 1999. Also available from: www.cdc.gov/od/ohs/biosfty/bmb14/bmb14toc.htm.
19. Sommers H. Special Mycobacterial Survey. Skokie, IL: College of American Pathologists; 1976.
20. Krasnow I, Wayne LG. Comparison of methods for tuberculosis bacteriology. Appl Microbiol. 1969;18:915-7.
21. Issac-Renton JL, Puselja BB, Allen EA, Grzybowski S, Black WA. Microscopic evaluation of sputum specimens submitted for *Mycobacterium tuberculosis* culture. Am J Clin Pathol. 1985;84(3):361-3.
22. Perkins MD, Cunningham J. Facing the crisis: improving the diagnosis of tuberculosis in the HIV era. J Infect Dis. 2007;196 Suppl 1:S15-27.
23. Watterson SA, Drobniewski FA. Modern laboratory diagnosis of mycobacterial infections. J Clin Pathol. 2000;53(10):727-32.
24. Kubica GP, David HL. The mycobacteria. In: Sonnenwirth AC, Jarett L, editors. Gradwohl's Clinical Laboratory Methods and Diagnosis. 8th ed. St. Louis: Mosby; 1980.
25. Sommers HM, Mc Clatchy JK. Laboratory Diagnosis of the Mycobacterioses. Cumitech 16. Washington, DC: American Society for Microbiology; 1983.
26. Kubica GP, Gross WM, Hawkins JE, Sommers HM, Vestal AL, Wayne LG. Laboratory services for mycobacterial diseases. Am Rev Respir Dis. 1975;112(6):773-87.
27. Kent PT, Kubica GP. Public Health Mycobacteriology: A Guide for the Level III Laboratory. Centers for Disease Control, Division of Laboratory Training and Consultation. Atlanta (GA): US Department of Health and Human Services; 1985.
28. Shah RR, Dye WE. The use of dithiothreitol to replace N-acetyl-L-cysteine for routine sputum digestion-decontamination for the culture of mycobacteria. Am Rev Respir Dis. 1966;94:454.
29. Smithwick RW, Stratigos CB, David HL. Use of cetylpyridinium chloride and sodium chloride for the decontamination of sputum specimens that are transported to the laboratory for the isolation of *Mycobacterium tuberculosis*. J Clin Microbiol. 1975;1:411-3.
30. Balows A, Hausler WJ Jr, Herrmann KL, Isenberg HD, Shadomy HJ, editors. Manual of Clinical Microbiology. 5th ed. Washington: American Society for Microbiology; 1991.
31. Rickman TW, Moyer NP. Increased sensitivity of acid-fast smears. J Clin Microbiol. 1980;11:618-20.
32. Knechel NA. Tuberculosis: pathophysiology, clinical features, and diagnosis. Crit Care Nurse. 2009;29(2):34-43.
33. Wilson ML. Recent advances in the laboratory detection of *Mycobacterium tuberculosis* complex and drug resistance. Clin Infect Dis. 2011;52(11):1350-5.
34. Hinson JM Jr, Bradsher RW, Bodner SJ. Gram-stain neutrality of *Mycobacterium tuberculosis*. Am Rev Respir Dis. 1981;123(4 Pt1):365-6.
35. Smithwick RW. Laboratory Manual for Acid-Fast Microscopy. 2nd ed. Atlanta, GA: Centers for Disease Control; 1976.
36. Saubolle MA, Sussland D. Nocardiosis: review of clinical and laboratory experience. J Clin Microbiol. 2003;41(10):4497-501.
37. Wayne LG, Kubica GP. Genus *Mycobacterium*. In: Sneath PH, Mair NS, Sharpe ME, Holt JG, editors. Bergey's Manual of Systematic Bacteriology. Baltimore: Williams & Wilkins; 1986. pp. 1436-57.
38. St Amand AL, Frank DN, De Groote MA, Basaraba RJ, Orme IM, Pace NR. Use of specific rRNA oligonucleotide probes for microscopic detection of *Mycobacterium tuberculosis* in culture and tissue specimens. J Clin Microbiol. 2005;43(10):5369-71.
39. Su WJ, Feng JY, Chiu YC, Huang SF, Lee YC. Role of 2-month sputum smears in predicting culture conversion in pulmonary tuberculosis. Eur Respir J. 2011;37(2):376-83.
40. Senkoro M, Mfinanga SG, Mørkve O. Smear microscopy and culture conversion rates among smear positive pulmonary tuberculosis patients by HIV status in Dar es Salaam, Tanzania. BMC Infect Dis. 2010;10:210.

41. Tenover FC, Crawford JT, Huebner RE, Geiter LJ, Horsburgh CR Jr, Good RC. The resurgence of tuberculosis: is your laboratory ready? J Clin Microbiol. 1993;31:767-70.
42. Cohn ML, Waggoner RF, McClatchy JK. The 7H11 medium for the cultivation of mycobacteria. Am Rev Respir Dis. 1968;98:295-6.
43. Irfan S, Hasan R, Kanji A, Hassan Q, Azam I. Evaluation of a microcolony detection method and phage assay for rapid detection of *Mycobacterium tuberculosis* in sputum samples. Southeast Asian J Trop Med Public Health. 2006;37(6):1187-95.
44. Gruft H. Isolation of acid-fast bacilli from contaminated specimens. Health Lab Sci. 1971;8(2):79-82.
45. Mitchison DA, Allen BW, Carrol L, Dickinson JM, Aber VR. A selective oleic acid albumin agar medium for tubercle bacilli. J Med Microbiol. 1972;5(2):165-75.
46. Abe C, Hosojima S, Fukasawa Y, et al. Comparison of MB-Check, BACTEC, and egg-based media for recovery of mycobacteria. J Clin Microbiol. 1992;30(4):878-81.
47. Bhattacharya S, Roy R, Chowdhury NR, Dasgupta A, Dastidar SG. Comparison of a novel bilayered medium with the conventional media for cultivation of *Mycobacterium tuberculosis*. Indian J Med Res. 2009;130(5):561-6.
48. Venkataraman P, Herbert D, Paramasivan CN. Evaluation of the BACTEC radiometric method in the early diagnosis of tuberculosis. Indian J Med Res. 1998;108:120-7.
49. Siddiqi SH, Rüsch-Gerdes S. MGIT Procedure Manual. Foundation for Innovative New Diagnostics, Geneva, Switzerland; 2006.
50. Tortoli E, Cichero P, Piersimoni C, Simonetti MT, Gesu G, Nista D. Use of BACTEC MGIT 960 for recovery of mycobacteria from clinical specimens: multicenter study. J Clin Microbiol. 1999;37(11):3578-82.
51. Rohner P, Ninet B, Metral C, Emler S, Auckenthaler R. Evaluation of the MB/BacT system and comparison to the BACTEC 460 system and solid media for isolation of mycobacteria from clinical specimens. J Clin Microbiol. 1997;35(12):3127-31.
52. Ramachandran R, Paramasivan C. What is new in the diagnosis of tuberculosis? Part 1: Techniques for diagnosis of tuberculosis. Ind J Tub. 2003;(50):133-41.
53. Williams-Bouyer N, Yorke R, Lee HI, Woods GL. Comparison of the BACTEC MGIT 960 and ESP culture system II for growth and detection of mycobacteria. J Clin Microbiol. 2000;38(11): 4167-70.
54. Fuller DD, Davis TE Jr, Denys GA, York MK. Evaluation of BACTEC MYCO/F Lytic medium for recovery of mycobacteria, fungi, and bacteria from blood. J Clin Microbiol. 2001;39(8):2933-6.
55. Laboratory Procedure. BBL SEPTI-CHEK AFB. Mycobacteria Culture System. [online] Available from: http://www.bd.com/ds/tecnicalcenter/clsi/clsi-sepchek AFB.pdf [Accessed January, 2016].
56. Ranjan K, Sharma M. An approach to the detection of mycobacteria in clinically suspected cases of urinary tract infection in immunocompromised patients. WebmedCentral BACTERIOLOGY. 2010;9(1):WMC00616.
57. Isenberg HD, D'Amato RF, Heifets L, et al. Collaborative feasibility study of a biphasic system (Roche Septi-Chek AFB) for rapid detection and isolation of mycobacteria. J Clin Microbiol. 1991;29(8):1719-22.
58. Barksdale L, Kim KS. *Mycobacterium*. Bacteriol Rev. 1977;41(1):217-372.
59. Tsukamura M. Niacin-negative *Mycobacterium tuberculosis*. Am Rev Respir Dis. 1974;110(1):101-3.
60. Gross WM, Hawkins JE. Radiometric selective inhibition tests for differentiation of *Mycobacterium tuberculosis*, *Mycobacterium bovis*, and other mycobacteria. J Clin Microbiol. 1985;21:565-8.
61. Chihota VN, Grant AD, Fielding K, et al. Liquid vs. solid culture for tuberculosis: performance and cost in a resource-constrained setting. Int J Tuberc Lung Dis. 2010;14(8):1024-31.
62. Brent AJ, Mugo D, Musyimi R, et al. Performance of the MGIT TBc identification test and meta-analysis of MPT64 assays for identification of the *Mycobacterium tuberculosis* complex in liquid culture. J Clin Microbiol. 2011;49(12):4343-6.
63. Ngamlert K, Sinthuwattanawibool C, McCarthy KD, et al. Diagnostic performance and costs of Capilia TB for *Mycobacterium tuberculosis* complex identification from broth-based culture in Bangkok, Thailand. Trop Med Int Health. 2009;14:748-53.
64. Ogbaini-Emovon E. Current trends in the laboratory diagnosis of tuberculosis. Benin J Postgrad Med. 2009;11:79-90.
65. Dalovisio JR, Montenegro-James S, Kemmerly SA, et al. Comparison of the amplified *Mycobacterium tuberculosis* (MTB) direct test, Amplicor MTB PCR, and IS6110-PCR for detection of MTB in respiratory specimens. Clin Infect Dis. 1996;23(5):1099-106.

66. Michos AG, Daikos GL, Tzanetou K, et al. Detection of *Mycobacterium tuberculosis* DNA in respiratory and nonrespiratory specimens by the Amplicor MTB PCR. Diagn Microbiol Infect Dis. 2006;54:121-6.
67. Ozkutuk A, Kirdar S, Ozden S, Esen N. Evaluation of Cobas Amplicor MTB test to detect *Mycobacterium tuberculosis* in pulmonary and extrapulmonary specimens. New Microbiol. 2006;29:269-73.
68. Piersimoni C, Scarparo C. Relevance of commercial amplification methods for direct detection of *Mycobacterium tuberculosis* complex in clinical samples. J Clin Microbiol. 2003;41:5355-65.
69. Abe C, Hirano K, Wada M, et al. Detection of *Mycobacterium tuberculosis* in clinical specimens by polymerase chain reaction and Gen-Probe Amplified *Mycobacterium Tuberculosis* Direct test. J Clin Microbiol. 1993;31:3270-4.
70. Centers for Disease Control and Prevention (CDC). Update: nucleic acid amplification tests for tuberculosis. MMWR Morb Mortal Wkly Rep. 2000;49:593-4.
71. Coll P, Garrigo M, Moreno C, Marti N. Routine use of Gen-Probe Amplified *Mycobacterium Tuberculosis* Direct (MTD) test for detection of *Mycobacterium tuberculosis* with smear-positive and smear-negative specimens. Int J Tuberc Lung Dis. 2003;7:886-91.
72. Bergmann JS, Woods GL. Clinical evaluation of the BDProbeTec strand displacement amplification assay for rapid diagnosis of tuberculosis. J Clin Microbiol. 1998;36:2766-8.
73. Pfyffer GE, Funke-Kissling P, Rundler E, Weber R. Performance characteristics of the BDProbeTec system for direct detection of *Mycobacterium tuberculosis* complex in respiratory specimens. J Clin Microbiol. 1999;37:137-40.
74. Rüsch-Gerdes S, Richter E. Clinical evaluation of the semiautomated BDProbeTec ET system for the detection of *Mycobacterium tuberculosis* in respiratory and nonrespiratory specimens. Diagn Microbiol Infect Dis. 2004;48:265-70.
75. Tortoli E, Mariottini A, Mazzarelli G. Evaluation of INNO-LiPA MYCOBACTERIA v2: improved reverse hybridization multiple DNA probe assay for mycobacterial identification. J Clin Microbiol. 2003;41:4418-20.
76. Richter E, Weizenegger M, Fahr AM, Rüsch-Gerdes S. Usefulness of the GenoType MTBC assay for differentiating species of the *Mycobacterium tuberculosis* complex in cultures obtained from clinical specimens. J Clin Microbiol. 2004;42:4303-6.
77. Richter E, Rüsch-Gerdes S, Hillemann D. Evaluation of the GenoType Mycobacterium assay for identification of mycobacterial species from cultures. J Clin Microbiol. 2006;44:1769-75.
78. Traore H, Fissette K, Bastian I, Devleeschouwer M, Portaels F. Detection of rifampicin resistance in *Mycobacterium tuberculosis* isolates from diverse countries by a commercial line probe assay as an initial indicator of multidrug resistance. Int J Tuberc Lung Dis. 2000;4:481-4.
79. De Beenhouwer H, Lhiang Z, Jannes G, et al. Rapid detection of rifampicin resistance in sputum and biopsy specimens from tuberculosis patients by PCR and line probe assay. Tuber Lung Dis. 1995;76:425-30.
80. Rossau R, Traore H, De Beenhouwer H, et al. Evaluation of the INNO-LiPA Rif TB assay, a reverse hybridization assay for the simultaneous detection of *Mycobacterium tuberculosis* complex and its resistance to rifampin. Antimicrob Agents Chemother. 1997;41:2093-8.
81. Morgan M, Kalantri S, Flores L, Pai M. A commercial line probe assay for the rapid detection of rifampicin resistance in *Mycobacterium tuberculosis*: a systematic review and meta-analysis. BMC Infect Dis. 2005;5:62.
82. Traore H, van Deun A, Shamputa IC, Rigouts L, Portaels F. Direct detection of *Mycobacterium tuberculosis* complex DNA and rifampin resistance in clinical specimens from tuberculosis patients by line probe assay. J Clin Microbiol. 2006;44:4384-8.
83. Hillemann D, Rüsch-Gerdes S, Richter E. Evaluation of the GenoType MTBDRplus assay for rifampin and isoniazid susceptibility testing of *Mycobacterium tuberculosis* strains and clinical specimens. J Clin Microbiol. 2007;45:2635-40.
84. Barnard M, Albert H, Coetzee G, O'Brien R, Bosman ME. Rapid molecular screening for multidrug-resistant tuberculosis in a high-volume public health laboratory in South Africa. Am J Respir Crit Care. 2008;177:787-92.
85. Boehme CC, Nabeta P, Hillemann D, et al. Rapid molecular detection of tuberculosis and rifampin resistance. N Engl J Med. 2010;363(11):1005-15.
86. Al-Ateah SM, Al-Dowaidi MM, El-Khizzi NA. Evaluation of direct detection of *Mycobacterium tuberculosis* complex in respiratory and nonrespiratory clinical specimens using the Cepheid Gene Xpert® system. Saudi Med J. 2012;33(10):1100-5.

87. Steingart KR, Schiller I, Horne DJ, Pai M, Boehme CC, Dendukuri N. Xpert® MTB/RIF assay for pulmonary tuberculosis and rifampicin resistance in adults. Cochrane Database Syst Rev. 2014;1:CD009593.
88. Denkinger CM, Schumacher SG, Boehme CC, Dendukuri N, Pai M, Steingart KR. Xpert MTB/RIF assay for the diagnosis of extrapulmonary tuberculosis: a systematic review and meta-analysis. Eur Respir J. 2014;44:435-46.
89. Porcel JM. Tuberculous pleural effusion. Lung. 2009;187:263-70.
90. Grosset J. Bacteriologic basis of short-course chemotherapy for tuberculosis. Clin Chest Med. 1980;1:231-41.
91. Woods GL, Brown-Elliott BA, Desmond EP, et al. Susceptibility testing of mycobacteria, nocardia, and other aerobic actinomycetes; approved standard. NCCLS Document M24-A. Wayne (PA): Clinical and Laboratory Standards Institute; 2003.
92. Pfyffer GE, Bonato DA, Ebrahimzadeh A, et al. Multicenter laboratory validation of susceptibility testing of *Mycobacterium tuberculosis* against classical second-line and newer antimicrobial drugs by using the radiometric BACTEC 460 technique and the proportion method with solid media. J Clin Microbiol. 1999;37:3179-86.
93. Bemer P, Palicova F, Rüsch-Gerdes S, Drugeon HB, Pfyffer GE. Multicenter evaluation of fully automated BACTEC Mycobacteria Growth Indicator Tube 960 system for susceptibility testing of *Mycobacterium tuberculosis*. J Clin Microbiol. 2002;40:150-4.
94. Rüsch-Gerdes S, Pfyffer GE, Casal M, Chadwick M, Siddiqi S. Multicenter laboratory validation of the BACTEC MGIT 960 technique for testing susceptibilities of *Mycobacterium tuberculosis* to classical second-line drugs and newer antimicrobials. J Clin Microbiol. 2006;44:688-92.
95. Lawn SD, Zumla AI, Tuberculosis. Lancet. 2011;378:57-72.
96. Nakamura RM, Einck L, Velmonte MA, et al. Detection of active tuberculosis by an MBP-64 transdermal patch: a field study. Scand J Infect Dis. 2001;33(6):405-7.
97. Pai M, Zwerling A, Menzies D. Systematic review: T-cell-based assays for the diagnosis of latent tuberculosis infection: an update. Ann Intern Med. 2008;149:177-84.
98. Adetifa IM, Ota MO, Walther B, et al. Decay kinetics of an interferon-γ release assay with anti-tuberculosis therapy in newly diagnosed tuberculosis cases. PLoS One. 2010;5(9):e12502.
99. Mazurek GH, Jereb J, Vernon A, LoBue P, Goldberg S, Castro K. Updated guidelines for using interferon-gamma release assays to detect *Mycobacterium tuberculosis* infection—United States, 2010. MMWR Recomm Rep. 2010;59(RR-5):1-25.
100. Tavast E, Salo E, Seppälä I, Tuuminen T. IGRA tests perform similarly to TST but cause no adverse reactions: pediatric experience in Finland. BMC Res Notes. 2009;2:9.
101. Menzies D, Pai M, Comstock G. Meta-analysis: new tests for the diagnosis of latent tuberculosis infection: areas of uncertainty and recommendations for research. Ann Intern Med. 2007;146(5):340-54.

CHAPTER 2

Epidemiology of Tuberculosis

Anna L Rich

INTRODUCTION

Despite being an ancient illness, with records dating back to the Egyptian mummies of 600 AD, as well as reference to an illness akin to tuberculosis (TB) in ancient Indian, Chinese, and Arabic literature; TB remains an important infectious disease and the second leading cause of death from a single infectious agent worldwide.[1] In 1993, the World Health Organization (WHO) declared a "global emergency", and set targets for the control of the disease by 2000.[2] Sadly these targets have not been met and in the 1990s, a resurgence of drug-resistant TB and subsequently multidrug-resistant TB (MDR-TB) has delayed progress in controlling the disease. At the start of the 21st century, the United Nations established eight Millennium Development Goals (MDGs) with targets set for the year 2015. Tuberculosis was included as part of MDG 6, and the targets included a fall in TB incidence, prevalence, and mortality rates. In addition, there should be an increase in the case detection rate and percentage of patients who complete treatment. Epidemiologists have used mathematical models to calculate that the requirements needed to reduce TB incidence, prevalence, and death are: a case detection rate of 70% with at least 85% of patients completing treatment. Table 1 illustrates the progress made so far.[3]

The WHO has produced a number of other documents in the past 10 years to support the implementation of Directly Observed Therapy (DOT) strategy, to help facilitate good TB control programs, and to address the problem of human immunodeficiency virus (HIV)/TB coinfection and the resurgence of drug-resistant TB.[4-6]

INCIDENCE AND PREVALENCE

The WHO estimates that about a third of the world's population is infected with TB, but only a few become ill with TB disease. In 2012, the WHO estimated that there were

TABLE 1	Global progress in tuberculosis care and control	
	2000	*2012*
Incidence (per 100,000 population per year)	148	122
Prevalence (per 100,000 population)	263	169
Mortality (per 100,000 population per year)	22	13
Case detection rate (%)	42	66
Treatment success rate (%)	69	87

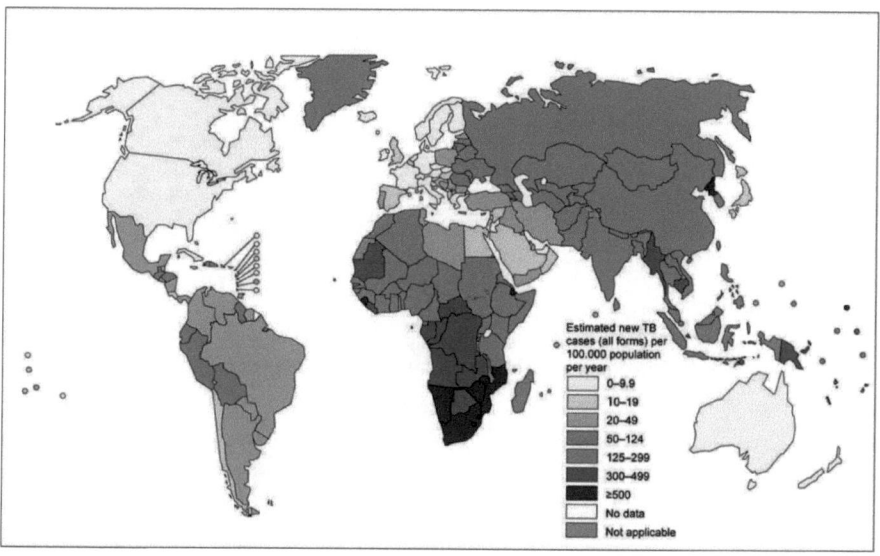

TB, tuberculosis.

FIG. 1: Estimated tuberculosis incidence rates worldwide in 2012. *(For color version, see Plate 2)*

Source: World Health Organization.

8.6 million incident cases of TB, although only 5.7 million (66%) were detected and notified to national TB programs. This leaves a group of patients, almost 3 million, who were either not diagnosed with TB disease, or were not notified.[3] There is a group of 22 countries, which together represent almost 80% of the disease burden worldwide, and they are referred to as high-burden countries. These countries can be grouped by continent; in Africa—Democratic Republic of the Congo, Ethiopia, Kenya, Mozambique, Nigeria, Tanzania, Uganda, South Africa, and Zimbabwe. In Asia, the countries are Afghanistan, Bangladesh, China, Indonesia, India, Cambodia, Myanmar, Pakistan, Philippines, Thailand, and Vietnam. The remaining countries are Brazil and the Russian Federation. Figure 1 illustrates the variation in estimated incidence of TB across the world.

MORTALITY

In 2012, there were 1.3 million deaths worldwide attributed to TB, which corresponds to 20 deaths per 100,000 population, and included 320,000 deaths due to TB/HIV coinfection.[7] Tuberculosis remains one of the top three causes of death in women aged 15–44 years, and kills more women than all causes of maternal mortality combined.[8] The burden of TB-related deaths (95%) is in low-middle income countries, and it has been reported that 26% of avoidable deaths in developing countries are due to TB.[8] However, there has been significant improvement in the mortality rate over the past 25 years, and in 2012, the mortality rate had fallen by 45% compared with 1990. The MDG was for this figure to have halved by 2015, and it looks as if this will be achieved.[3] Although TB mortality rates have fallen in every region, the fall has been relatively little in sub-Saharan Africa, due to the sharp rise in HIV-related disease since 1990. As a result of this HIV epidemic, the incidence and mortality of TB in Africa only began to fall in 2004.[9] Figure 2 illustrates the variation in estimated TB mortality rates worldwide.

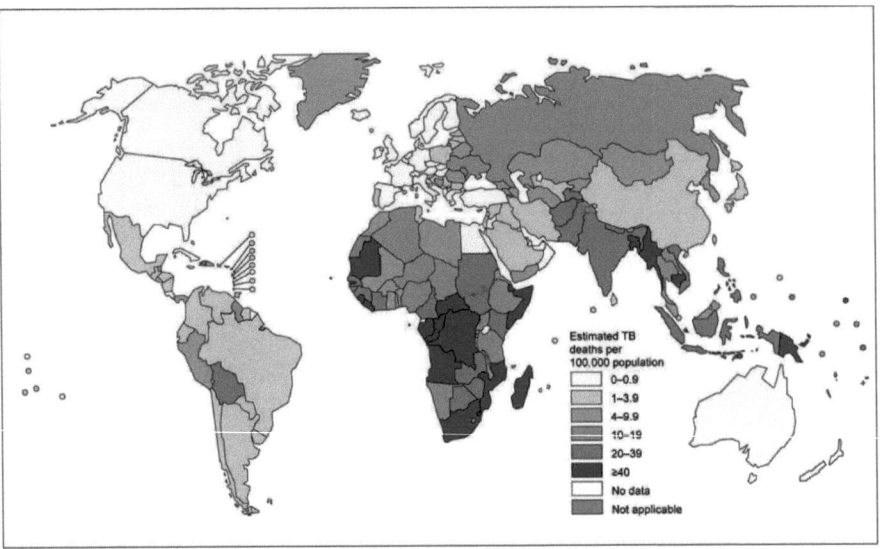

TB, tuberculosis.

FIG. 2: Estimated tuberculosis mortality rates excluding tuberculosis deaths among human immunodeficiency virus-positive people, 2012. *(For color version, see Plate 2)*

Source: World Health Organization.

AGE

In the developing world, TB is more prevalent in children and young adults, which reflects primary transmission. It can be difficult to diagnose and treat children, and this can lead to TB meningitis and miliary TB. In 2012, the WHO reported 74,000 deaths in HIV-negative children.[7] In developed countries, the rate of TB is higher amongst older adults, compared with young adults,[10] and this is thought to be due to reactivation of latent infection.[11] Reactivation may occur due to impaired host immunity with increasing age. Hochberg reported 22% of patients with TB in the United States of America were over 65 years of age, and within this population there were subgroups who were at increased risk; namely men, non-Caucasians, and those in long-term institutionalized care.[12] The elderly are known to have an increased mortality rate from TB; therefore, it is important to try and prevent reactivation in this subgroup of adults in order to prevent avoidable deaths.[10,13]

SEX

Globally, the prevalence of TB is equal amongst men and women up to adolescence. From 15 years upward, there is a higher rate of TB in men compared with women. One suggestion is that this reflects a greater burden of disease in adult men, due to a higher number of social contacts outside the home and exposure to infection.[14] But it may simply represent a higher notification rate in men, given there is an estimated 2:1 (male:female) ratio of cases notified to public health authorities worldwide.[15] This under notification of disease in women compared to men has been observed in other infections too, including malaria and leishmaniasis.[16,17] In 2012, the WHO reported that more than half the estimated cases of TB in women went undetected, compared with less than 40% of the total population.[18]

There is also evidence that women of childbearing age are more likely to progress from infection to disease, compared with men of a similar age;[8,19] and women are more likely to have extrapulmonary TB compared with men. Yang et al. reported the results of a retrospective case control study in Arkansas, United States, which found that 17% of the women with TB had extrapulmonary disease compared with only 9% of the men.[20] Extrapulmonary disease has been linked with a weakened immune system, which may be relevant given women are known to have a higher mortality rate from TB.[14,18] Active case finding of adult women is an important public health control measure to try and find and treat these individuals and reduce the disease burden.

RACE

Given the geographical variation in the prevalence of TB worldwide, individuals who are born or spend their childhood in countries where TB is highly prevalent are observed to have an increased likelihood of developing TB later in life. This can be most striking in low-incidence countries, like the United Kingdom and the United States of America. Almost three quarters (73%) of the patients diagnosed with TB in the United Kingdom in 2013 were born abroad.[21] Since 1986, the percentage of patients in America who were born in endemic countries has increased from 22 to 58%.[22] Asghar et al. reported an independent association between extrapulmonary TB, often a marker of disseminated disease, and origin in Southeast Asia, compared to immigrants from other areas of the world.[23] Asian patients are also less likely to be part of a cluster, which implies disease reactivation, in contrast to Black Americans who are often part of a cluster group reflecting recent transmission.[24] Fiske reported that Black men were almost six times more likely to develop extrapulmonary TB than non-Black men.[25] Black Americans developing TB were more likely to be young, from an inner city background (reflecting low socioeconomic status), be HIV-positive and have drug-resistant disease.[24] Mexicans account for 25% of the migrant TB population of America. Joseph et al. reported an ethnographic study looking at the sociocultural aspects of TB in this population.[26] They reported significant misconceptions regarding disease transmission, low perception of risk and stigma amongst those who had TB. Tuberculosis control programs need to be aware of these cultural differences and how they might lead to barriers in accessing health care and completing treatment.

In 2013, Tollefson published a literature review to summarize the burden of disease amongst indigenous people. The United Nations defines an indigenous group as being any group of people who self-identify as indigenous. The majority of the published literature relates to the Aborigines of Australia, the Inuits of Canada, and the Indians of North America. However, there are indigenous people in every continent of the world. Although there is a paucity of data, and some papers are more than 25 years old; it does appear as if the rate of TB in indigenous people is often higher than the nonindigenous people in the same country.[27] The reason for this is unclear, and more research is required.

SOCIOECONOMIC STATUS

Tuberculosis has long been regarded as a disease of the poor, with overcrowding, malnutrition, and poor sanitation contributing to its prevalence. Efforts to improve these social factors have led to success in reducing the prevalence rate, but they rely on political and cultural change. The role of the health service, and in particular the TB control program, has been highlighted in New York and the United States of America as a whole.[28] In the 1980s, the incidence of TB had been falling for several decades, and TB services had been cut back. However, what followed was a steep rise in the incidence, which peaked in 1992. This was attributed to a number of factors, including the epidemic of HIV/AIDS, immigration of individuals from endemic countries, and the dismantling of public health infrastructure. Since 1992, there has been a substantial reduction in the incidence of TB in the United States of America, which has been achieved by improved public health efforts, infection control measures, and the use of DOT, as well as public education programs.[29,30] In Eastern Europe, a socioeconomic crisis followed the dismantling of the former Soviet Union, and this led to struggling public health systems which have undoubtedly contributed to the increase in the incidence and prevalence of TB including MDR-TB.[6]

There is evidence that aspects of an individual's socioeconomic status will affect the likelihood of them developing TB, and these include wealth, education, smoking, alcohol consumption, and drug use. However, many of these factors are related, and often an individual with a poor education record, will find themselves unemployed or homeless, resulting in malnutrition, perhaps overcrowding and at risk of coinfections. Khan et al. reported that those individuals below the poverty line were twice as more likely to develop TB than those above it, and those with less than a high school education were also more likely to develop TB than those with higher education.[30] A systematic review by Lonnroth reported an almost threefold increased relative risk of developing TB if an individual had an alcohol-related disorder, or drank more than 40 g of alcohol per day.[31] However, it is not possible to determine whether this is a direct link between excess alcohol and a reduced immunity or the social implications of drinking excess alcohol, such as an increased likelihood of smoking cigarettes, and low income. Several papers have reported a link between tobacco smoking and an increased likelihood of developing TB.[32-35] Lin performed a prospective cohort study, and reported an almost twofold increased odds ratio amongst those who smoked, compared with nonsmokers.[33] The greater the tobacco consumption, the higher the odds ratio for developing TB. Bates et al. performed a meta-analysis and discovered that smoking is a risk factor for TB infection and disease, but there was no definite increased mortality from TB amongst tobacco smokers.[34] Individuals who use recreational or illicit drugs are at increased risk of developing TB, and they put themselves at risk of coinfection with hepatitis and HIV, and require specialist management in terms of drug interactions.[36-38]

The prison community is the perfect setting for an outbreak of TB, with large numbers of usually young men living in close communities, and often with concomitant risk factors, such as HIV infection, smoking, malnutrition, etc. Several studies from Africa have looked at this setting and confirmed that there is a high prevalence of HIV infection, 25–27%, and that prospective case finding has identified between 4 and 8% of the prisoners screened had active TB.[39,40] Screening for latent TB infection (LTBI) has also been studied, and rates vary depending on location; 73% of inmates in a Brazilian prison were tuberculin skin test (TST)-positive.[41] Two studies from Europe, in Switzerland and Spain, used the TST to assess prisoners on arrival and found between 40 and 47% had LTBI; and the rate was greatest amongst those originally from sub-Saharan Africa.[42,43] In order to prevent outbreaks of active TB in prisons, screening for LTBI should be routine practice, and chemoprophylaxis given.

Malnutrition profoundly affects cell-mediated immunity which is the principle mechanism employed in the defense against TB. Individuals who are underweight are more likely to develop TB than those with a good nutritional status, and are more likely to die of the disease.[44,45] Patients who have had gastric surgery, including jejunoileal bypass are reported to have an increased risk of developing TB,[46] as are those with celiac disease.[47] The mechanism for the latter association may be related to malabsorption.

PREDISPOSING HUMAN FACTORS

There are a number of conditions which are linked to an increased risk of developing TB, which are usually attributed to a change in the host immune system and reactivation of latent infection. Diabetes is one such disease and poor diabetic control along with an increasing number of complications secondary to diabetes have been linked to an increased likelihood of developing TB.[48-51] Jeon et al. reviewed 13 observational studies and reported a threefold increased risk of developing TB in those individual with diabetes.[49] Chronic renal disease is another condition related to a significant increase in the likelihood of developing TB. In 2003, Hussein et al. summarized the published literature to date, and reported a range of 5.9–52.5 increased risk of developing TB in individuals with chronic renal disease.[52] The association is greatest in those patients on hemodialysis. Liver cirrhosis has also been reported as an independent risk factor for TB, and one with a poor prognosis. A cohort review of patients entered into the Danish registry with liver cirrhosis revealed that over a 16-year period, and more than 20,000 patients, 151 cases of TB were identified. This equated to an incidence rate of more than 160/100,000 person-years. Sadly the 30-day mortality for those with TB was very high at 27%.[53] Individuals with cancer are also thought to be at increased risk, but this risk is not uniform. Hematological malignancies or those of the head and neck have been found to be particularly relevant to the development of TB. Kamboj et al. performed a 25-year review of cancer patients in the United States of America, and reported a rate of TB in those with a hematological malignancy as more than 200/100,000. This is 40 times the rate in the general population. Among patients with cancer of the head and neck, the rate was more than 100/100,000; whilst no increased risk was observed in solid tumors that were not in the head and neck.[54]

There are certain situations in which the immune status of an individual is directly suppressed, either deliberately or inadvertently. The risk of HIV coinfection with TB is discussed in a separate section below. Patients who have had a solid organ transplant are deliberately immunosuppressed to avoid rejection of the donor organ, but screening should be done before this, in order to treat LTBI and avoid reactivation.[55,56] Several chronic systemic diseases have previously relied upon long-term use of glucocorticoids, which are known to increase the risk of TB reactivation;[57] and now use anti-tumor necrosis factor (anti-TNF) agents as disease-modifying drugs, and these patients should be screened and treated for LTBI, before anti-TNF agents are started.

HUMAN IMMUNODEFICIENCY VIRUS/TUBERCULOSIS COINFECTION

The WHO reports that a third of the 35 million people living with HIV worldwide are infected with LTBI. Those diagnosed with HIV have a significantly increased risk of acquiring primary TB infection and reactivation of latent infection. The size of the risk of acquiring TB in those who are HIV-positive has been reported between 9 and 30 times the risk in HIV-negative individuals.[58-60] There is strong evidence that a fall in CD4 count and a rise in viral load are risk factors for disease, and antiretroviral therapy (ART)

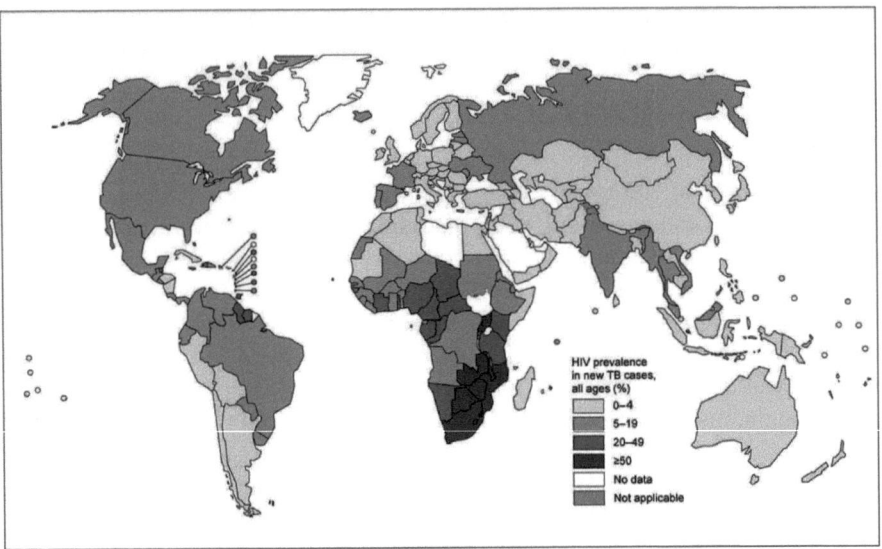

HIV, human immunodeficiency virus; TB, tuberculosis.

FIG. 3: Human immunodeficiency virus prevalence in new cases of tuberculosis in 2012. *(For color version, see Plate 3)*

Source: World Health Organization.

reduces the risk of TB.[61,62] Tuberculosis is the most common presenting illness in individuals living with HIV, with and without ART. There were 1.1 million new cases of TB in HIV-positive patients in 2012, and 75% of these were in sub-Saharan Africa.[60] Approximately, 1 in every 15 new patients with TB is already HIV-positive.[5] Figure 3 illustrates the variation in estimated HIV prevalence in new cases of TB across the world.

Tuberculosis is the leading cause of death for individuals with HIV, and it accounts for 20% of HIV-related deaths, and the reverse is also true. An extra 25% of deaths amongst patients with TB is attributable to coinfection with HIV.[63] A retrospective cohort study from Ethiopia, comparing the mortality rate in HIV-positive compared with HIV-negative patients, confirmed the increased mortality rate in those with coinfection, but reported that this was more likely in the self-administered continuation phase, rather than the initiation phase which was under DOT.[64] Globally, there is no difference between men and women with regard to HIV/TB-related deaths; but in sub-Saharan Africa, there is a female predominance.[60] In response to the synergy between HIV and TB, leading to increasing levels of disease and death, the WHO has set several targets related to HIV/TB coinfection—universal HIV testing amongst patients with TB, provision of ART to HIV-positive patients with TB, and the provision of chemoprophylaxis to those people living with HIV.[3] The data currently suggests that less than 50% of patients with TB are tested for HIV infection (46% in 2012); and only 57% of the TB patients know to be HIV-positive were receiving ART, although 80% were had been enrolled on to a program of cotrimoxazole preventive therapy.[60]

MULTIDRUG-RESISTANT TUBERCULOSIS

The primary cause of MDR-TB is inappropriate, incorrect, or inadequate use of antituberculous therapy to treat susceptible TB. Cases have been reported in every country but there are certain areas which have a higher percentage of the TB burden who are multidrug resistant. This is illustrated in figure 4, which identifies the former Union of Soviet Socialist Republics, and parts of Eastern Europe, and China as being the worst affected areas. The WHO is concerned that there is significant underreporting of cases with MDR-TB and that clinical outcomes are very poor in this patient group, with a high-mortality rate, and successful completion of treatment in only 50% of patients.[3] Makinen et al. report a population-based study in the Murmansk region of the Russian Federation between 2003 and 2004.[65] In total 1,226 patients were diagnosed with TB, of whom 688 (56%) had MDR-TB. The majority of the patients with MDR-TB had been treated for TB in the past. Of those previously treated for TB, 73% had MDR disease, in contrast to 26% of those who had not been treated before. This highlights the need for good education and support from a designated key worker, or TB specialist nurse, to ensure compliance with the regime and high TB treatment completion rates first time. The WHO reports that global treatment success rates in MDR-TB are less than 50%, due to the high-mortality rate and large numbers of patients who are simply lost to follow-up.[3]

In 2006, it became clear that a new problem had emerged, extensively drug-resistant TB (XDR-TB). This is defined as resistance to rifampicin and isoniazid, but in addition resistance to a fluoroquinolone and also to an injectable agent. A mission hospital in

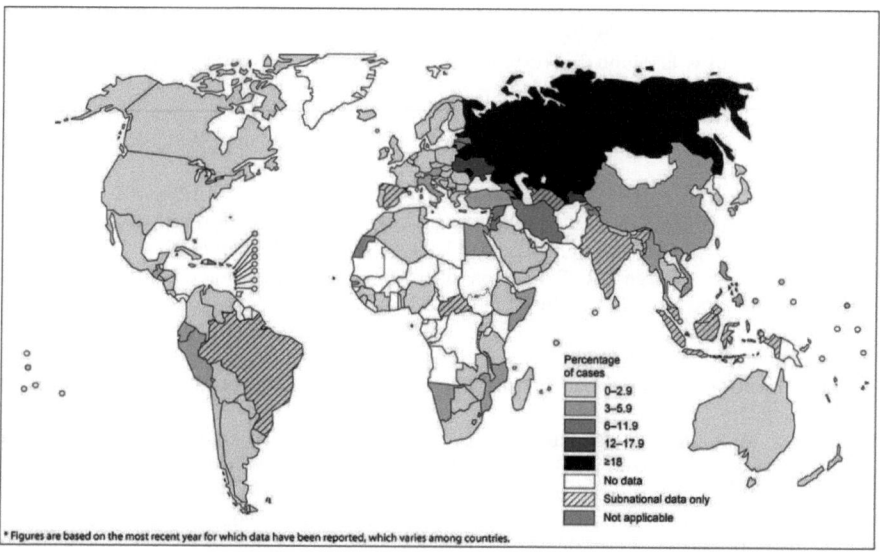

Note: Figures are based on the most recent year for which data has been reported, which varies among countries.

FIG. 4: Percentage of new cases of tuberculosis with multidrug-resistant tuberculosis. *(For color version, see Plate 3)*

Source: World Health Organization.

Tugela Ferry, KwaZulu-Natal province, South Africa reported 53 cases with XDR-TB, all of whom were coinfected with HIV. Sadly the mortality rate was 98%, and the median survival time from sputum collection was a mere 16 days.[66] Since then the situation in Tugela Ferry has improved. There have been a total of 463 patients with XDR-TB between 2005 and the end of 2008, of whom 69 have survived more than 6 months. This subgroup of survivors had less advanced TB at diagnosis, and it was more likely to be their first episode of TB. Although rates of HIV coinfection were similar between the survivors and those who died, the CD4 count was significantly higher in the group that survived.[67] There was no significant variation in sex or age in these two patient groups. Although South Africa remains a country severely affected by drug-resistant disease, cases of XDR-TB have been reported in almost 100 countries.[3]

REFERENCES

1. Sharma SK, Mohan A. Tuberculosis: from an incurable scourge to a curable disease—journey over a millennium. Indian J Med Res. 2013;137(3):455-93.
2. World Health Organization. TB—A Global Emergency: WHO Report on the TB Epidemic. Geneva: WHO; 1994.
3. World Health Organization. Countdown to 2015: Global Tuberculosis Report 2013. Supplement. Geneva: WHO; 2013.
4. World Health Organization. Stop TB Partnership. The Global Plan to Stop TB 2006–2015. Geneva: WHO; 2006.
5. World Health Organization. Global Tuberculosis Control. Geneva: WHO; 2008.
6. World Health Organization. The Stop TB Strategy: Building on and Enhancing DOTS to meet the TB-Related Millennium Development Goals. Geneva: WHO; 2006.
7. World Health Organization. 10 facts about tuberculosis. (2014). [online] Available from: http://www.who.int/features/factfiles/tb_facts/en/ [Accessed January, 2016].
8. Holmes CB, Hausler H, Nunn P. A review of sex differences in the epidemiology of tuberculosis. Int J Tuberc Lung Dis. 1998;2(2):96-104.
9. Glaziou P, Floyd K, Korenromp EL, et al. Lives saved by tuberculosis control and prospects for achieving the 2015 global target for reducing tuberculosis mortality. Bull World Health Organ. 2011;89(8):573-82.
10. Davies PD. TB in the elderly in industrialised countries. Int J Tuberc Lung Dis. 2007;11(11):1157-9.
11. Horsburgh CR, O'Donnell M, Chamblee S, et al. Revisiting rates of reactivation tuberculosis: a population-based approach. Am J Respir Crit Care Med. 2010;182(3):420-5.
12. Hochberg NS, Horsburgh CR. Prevention of tuberculosis in older adults in the United States: obstacles and opportunities. Clin Infect Dis. 2013;56(9):1240-7.
13. Chan-Yeung M, Noertjojo K, Tan J, Chan SL, Tam CM. Tuberculosis in the elderly in Hong Kong. Int J Tuberc Lung Dis. 2002;6(9):771-9.
14. Hudelson P. Gender differentials in tuberculosis: the role of socio-economic and cultural factors. Tuber Lung Dis. 1996;77(5):391-400.
15. Kumaresan JA, Raviglione MC, Murray CJL, editors. The global burden of disease and risk factors in 1990: Geneva, Switzerland: World Health Organization and the World Bank; 1996.
16. World Health Organization. Gender and Leishmaniasis in Colombia: a redefinition of existing concepts? (Gender and tropical diseases resource paper no. 2). 1996.
17. Ettling MB, Thimasarn K, Krachaiklin S, Bualombai P. Evaluation of malaria clinics in Maesot, Thailand: use of serology to assess coverage. Trans R Soc Trop Med Hyg. 1989;83(3):325-30.
18. World Health Organization. Tuberculosis in women. Geneva: WHO; 2014.
19. Murray CJ. Social, economic and operational research on tuberculosis: recent studies and some priority questions. Bull Int Union Tuberc Lung Dis. 1991;66(4):149-56.
20. Yang Z, Kong Y, Wilson F, et al. Identification of risk factors for extrapulmonary tuberculosis. Clin Infect Dis. 2004;38(2):199-205.
21. Public Health England. Tuberculosis in the UK 2014 report. 2014.

22. Cain KP, Haley CA, Armstrong LR, et al. Tuberculosis among foreign-born persons in the United States: achieving tuberculosis elimination. Am J Respir Crit Care Med. 2007;175(1):75-9.
23. Asghar RJ, Pratt RH, Kammerer JS, Navin TR. Tuberculosis in South Asians living in the United States, 1993-2004. Arch Intern Med. 2008;168(9):936-42.
24. Serpa JA, Teeter LD, Musser JM, Graviss EA. Tuberculosis disparity between US-born blacks and whites, Houston, Texas, USA. Emerg Infect Dis. 2009;15(6):899-904.
25. Fiske CT, Griffin MR, Erin H, et al. Black race, sex, and extrapulmonary tuberculosis risk: an observational study. BMC Infect Dis. 2010;10:16.
26. Joseph HA, Waldman K, Rawls C, Wilce M, Shrestha-Kuwahara R. TB perspectives among a sample of Mexicans in the United States: results from an ethnographic study. J Immigr Minor Health. 2008;10(2):177-85.
27. Tollefson D, Bloss E, Fanning A, Redd JT, Barker K, McCray E. Burden of tuberculosis in indigenous peoples globally: a systematic review. Int J Tuberc Lung Dis. 2013;17(9):1139-50.
28. Frieden TR, Fujiwara PI, Washko RM, Hamburg MA. Tuberculosis in New York City—turning the tide. N Engl J Med. 1995;333(4):229-33.
29. Burzynski J, Schluger NW. The epidemiology of tuberculosis in the United States. Semin Respir Crit Care Med. 2008;29(5):492-8.
30. Khan K, Wang J, Hu W, Bierman A, Li Y, Gardam M. Tuberculosis infection in the United States: national trends over three decades. Am J Respir Crit Care Med. 2008;177(4):455-60.
31. Lonnroth K, Williams BG, Stadlin S, Jaramillo E, Dye C. Alcohol use as a risk factor for tuberculosis—a systematic review. BMC Public Health. 2008;8:289.
32. Rao VG, Bhat J, Yadav R, Muniyandi M, Bhondeley MK, Sharada MA, et al. Tobacco smoking: a major risk factor for pulmonary tuberculosis—evidence from a cross-sectional study in central India. Trans R Soc Trop Med Hyg. 2014;108(8):474-81.
33. Lin HH, Ezzati M, Chang HY, Murray M. Association between tobacco smoking and active tuberculosis in Taiwan: prospective cohort study. Am J Respir Crit Care Med. 2009;180(5):475-80.
34. Bates MN, Khalakdina A, Pai M, Chang L, Lessa F, Smith KR. Risk of tuberculosis from exposure to tobacco smoke: a systematic review and meta-analysis. Arch Intern Med. 2007;167(4):335-42.
35. Slama K, Chiang CY, Enarson DA, et al. Tobacco and tuberculosis: a qualitative systematic review and meta-analysis. Int J Tuberc Lung Dis. 2007;11(10):1049-61.
36. Deiss RG, Rodwell TC, Garfein RS. Tuberculosis and illicit drug use: review and update. Clin Infect Dis. 2009;48(1):72-82.
37. Durante AJ, Selwyn PA, O'Connor PG. Risk factors for and knowledge of Mycobacterium tuberculosis infection among drug users in substance abuse treatment. Addiction. 1998;93(9):1393-401.
38. Pevzner ES, Robison S, Donovan J, et al. Tuberculosis transmission and use of methamphetamines in Snohomish County, WA, 1991-2006. Am J Public Health. 2010;100(12):2481-6.
39. Telisinghe L, Fielding KL, Malden JL, et al. High tuberculosis prevalence in a South African prison: the need for routine tuberculosis screening. PLoS One. 2014;9(1):e87262.
40. Henostroza G, Topp SM, Hatwiinda S, et al. The high burden of tuberculosis (TB) and human immunodeficiency virus (HIV) in a large Zambian prison: a public health alert. PLoS One. 2013;8(8):e67338.
41. Nogueira PA, Abrahao RM, Galesi VM. Tuberculosis and latent tuberculosis in prison inmates. Rev Saude Publica. 2012;46(1):119-27.
42. Ritter C, Elger BS. Prevalence of positive tuberculosis skin tests during 5 years of screening in a Swiss remand prison. Int J Tuberc Lung Dis. 2012;16(1):65-9.
43. Marco A, Sole N, Orcau A, et al. Prevalence of latent tuberculosis infection in inmates recently incarcerated in a men's prison in Barcelona. Int J Tuberc Lung Dis. 2012;16(1):60-4.
44. Cegielski JP, McMurray DN. The relationship between malnutrition and tuberculosis: evidence from studies in humans and experimental animals. Int J Tuberc Lung Dis. 2004;8(3):286-98.
45. Tverdal A. Body mass index and incidence of tuberculosis. Eur J Respir Dis. 1986;69(5):355-62.
46. Bruce RM, Wise L. Tuberculosis after jejunoileal bypass for obesity. Ann Intern Med. 1977;87(5):574-6.
47. Ludvigsson JF, Wahlstrom J, Grunewald J, Ekbom A, Montgomery SM. Coeliac disease and risk of tuberculosis: a population based cohort study. Thorax. 2007;62(1):23-8.
48. Baker MA, Lin HH, Chang HY, Murray MB. The risk of tuberculosis disease among persons with diabetes mellitus: a prospective cohort study. Clin Infect Dis. 2012;54(6):818-25.

49. Jeon CY, Murray MB. Diabetes mellitus increases the risk of active tuberculosis: a systematic review of 13 observational studies. PLoS Med. 2008;5(7):e152.
50. Pablos-Mendez A, Blustein J, Knirsch CA. The role of diabetes mellitus in the higher prevalence of tuberculosis among Hispanics. Am J Public Health. 1997;87(4):574-9.
51. Stevenson CR, Forouhi NG, Roglic G, et al. Diabetes and tuberculosis: the impact of the diabetes epidemic on tuberculosis incidence. BMC Public Health. 2007;7:234.
52. Hussein MM, Mooij JM, Roujouleh H. Tuberculosis and chronic renal disease. Semin Dial. 2003;16(1):38-44.
53. Thulstrup AM, Molle I, Svendsen N, Sorensen HT. Incidence and prognosis of tuberculosis in patients with cirrhosis of the liver. A Danish nationwide population based study. Epidemiol Infect. 2000;124(2):221-5.
54. Kamboj M, Sepkowitz KA. The risk of tuberculosis in patients with cancer. Clin Infect Dis. 2006;42(11):1592-5.
55. Munoz P, Palomo J, Munoz R, Rodriguez-Creixems M, Pelaez T, Bouza E. Tuberculosis in heart transplant recipients. Clin Infect Dis. 1995;21(2):398-402.
56. Meyers BR, Halpern M, Sheiner P, Mendelson MH, Neibart E, Miller C. Tuberculosis in liver transplant patients. Transplantation. 1994;58(3):301-6.
57. Jick SS, Lieberman ES, Rahman MU, Choi HK. Glucocorticoid use, other associated factors, and the risk of tuberculosis. Arthritis Rheum. 2006;55(1):19-26.
58. Antonucci G, Girardi E, Raviglione MC, Ippolito G. Risk factors for tuberculosis in HIV-infected persons. A prospective cohort study. The Gruppo Italiano di Studio Tubercolosi e AIDS (GISTA). J Am Med Assoc. 1995;274(2):143-8.
59. Guelar A, Gatell JM, Verdejo J, et al. A prospective study of the risk of tuberculosis among HIV-infected patients. AIDS. 1993;7(10):1345-9.
60. World Health Organization. (2013). HIV-associated TB. Facts 2013. [online] Available from: http://www.who.int/tb/challenges/hiv/tbhiv_factsheet_2013_web.pdf?ua=1 [Accessed January, 2016].
61. Sharma SK, Mohan A, Kadhiravan T. HIV-TB co-infection: epidemiology, diagnosis and management. Indian J Med Res. 2005;121(4):550-67.
62. Padmapriyadarsini C, Narendran G, Swaminathan S. Diagnosis and treatment of tuberculosis in HIV co-infected patients. Indian J Med Res. 2011;134(6):850-65.
63. World Health Organization. Global tuberculosis control: epidemiology, strategy, financing: WHO report 2009.
64. Shaweno D, Worku A. Tuberculosis treatment survival of HIV positive TB patients on directly observed treatment short-course in Southern Ethiopia: a retrospective cohort study. BMC Res Notes. 2012;5:682.
65. Makinen J, Marjamaki M, Haanpera-Heikkinen M, et al. Extremely high prevalence of multidrug resistant tuberculosis in Murmansk, Russia: a population-based study. Eur J Clin Microbiol Infect Dis. 2011;30(9):1119-26.
66. Gandhi NR, Shah NS, Andrews JR, et al. HIV coinfection in multidrug-and extensively drug-resistant tuberculosis results in high early mortality. Am J Respir Crit Care Med. 2010;181(1):80-6.
67. Shenoi SV, Brooks RP, Barbour R, et al. Survival from XDR-TB is associated with modifiable clinical characteristics in rural South Africa. PLoS One. 2012;7(3):e31786.

CHAPTER 3

Latent Tuberculosis

Hannah Jarvis, Onn M Kon

INTRODUCTION

The World Health Organization estimates that 2 billion people, one-third of the world's population, are infected with *Mycobacterium tuberculosis*.[1] Of these, only about 5–10% will go on to develop active disease during their lifetime,[2] causing individual morbidity and mortality and acting as agents of transmission. It is this cohort of latency that acts as the greatest reservoir for the tubercle bacilli and much interest has focused on the value, both for the individual and for global attempts at eradication of identification, and treatment of infected persons.[3]

Clemens von Pirquet first coined the term latent tuberculosis (LTB) to describe the observation that asymptomatic children previously exposed to tuberculosis (TB) developed skin reactions when inoculated with tuberculin,[4] a heat-killed filtrate of mycobacterial culture. These individuals did not have the clinical or radiological features of active disease but clearly had an immune response to the presence of antigenic stimuli suggestive of occult disease.

Over the decades, we have developed our understanding of the term to denote those who have been infected by mycobacteria but instead of progressing to active (primary) disease, have contained it in a state whereby the bacilli persist in a dormant form not causing disease but maintaining the potential to reactivate, replicate, and cause pathology at a later stage (latent infection).

In a small percentage of individuals with LTB, this reactivation occurs, particularly in the context of deficits in host immunity, namely acquired immunodeficiency states related to illness, malnutrition, or drugs. Most commonly reactivation is seen within the first 5 years[2] following exposure although reports have documented a latency period of up to 30 years.[5] The challenge to physicians has been to identify those at higher risk of activation and facilitate a treatment which would be acceptable to those healthy, asymptomatic individuals. The nature of a paucibacillary disease with dormant organisms, evolved to evade host clearance, has made this a challenging task.

By definition, the diagnosis of LTB is reliant on proving that active disease does not exist whilst simultaneously demonstrating evidence of ongoing immune containment.

The inherent problem with such a diagnosis is the reliance on surrogates of latency; biomarkers which indicate exposure to tuberculous pathogens rather than definite infection. Historically, this has meant a positive tuberculin skin test (TST) and more recently the interferon-γ release assays (IGRAs) which detect interferon release to stimulation with *M. tuberculosis*-specific antigens.

Despite these advances, clinically available biomarkers are still unable to distinguish active from latent disease or identify those with latent disease with a higher risk of progression to active disease. In addition, it is also unclear if a positive immune test reflects true latency or merely the memory of an exposure now completely eradicated. In fact, the true sensitivity of the TST or even an IGRA is not definable as there is no gold standard for LTB apart from our prior understanding embedded in the historic definition by use of the TST itself.

This issue will be discussed further in a later section including the future development of more specific biomarkers. Currently, the clinical assessment of individuals is, therefore, limited to imprecise tests of exposure and state of TB infection. This is then combined with an assessment of the risk of reactivation in each individual, including an assessment of when they acquired the infection.

A balance then must be made between the risks of developing active disease versus the risks from potentially unnecessary treatment. This balance is particularly difficult, as there remain significant issues with available treatment options both in terms of practicalities such as length of treatment and also potential serious adverse effects. In addition, there needs to be an assessment of the risks to the general population of leaving untreated latent disease.

Lastly, commentators are increasingly moving toward the idea that TB exists as more of a spectrum than had previously been conceptualized;[6-8] with active disease, latent disease, and no disease existing in a continuum rather than the discrete entities they were once thought to be. The implications of this reach further than academic definitions, as treatment for active and latent disease vary, not least in the use of mono- versus polytherapies to prevent pathogen resistance.

In order to address the challenges faced by clinicians in diagnosis and treatment of LTB, a consideration of the pathogenesis of LTB must be made to better understand the points at which future research and intervention can be targeted.

PATHOGENESIS

The ability of *M. tuberculosis* to provoke a range of responses in different individuals—with some developing rapidly disseminating active disease, others contained latent disease, and some complete eradication—is well documented.[9]

Mycobacterium tuberculosis is contracted following the inhalation of infected particles transmitted via the aerosol route. Once inhaled, the bacilli are engulfed by alveolar macrophages whereupon further degradation is inhibited.[10] These infected macrophages then interact with T cells and a subsequent cascade of cell-mediated immune responses occurs. In the immunocompetent host, a T helper (Th)-1 lead response begins with the activation of a variety of other cellular components of the immune system including other T cells, alveolar macrophages, and dendritic cells. The activation of these results in the subsequent release of immune mediators including proinflammatory cytokines [such as interleukins (ILs) and interferons] and chemokines leading to the recruitment of further cells (both B and T cells, NK cells, and fibroblasts).[3] These cells interact to form granulomas, encasing the offending bacilli in an attempt to facilitate its destruction.[11] In some instances, the balance between host response and pathogen virulence is over- or underactive, resulting in necrosis within the granuloma, tissue destruction, and disease dissemination.[6]

In most cases, this response is sufficient to wall off infection and drive the mycobacteria into a state of dormancy required to survive the inhospitable environment of the granuloma.[12] In order to achieve this conversion, the bacillus undergoes a wide range of metabolic adaptations.[13] In addition to hypoxia, the granuloma exerts a number of other toxic influences upon the mycobacteria including acidity, nitric oxide, and nutrient deprivation.[14]

A range of studies have been performed to elucidate the mechanisms for some of the changes made by mycobacteria during the switch to a dormant state.[13] Although many of these remain poorly understood, several processes have been identified. These include the dormancy survival regulon (DosR) portion of mycobacterial genome which, in response to hypoxia, encodes for the transcription of genes thought to be used to alter cellular metabolic demands.[15] Prolonged hypoxic exposure then stimulates the induction of a further group of genes named the enduring hypoxic response.[16] These genes have been implicated in a variety of downstream changes including cell wall remodeling, fatty acid metabolism, and anaerobic respiration.[17] One possible result of cell wall changes is the stimulation of macrophages to become foamy macrophages, which in turn have been demonstrated to act as a source of nutrition for the bacilli.[18] In addition to changes encoded for in the DosR, mechanisms have been identified in *in vitro* studies for the stimulation of nitrates as a substrate for respiration in hypoxic environments by mycobacteria.[12] In turn this form of respiration has been shown to confer a degree of protection to the bacilli against damage from acidity.[19]

Less well understood are the mechanisms for reactivation of the bacilli to an active state. Risks for reactivation have been identified however and include human immunodeficiency virus (HIV) infection, treatment with immunosuppressants [including anti-tumor necrosis factor (anti-TNF) regimens in rheumatological disorders, transplant antirejection drugs, and corticosteroids], chronic kidney disease and hemodialysis, silicosis, hematological malignancies, and gastrectomy and jejunal bypass surgery.[3,20] It is likely that the immunocompromise resulting from these situations aids breakdown of the immune processes maintaining the integrity of the granuloma, signaling to the bacilli the opportunity to upregulate to an active state. Indeed several studies have identified that reduced expression of Th17 responses through downregulation of IL-6 receptor have been associated with reactivation.[21,22]

It has also been noted that calcified granulomas are less likely to yield viable bacilli than those of cellular or caseous consistency again supporting the concept of the granulomas as the key structure in prevention of disease progression.[23]

Commentators have emphasized that the study of dormant state bacilli within granuloma will enable our understanding of the resilience mechanisms of the pathogen and may yield future targets for intervention.[6] The details of such foci for future research are discussed in more detail later in the chapter.

IMMUNOLOGICAL TESTING

Tuberculin Skin Tests

Historically, the diagnosis of LTB has relied on the use of TSTs. First derived by Robert Koch at the end of the 19th century as a possible treatment for TB, tuberculin is an extract from the filtrate of mycobacterial culture.[24] When injected intradermally, it generates a delayed hypersensitivity reaction within the skin of individuals who have previously been exposed to TB, a surrogate of latent disease. Current clinical practice is to use purified protein derivative (PPD) extract for the procedure (the Mantoux procedure), a standardized mixture of over 200 mycobacterial proteins. Conventional understanding of the mechanism of the TST is that skin induration reflects the influx of T cells in response to the tuberculin stimulus.[6] Recent studies using intravital imaging have demonstrated that lymphocytic infiltrates found in the indurated skin contain CD4 cells with a memory phenotype.[25] Further studies using rat models have demonstrated an interaction between memory T cells with skin specificity and antigen presenting cells within 3 hours of a PPD challenge.[26] Interestingly, Walrath et al. have demonstrated a similar response of memory cells when PPD is instilled bronchoscopically in TST-positive individuals, although not in those with negative skin tests.[27]

Although there are international variations to the method used, primarily relating to the dose of PPD injected, the general procedure is the same. A small quantity of PPD is injected into the skin of the subject and then measured at 48 and 72 hours. The borders of the reaction are defined by visual inspection and palpation and then measured (Fig. 1).

Definitions of a positive reaction are determined by the dose and type of PPD used. In the United Kingdom, for instance, a dose is of 2 international units (IU) of RT 23 is used and a positive reaction is seen when the skin induration is greater than or equal to 5 mm irrespective of Bacillus Calmette–Guérin (BCG) status (new version of NICE guidelines)[47].

Internationally, including in the United States, 0.1 mL of PPD 5 tuberculin units (TUs) is used for tuberculin skin testing. The size definitions for a positive reaction are determined in conjunction with the individual's risk. Those people who are, high risk for TB (HIV-positive status, recent contacts, fibrotic or nodular changes on chest radiograph, organ transplant recipients) are considered to have a positive TST with an induration of greater than or equal to 5 mm. Those with intermediate risk of TB (entrants within the last 5 years; intravenous drug users; residents and personnel in high risk settings such as prisons, hospitals, homeless shelters, and staff in mycobacterial laboratories, people with high risk chronic conditions such as diabetes, chronic kidney disease, silicosis, and malnutrition; and children under the age of 4) are deemed to have a positive response at

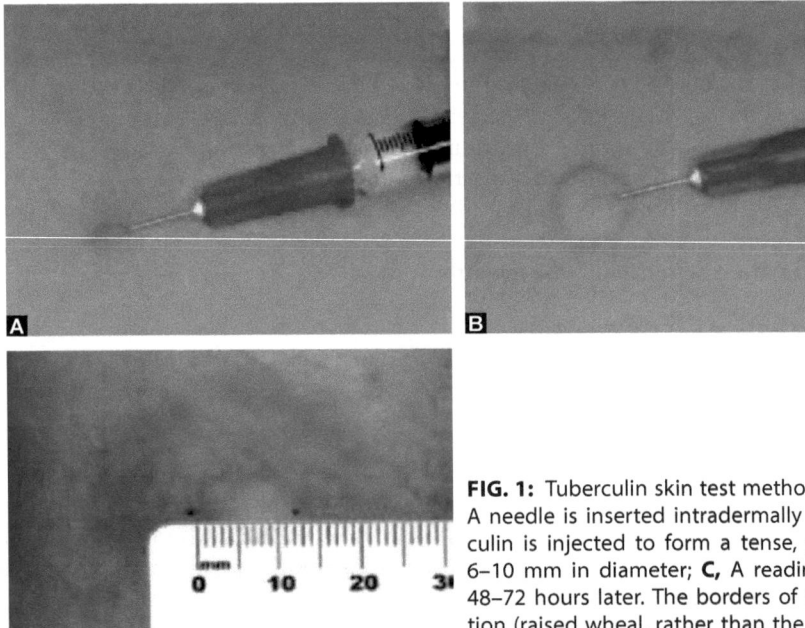

FIG. 1: Tuberculin skin test method. **A** and **B**, A needle is inserted intradermally and tuberculin is injected to form a tense, pale wheal 6–10 mm in diameter; **C,** A reading is made 48–72 hours later. The borders of the induration (raised wheal, rather than the larger area of erythema) are marked and the diameter is measured. *(For color version, see Plate 4)*

greater than or equal to 10 mm. All other individuals with no risk factors are classified as having positive skin tests at greater than or equal to 15 mm.[29]

The phenomenon of boosting can also be seen with TSTs.[30] This describes the finding of increased skin induration on serial testing. This must be differentiated from random biologic variation between tests (which is expected to result in differences of <6 mm, or 2 standard deviations, in 95% of subjects) and conversion of a skin test from negative to positive due to a recent infection with *M. tuberculosis*.[31] Reversion of a previously positive test can also be seen. The rate at which reversion occurs following treatment varies significantly but tends to be more common in older adults, those who experience boosting of their initial TST reaction and in people with reactions greater than 10 mm.[32] The phenomena of boosting and reversion emphasize the difficulty faced when interpreting repeated skin testing.[31]

The variance seen in those with and without BCG vaccination highlights the main concern with TST as a test, namely its lack of specificity. Skin reactions can be seen with other environmental mycobacteria, including the *M. bovis* used in BCG vaccinations. A review of 20 studies by Pai et al. in 2008[33] reported a pooled sensitivity of 77% (CI 71-82%) with a specificity of only 59% (CI 46-73%) in BCG-vaccinated individuals. The specificity was improved in a non-BCG-vaccinated population to 97% (CI 95-99%), with absolute values for specificity affected by the cutoff for induration size, with lower cutoffs more sensitive for latent disease. In addition to the effect of BCG, immunocompetence also plays a role in the reliability of the TST, with immunodeficiency resulting in a higher likelihood of a false negative due to the need for adequate T-cell activation.[34]

As with all currently available methods for diagnosing LTB, the TST acts as surrogate for latent infection. In the 1960s, Riley et al. performed a series of experiments examining the rates of TB transmission in exposed guinea pigs.[35] In these, guinea pigs (who have no latent phase of disease) were exposed to air from wards containing cases of active human TB. Tuberculin skin tests were performed and correlated to autopsy findings. The results showed that 0% of guinea pigs with TST reaction 0-5 mm had evidence of infection at necropsy, however, 25% of guinea pigs with a TST between 6 and 13 mm and 92% of those with a TST of 14 mm or more had evidence of infection. This finding confirmed that not all guinea pigs with positive TSTs had evidence of disease. An explanation for this was found in the subsequent studies which showed that the majority of TSTs remain positive even following successful treatment,[36] thus confirming that skin tests are unable to distinguish between immune sensitization with bacilli clearance and true latency.

Other issues with skin testing include the need for two visits to complete the test, the first to instill the antigen and the second to read the test. This is a particularly a problem in hard to reach patients and those with compliance issues. Severe localized skin reactions including blistering and edema can also occur and cause significant discomfort for the individual. Lastly, the test is operator dependent in terms of instillation and reading, and therefore, subject to a degree of potential error.

All of the above have fuelled a need to develop more accurate, objective measures of LTB although the TST has the advantage of being relatively cheap and has the wealth of many decades of experience and epidemiological data to allow for prognostication.

Interferon-γ Release Assays

The development of IGRAs reflects a recent improvement in our understanding and knowledge of the genetics of TB.

The two commercially available assays (QuantiFERON assays and T-SPOT.TB assay) detect *ex vivo* release of cytokines in response to stimulation of the peripheral blood with antigens from *M. tuberculosis*. These antigens, early secreted antigen target-6 and culture filtrate protein-10, are encoded for in the RD1 region of the TB genome.[30] The original QuantiFERON assay also employed a further antigen TB 7.7 (p4), although this has recently been replaced with the QuantiFERON plus which uses short CD8 specific peptides instead.[3,37] Importantly, the RD1 region is not present in the *M. bovis* species used in BCG vaccinations, and therefore, allows a significant specificity advantage over the TST. Only four other mycobacteria species have been identified which contain this segment of genome (*M. riyadhense, M. marinum, M. kansasii,* and *M. szulgai*) and the rarity of these pathogens has meant that problems with false positives to other species have not been an important issue clinically.[38,39]

The test is performed under laboratory conditions in a controlled, reproducible setting. The blood of *in vivo* sensitized individuals produces an *ex vivo* interferon-γ response when stimulated by the antigens which can be measured by enzyme-linked immunosorbent assay or by counting the number of interferon-producing cells.[34]

The development of these new tests has generated much interest and numerous studies have been performed to assess their relative efficacies. These reviews have however encountered a fundamental difficulty, namely the lack of a gold standard for TB exposure or infection to which to compare the new assays. Surrogates of infection have therefore been used including cases of active disease, correlation with clinical assessment of exposure, and some longitudinal studies examining the development of active disease in IGRA-positive-untreated cohorts.[30,34]

Several meta-analyses and reviews have concluded that the specificity of IGRAs ranges from 96 to 99% for the QuantiFERON test and between 86 and 93% for the T-SPOT for immunocompetent adults. Sensitivity has been quoted as ranging from 61 to 84% in the QuantiFERON test and between 67 and 89% in the T-SPOT.[30]

Unfortunately, despite their initial promise, IGRAs are still subject to a number of limitations. Firstly, they are more expensive than TST. Despite this, in high-income, low-incidence countries, cost-effectiveness has been proven and various national clinical bodies have accepted their use. Secondly, the cytokine response is subject to a functioning immune system; therefore, those individuals with immunodeficiency have an increased risk of a falsely negative test result or of an indeterminate reading.[40] This is compounded by the relative paucity of large studies specifically examining immunocompromised groups such as HIV-positive patients. Those studies that have been performed demonstrate an equivalent sensitivity between IGRAs and TST, but overall lower sensitivities are seen in HIV-negative patents.[41-43] Greater caution is therefore required when interpreting IGRAs in nonimmunocompetent adults.

In contrast to the TST though they avoid the issues of cross-reactivity with the BCG, do not require two visits for the patient and eliminate the need for skilled personnel to administer the skin test and the subsequent inevitable degree of observer error present in the interpretation. Interferon-γ release assays are also not subject to the phenomena of boosting which as described above, is seen in repeated TST where the skin reaction gets larger with each test, leading potentially to false positives. However, caution is required when performing an IGRA after a TST as boosting of the IGRA post TST is now recognized.[44]

Unfortunately, both IGRAs and TSTs are suboptimal at the most clinically relevant question; identifying those people with latent disease who will go on to develop active disease in the future. This so-called positive predictive value (PPV) for progression to active disease is low for both IGRAs and TST. A recent meta-analysis by Diel et al. concluded that the pooled PPV from the 28 studies it reviewed was 2.7% for IGRAs and 1.5% for TST, although these values rose when analysis was restricted to only those individuals clinically felt to be high risk for active disease development. The negative predictive value, or the likelihood of a person with a negative test not developing active disease, was almost 100% (99.7% for IGRAs and 99.4% for TST).[45]

The uptake of IGRAs for the diagnosis of LTB has been varied between countries. The WHO states that in resource-poor, high-prevalence countries, TST is the preferred option.[46] The high pretest probability of latent disease or a positive test in these settings makes the sensitivity of the tests equivalent, and therefore, the cheaper option is preferable.[47] In low-incidence countries, the opposite is true. For this reason, many low-incidence countries routinely employ IGRAs in the diagnosis of latent disease.

In the United States, IGRAs are often used as the primary test for latent infection, replacing the previously used TST. This is the case for all screening—contacts, immigrants, preimmunosuppression, and healthcare workers.[34]

In the United Kingdom, Canada and most European countries, guidance is to use IGRAs to confirm positive TSTs in a dual strategy.[28,30] In this situation, those being screened routinely undergo both TST and IGRA testing. If both screens are negative then LTB is felt to be unlikely and the patient can be discharged. If both tests are positive then a diagnosis of LTB is confirmed (provided active disease has been excluded) and treatment should be offered if appropriate. If either test is positive (with the other being negative) then provided the clinical presentation is supportive of a diagnosis of LTB, treatment should be considered. In this way, the rationale is to reduce the number of people in whom a diagnosis of LTB is missed. Flowchart 1 gives an example algorithm for the use of a dual testing strategy.

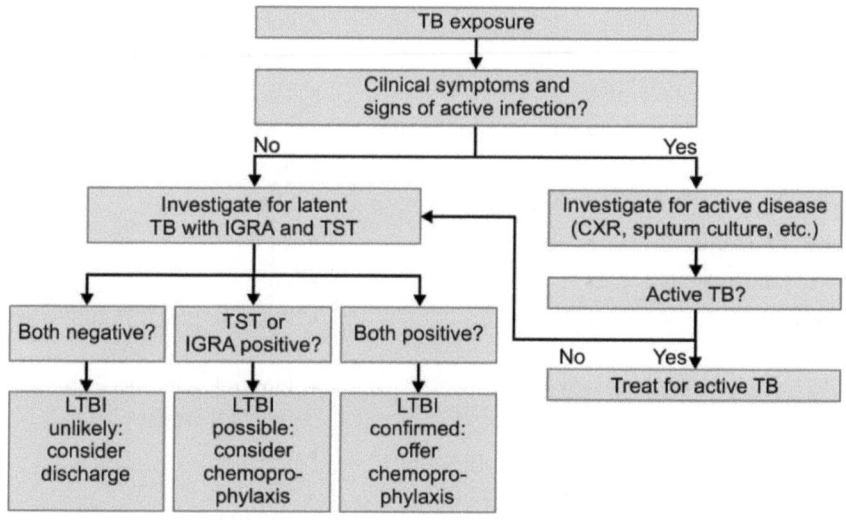

Note:
- Chemoprophylaxis decisions based on risk stratification and age
- In the event of discordance between IGRA and TST positivity, see text for suggestion on possible diagnostic strategy.

TB, tuberculosis; IGRA, interferon-γ release assay; TST, tuberculin skin test; CXR, chest X-ray; LTBI, latent tuberculosis infection.

FLOWCHART 1: Algorithm for diagnosis of latent tuberculosis in immunocompetent patients.

A more complicated situation arises when there is discordance between the results of the TST and IGRA. Although there exists minimal guidance for clinicians in this situation,[47] a sensible approach is often to repeat the dual screen at 6 weeks (if the initial TST was negative and IGRA positive) or to repeat the IGRA alone if the initial TST was positive. This, along with a clinical assessment for the development of active disease and risk stratification for the likelihood of TB exposure, can help clinicians determine the need for treatment. The repeating of skin tests, as described earlier, does incur the possibility of boosting phenomena which increases the difficulty of interpretation.[31]

The complexity of a single "one size fits all" strategy for screening is highlighted in the most recent set of guidance produced by the National Institute for Clinical Excellence (NICE) in the United Kingdom. In this document, there is an acknowledgment that patients at risk of TB can often be challenging to engage and as such recommendations are made for the use of IGRA screening alone in certain groups such as hard-to-reach people for whom the two visits needed for TST screening might be a challenge, in the case of large scale outbreaks, and in some instances in immunosuppressed individuals.[28]

Further research is currently underway to refine immunological testing mechanisms to overcome the issues described and to improve their PPV.

Different features of the TST and IGRA have been shown in table 1.

TABLE 1	Comparing different features of tuberculin skin test and interferon-γ release assay	
Feature	**TST**	**IGRA**
Technique	• In vivo • Skin prick test	• Ex vivo • ELISPOT (T-Spot) • ELISA (QFT)
Antigen	• PPD	• ESAT-6, CFP-10 (both) • TB 7.7 (p4)/CD8 peptides (QFT)
Results reported as	• Skin induration (mm)	• Number of spots (T-spot) • IFN-γ concentration (QFT)
Interpretation	• Subjective	• Objective
Time taken for results	• 48–72 h	• 24 h
Number of patient visits	• 2	• One
Booster effect?	• Yes	• Possible post TST (not seen within first 3 days)
Cross-reactivity with NTM?	• Yes	• Limited, with less clinically relevant species
Influenced by BCG?	• Yes	• No
Sensitivity (HIV negative)*	• 65–77%	• 61–84% (QFT) • 67–89% (T-spot)
Specificity (HIV negative)*	• 65–70%	• 96–99% (QFT) • 86–93% (T-spot)
PPV (for progression to active disease)†	• 2.4%	• 2.7%

Continued

Continued

TABLE 1	Comparing different features of tuberculin skin test and interferon-γ release assay	
Feature	TST	IGRA
NPV (for progression to active disease)†	• 99.4%	• 99.7%

*Thillai M, Pollock K, Pareek M, Lalvani A. Interferon-γ release assays for tuberculosis: current and future applications. Expert Rev Respir Med. 2014;8(1):67-78.
†Diel R, Loddenkemper R, Nienhaus A. Predictive value of interferon-γ release assays and tuberculin skin testing for progression from LTB infection to disease state: a meta-analysis. Chest. 2012;142(1):63-75.

TST, tuberculin skin test; IGRA, interferon-γ release assay; NTM, nontuberculous mycobacteria; HIV, human immunodeficiency virus; PPV, positive predictive value; NPV, negative predictive value; BCG, Bacillus Calmette–Guérin; PPD, purified protein derivative; ELISA, enzyme-linked immunosorbent assay; QFT, QuantiFERON-TB; ESAT-6, early secreted antigen target-6; CFP-10, culture filtrate protein-10; IFN, interferon.

RADIOLOGY OF LATENT TUBERCULOSIS

The most recently published guidelines from the WHO highlight the continuing importance of the chest radiograph in the diagnosis and stratification of patients with LTB.[46] This simple test remains a key tool for clinicians both in helping to exclude active disease and also in identifying latently infected individuals with a higher risk of progression. The features of the chest X-ray in latent disease can range considerably, from entirely normal to significant scarring and calcification consistent with healed TB. Some features are highly indicative of previous TB including calcification with nodules and fibrosis in a hilar or upper lobe distribution. These lesions tend to be well demarcated with sharp margins. There may be associated volume loss in the upper lobes. Other nonspecific findings can include upper lobe bronchiectasis and pleural scarring and thickening. Evidence suggests that those with nodules and fibrosis are at higher risk of disease reactivation, whereas, calcification and pleural thickening tend to be associated with lower risk.[29] These associations form the basis of the recommendations of the Centers for Disease Control and Prevention (CDC) for the stratification of TST results and subsequent guidance on whom to consider for treatment for latent disease.

TREATMENT

The first challenge facing clinicians in the treatment of LTB is the question of whom to treat. Studies have shown that approximately only 10% of those with latent infection progress to active disease.[2] Treatment is protracted, potentially harmful, and requires good compliance. The decision of which people to treat is, therefore, a balance between identifying those at most risk of reactivation, both to avoid their own morbidity related to active disease and to prevent them acting as a source for transmission, whilst balancing the risk to their health of treatment. As this balance is a difficult one, it is argued that only those for whom treatment is a sensible option should be screened for LTB.

Whilst in high-incidence countries, the focus remains on treatment of active cases, in low-incidence countries, reactivation of latent infection accounts for a much more significant proportion of active disease burden, and therefore, screening for latent infection is a greater priority. In resource-poor countries with high incidence, even the screening of high-risk individuals without evidence of active disease, such as those with HIV infection, has not been recommended. Instead the WHO recommends that these individuals are assumed to have latent infection and are given treatment accordingly.[1]

Studies have identified a number of higher risk groups, more likely to reactivate latent infection.[3,20] These groups along with healthcare workers and new entrants form the basis for the rationale behind many screening programs in place, particular in low-incidence settings.

The question of how to treat has also been subject to debate. Many studies have looked at the optimum treatment regimen for latent disease. The ideal would, of course, be the least toxic and most brief regimen. The standard globally has been to use 6–9 months of treatment with isoniazid.[48] This recommendation is based on a study performed in the 1970s by the International Union Against Tuberculosis who compared treatment in a group of 28,000 people from Eastern Europe with fibrotic lesions on chest radiograph and positive TSTs.[49] Patients were randomized to receive either placebo, 12, 24, or 52 weeks of isoniazid treatment. They found that treatment with isoniazid monotherapy significantly reduced the probability of developing culture-positive TB compared to placebo (by 21% in the 12-week arm, 65% in the 24-week arm, and 75% in the 52-week arm). They further reported that in those with good compliance and therapy completion these rates were even better at 30, 69, and 93%, respectively for the three time points.

Comstock et al. subsequently reviewed this data in 1999 and concluded that the optimal protection was conferred with 9 months of therapy.[50] On this basis, the CDC and the American Thoracic Society (ATS) made this their first line treatment recommendation in their 2000 guidelines.[29]

The mechanism of action of isoniazid is via inhibition of cell wall synthesis.[6] This allows effective treatment of rapidly dividing bacilli and explains an early peak in its effectiveness at the start of treatment. Unfortunately, although it has these rapidly bactericidal properties, it is not a good sterilizing agent, and hence the need for prolonged treatment courses.[6] Protracted therapy increases the possibility of noncompliance, a finding which has been confirmed by a number of authors.[51] It does not, however, increase the likelihood of adverse effects, namely hepatotoxicity, as most of these occur within the first few months of treatment initiation.[52]

To quantify the risk of hepatic injury, the United States Public Health Service undertook an audit and concluded that isoniazid regimens were associated with a 1% rate of hepatitis.[53] Subsequent studies have quoted this as less, at a value of 0.1% and have found that the risk of hepatitis increases with age and alcohol consumption.[54]

For a number of reasons, isoniazid treatment for 9–12 months has not been universally accepted as the treatment of choice. In the United Kingdom for instance, guidelines from the NICE recommend the use of dual therapy with rifampicin and isoniazid for a shorter, 3-month duration.[28] The evidence base for this regimen is a trial performed in men in Hong Kong with a diagnosis of silicosis.[55] This study compared development of TB in four randomized groups—placebo, 3 months of rifampicin, 3 months of rifampicin and isoniazid, and 6 months of isoniazid. The results demonstrated that the shorter treatment regimens were as effective as standard treatment with isoniazid. The United Kingdom advocates that duration of therapy of isoniazid alone is 6 months as the additional benefit of 9 months duration is minimal.[49]

A subsequent Spanish study confirmed these findings, concluding that 6–12 months of isoniazid monotherapy was equivalent to 3–4 months of rifampicin and isoniazid dual therapy in a cohort of both HIV-negative and HIV-positive patients.[56]

In addition to a shorter regimen, and therefore potentially improved completion rates, there is the theoretical advantage of reducing the possibility of producing a drug-resistant organism in the circumstance of latent disease being mistaken for minimally active disease. Some commentators have argued that this rationale is not justified against the increased risk of hepatotoxicity that a dual-medication regimen brings.[51]

Other treatment strategies have also been examined using combinations of standard TB antibiotics. In 2000, the ATS recommended a combination of rifampicin and pyrazinamide for a 2-month period particularly in patients with HIV coinfection.[29] These recommendations were based on a number of studies which showed equal efficacy of this regimen at preventing the development of active TB infection in both mouse models[57] and human trials.[58] Unfortunately, a significant increase in hepatotoxicity was observed including some deaths and as a result this recommendation was withdrawn. This event highlighted the need for stringent safety profiling of new proposed regimens.

More recently, studies have investigated the use of the long-acting rifamycin, rifapentine.[59] Due to its half-life, rifapentine requires administration only once a week. Sterling et al. demonstrated that a 12-week course of directly observed once weekly regimen in combination with isoniazid is as efficacious as standard therapy with 9 months of isoniazid[59] with higher completion rates. These findings have been replicated and data suggest hepatotoxicity is less with this regimen although other adverse effects may be higher.[60]

Stagg et al. in their 2014 meta-analysis of LTB treatment options concluded that regimens containing at least 3 months of treatment with rifamycins were efficacious standard treatment with isoniazid.[48] This review looked at randomized control studies that evaluated LTB treatment in humans and looked at 1 or 2 of the primary endpoints of preventing TB or hepatotoxicity. They identified 1,516 articles and of these 53 met the studies inclusion criteria. The authors postulated that from an efficacy and safety perspective most of the available regimens were equivalent. They argued therefore that choice should be made based on the specifics of the individual being treated including their personal likelihood of compliance with a given regimen and their individual risk of developing adverse effects.

Most commentators agree, however, on the need for further research into shorter, more efficacious, and better tolerated regimens.

In those people with exposure to multidrug-resistant TB (MDR-TB), the strategy for chemoprophylaxis and treatment of latent disease is variable. In the United States, recommendations are to treat as presumed MDR disease with pyrazinamide and a quinolone.[29] In the United Kingdom and European countries, consensus is to adopt a "watch and wait" policy and treat according to sensitivities if active disease develops. The concern being that empirical treatment in the context of drug resistance may theoretically increase the likelihood of further resistance developing and may be unsuccessful at clearance of the latent infection.

Different available treatment regimens for LTB have been shown in table 2.

LATENT TUBERCULOSIS AS PART OF A SPECTRUM OF DISEASE

Historically, the natural history of TB exposure has been described as resulting in one of two outcomes—initial progression to active disease or development of latent infection with an overall low lifetime risk of reactivation. More recently, experts have argued that this binary conceptualization of active and latent disease is likely to be an oversimplification.[30]

TABLE 2	Comparing different available treatment regimens for latent tuberculosis		
Drug	Dose and frequency	Duration	Comment
Isoniazid	300 mg OD (5 mg/kg for adults or 10 mg/kg for children)	6 months	• NICE • WHO
Isoniazid	300 mg OD (5 mg/kg for adults or 10 mg/kg for children) or 900 mg twice* weekly (DOT)	9 months	• WHO • ATS/CDC*
Rifampicin	600 mg OD	6 months	• NICE INH-resistant or intolerant
Rifampicin	600 mg OD (10 mg/kg)	3–4 months	• ATS/CDC • WHO
Rifampicin + isoniazid	600 mg OD (10 mg/kg) + 300 mg OD (5 mg/kg adults and 10 mg/kg children)	3 months	• NICE • WHO
Rifapentine + isoniazid	By body weight + 900 mg (15 mg/kg) once weekly	3 months	• ATS/CDC • WHO • Not in pregnancy or children <2 years

*The ATS/CDC offer the option of a twice weekly regime which should be given via DOT.
ATS, American Thoracic Society, CDC, Centers for Disease Control and Prevention; WHO, World Health Organization; NICE, National Institute for Clinical Excellence.

The advances in modern diagnostics have provided evidence of a more fluid state of affairs controlled by a dynamic interaction between host and pathogen.

The role out of chest X-ray screening programs in the last century identified a cohort of individuals with no symptoms of active disease and no knowledge of previous TB infection, with signs of apical calcification and scarring. The presence of such parenchymal changes suggests a degree of active disease which was halted in its course; either contained by the host immune system or cleared entirely.[61]

The advent of more sensitive immunological markers of infection such as the IGRAs has added further support to this theory by allowing us to perform longitudinal follow-up of exposed individuals, mapping both their clinical course as well as the serum immune response. Sridhar et al.[62] propose a new envisaging of infection based on this evidence. They describe three outcomes to infection with bacilli aside from progression to active disease. The first outcome they describe as "resistance". This is likely to be mediated by the innate immune system with immediate and complete clearance of the bacilli. These individuals, despite exposure, do not show any evidence of a detectable immune response, in the form of a positive IGRA or TST and remain asymptomatic. A second group is described as "eliminating infection". Evidence for the existence of this group comes from studies which demonstrate a conversion from initially positive TST/IGRA tests following an exposure, to negative tests at 6 months.[63] This transient response has subsequently been replicated by a number of studies in a variety of different settings.

Lastly, there is the group with "contained infection", those who exist with quiescent infection with the potential for reactivation. They argue, that even within this group, the balance between host immunity and pathogen activity is dynamic. Other commentators have also supported a state of "waxing and waning" subclinical infection.[61] Evidence from studies in macaques has shown a state of "percolating" infection in some asymptomatic individuals infected with *M. tuberculosis* who intermittently shed bacilli during periods of asymptomatic, minimally active disease, whilst at other times remain clinically in a state of true latency.[64] Similar situations have also been described in humans, most notably in conjunction with HIV infection, where a number of TB screening studies have identified small, but significant proportions of asymptomatic individuals with normal chest radiographs who grow *M. tuberculosis* from sputum culture.[65]

Further longitudinal research is needed to confirm if such patients, with periods of subclinical disease, always progress to active disease (provided they remain grossly immunocompetent) or avoid the development to true active TB.

The concept of a spectrum of disease also raises questions as to the mechanisms of control between the host and pathogen. Many of these factors are well known; including HIV infection and anti-TNF medications, but others remain undefined. In particular, the role of more subtle immunomodulators, such as vitamin D, which has been linked to TB on the basis of a winter peak in notifications[66] and the observation of a spike in TB following influenza outbreaks.[67] Likewise, understanding pathogen factors, including the ability of the bacilli to adapt itself and its genetic expression in certain situations, is likely to be as relevant to the overall balance as host factors.

POTENTIALS FOR FUTURE RESEARCH

Moving forward, clinicians and researchers have a number of questions left to answer; both about the natural history of LTB and where medical interventions may be targeted. In this final section, we will outline a number of areas for future research.

First, more accurate diagnostic tests are required to help identify cases of LTB.

Although IGRAs have proved useful tools, especially in low-incidence environments, they are limited by their lack of PPV, their inability to distinguish between active and latent disease, and their reduced efficacy in those with immunodeficiency. There remains, therefore, a need for a cheap, reliable, easily implementable diagnostic test which is able to overcome some of these issues.

Research has been conducted on a number of avenues in immunodiagnostics including the development of more specific and sensitive IGRAs by incorporating further mycobacterial antigens.[30] Some of these antigens (Rv3879 and Rv3873) have been shown to be present prior to TST conversion, suggesting a possible biomarker for progression from latent to active disease.[30,68] Much interest has also been generated by the discovery of "dormancy and resuscitation antigens" which may enable distinction between cleared and active infection.[30] Such immune signatures, if reliably established, would enable focused treatment in only those whom the risk of reactivation is high, thereby avoiding unnecessary and potentially harmful therapy.

The difficulties faced in the management of LTB do not end with a diagnosis. Treatment options continue to be suboptimal and regimens with shorter durations that are efficacious, tolerable, and conducive to patient compliance are needed. Several new drugs are currently undergoing development including some specifically focused on targeting dormant bacilli.[6]

As with diagnosis, a clearer understanding of the immunopathology of TB and how the host immune system interacts with pathogen to enable a variety of clinical outcomes is key. By understanding this, it is possible that some of the mechanisms used by the host immune system can be harnessed to improve treatment outcomes and shorten treatment duration. One possibility of such a treatment is the use of vaccines in conjunction with standard treatment.[68] A novel vaccine (RUTI) is currently in development and contains heat inactivated fragments of *M. tuberculosis*. If administered after 1 month of therapy, it may be able to assist the immune clearance of persisting bacilli.[69]

In addition, new vaccines are in development for both pre- and postexposure, with the aim of preventing infection occurring and preventing latency progressing respectively. Unfortunately, to date, no vaccines have been successfully proven to achieve these aims.[61]

Lastly, as with the treatment and management of any disease, a population-wide perspective is needed. Public health interventions, ranging from better housing and ventilation to prevent primary infection and to the prioritization of funding to support active case finding and identification and treatment of HIV infection, are crucial.

CONCLUSION

The diagnosis and treatment of LTB remains a key challenge facing clinicians and policy-makers working toward the WHO aim of eradication of TB.[46] As the largest source of bacilli, clearly targeting this cohort is vital to controlling the disease. Our improved understanding of the pathology, clinical course, and diagnostics of LTB has enabled the development of more robust protocols for addressing the problem but clearly much more needs to be achieved. In particular, improved diagnostics to facilitate the identification of those who will develop active disease to enable focused treatment of only those individuals for whom it is necessary. Parallel to this, improved drug regimens, perhaps targeted at those mechanisms which enable bacilli to remain suspended in a state of latency, which are more tolerable and acceptable to asymptomatic individuals, are required. Without these, the challenge to eliminate the globally vast reservoir of LTB will remain an uphill battle.

REFERENCES

1. Dye C, Scheele S, Dolin P, Pathania V, Raviglione MC. Consensus statement. Global burden of tuberculosis: estimated incidence, prevalence, and mortality by country. WHO Global Surveillance and Monitoring Project. JAMA. 1999;282:677-86.
2. Comstock GW, Livesay VT, Woolpert SF. The prognosis of a positive tuberculin reaction in childhood and adolescence. Am J Epidemiol. 1974;99:131-8.
3. Druszczynska M, Kowalewicz-Kulbat M, Fol M, Wlodarczyk M, Rudnicka W. Latent M. tuberculosis infection—pathogenesis, diagnosis, treatment and prevention strategies. Pol J Microbiol. 2012;61:3-10.
4. Wagner R. Clemens von Pirquet, discoverer of the concept of allergy. Bull N Y Acad Med. 1964;40:229-35.
5. Lillebaek T, Dirksen A, Baess I, Strunge B, Thomsen V, Anderson A. Molecular evidence of endogenous reactivation of Mycobacterium tuberculosis after 33 years of latent infection. J Infect Dis. 2002;185(3):401-4.
6. Esmail H, Barry CE 3rd, Wilkinson RJ. Understanding latent tuberculosis: the key to improved diagnostic and novel treatment strategies. Drug Discov Today. 2012;17(9-10):514-21.
7. Barry CE 3rd, Boshoff HI, Dartois V, et al. The spectrum of latent tuberculosis: rethinking the biology and intervention strategies. Nat Rev Microbiol. 2009;7:845-55.
8. Robertson BD, Altmann D, Barry C, et al. Detection and treatment of subclinical tuberculosis. Tuberculosis. 2012;92:447-52.
9. Lin PL, Flynn JL. Understanding latent tuberculosis: a moving target. J Immunol. 2010;185:15-22.
10. Hernandez-Pando R, Orozco H, Aguilar D. Factors that deregulate the protective immune response in tuberculosis. Arch Immunol Ther Exp. 2009;57:355-67.
11. Day TA, Koch M, Nouailles G, et al. Secondary lymphoid organs are dispensable for the development of T-cell-mediated immunity during tuberculosis. Eur J Immunol. 2010;40:1663-73.
12. Saunders BM, Cooper AM. Restraining mycobacteria: role of granulomas in mycobacterial infections. Immunol Cell Biol. 2000;78(4):334-41.

13. Chao MC, Rubin EJ. Letting sleeping dos lie: does dormancy play a role in tuberculosis? Annu Rev Microbiol. 2010;64:293-311.
14. Gideon HP, Flynn JL. Latent tuberculosis: what the host "sees"? Immunol Res. 2011;50:202-12.
15. Park HD, Guinn KM, Harrell MI, et al. Rv3133c/dosR is a transcription factor that mediates the hypoxic response of Mycobacterium tuberculosis. Mol Microbiol. 2003;48(3):833-43.
16. Rustad TR, Harrell MI, Liao R, Sherman DR. The enduring hypoxic response of Mycobacterium tuberculosis. PLoS One. 2008;3(1):e1502.
17. Schnappinger D, Ehrt S, Voskuil MI, et al. Transcriptional adaptation of Mycobacterium tuberculosis within macrophages: insights into the phagosomal environment. J Exp Med. 2003;198(5):693-704.
18. Peyron P, Vaubourgeix J, Poquet Y, et al. Foamy macrophages from tuberculous patients' granulomas constitute a nutrient-rich reservoir for M. tuberculosis persistence. PLoS Pathog. 2008;4:el1000204.
19. Tan MP, Sequeira P, Lin WW, et al. Nitrate respiration protects hypoxic Mycobacterium tuberculosis against acid and reactive nitrogen species stresses. PLoS One. 2010;5(10):e13356.
20. Chee CB, Sester M, Zhang W, Lange C. Diagnosis and treatment of latent infection with Mycobacterium tuberculosis. Respirology. 2013;18:205-16.
21. Chen X, Zhang M, Liao M, et al. Reduced Th17 response in patients with tuberculosis correlates with IL-6R expression on CD4+ T cells. Am J Respir Crit Care Med. 2010;181:734-42.
22. Marin ND, Paris SC, Velez WM, Rojas CA, Rojas M, García LF. Regulatory T cell frequency and modulation of IFN-gamma and IL-17 in active and latent tuberculosis. Tuberculosis (Edinb). 2010;90:252-61.
23. Opie EL, Aronson JD. Tubercle bacilli in latent tuberculosis lesions and in lung tissue without tuberculous lesions. Arch Pathol Lab Med. 1927;4(1):1-21.
24. Koch R. A further communication on a remedy for tuberculosis. Br Med J. 1891;1(1568):125-7.
25. Sarrazin H, Wilkinson KA, Andersson J, et al. Association between tuberculin skin test reactivity, the memory CD4 cell subset, and circulating FoxP3-expressing cells in HIV-infected persons. J Infect Dis. 2009;199(5):702-10.
26. Matheu MP, Beeton C, Garcia A, et al. Imaging of effector memory T cells during a delayed-type hypersensitivity reaction and suppression by Kv1.3 channel block. Immunity. 2008;29(4):602-14.
27. Walrath J, Zukowski L, Krywiak A, Silver RF. Resident Th1-like effector memory cells in pulmonary recall response to Mycobacterium tuberculosis. Am J Resp Cell Mol Biol. 2005;33(1):48-55.
28. Tuberculosis (NG33) NICE Guideline. 2016 (online) Available from https://www.nice.org.uk/guidance/ng33/resources/tuberculosis-1837390683589 [Accessed March, 2017].
29. Targeted tuberculin testing and treatment of latent tuberculosis infection. American Thoracic Society. MMWR Recomm Rep. 2000;49(RR-6):1-51.
30. Thillai M, Pollock K, Pareek M, Lalvani A. Interferon-gamma release assays for tuberculosis: current and future applications. Expert Rev Respir Med. 2014;8(1):67-78.
31. Menzies D. Interpretation of repeated tuberculin tests. Boosting, conversion, and reversion. Am J Respir Crit Care Med. 1999;159(1):15-21.
32. Gordin FM, Perez-Stable EJ, Reid M, et al. Stability of positive tuberculin tests: are boosted reactions valid? Am Rev Respir Dis. 1991;144:560-3.
33. Pai M, Zwerling A, Menzies D. Systematic review: T-cell-based assays for the diagnosis of latent tuberculosis infection: an update. Am Intern Med. 2008;149:177-84.
34. Schluger NW. Advances in the diagnosis of latent tuberculosis infection. Semin Respir Crit Care Med. 2013;34(1):60-6.
35. Mills CC, O'Grady F, Riley RL. Tuberculin conversion in the "naturally infected" guinea pig. Bull Johns Hopkins Hosp. 1960;106:36-45.
36. Ferebee SH. Controlled chemoprophylaxis trials in tuberculosis. A general review. Bibl Tuberc. 1970;26:28-106.
37. QuantiFERON-TB Gold Package Insert. March 2013. US05990301L.
38. van Ingen J, de Zwaan R, Dekhuijzen R, Boeree M, van Soolingen D. Region of difference 1 in nontuberculous Mycobacterium species adds a phylogenetic and taxonomical character. J Bacteriol. 2009;191(18):5865-7.
39. Holland SM. Nontuberculous mycobacteria. Am J Med Sci. 2001;321(1):49-55.
40. Oni T, Gideon HP, Bangani N, et al. Risk factors associated with indeterminate gamma interferon responses in the assessment of latent tuberculosis infection in a high incidence environment. Clin Vaccine Immunol. 2012;19(8):1243-7.

41. Vincenti D, Carrara S, Butera O, et al. Response to region of difference 1 (RD1) epitopes in human immunodeficiency virus (HIV)-infected individuals enrolled with suspected active tuberculosis: a pilot study. Clin Exp Immunol. 2007;150(1):91-8.
42. Clark SA, Martin SL, Pozniak A, et al. Tuberculosis antigen-specific immune responses can be detected using enzyme-linked immunospot technology in human immunodeficiency virus (HIV)-1 patients with advanced disease. Clin Exp Immunol. 2007;150(2):238-44.
43. Aabye MG, Ravn P, PrayGod G, et al. The impact of HIV infection and CD4 cell count on the performance of an interferon-gamma release assay in patients with pulmonary tuberculosis. PLoS One. 2009;4(1):e4220.
44. Naseer A, Naqvi S, Kampmann B. Evidence for boosting Mycobacterium tuberculosis-specific IFN-gamma responses at 6 weeks following tuberculin skin testing. Eur Respir J. 2007;29(6):1282-3.
45. Diel R, Loddenkemper R, Nienhaus A. Predictive value of interferon-gamma release assays and tuberculin skin testing for progression from latent TB infection to disease state: a meta-analysis. Chest. 2012;142(1):63-75.
46. WHO. Guidelines on the management of latent tuberculosis infection. The end TB strategy. WHO; 2015.
47. Denkinger CM, Dheda K, Pai M. Guidelines on interferon-gamma release assays for tuberculosis infection: concordance, discordance or confusion? Clin Microbiol Infect. 2011;17(6):806-14.
48. Stagg HR, Zenner D, Harris R, Munoz L, Lipman MC, Abubakar I. Treatment of latent tuberculosis infection: a network meta-analysis. Ann Intern Med. 2014;161:419-28.
49. Efficacy of various durations of isoniazid preventive therapy for tuberculosis: five years of follow up in the IUAT trial. International Union Against Tuberculosis Committee on Prophylaxis. Bull World Health Organ. 1982;60:555-64.
50. Comstock GW. How much isoniazid is needed for prevention of tuberculosis among immunocompetent adults? Int J Tuberc Lung Dis. 1999;3:847-50.
51. Menzies D, Al Jahdali H, Al Otaibi B. Recent developments in the treatment of latent tuberculosis infection. Indian J Med Res. 2011;133:257-66.
52. Tedla Z, Nguyen ML, Sibanda T, et al. Isoniazid-associated hepatitis in adults infected with HIV receiving 36 months of isoniazid prophylaxis in Botswana. Chest. 2015;147(5):1376-84.
53. Kopanoff DE, Snider DE Jr, Caras GJ. Isoniazid-related hepatitis: a US Public Health Service cooperative surveillance study. Am Rev Respir Dis. 1978;117:991-1001.
54. LoBue PA, Moser KS. Use of isoniazid for latent tuberculosis infection in a public health clinic. Am J Respir Crit Care Med. 2003;168:443-7.
55. A double-blind placebo-controlled clinical trial of three antituberculous chemoprophylaxis regimens in patients with silicosis in Hong Kong. Hong Kong Chest Service/Tuberculosis Research Centre, Madras/British Medical Research Council. Am Rev Respir Dis. 1992;145:36-41.
56. Ena J, Valls V. Short-course therapy with rifampicin plus isoniazid, compared with standard therapy with isoniazid, for latent tuberculosis infection: a meta-analysis. Clin Infect Dis. 2005;40:670-6.
57. Lecoeur HF, Truffot-Pernot C, Grosset JH. Experimental short-course preventive therapy of tuberculosis with rifampin and pyrazinamide. Am Rev Respir Dis. 1989;140:1189-93.
58. Gao XF, Wang L, Liu GJ, et al. Rifampicin plus pyrazinamide versus isoniazid for treating latent tuberculosis infection: a meta-analysis. Int J Tuberc Lung Dis. 2006;10:1080-90.
59. Sterling TR, Villarino ME, Borisov AS, et al. Three months of rifapentine and isoniazid for latent tuberculosis infection. N Engl J Med. 2011;365:2155-66.
60. Sharma SK, Sharma A, Kadhiravan T, Tharyan P. Rifamycins (rifampicin, rifabutin and rifapentine) compared to isoniazid for preventing tuberculosis in HIV-negative people at risk of active TB. Evid Based Child Health. 2014;9(1):169-294.
61. Esmail H, Barry CE 3rd, Young DB, Wilkinson RJ. The ongoing challenge of latent tuberculosis. Philos Trans R Soc Lond B Biol Sci. 2014;369(1645):20130437.
62. Sridhar S, Pollock K, Lalvani A. Redefining latent tuberculosis. Future Microbiol. 2011;6(9):1021-35.
63. Ewer K, Millington KA, Deeks JJ, Alvarez L, Bryant G, Lalvani A. Dynamic antigen-specific T-cell responses after point-source exposure to Mycobacterium tuberculosis. Am J Respir Crit Care Med. 2006;174(7):831-9.
64. Lin PL, Rodgers M, Smith L, et al. Quantitative comparison of active and latent tuberculosis in the cynomolgus macaque model. Infect Immun. 2009;77(10):4631-42.

65. Achkar JM, Jenny-Avital ER. Incipient and subclinical tuberculosis: defining early disease states in the context of host immune response. J Infect Dis. 2011;204:S1179-86.
66. Martineau AR, Nhamoyebonde S, Oni T, et al. Reciprocal seasonal variation in vitamin D status and tuberculosis notifications in Cape Town, South Africa. Proc Natl Acad Sci U S A. 2011;108:19013-7.
67. Oei W, Nishiura H. The relationship between tuberculosis and influenza death during the influenza (H1N1) pandemic from 1918-19. Comput Math Methods Med. 2012;2012:124861.
68. Dosanjh DP, Bakir M, Millington KA, et al. Novel M. tuberculosis antigen-specific T-cells are early markers of infection and disease progression. PLoS One. 2011;6(12):e28754.
69. Vilaplana C, Montane E, Pinto S, et al. Double-blind, randomized, placebo-controlled phase I clinical trial of the therapeutical antituberculous vaccine RUTI. Vaccine. 2009;28:1106-16.

CHAPTER 4

Diagnosis of Tuberculosis

Violeta V Mihailovic Vucinic, Dragana M Jovanovic

INTRODUCTION

Assessing the diagnosis of tuberculosis (TB) includes:
- Clinical manifestations TB infection
- History of previous TB infection
- Possible exposure to TB infection
- Radiographic features
- Clinical specimen analysis
- Molecular tests.

CLINICAL MANIFESTATIONS OF TUBERCULOSIS INFECTION

The clinical manifestations of primary TB vary but symptoms and signs characterizing lung disease are present in approximately 30% of patients. The most common symptom is fever occurring in approximately 70% of patients. Fever is not obviously accompanied by other symptoms, although some patients may develop pleuritic or retrosternal pain. Most frequently, patients with pleuritic chest pain have evidence of a pleural effusion. Some patients develop retrosternal pain due to enlarged bronchial lymph nodes. The pain worsens with swallowing.[1]

Clinical Manifestations of Primary Tuberculosis

Primary TB infection is characterized by general symptoms like fatigue, malaise, and weight loss; respiratory symptoms are represented with most frequently cough and chest pain.

Chest X-ray

In primary TB, chest X-ray is often normal. Chest X-ray abnormality most frequently seen in primary TB is hilar adenopathy.[1]

This radiographic finding usually resolves slowly over a period of 1 year or even longer.

About 30% of tuberculin converters in one study[1] developed pleural effusion within 3–4 months after TB infection. In a Canadian study,[2] pulmonary infiltrates were present in about 60% of patients. About 85% of patients had infiltrates in the middle or lower lung fields; cavitations and endobronchial spread were rare.[2]

After primary infection, 90% of infected population with adequate immune system manages to control *Mycobacterium tuberculosis* replication. This probably means the beginning of a latent phase (Fig. 1).

The remaining 10% of the infected population develop TB pneumonia with spreading out of pulmonary infiltrates at the site of initial beginning of the infection next to the hilar region with hilar adenopathy as well (Fig. 2).

Some of the infected individuals may develop TB disease at distant sites with cervical lymph nodes involvement, meningitis, pericarditis, or miliary dissemination.

Progressive disease occurs in those with poor immune response [human immunodeficiency virus (HIV)-positive, chronic kidney insufficiency, diabetes mellitus, and

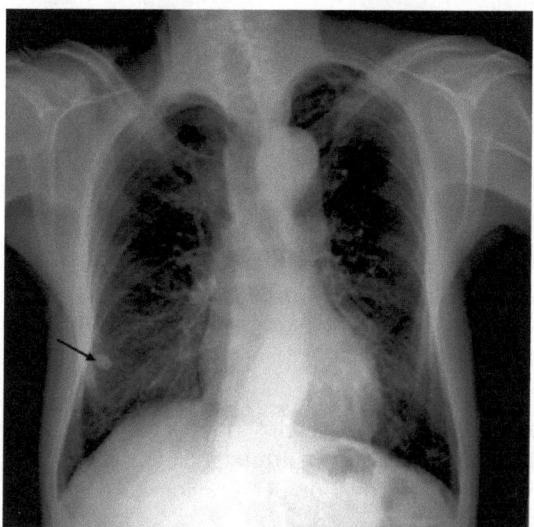

FIG. 1: Some individuals may have very prominent calcification at the chest X-ray with prominent calcification at the place of the primary infection (arrow) place of the primary infection.
Courtesy: Professor R Stevic, Radiologist, Clinical Center of Serbia, Belgrade.

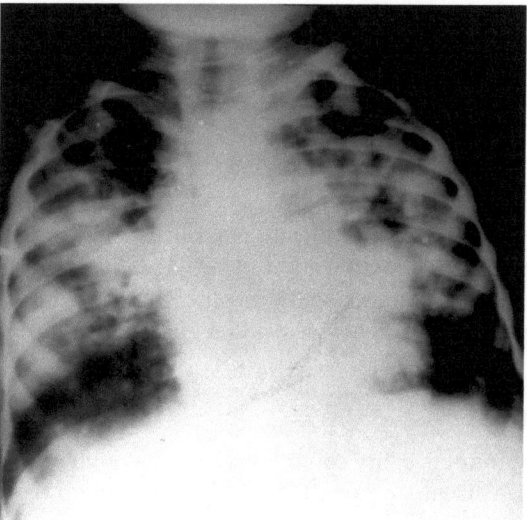

FIG. 2: Chest X-ray presenting caseous bronchopneumonia with hilar lymph nodes enlargement in primary tuberculosis.

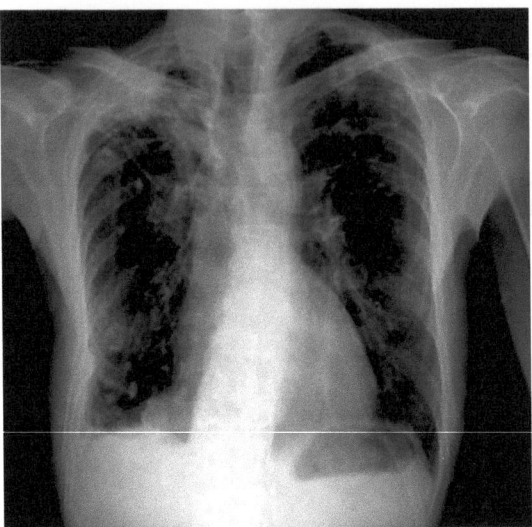

FIG. 3: Patients with upper lobe fibrotic lesions are often thought to have healed primary tuberculosis infection. However, these patients should be always evaluated for active tuberculosis.
Courtesy: Professor R Stevic, Radiologist, Clinical Center of Serbia, Belgrade.

older adults]. This phase of TB infection is described as chronic TB, postprimary disease, recrudescent TB, endogenous infection, or adult type of progressive TB. In 90% of adult TB cases, the disease is a result of reactivation of a previously "dormant" focus from the time of the primary infection (Fig. 3).

Clinical Manifestations of Postprimary Tuberculosis Disease

This form of TB infection may be asymptomatic at the beginning, thus remaining undiagnosed and potentially infectious for years. Symptoms may develop in the late phase during the natural course in uncured patients. Most of the patients develop cough, weight loss, and sensation of extreme fatigue. Fever and night sweats are present in approximately 50% of patients.[3-5]

General Symptoms

Low-grade fever with characteristic diurnal rhythm is often present (gradually rising throughout the day with the late afternoon peak). The two symptoms fever and night sweats are typical among patients with advanced pulmonary TB.[6] Consumption, appetite loss, and consecutive weight loss, and fatigue are common features of advanced TB infection.

Respiratory Symptoms

Cough initially is nonproductive, dry cough; this kind of cough may be present only in the morning. In progressive disease, productive yellow-green cough is present throughout the day. Sputum is smear-positive.[7,8]

Hemoptysis occurs later in the course of disease due to caseous necrosis or endobronchial erosion.

Dyspnea may occur in cases with extensive parenchymal disease, pleural effusion, or pneumothorax. Pleuritic chest pain may indicate inflammation of the pleura with or without effusion.

Physical Examination

Physical findings of pulmonary TB are not specific and usually they are absent in mild or moderate disease. Large parenchymal infiltrates due to TB infection may cause typical signs of consolidations. In patients with cavitary lesions, typical amphoric soundsare found.

Laboratory Findings

Routine laboratory findings are usually normal in pulmonary TB, although C-reactive protein can be elevated in more than 80% of patients.[9]

Radiographic Abnormalities

Majority of patients with respiratory TB have chest X-ray abnormalities, even if the prominent respiratory symptoms are not present.[3,10]

In approximately 80–90% of patients, the reactivation TB (postprimary TB) typically involves the apical-posterior segments of the upper lobes, superior segments of the upper lobes, and/or anterior segments of the upper lobes (Fig. 4).

Approximately 30% of cases with postprimary TB have atypical radiographic patterns. The term "atypical" here includes hilar adenopathy and/or associated with right middle lobe affection, infiltrates or cavities in the middle or lower lobes, pleural effusion.[11-13]

At last, approximately 5% of patients with active TB have normal chest X-rays with or without respiratory symptoms.[14]

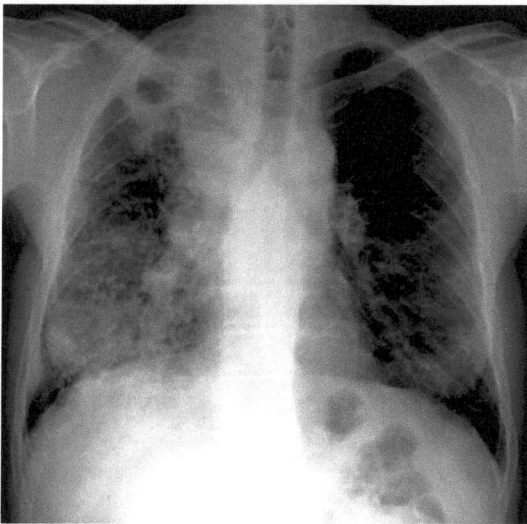

FIG. 4: Chest X-ray with cavitary formation (upper lobe right lung) typical finding in patient with pulmonary tuberculosis.
Courtesy: Professor R Stevic, Radiologist, Clinical Center of Serbia, Belgrade.

Computed Tomography Scan in Pulmonary Tuberculosis

Computed tomography (CT) scan is more sensitive than chest radiography for diagnosis of postprimary TB lesions especially located in the upper lobes of the lung (apical lesions).

Thoracic CT scan may represent a cavity or infiltrates of the apicoposterior segments, or fibrotic lesions with parenchymal distortion and consecutive traction bronchiectasis.

High-resolution CT scan can detect early bronchogenic TB spread (Fig. 5).[15]

Magnetic Resonance Imaging

Magnetic resonance imaging is a technique used to detect intrathoracic lymphadenopathy, pericardial thickening, or pericardial effusion and/or pleural effusion.[16]

Atypical Tuberculosis Presentations—Lower Lung Field Tuberculosis

This is the disease with lesions located below the hilar regions, as presented on chest X-ray.[17]

Consolidations in the lower fields of the lungs are more extensive compared to the upper lobe TB consolidations. Even very large cavities have been described in this area of the lungs (Fig. 6).[18-20]

Symptoms of TB infection in patients with lower lobe TB are often subacute in onset or even chronic. This presentation of TB infection is sometimes misdiagnosed initially as viral or bacterial pneumonia.

Older, adult patients, HIV-positive individuals, patients with chronic renal or hepatic disease, patients receiving corticosteroids, or those with silicosis are at highest risk for lower TB.

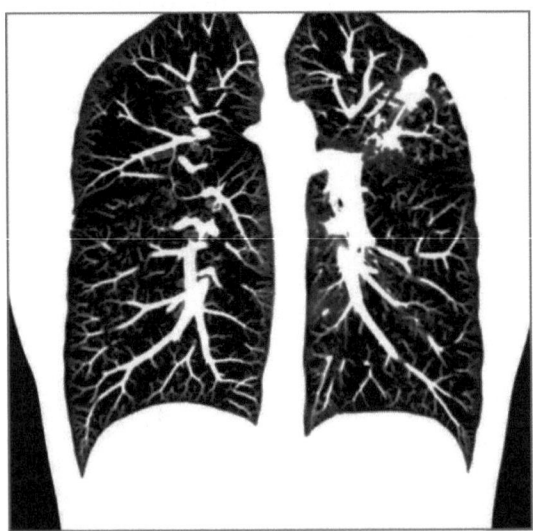

FIG. 5: Computed tomography scan: Tree-in-bud finding, usually indicating the presence of infection in this case tuberculosis infection. The tree-in-bud pattern is caused by demarcation of the normally invisible branching course of the peripheral airways, which usually results from bronchial impaction with mucus, or pus, or even fluid.
Courtesy: Professor R Stevic, Radiologist, Clinical Center of Serbia, Belgrade.

Tuberculoma

This round lesion can develop during primary TB infection or when a focus of postprimary TB becomes encapsulated (Fig. 7).[20]

The diagnosis sometimes can be very difficult since sputum Lowenstein cultures are frequently negative.

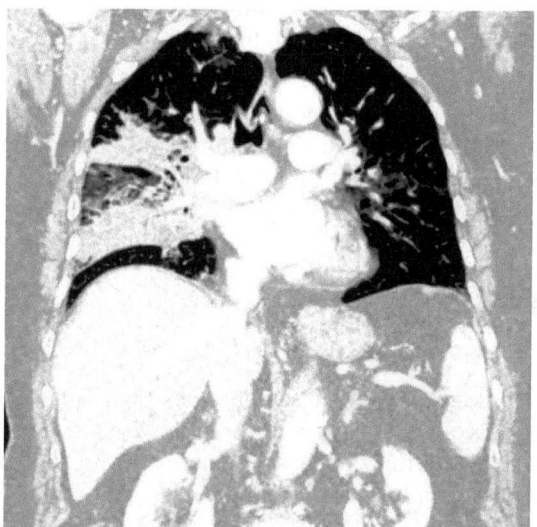

FIG. 6: Pulmonary tuberculosis infection as presented on this computed tomography scan with lesions not quite typical for reactivation tuberculosis. In this patient, apical segments of the upper lobes are not involved.
Courtesy: Professor R Stevic, Radiologist, Clinical Center of Serbia, Belgrade.

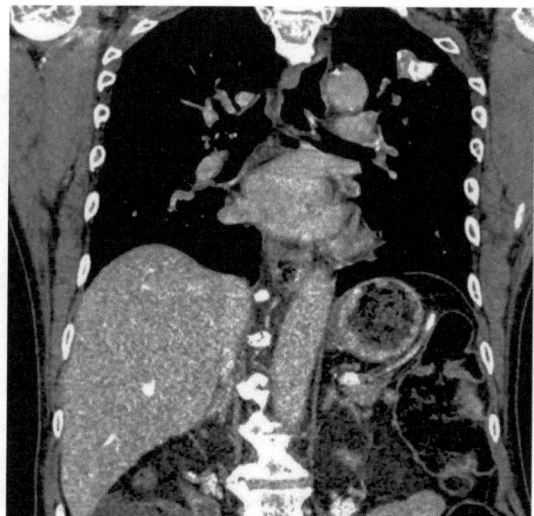

FIG. 7: Resembling tuberculoma in the upper lobe left lung.
Courtesy: Professor R Stevic, Radiologist, Clinical Center of Serbia, Belgrade.

HISTORY OF PREVIOUS INFECTION

In suspected case of TB infection, tuberculin skin test (TST) and/or interferon-gamma release assay (IGRA) should be performed. Of note, negative test does not exclude disease, while positive tests support diagnosis.

POSSIBLE EXPOSURE TO TUBERCULOSIS INFECTION

History of any contacts with TB patients or history of traveling to high-incidence countries can support the assessment of new case of TB infection.

CHEST X-RAY

Chest radiography is initial approach to the diagnosis of many pulmonary diseases and suspected TB. Active TB is represented with focal infiltration of the upper lobe(s) or the upper segments of the lower lobes. In some cases, cavitations may be seen as well as enlarged lymph nodes.

CLINICAL SPECIMENS

Sputum

Sputum samples for *M. tuberculosis* might be obtained by coughing or the sputum might be induced for the analysis. A series of at least three single specimens should be collected (suggestion is early morning sputum—at least one sample). Three specimens are important for culture, even if the first sample is smear positive.

Patients with dry, nonproductive cough should be inhaled by hypertonic saline solution.

Bronchoscopy

Bronchoscopy with bronchoalveolar lavage and/or biopsy should be performed if the patient:
- Failed to produce adequate sputum sample
- Negative sputum findings in cases with high clinical suspicion for TB infection
- In cases when alternative diagnosis different from TB is highly suspected (Fig. 8).

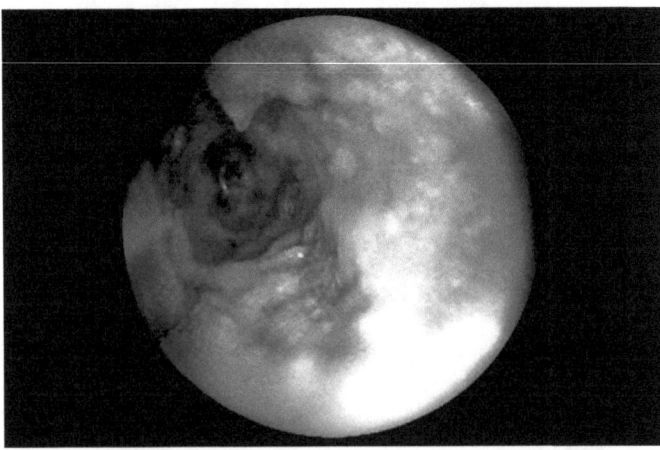

FIG. 8: Extensive pulmonary distraction (bronchopulmonary communication) due to progressive tuberculosis. *(For color version, see Plate 4)*

Courtesy: Dr Spasoje Popevic, Bronchologist, University Clinic of Pulmonology, Clinical Center of Serbia, Belgrade.

Tissue biopsy may establish definite diagnosis of TB when noninvasive diagnostics failed. Histology of tissue biopsy represents typical granulomatous inflammation with central parts representing characteristic (cheese-like), caseous necrosis finding unique for TB granulomas.

Diagnostic Microbiology

Stained Smear

Acid-fast bacilli (AFB) on stained smear analysis may represent *M. tuberculosis* but also nontuberculous mycobacteria (NTM), so this procedure cannot show definitive diagnosis of TB case.

Sputum Culture

Sputum samples obtained from patients suspected for active TB disease should be cultured. Culture can detect 10–100 bacilli/mL while stained smear needs at least 5,000–10,000 bacilli/mL.[21] Culture is required for drug susceptibility tests.

Sputum samples should be obtained from patients with pulmonary TB at least monthly until two (at least) chronological sputum cultures are negative in order to confirm the efficiency of the therapy.

MOLECULAR TESTS

Nucleic Acid Amplification

This molecular test can be used in individuals with high suspicion for TB infection. Nucleic acid amplification (NAA) is rapid test used to define organism belonging to the *M. tuberculosis* complex within 24–48 hours.

Only up to 10 microorganisms/mL is enough to gain positive result.[22-26]

In AFB smear-positive patients, NAA test has positive predictive value in distinguishing TB from NTM.[27]

The test is based on amplification of a specific ribonucleic acid or deoxyribonucleic acid sequence that is detected via a nucleic acid probe.[28,29] Nucleic acid amplification test results must be interpreted in the context of clinical manifestation and epidemiological conditions. Of note, NAA test can detect nucleic acid from dead and live organisms, so the testing can remain positive even after the treatment, so this method is only reliable for initial diagnosis.

Xpert MTB/RIF Assay

This is a type of NAA test that can identify *M. tuberculosis* and rifampin resistance at the same time.[30,31]

Boehme and coworkers conducted a study on 1,730 patients with suspected TB infection, the test was positive in 98% of patients with smear-positive TB and 72% of patients with AFB negative/culture-positive patients. The reliability of rifampin resistance detection was 98%.[30] In conditions when it is not possible to established prompt and accurate laboratory diagnosis, clinical diagnosis based on positive history of exposure, positive TST or IGRA, with adequate clinical and radiological findings, it is advised to initiate the treatment.

In a minority of TB patients, this is predominantly case in children under 5 years of age; laboratory diagnosis of TB is never established.[32]

In such cases, the diagnosis of TB can be establish based on clinical and radiological presentations as well as on positive response to empiric treatment.

For certain specific forms of TB (pleural TB) refer to Chapter "Tuberculosis Effusion and the Role of Closed Pleural Biopsy and Pleuroscopy".

COMPLICATIONS OF TUBERCULOSIS

Complications of TB and their characteristics, causes, and therapy have been shown in table 1.

TABLE 1	Complications of tuberculosis[33-39]		
Complications	*General characteristics*	*Causes*	*Therapy*
Hemoptysis	• Massive hemoptysis is rare complication • Sources of massive hemoptysis include pulmonary artery, bronchial arteries, intercostal arteries	• Active TB infection • Patients are often acid-fast positive • Cavitary disease • TB relapse after completion of therapy	• Conservative • Surgery in patients with failure of conservative therapy
Pneumothorax	• Spontaneous pneumothorax associated with TB has been reported in 1–2% of patients since the therapy era	• Rupture of peripheral cavity or subpleural caseous lesions with bronchopleural fistula	• Spontaneous remission of bronchopleural fistula and the lung expansion • Thoracic drainage
Bronchiectasis	–	• Progressive chronic lung TB with fibrosis of the lung parenchyma	–
Extensive pulmonary destruction	• Nowadays rare	• Progressive TB, absence of effective therapy	–
Pulmonary gangrene	• Nowadays rare	• Progressive TB with arteritis and thrombosis of the vessels supplying necrotic lung	• Mortality high 75%
Aspergillosis (Fig. 9)	• Sequela of pulmonary TB		• Antimycotics or surgery
Malignancy	• The possible cause: Cell components of the mycobacteria can cause deoxyribonucleic acid damage leading to cancerogenesis • Chronic inflammation enhancing mutagenesis		–

TB, tuberculosis.

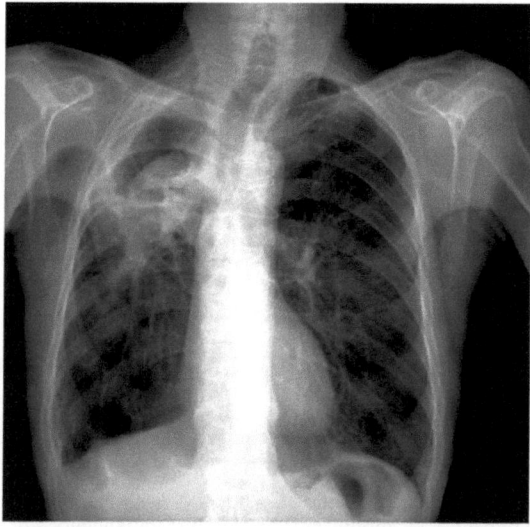

FIG. 9: Aspergillosis in the tuberculosis cavity in the upper lobe right lung.
Courtesy: Professor R Stevic, Radiologist, Clinical Center of Serbia, Belgrade.

REFERENCES

1. Poulsen A. Some clinical features of tuberculosis. Acta Tuberc Scand. 1957;33:37-92.
2. Krysl J, Korzeniewska-Kosela M, Müller NL, FitzGerald JM. Radiologic features of pulmonary tuberculosis: an assessment of 188 cases. Can Assoc Radiol J. 1994;45:101-7.
3. Barnes PF, Verdegem TD, Vachon LA, Leedom JM, Overturf GD. Chest roentgenogram in pulmonary tuberculosis. New data on an old test. Chest. 1988;94:316-20.
4. Arango L, Brewin AW, Murray JF. The spectrum of tuberculosis as currently seen in a metropolitan hospital. Am Rev Respir Dis. 1973;108:805-12.
5. MacGregor RR. A year's experience with tuberculosis in a private urban teaching hospital in the postsanatorium era. Am J Med. 1975;58:221-8.
6. Mayock RL, MacGregor RR. Diagnosis, prevention and early therapy of tuberculosis. Dis Mon. 1976;22:1-60.
7. Verver S, Bwire R, Borgdorff MW. Screening for pulmonary tuberculosis among immigrants: estimated effect on severity of disease and duration of infectiousness. Int J Tuberc Lung Dis. 2001;5:419-25.
8. Miller LG, Asch SM, Yu EI, Knowles L, Gelberg L, Davidson P. A population-based survey of tuberculosis symptoms: how atypical are atypical presentations? Clin Infect Dis. 2000;30:293-9.
9. Breen RA, Leonard O, Perrin FM, et al. How good are systemic symptoms and blood inflammatory markers at detecting individuals with tuberculosis? Int J Tuberc Lung Dis. 2008;12:44-9.
10. Day JH, Charalambous S, Fielding KL, Hayes RJ, Churchyard GJ, Grant AD. Screening for tuberculosis prior to isoniazid preventive therapy among HIV-infected gold miners in South Africa. Int J Tuberc Lung Dis. 2006;10:523-9.
11. Choyke PL, Sostman HD, Curtis AM, et al. Adult-onset pulmonary tuberculosis. Radiology. 1983;148:357-62.
12. Miller WT, MacGregor RR. Tuberculosis: frequency of unusual radiographic findings. AJR Am J Roentgenol. 1978;130:867-75.
13. Woodring JH, Vandiviere HM, Fried AM, Dillon ML, Williams TD, Melvin IG. Update: the radiographic features of pulmonary tuberculosis. AJR Am J Roentgenol. 1986;146:497-506.
14. Marciniuk DD, McNab BD, Martin WT, Hoeppner VH. Detection of pulmonary tuberculosis in patients with a normal chest radiograph. Chest. 1999;115:445-52.

15. Im JG, Itoh H, Han MC. CT of pulmonary tuberculosis. Semin Ultrasound CT MR. 1995;16:420-34.
16. De Backer AI, Mortelé KJ, De Keulenaer BL, Parizel PM. Tuberculosis: epidemiology, manifestations, and the value of medical imaging in diagnosis. JBR-BTR. 2006;89:243-50.
17. Segarra F, Sherman DS, Rodriguez-Aguero J. Lower lung field tuberculosis. Am Rev Respir Dis. 1963;87:37-40.
18. Chang SC, Lee PY, Perng RP. Lower lung field tuberculosis. Chest. 1987;91:230-2.
19. Parmar MS. Lower lung field tuberculosis. Am Rev Respir Dis. 1967;96:310-3.
20. Steele JD. The solitary pulmonary nodule. Report of a cooperative study of resected asymptomatic solitary pulmonary nodules in males. J Thorac Cardiovasc Surg. 1963;46:21-39.
21. Hobby GL, Holman AP, Iseman MD, Jones JM. Enumeration of tubercle bacilli in sputum of patients with pulmonary tuberculosis. Antimicrob Agents Chemother. 1973;4:94-104.
22. Cheng VC, Yew WW, Yuen KY. Molecular diagnostics in tuberculosis. Eur J Clin Microbiol Infect Dis. 2005;24:711-20.
23. Catanzaro A, Perry S, Clarridge JE, et al. The role of clinical suspicion in evaluating a new diagnostic test for active tuberculosis: results of a multicenter prospective trial. JAMA. 2000;283:639-45.
24. Conaty SJ, Claxton AP, Enoch DA, Hayward AC, Lipman MC, Gillespie SH. The interpretation of nucleic acid amplification tests for tuberculosis: do rapid tests change treatment decisions? J Infect. 2005;50:187-92.
25. Lim TK, Mukhopadhyay A, Gough A, Khoo KL, Khoo SM, Lee KH, et al. Role of clinical judgment in the application of a nucleic acid amplification test for the rapid diagnosis of pulmonary tuberculosis. Chest. 2003;124:902-8.
26. Wiener RS, Della-Latta P, Schluger NW. Effect of nucleic acid amplification for Mycobacterium tuberculosis on clinical decision making in suspected extrapulmonary tuberculosis. Chest. 2005;128:102-7.
27. Centers for Disease Control and Prevention (CDC). Updated guidelines for the use of nucleic acid amplification tests in the diagnosis of tuberculosis. MMWR Morb Mortal Wkly Rep. 2009;58:7-10.
28. Cohen RA, Muzaffar S, Schwartz D, Bashir S, Luke S, McGartland LP, et al. Diagnosis of pulmonary tuberculosis using PCR assays on sputum collected within 24 hours of hospital admission. Am J Respir Crit Care Med. 1998;157:156-61.
29. Centers for Disease Control and Prevention (CDC). Nucleic acid amplification tests for tuberculosis. MMWR Morb Mortal Wkly Rep. 1996;45:950-2.
30. Boehme CC, Nabeta P, Hillemann D, Nicol MP, Shenai S, Krapp F, et al. Rapid molecular detection of tuberculosis and rifampin resistance. N Engl J Med. 2010;363:1005-15.
31. Steingart KR, Sohn H, Schiller I, Kloda LA, Boehme CC, Pai M, et al. Xpert® MTB/RIF assay for pulmonary tuberculosis and rifampicin resistance in adults. Cochrane Database Syst Rev. 2013;1:CD009593.
32. Centers for Disease Control and Prevention. Reported tuberculosis in the United States, 2008. [online] Available from www.cdc.gov/tb/statistics/reports/2008/default.htm [Accessed January, 2016].
33. Johnston H, Reisz G. Changing spectrum of hemoptysis. Underlying causes in 148 patients undergoing diagnostic flexible fiberoptic bronchoscopy. Arch Intern Med. 1989;149:1666-8.
34. McGuinness G, Beacher JR, Harkin TJ, Garay SM, Rom WN, Naidich DP. Hemoptysis: prospective high-resolution CT/bronchoscopic correlation. Chest. 1994;105:1155-62.
35. Conlan AA, Hurwitz SS, Krige L, Nicolaou N, Pool R. Massive hemoptysis. Review of 123 cases. J Thorac Cardiovasc Surg. 1983;85:120-4.
36. Wilder RJ, Beacham EG, Ravitch MM. Spontaneous pneumothorax complicating cavitary tuberculosis. J Thorac Cardiovasc Surg. 1962;43:561-73.
37. Ihm HJ, Hankins JR, Miller JE, McLaughlin JS. Pneumothorax associated with pulmonary tuberculosis. J Thorac Cardiovasc Surg. 1972;64:211-9.
38. Khan FA, Rehman M, Marcus P, Azueta V. Pulmonary gangrene occurring as a complication of pulmonary tuberculosis. Chest. 1980;77:76-80.
39. Falagas ME, Kouranos VD, Athanassa Z, Kopterides P. Tuberculosis and malignancy. QJM. 2010;103:461-87.

CHAPTER 5

Lymph Node Tuberculosis

Anand Jaiswal, Dipti Gothi

INTRODUCTION

Tuberculosis (TB) has been a major cause of suffering and death since time immemorial.[1] India, China, Indonesia, South Africa, and Nigeria from rank first to fifth respectively in terms of absolute number of cases.[2] Tuberculosis is primarily considered to be a pulmonary disease.[3] Hence, the term "extrapulmonary TB" has been used to describe the occurrence of TB at body sites other than the lung. Lymph node (LN) is one of the most common, easily diagnosable, easily treatable, and least complicated forms of extrapulmonary TB.[1] The field of molecular diagnosis has improved our understanding of different strains of TB and enhanced the diagnosis of lymph node tuberculosis (LNTB).[4] Recent years have witnessed a dramatic upsurge in cases of drug-resistant *Mycobacterium tuberculosis*, molecular diagnosis has been useful in that as well.[1] Knowledge about differential diagnosis and paradoxical reaction (PR) are essential tools for the management of LNTB. Short-course chemotherapy is the standard of care for this form of extrapulmonary TB, which is usually paucibacillary.

HISTORY

Isolated peripheral tuberculous lymphadenitis has afflicted mankind for thousands of years. Tuberculous lymphadenitis in the cervical region is known as scrofula, a term derived from Latin for "glandular swelling". The disease was also known as the "King's Evil" in the Middle Ages because of the widespread belief that it could be cured when the affected individual was touched by royalty.[1,5]

EPIDEMIOLOGY

Extrapulmonary TB comprises 10–50% of all TB in human immunodeficiency virus (HIV)-negative patients and about 35–80% in HIV-infected patients. Tuberculosis lymphadenitis is seen in nearly 40% of extrapulmonary TB,[6-8] which constitutes about 15–20% of all cases of TB in India.[9-12] Overall amongst cases of LNTB, in HIV-positive as well as HIV-negative patients, the most common nodes to be involved are cervical LNs, followed by the mediastinal and axillary nodes.[13,14] Cervical and mediastinal group of LNs[8] are involved in about 70% of cases.[7]

PATHOGENESIS

Clinicopathologically, TB lymphadenitis cannot be distinguished from lymphadenitis due to nontuberculous mycobacteria (NTM). Though, the pathogenesis and management remain diverse, it is important to know the pathogenesis of both for an appropriate management of tuberculous lymphadenitis. Tuberculous lymphadenitis is considered to be a local manifestation of the systemic disease, whereas lymphadenitis due to NTM is truly a localized disease.[6]

Tuberculous Lymphadenitis

Tuberculous lymphadenitis may occur due to:
- Reactivation of healed focus involved during primary infection
- Progressive primary TB, i.e., spread from lung into mediastinal LN
- Spread from tonsil
- Hematogenous spread due to miliary TB.

The most common mode of development of tuberculous lymphadenitis is reactivation of healed focus and progressive primary TB. Both these modes of spread are due to systemic dissemination of *M. tuberculosis*.[15] *Mycobacterium tuberculosis* usually enters the human body via the respiratory tract and forms primary complex or Ghon's complex in the posterior segment of upper lobe. The organisms within the Ghon's focus gain an access to the bloodstream and may disseminate to extrathoracic organs. Usually the host defense curtails the organisms both at primary site and the extrapulmonary sites. The bacteria remains dormant but may serve as nidus for reactivation. Lymph node tuberculosis may also occur at the time of initial infection (progressive primary disease). Rarely, LN involvement may occur via spread from tonsils and adenoids,[16,17] providing an early portal of entry or via hematogenous spread of TB bacilli as seen in miliary TB.

Lymphadenitis due to Nontuberculous Mycobacteria

Nontuberculous mycobacteria known to cause lymphadenitis are *M. scrofulaceum*, *M. avium-intracellulare* complex, and *M. kansasii*. Unlike tuberculous lymphadenitis, NTM lymphadenitis appears to be a truly localized disease. The pathogens usually enter the LNs directly via oropharyngeal mucosa, salivary glands, tonsils, gingiva, or conjunctiva. It is particularly an important mode of entry in children because of deciduous teeth harbor NTM. Nontuberculous mycobacteria may reach LNs in the neck via lymphatics leading to nontuberculous involvement of LN, which is difficult to differentiate from tuberculous lymphadenitis.[1,18]

CLINICAL FEATURES

Tuberculous lymphadenitis most frequently involves the cervical LNs (Fig. 1) followed in frequency by mediastinal, axillary, mesenteric, hepatic portal, perihepatic, and inguinal LNs.[4,13,19] It may present as a unilateral single or multiple painless slow growing mass or masses developing over weeks to months, mostly located in the posterior cervical, and less commonly in supraclavicular region.[20] Classically, patients present with low-grade fever, weight loss, and fatigue and somewhat less frequently with night sweats.[21,22] Cough is not a prominent feature of tuberculous lymphadenitis.[21] Upto 57% of patients have no systemic symptoms.[21,23] Sinus formation is seen in nearly 10% of the mycobacterial cervical lymphadenitis (Fig. 2).[18,24]

Jones and Campbell in 1962 described the stages of tuberculous lymphadenitis. These are as follows:[25]
- Enlarged, firm, mobile, discrete nodes
- Large rubbery nodes fixed to surrounding tissue

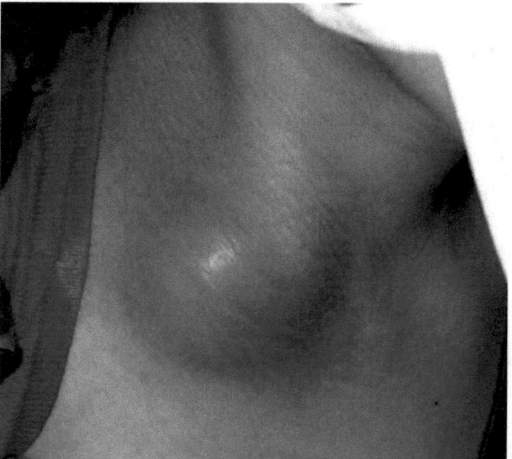

FIG. 1: Cervical lymph node with abscess formation. *(For color version, see Plate 5)*

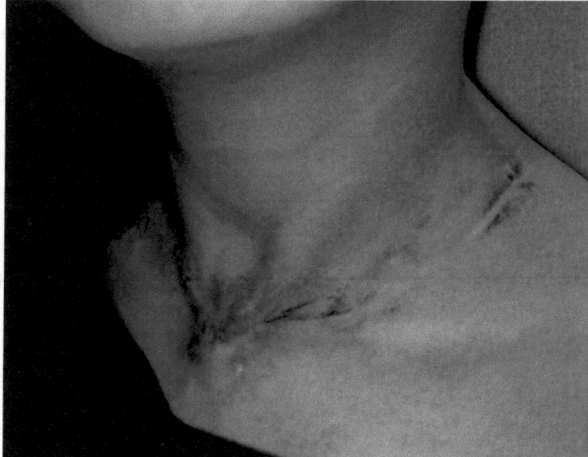

FIG. 2: Multiple scar formation, a complication of cervical lymph node tuberculosis. *(For color version, see Plate 5)*

- Central softening-abscess
- Collar-stud formation
- Sinus tract formation

Human Immunodeficiency Virus and Tuberculous Lymphadenitis

Tuberculous lymphadenitis is the most common form of extrapulmonary TB in HIV-positive patients.[26] These patients are often older and males with involvement of multiple sites. Tender lymphadenopathy, fever, weight loss, and coexisting pulmonary TB are more common in HIV seropositive patients as compared to HIV seronegatives.[27]

Differential Diagnosis

Tuberculous lymphadenitis needs to be differentiated from lymphadenopathy due to other causes. These include granulomatous lymphadenopathy like NTM, sarcoidosis, lymphoma, berylliosis, tularemia lymphadenitis, cat-scratch lymphadenitis, Yersinia lymphadenitis, lymphogranuloma venereum, fungal infection, toxoplasma lymphadenitis (Piringer-Kuchinka lymphadenopathy), leprosy, syphilis, and brucellosis.[28-30] In general, multiplicity, matting, and caseation of the LNs are features of tuberculous lymphadenitis but these are neither specific nor sensitive enough to be pathognomonic.

DIAGNOSIS

The diagnostic modalities can be divided into primary diagnostic studies and ancillary diagnostic studies.[30]

Primary Diagnostic Studies

Fine Needle Aspiration Cytology

Fine needle aspiration cytology (FNAC) is safe, quick, easily available, relatively less invasive, practical, and fairly reliable test for the diagnosis of peripheral LNTB.[30] It has emerged as a first-line diagnostic technique, especially in TB-endemic countries.[30-32] Caseating granuloma with acid-fast bacilli (AFB) positivity is fairly sensitive and specific for the diagnosis of TB. Although, caseating granuloma alone may not be very specific because caseation can mimic necrosis and needs to be differentiated by special stains for collagen and reticulin.[32] Caseation has presence of reticulin whereas necrosis does not. This necrosis which can mimic "caseation" along with granuloma can be seen in many diseases like lymphoma, sarcoidosis. On the contrary, positive AFB stain result has excellent specificity for *M. tuberculosis* in adults since AFB positivity can only be due to tuberculous or NTM, and NTM usually affects children.[30] Apart from the Ziehl-Neelsen stain, fluorescence microscopy using light-emitting diodes can also be used as inexpensive yet robust method of AFB smear analysis of FNAC specimens.[33] Overall, the diagnostic accuracy of LN FNAC ranges from 71.3 to 97%.[34-42] Histologic features, such as nonspecific lymphoid infiltrates, noncaseating granulomas, or Langhans giant cells in areas of extensive caseous necrosis, support a diagnosis of probable TB.[30]

Lymph Node Biopsy

The open biopsies with tissue culture are accepted as the gold standard to diagnose TB lymphadenitis.[30,43] However, excisional biopsy is the most invasive approach to diagnosis. It has the highest sensitivity and has been recommended in cases involving multiple nodes, when the diagnosis is doubtful on FNAC or when drug resistance is suspected.[30,44] The surgical biopsy specimen should be collected both in saline and formalin separately. If care is not taken to send the sample separately into saline, culture would be negative and sensitivity report will be missed. Complications of biopsy include postsurgical pain, wound infection, sinus formation, and scar.[30]

Culture

Isolation of mycobacteria by culture still represents the cornerstone on which the definitive diagnosis is based. The culture can be performed with both FNAC and biopsy material. It has been shown that when combined with microscopy and culture, the diagnostic accuracy of FNAC improves significantly.[45] Although culture can be performed with aspirated specimen, the positive rates are at times significantly lower in aspirated specimen as compared to biopsy specimen (17% vs. 80% respectively in a study from Hong Kong).[46] Although, culture establishes the diagnosis most definitively, the time consumed to grow mycobacteria makes it unsuitable for routine use. Hence, a few modern rapid methods have been developed.[1] These include microcolony detection on solid media, Septi-Check AFB method, microscopic observation of broth culture, the BACTEC 460 radiometric system, BACTEC MGIT 960 system, MB/BacT system, and ESP II culture system.[1,47]

Molecular Tests

Molecular diagnosis or nucleic acid amplification (NAA) to detect mycobacterial deoxyribonucleic acid (DNA) instead of detection of mycobacteria by traditional microbiological methods holds a promise in the diagnosis of TB. This is because they have higher sensitivity, are quicker, and allow identification of the species and drug resistance earlier compared to conventional methods.[1] They have been available for diagnosis of pulmonary TB since the 1990s. Gen-Probe test was the first NAA test to get the United States Food and Drug Administration approval for detection of pulmonary TB. Many other tests have been subsequently approved. Early molecular methods were polymerase chain reaction (PCR) designed to detect the *M. tuberculosis* complex only. Subsequently, line probe assays (LPAs) have been developed which combine NAA with hybridization. These can even detect drug resistance.[48] Guidelines for the use of NAA tests for the diagnosis of TB were published in 1996 and updated in 2000 and 2009.[49,50] Since then, NAA testing has become a routine procedure in many settings. The role of molecular tests or NAA in the diagnosis of LNTB is being discussed under following subtitles:
- Amplified molecular tests for detecting *M. tuberculosis*
- Test for detecting drug resistance to *M. tuberculosis*.

Amplified molecular tests for detecting *M. tuberculosis*: These are PCR-based fast and useful techniques for the demonstration of mycobacterial DNA fragments in patients with clinically suspected mycobacterial lymphadenitis. The most common target used in PCR is IS6110. Although tissue PCR is a less time-consuming test (1 week) compared to the culture technique (MGIT about 3 weeks), PCR cannot give information about susceptibility to antimicrobial agents.[6] A systematic review of NAA using PCR technique in tuberculous lymphadenitis revealed highly variable and inconsistent results (sensitivity, 2–100%; specificity, 28–100%), with more favorable performance from commercial assays and with sample sizes of more than 0.20 uL. The systemic review had included commercial PCR probes and in-house PCR tests and possibly because of in-house PCR, the specificity was variable.[49] Overall, PCR with biopsy specimen has much higher sensitivity and specificity compared to FNAC.[51] Real-time PCR assay for detecting the 16S ribosomal ribonucleic acid gene of *M. tuberculosis* also shows results similar to non-real-time PCR both with FNAC and biopsy specimens. For biopsy specimens, the sensitivity of real-time PCR in one of the reported studies is 63.4%, and the specificity is 96.9%. For FNAC specimens, the sensitivity was 17.1%, and the specificity was 100% in the same study.[52] If FNAC samples are processed by combining microbiological (rapid culture) and molecular technique (PCR), the sensitivity and specificity improve significantly, and biopsy can be avoided for confirmatory diagnosis of tuberculous lymphadenitis.[43]

Test for detecting drug resistance to *M. tuberculosis*:[53] Advances in molecular technique beyond PCR allow simultaneous detection of *M. tuberculosis* DNA and drug-resistant gene. They can be performed on cultured TB isolates or directly on pretreated primary

specimens. Some assays (Cepheid Xpert and INNOLIPA) have been designed to detect TB and resistance to rifampicin only, while others (GenoType MTBDRplus) are able to detect both isoniazid and rifampicin-resistance in primary specimens and cultures. Cepheid GeneXpert® MTB/RIF assay 4th edition has been developed using semiquantitative nested real-time PCR technique with facility of automated sample processing, and real-time-based molecular beacon assay. The commercially available INNO-LiPA Rif.TB kit is also an LPA, which is able to identify the *M. tuberculosis* complex and simultaneously detect genetic mutations in the region of the *rpoB* gene associated with rifampicin resistance. The GenoType MTBDRplus is LPA and includes three steps:
1. DNA extraction
2. Multiplex PCR amplification
3. Reverse hybridization.

The Cepheid GeneXpert®, INNO-LiPA Rif.TB, and GenoType MTBDRplus system have all been approved for TB detection in sputum by regulatory agencies.[54-56] Though all have not been approved for use in extrapulmonary TB, in 2013 the World Health Organization (WHO) endorsed the use Cepheid GeneXpert® for diagnosis of extrapulmonary TB.[57,58] There are multiple studies to assess the utility. A meta-analysis of FNAC samples for Cepheid GeneXpert® has shown a sensitivity of 50–100% with pooled sensitivity of 83.1% (95% CI 71.4–90.7%) and pooled specificity of 93.6% (95% CI 87.9–96.8%).[59] The pooled sensitivity for INNOLIPA for extrapulmonary sample is somewhat lower at 63–68%.[53] For the GenoType MTBDRplus assay, only one study analyzed the sensitivity of TB identification and found a sensitivity of 91% (n = 10).[60] Thus, molecular diagnosis especially for Cepheid GeneXpert® system shows reasonable sensitivity and specificity. If, due to feasibility, they cannot be used for rapid diagnosis of LNTB, they can definitely be very useful for rapid diagnosis of drug-resistant LNTB.

Ancillary Diagnostic Tests

Tuberculin Skin Test

Tuberculin skin test (Mantoux test) is useful to show delayed type hypersensitivity reactions against mycobacterial antigens. Positive reactions (>10 mm induration) can occur in *M. tuberculosis* infections. Intermediate reactions (5–9 mm induration) can occur after bacillus Calmette-Guérin (BCG) vaccination, *M. tuberculosis* infection, or NTM infections. Negative reactions (≤4 mm induration) represent a lack of tuberculin sensitization.[23] The sensitivity and specificity of tuberculin skin test are 86 and 67%, respectively.[61] Though, tuberculin test is not useful in distinguishing prior BCG or prior infections or latent infection versus active disease, it is useful as an ancillary diagnostic test. It helps in differentiating tuberculous lymphadenitis from sarcoidosis and lymphoma because of anergy. Since there are no specific features on FNAC to differentiate the two conditions from TB with certainty, except a positive culture of *M. tuberculosis*,[62-64] tuberculin anergy is useful in distinguishing sarcoidosis and lymphoma from TB.[62-65]

Interferon-gamma Release Assays

The interferon-γ release assays (IGRAs) available are TB Gold and TB Platinum. They are useful for diagnosing latent TB infection like tuberculin testing, but unlike tuberculin test they can also be used to distinguish latent infection from BCG vaccination and NTM.[66,67] However, they cannot be used for the diagnosis of active TB. The Indian government banned serological antibody tests in 2012, and both the Standards for TB

Care in India and the International Standards for TB Care discourage the use of IGRAs for the diagnosis of active TB.[68,69]

Diagnosis of Mediastinal Lymphadenitis

Mediastinal lymphadenopathy commonly presents with fever and cough.[9] It may also present with one of the complications like compression of one of the bronchus leading to atelectasis (Fig. 3), lung infection, and bronchiectasis or thoracic duct leading to chylous effusion. Other intrathoracic complications include dysphagia, esophagomediastinal fistula, and tracheoesophageal fistula.[9] Lone mediastinal LN enlargement due to TB is a rare manifestation.[70] Hence, accompanying manifestations like lung involvement are useful for diagnosis. Contrast-enhanced computed tomography (CT) is a viable noninvasive cost-effective option for the diagnosis of tuberculous mediastinal LN. Peripheral enhancement (rim enhancement) or multilocular (a subtype of peripheral enhancement) appearance (Fig. 4) is useful in differentiating tuberculous mediastinal LN from other causes like lymphoma sarcoidosis.[71-73] Homogeneous enhancement or absence of "classical" finding needs further differentiation with positron emission tomography (PET) scan or endobronchial ultrasound (EBUS). Both PET scan and EBUS are not easily available and are expensive. Judicious application of PET is helpful for differentiating tuberculous LN from sarcoidosis in cases with homogeneously enhancing LN for detecting unsuspected sites and identifying potential site for tissue biopsy.[74] In the present era of evidence-based medicine, EBUS is a very useful tool for an accurate diagnosis of tuberculous mediastinal LN.[75,76] In a study by Sun et al. on EBUS-guided transbronchial needle aspiration for intrathoracic TB lymph node, the sensitivity was 85%, specificity was 100%, positive and negative predictive values were 100% and 75%, respectively, with the accuracy of 90%.[75] In a multicenter study of 156 patients, by Navani et al., EBUS-TBNA was diagnostic of TB in 146 patients (94%; 95% CI 88–97%).[77] Endobronchial ultrasound-TBNA has been shown to have high-negative predictive value and avoids use of more invasive mediastinoscopy for the diagnosis of mediastinal LN.[77]

TREATMENT

The Infectious Diseases Society of America and the WHO recommend 6 months of treatment for drug-susceptible disease, i.e., 2 months of isoniazid (H), rifampicin (R), pyrazinamide (Z), and ethambutol (E) in intensive phase followed by 4 months of rifampicin and isoniazid in continuation phase (2HRZE/2HR). In areas with high prevalence of isoniazid resistance, the WHO has recommended a regimen of 2HRZE/4HRE.[78,79] The 6-month recommendation is supported by studies that showed no difference between 6 months and 9 months of treatment in cure rates (89–94%)[80,81] or relapse rates (3%).[82] Human immunodeficiency virus testing is recommended as part of the evaluation of all TB patients and patients in whom the disease is suspected. Human immunodeficiency virus testing is especially important in persons with extrapulmonary tuberculosis because of the increased frequency of extrapulmonary involvement in persons with immunosuppression. Daily dosing is strongly recommended during the intensive phase for TB patients with known positive HIV status.[79]

Paradoxical Reaction

A PR in a patient infected with TB is defined as the clinical (Fig. 5) and/or radiological worsening (Fig. 6) of preexisting tuberculous lesions or the development of new lesions

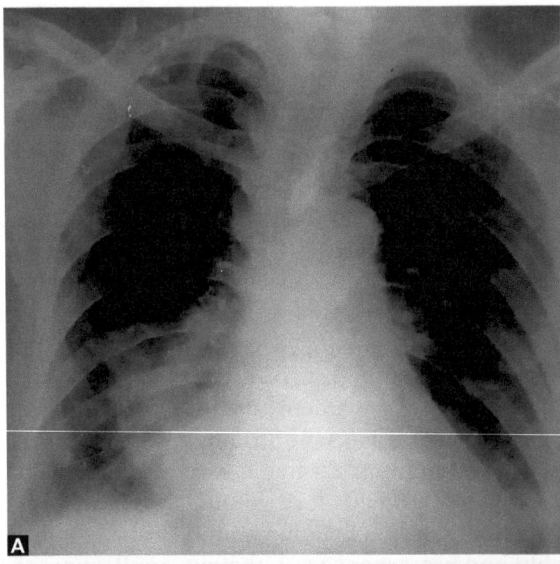
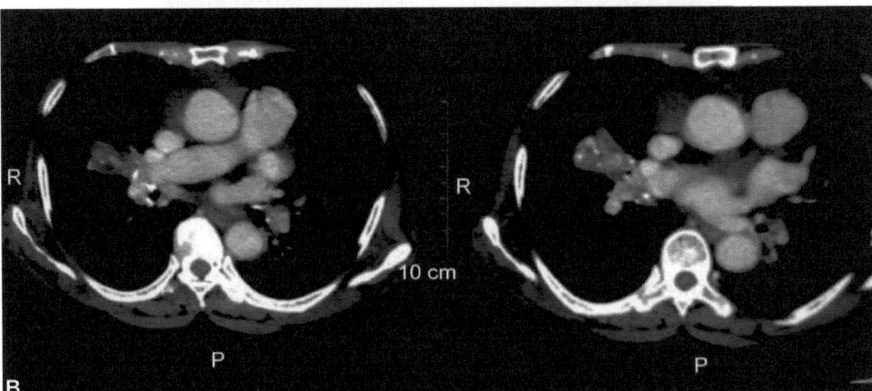
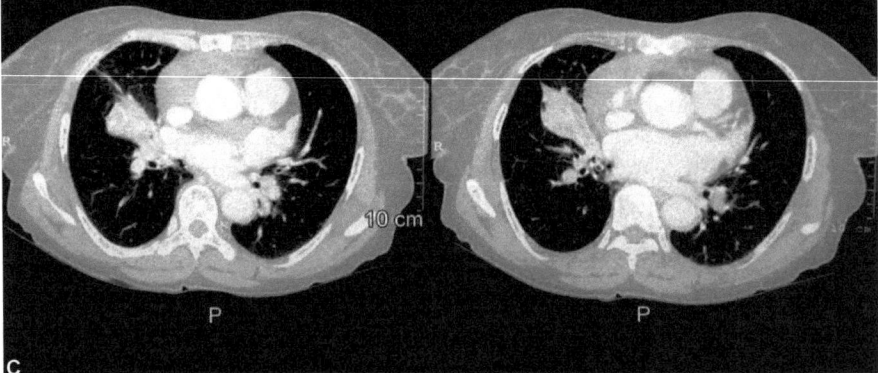

FIG. 3: A, Chest radiograph showing collapse of right middle lobe; **B,** Computed tomography (CT) chest in mediastinal widow axial cut showing mediastinal lymph node with calcification causing obstruction of middle lobe bronchus; **C,** CT chest lung window showing collapse of right middle lobe (Brock syndrome).

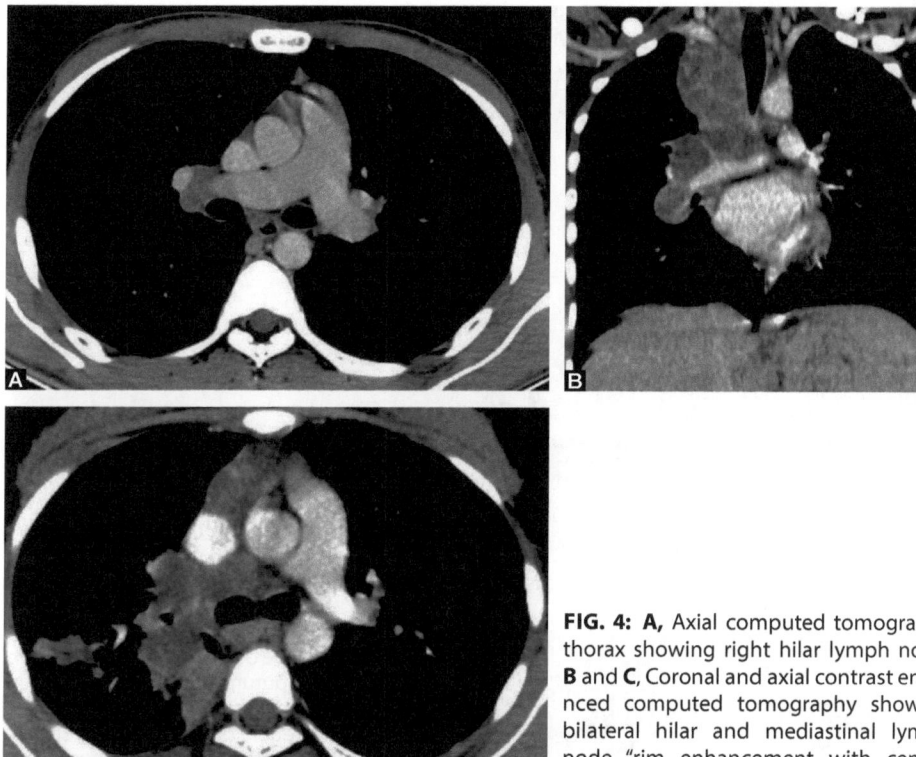

FIG. 4: A, Axial computed tomography thorax showing right hilar lymph node; **B** and **C,** Coronal and axial contrast enhanced computed tomography showing bilateral hilar and mediastinal lymph node "rim enhancement with central caseation" suggestive of tuberculosis.

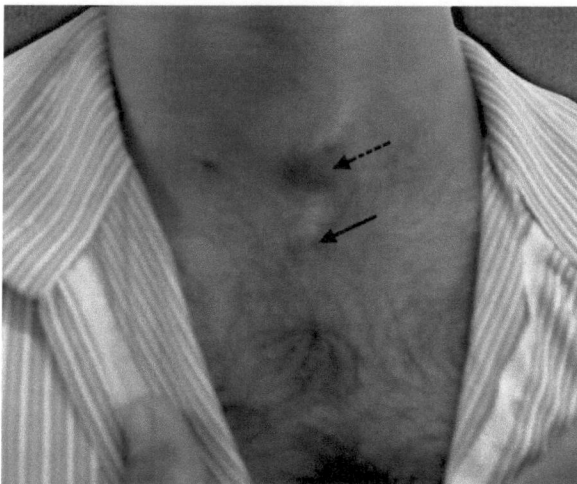

FIG. 5: A 36-year-old man with paradoxical reaction. The solid arrow shows suprasternal lymph node for which he was started on antituberculosis treatment based on cytology showing acid-fast bacilli (AFB). Two months later another lymph node shown by dotted arrow appeared. The culture for AFB was negative confirming paradoxical reaction. *(For color version, see Plate 5)*

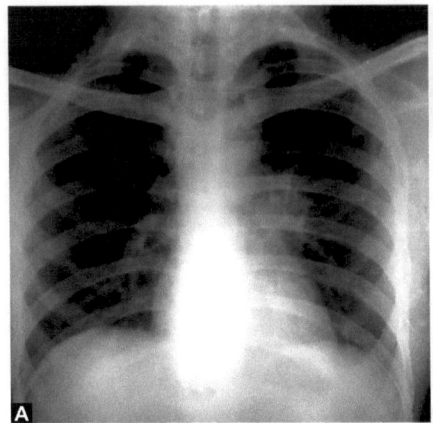
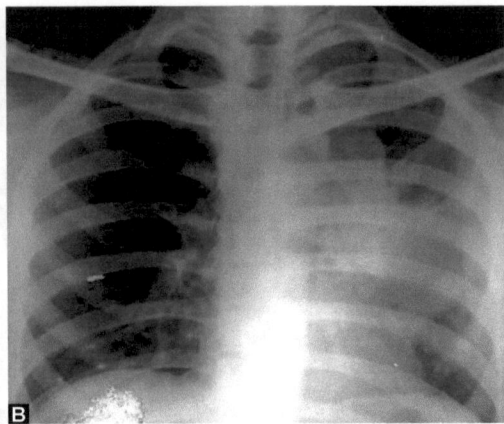
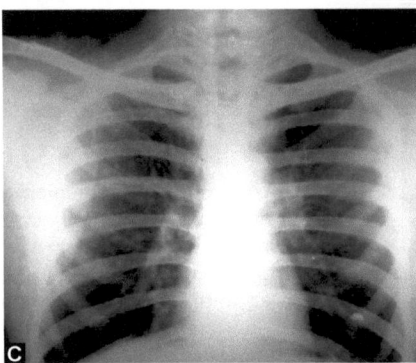

FIG. 6: A, Chest radiograph showing left hilar and paratracheal lymphadenopathy in a patient with cervical lymph node. The diagnosis of tuberculosis was proven on cervical lymph node fine needle aspiration cytology (FNAC); **B,** Two months after starting treatment, the patient had clinically improved but the chest radiograph showed paradoxical worsening. The chest radiograph shows collapse of left upper lobe due to enlargement of left hilar lymph node. The sputum and lymph node acid-fast bacilli (AFB) culture was negative; **C,** The chest radiograph on completion of treatment. It shows significant regression of hilar enlargement compared to Figure 6A when the treatment was initiated.

in a patient who initially improves with antituberculosis therapy (ATT).[83] Most reported cases are of TB lymph node or central nervous system.[84] It occurs in about 10–15% of immunocompetent[84] and 22–60% with HIV-positive patients treated for tuberculous lyphadenitis.[85,86] The median time to development of a PR in HIV-negative patients is 60 days (14–270 days).[87] In HIV-positive patients, 90% of cases occur within 3 months after starting antiretroviral therapy (ART).[88]

The exact mechanism of PR remains uncertain. Immune reconstitution phenomenon has been suggested as a possible explanation. In HIV-positive patients, a paradoxical response may occur during reversal of the immunosuppressive state when highly active antiretroviral therapy (HAART) is coadministered within 2 months of anti-TB treatment. This phenomenon appears more frequently in those patients with a significant reduction in HIV viral load and an increase in CD4 lymphocyte count after HAART.[89] Management primarily consists of differentiating PR from treatment failure, drug resistance or another infection. Fine needle aspiration culture or biopsy culture is useful in differentiating PR from drug resistance if definitive diagnosis was made at the time of initial evaluation. The use of aspiration has been reported to be a successful therapeutic intervention for suppurative tuberculous lymphadenitis.[90] Otherwise, reassurance is the single most important intervention required for the management of PR. Steroids have been considered as a means to reduce the robust immune response in PR in general, but their use is controversial in LNTB.[76] Some authors report benefit,[91,92] but retrospective studies have shown that steroids do not prevent PR if steroids have been given since the beginning of treatment.[93] Also, steroids do not have any effect on the duration of PR.[94,95]

Nontuberculous Lymph Node Tuberculosis

The most important alternative diagnosis of tuberculous lymphadenitis is NTM lymphadenitis.[96] If culture is not performed on LN, it is not possible to diagnose nontuberculous LN. The presumptive diagnosis of NTM lymphadenitis is based on the histopathologic appearance of the LN showing caseating granulomata with or without AFB and, in the majority of cases, a negative tuberculin skin test. In the United States, only about 10% of the culture-proven mycobacterial cervical lymphadenitis in children has been reported to be due to *M. tuberculosis*.[97] In contrast, in adults, more than 90% of the culture-proven mycobacterial lymphadenitis is due to *M. tuberculosis*.[98] There are no formal studies done on prevalence of NTM from India. In absence of formal studies, it is important to note that patients with nonresolving, suspected resistant lymphadenitis, diagnosis of NTM should be considered. The guiding principle for most localized NTM lymphadenitis that occurs in immunocompetent patients, due to any NTM species, is complete surgical excision of the involved LNs.[96]

Surgical Management

The indications for surgical management of TB lymphadenitis are:[30]
- Treatment failure: Surgical treatment is beneficial to establish the diagnosis and management of drug-resistant organisms
- Adjuvant treatment for drug-sensitive cases: For patients who have discomfort from tense, fluctuant LN surgical treatment is beneficial
- Paradoxical reaction: In a retrospective review, aspiration, incision and drainage, or excision were associated with a trend toward a shorter duration of PR[95]
- Nontuberculous mycobacteria: In children with NTM, LN removal has been associated with better outcomes.

Problems in the Management of TB Lymphadenitis

- Appearance of new nodes/enlargement of existing nodes:[26] Appearance of new nodes is due to PR, drug resistance, erroneous diagnosis, or disease caused by NTM. Most nodes that enlarge during therapy are due to PR. These ultimately respond to treatment. However, it is important to assess the patients for drug resistance if the history of irregularity in treatment is suspected or assess for revision of diagnosis if microbiological diagnosis was not performed during initial evaluation. Biopsy of LN with molecular/microbiological investigation may be required for the final confirmation
- Development of fluctuation: Appearance of fluctuation in one or more LNs calls for aspiration under all aseptic precautions[26]
- Appearance of sinus tracts: Any worsening after 8 weeks of therapy calls for en block resection of the involved LN chain to avoid appearance of ugly sinus tracts[26]
- Residual LNs after completion of treatment: At the end of therapy, about 10% of cases may be left with residual nodes.[99] Biopsy from these residual nodes often shows caseating granuloma but culture would be negative. Presence of residual LN after ATT does not merit continuation of treatment unless the microbiological evidence (culture) supports persistence of viable organisms

- Relapse: Relapse rates of up to 3.5% have been reported in patients treated for tuberculous lymphadenitis.[83] This should be treated with the same drugs but culture or molecular diagnostic test must be performed to rule out resistance or NTM disease
- Drug resistance: Though it is at times difficult to confirm drug-resistance in LNTB, it is essential to demonstrate drug resistance prior to starting multidrug-resistant regimen. Similarly, single agent (fluoroquinolones or others) should never be introduced even if response to treatment is not appropriate. Each case should be reasonably investigated with culture or molecular diagnostic tools. Also, appropriate measures should be taken to prevent the use of second-line drugs in unproven cases.

CLINICAL PEARLS

- Lymph node enlargement due to TB is frequently seen in young population
- One must look for other concurrent TB foci in the body, e.g., in a patient with cervical lymphadenopathy, chest radiograph, and ultrasound abdomen/pelvis are important for providing information regarding the other disease sites. This is also helps in monitoring other foci also
- Microbiological and molecular tests provide diagnostic certainty and confidence of response if a sensitive strain is identified
- If abscess formation occurs, it should be either aspirated to dryness (each time it recurs) or excised surgically. Otherwise, scar and sinus often cause cosmetic disfigurement. Steroid should not be used if abscess formation has occurred
- As a personal observation of authors if multifocal or late paradoxical responses occurs without demonstration of drug resistance addition of injection of streptomycin in the regimen is often helpful
- For mediastinal LN, CT scan should not be used as routine follow-up tool. Computed tomography scan should be reserved for initial and final assessment as radiation exposure risk is significant. Chest radiograph remains a useful tool. A good magnetic resonance imaging may also help in a particular case especially if abdominal gland has been involved.

REFERENCES

1. Handa U, Mundi I, Mohan S. Nodal tuberculosis revisited: a review. J Infect Dev Ctries. 2012;6:6-12.
2. World Health Organization. Global tuberculosis control: surveillance, planning, financing. Geneva: WHO; 2008.
3. Beyene D, Bergval I, Hailu E, et al. Identification and genotyping of the etiological agent of tuberculous lymphadenitis in Ethiopia. J Infect Dev Ctries. 2009;3:412-9.
4. Mathema B, Kurepina NE, Bifani PJ, Kreiswirth BN. Molecular epidemiology of tuberculosis: current insights. Clin Microbiol Rev. 2006;19:658-85.
5. Artenstein AW, Kim JH, Williams WJ, Chung RC. Isolated peripheral tuberculous lymphadenitis in adults: current clinical and diagnostic issues. Clin Infect Dis. 1995;20:876-82.
6. Peto HM, Pratt RH, Harrington TA, LoBue PA, Armstrong LR. Epidemiology of extrapulmonary tuberculosis in the United States, 1993-2006. Clin Infect Dis. 2009;49:1350-7.
7. Dandapat MC, Mishra BM, Dash SP, Kar PK. Peripheral lymph node tuberculosis: a review of 80 cases. Br J Surg. 1990;77:911-2.
8. Gothi D, Joshi JM. Clinical and laboratory observations of tuberculosis at a Mumbai (India) clinic. Postgrad Med J. 2004;80:97-100.
9. Sharma SK, Mohan A. Extrapulmonary tuberculosis. Indian J Med Res. 2004;120:316-53.
10. Aaron L, Saadoun D, Calatroni I, Launay O, Mémain N, Vincent V, et al. Tuberculosis in HIV-infected patients: a comprehensive review. Clin Microbiol Infect. 2004;10:388-98.

11. Aguado JM, Castrillo JM. Lymphadenitis as a characteristic manifestation of disseminated tuberculosis in intravenous drug abusers infected with human immunodeficiency virus. J Infect. 1987;14:191-3.
12. Finfer M, Perchick A, Burstein DE. Fine needle aspiration biopsy diagnosis of tuberculous lymphadenitis in patients with and without the acquired immune deficiency syndrome. Acta Cytol. 1991;35:325-32.
13. Thompson MM, Underwood MJ, Sayers RD, Dookeran KA, Bell PR. Peripheral tuberculous lymphadenopathy: a review of 67 cases. Br J Surg. 1992;79:763-4.
14. Geldmacher H, Taube C, Kroeger C, Magnussen H, Kirsten DK. Assessment of lymph node tuberculosis in northern Germany: a clinical review. Chest. 2002;121:1177-82.
15. Kent DC. Tuberculous lymphadenitis: not a localized disease process. Am J Med Sci. 1967;254:866-74.
16. Chavollo R, Dolci GF, Hernandez JF, et al. Primary tuberculosis of tonsil. Int J Pediatr Otorhinolaryngol Extra. 2006;1:150-3.
17. Belizna C, Kerleau JM, Heron F, Lévesque H. Tonsillar and lymph node tuberculosis revealing asymptomatic pulmonary tuberculosis. QJM. 2007;100:800-1.
18. Kanlikama M, Mumbuc S, Bayazit Y, Sirikci A. Management strategy of mycobacterial cervical lymphadenitis. J Laryngol Otol. 2000;114:274-8.
19. Brizi MG, Celi G, Scaldazza AV, Barbaro B. Diagnostic imaging of abdominal tuberculosis: gastrointestinal tract, peritoneum, lymph nodes. Rays. 1998;23:115-25.
20. Penfold CN, Revington PJ. A review of 23 patients with tuberculosis of the head and neck. Br J Oral Maxillofac Surg. 1996;34:508-10.
21. Kvaerner KJ, Kvestad E, Orth M. Surgery required to verify atypical mycobacterial infections. Int J Pediatr Otorhinolaryngol. 2001;61:121-8.
22. Lee KC, Tami TA, Lalwani AK, Schecter G. Contemporary management of cervical tuberculosis. Laryngoscope. 1992;102:60-4.
23. Mohapatra PR, Janmeja AK. Tuberculous lymphadenitis. J Assoc Physicians India. 2009;57:585-90.
24. Konishi K, Yamane H, Iguchi H, et al. Study of tuberculosis in the field of otorhinolaryngology in the past 10 years. Acta Otolaryngol Suppl. 1998;538:244-9.
25. Jones PG, Campbell PE. Tuberculous lymphadenitis in childhood: the significance of anonymous mycobacteria. Br J Surg. 1962;50:302-14.
26. Gupta PR. Difficulties in managing lymph node tuberculosis. Lung India. 2004;21:50-3.
27. Bem C. Human immunodeficiency virus-positive tuberculosis lymphadenitis in Central Africa: clinical presentation of 157 cases. Int J Tuberc Lung Dis. 1997;1:215-9.
28. Asano S. Granulomatous lymphadenitis. J Clin Exp Hematop. 2012;52:1-16.
29. Al-Maghrabi JA, Sawan AS, Kanaan HD. Hodgkin's lymphoma with exuberant granulomatous reaction. Saudi Med J. 2006;27:1905-7.
30. Fontanilla JM, Barnes A, von Reyn CF. Current diagnosis and management of peripheral tuberculous lymphadenitis. Clin Infect Dis. 2011;53(6):555-62.
31. Ellison E, Lapuerta P, Martin SE. Fine needle aspiration diagnosis of mycobacterial lymphadenitis. Sensitivity and predictive value in the United States. Acta Cytol. 1999;43:153-7.
32. Wright CA, van der Burg M, Geiger D, Noordzij JG, Burgess SM, Marais BJ. Diagnosing mycobacterial lymphadenitis in children using fine needle aspiration biopsy: cytomorphology, ZN staining and autofluorescence—making more or less. Diagn Cytopathol. 2008;36:245-51.
33. van Wyk AC, Marais BJ, Warren RM, van Wyk SS, Wright CA. The use of light-emitting diode fluorescence to diagnose mycobacterial lymphadenitis in fine-needle aspirates from children. Int J Tuberc Lung Dis. 2011;15(1):56-60.
34. Goel MM, Ranjan V, Dhole TN, et al. Polymerase chain reaction vs. conventional diagnosis in fine needle aspirates of tuberculous lymph nodes. Acta Cytol. 2001;45:333-40.
35. Chao SS, Loh KS, Tan KK, Chong SM. Tuberculous and nontuberculous cervical lymphadenitis: a clinical review. Otolaryngol Head Neck Surg. 2002;126:176-9.
36. Gupta AK, Nayar M, Chandra M. Reliability and limitations of fine needle aspiration cytology of lymphadenopathies. An analysis of 1,261 cases. Acta Cytol. 1991;35:777-83.
37. Gupta AK, Nayar M, Chandra M. Critical appraisal of fine needle aspiration cytology in tuberculous lymphadenitis. Acta Cytol. 1992;36:391-4.
38. Das DK, Pant JN, Chachra KL, et al. Tuberculous lymphadenitis: correlation of cellular components and necrosis in lymph node aspirate with A.F.B. positivity and bacillary count. Indian J Pathol Microbiol. 1990;33:1-10.

39. Kumar N, Tiwari MC, Verma K. AFB staining in cytodiagnosis of tuberculosis without classical features: a comparison of Ziehl-Neelsen and fluorescent methods. Cytopathology. 1998;9:208-14.
40. Pandit AA, Khilnani PH, Prayag AS. Tuberculous lymphadenitis: extended cytomorphologic features. Diagn Cytopathol. 1995;12:23-7.
41. Clarridge JE, Shawar RM, Shinnick TM, Plikaytis BB. Large-scale use of polymerase chain reaction for detection of Mycobacterium tuberculosis in a routine mycobacteriology laboratory. J Clin Microbiol. 1993;31:2049-56.
42. Goel MM, Budhwar P, Jain A. Immunocytochemistry versus nucleic acid amplification in fine needle aspirates and tissues of extrapulmonary tuberculosis. J Cytol. 2012;29:157-64.
43. Supiyaphun P, Tumwasorn S, Udomsantisuk N, Keelawat S, Songsrisanga W, Prasurthsin P, et al. Diagnostic tests for tuberculous lymphadenitis: fine needle aspirations using tissue culture in mycobacteria growth indicator tube and tissue PCR. Asian Biomed. 2010;4:787-92.
44. Blaikley JF, Khalid S, Ormerod LP. Management of peripheral lymph node tuberculosis in routine practice: an unselected 10-year cohort. Int J Tuberc Lung Dis. 2011;15:375-8.
45. Gadre DV, Singh UR, Saxena K, Bhatia A, Talwar V. Diagnosis of tubercular cervical lymphadenitis by FNAC, microscopy and culture. Indian J Tuberc. 1991;38:25-7.
46. Lau SK, Wei WI, Hsu C, Engzell UC. Efficacy of fine needle aspiration cytology in the diagnosis of tuberculous cervical lymphadenopathy. J Laryngol Otol. 1990;104:24-7.
47. Indian Council of Medical Research. What is new in the diagnosis of tuberculosis? Part I: techniques for diagnosis of tuberculosis. ICMR Bulletin. 2002;32(8).
48. Bateson A, Reddington K, O'Grady J. Molecular diagnosis of active pulmonary tuberculosis. In: McHugh TD (Ed). Tuberculosis: Laboratory Diagnosis and Treatment Strategies (Advances in Molecular and Cellular Microbiology). Boston, USA: CABI; 2013.
49. Daley P, Thomas S, Pai M. Nucleic acid amplification tests for the diagnosis of tuberculous lymphadenitis: a systematic review. Int J Tuberc Lung Dis. 2007;11:1166-76.
50. Centers for Disease Control and Prevention (CDC). Updated guidelines for the use of nucleic acid amplification tests in the diagnosis of tuberculosis. MMWR Morb Mortal Wkly Rep. 2009;58:7-10.
51. Derese Y, Hailu E, Assefa T, et al. Comparison of PCR with standard culture of fine needle aspiration samples in the diagnosis of tuberculosis lymphadenitis. J Infect Dev Ctries. 2012;6:53-7.
52. Linasmita P, Srisangkaew S, Wongsuk T, Bhongmakapat T, Watcharananan SP. Evaluation of real-time polymerase chain reaction for detection of the 16S ribosomal RNA gene of Mycobacterium tuberculosis and the diagnosis of cervical tuberculous lymphadenitis in a country with a high tuberculosis incidence. Clin Infect Dis. 2012;55(3):313-21.
53. European Centre for Disease Prevention and Control. (2013). ERLN-TB expert opinion on the use of the rapid molecular assays for diagnosis of tuberculosis and detection of drug resistance. [online] Available from www.ecdc.europa.eu [Accessed January, 2016].
54. World Health Organization. Automated real-time nucleic acid amplification technology for rapid and simultaneous detection of tuberculosis and rifampicin resistance: Xpert MTB/RIF system, Geneva: WHO; 2011.
55. US Food and Drug Administration. (2013). Press release: FDA permits marketing of first U.S. test labeled for simultaneous detection of tuberculosis bacteria and resistance to the antibiotic rifampin. [online] Available from www.fda.gov/NewsEvents/Newsroom/PressAnnouncements/ucm362602.htm [Accessed January, 2016].
56. Weyer K, Mirzayev F, Migliori GB, et al. Rapid molecular TB diagnosis: evidence, policy making and global implementation of Xpert MTB/RIF. Eur Respir J. 2013;42:252-71.
57. World Health Organization. (2013). Policy update: automated real-time nucleic acid amplification technology for rapid and simultaneous detection of tuberculosis and rifampicin resistance: Xpert MTB/RIF system for the diagnosis of pulmonary and extrapulmonary TB in adults and children. [online] Available from http://apps.who.int/iris/bitstream/10665/112472/1/9789241506335_eng.pdf?ua=1 [Accessed January, 2016].
58. Pai M, Nathavitharana R. Extrapulmonary tuberculosis: new diagnostics and new policies. Indian J Chest Dis Allied Sci. 2014;56:71-3.
59. Denkinger CM, Schumacher SG, Boehme CC, Dendukuri N, Pai M, Steingart KR. Xpert MTB/RIF assay for the diagnosis of extrapulmonary tuberculosis: a systematic review and meta-analysis. Eur Respir J. 2014;44(2):435-46.
60. Neonakis IK, Gitti Z, Baritaki S, Petinaki E, Baritaki M, Spandidos DA. Evaluation of GenoType mycobacteria direct assay in comparison with Gen-Probe Mycobacterium tuberculosis amplified

direct test and GenoType MTBDRplus for direct detection of Mycobacterium tuberculosis complex in clinical samples. J Clin Microbiol. 2009;47:2601-3.
61. Song KH, Jeon JH, Park WB, et al. Usefulness of the whole-blood interferon-gamma release assay for diagnosis of extrapulmonary tuberculosis. Diagn Microbiol Infect Dis. 2009;63:182-7.
62. Zhao NA, Yang JJ, Zhang GS. Differential diagnosis between AML infiltration, lymphoma and tuberculosis in a patient presenting with fever and mediastinal lymphadenopathy: a case report. Oncol Lett. 2014;7:705-8.
63. Babu K. Sarcoidosis in tuberculosis-endemic regions: India. J Ophthalmic Inflamm Infect. 2013;3:53.
64. Xiong L, Mao X, Li C, Liu Z, Zhang Z. Posterior mediastinal tuberculous lymphadenitis with dysphagia as the main symptom: a case report and literature review. J Thorac Dis. 2013;5(5):E189-94.
65. Smith-Rohrberg D, Sharma SK. Tuberculin skin test among pulmonary sarcoidosis patients with and without tuberculosis: its utility for the screening of the two conditions in tuberculosis-endemic regions. Sarcoidosis Vasc Diffuse Lung Dis. 2006;23:130-4.
66. Metcalfe JZ, Everett CK, Steingart KR, et al. Interferon-gamma release assays for active pulmonary tuberculosis diagnosis in adults in low- and middle-income countries: systematic review and meta-analysis. J Infect Dis. 2011;204(suppl 4):S1120-9.
67. Fan L, Chen Z, Hao XH, Hu ZY, Xiao HP. Interferon-gamma release assays for the diagnosis of extrapulmonary tuberculosis: a systematic review and meta-analysis. FEMS Immunol Med Microbiol. 2012;65:456-66.
68. TB CARE I. (2014). International Standards for Tuberculosis Care. 3rd ed. [online] Available from www.istcweb.org [Accessed January, 2016].
69. World Health Organization (Country Office for India). (2014). Standards for TB Care in India. [online] Available from http://www.tbcindia.nic.in/pdfs/stci%20Bookfinal%20%20060514.pdf [Accessed January, 2016].
70. Kumar N, Gera C, Philip N. Isolated mediastinal tuberculosis: a rare entity. J Assoc Physicians India. 2013;61:202-3.
71. Chen J, Yang ZG, Shao H, Xiao JH, Deng W, Wen LY, et al. Differentiation of tuberculosis from lymphomas in neck lymph nodes with multidetector-row computed tomography. Int J Tuberc Lung Dis. 2012;16(12):1686-91.
72. Evison M, Crosbie PA, Morris J, Martin J, Barber PV, Booton R. A study of patients with isolated mediastinal and hilar lymphadenopathy undergoing EBUS-TBNA. BMJ Open Respir Res. 2014;1:e000040.
73. Jaiswal A, Khanna SP, Menon MP. Computed tomography features of tuberculous mediastinal lymphadenopathy. Indian J Tuberc. 1992;59:229.
74. Wong ML. PET/CT scans in sarcoidosis: a review. South African Respir J. 2014;20:7-16.
75. Vaidya PJ, Kate AH, Chhajed PN. Endobronchial ultrasound-guided transbronchial needle aspiration: the standard of care for evaluation of mediastinal and hilar lymphadenopathy. J Cancer Res Ther. 2013;9:549-51.
76. Sun J, Teng J, Yang H, et al. Endobronchial ultrasound-guided transbronchial needle aspiration in diagnosing intrathoracic tuberculosis. Ann Thorac Surg. 2013;96:2021-7.
77. Navani N, Molyneaux PL, Breen RA, et al. Utility of endobronchial ultrasound-guided transbronchial needle aspiration in patients with tuberculous intrathoracic lymphadenopathy: a multicentre study. Thorax. 2011;66:889-93.
78. American Thoracic Society; CDC; Infectious Diseases Society of America. Treatment of tuberculosis. MMWR Recomm Rep. 2003;52:1-77.
79. Treatment of tuberculosis: guidelines. 4th ed. Geneva: WHO; 2009 (WHO/HTM/TB/2009.420).
80. Campbell IA, Ormerod LP, Friend JA, Jenkins PA, Prescott RJ. Six months versus nine months chemotherapy for tuberculosis of lymph nodes: final results. Respir Med. 1993;87:621-3.
81. Yuen AP, Wong SH, Tam CM, Chan SL, Wei WI, Lau SK. Prospective randomized study of thrice weekly six-month and nine-month chemotherapy for cervical tuberculous lymphadenopathy. Otolaryngol Head Neck Surg. 1997;116:189-92.
82. van Loenhout-Rooyackers JH, Laheij RJ, Richter C, Verbeek AL. Shortening the duration of treatment for cervical tuberculous lymphadenitis. Eur Respir J. 2000;15:192-5.
83. Breen RA, Smith CJ, Bettinson H, et al. Paradoxical reactions during tuberculosis treatment in patients with and without HIV co-infection. Thorax. 2004;59:704-7.
84. Cheng VC. Paradoxical response during anti-tuberculosis therapy. Medical Bulletin. 2006;11:20-1.

85. Narita M, Ashkin D, Hollender ES, Pitchenik AE. Paradoxical worsening of tuberculosis following antiretroviral therapy in patients with AIDS. Am J Respir Crit Care Med. 1998;158:157-61.
86. Wendel KA, Alwood KS, Gachuhi R, Chaisson RE, Bishai WR, Sterling TR. Paradoxical worsening of tuberculosis in HIV-infected persons. Chest. 2001;120:193-7.
87. Cheng VC, Ho PL, Lee RA, et al. Clinical spectrum of paradoxical deterioration during antituberculosis therapy in non-HIV-infected patients. Eur J Clin Microbiol Infect Dis. 2002;21(11):803-9.
88. Breton G, Duval X, Estellat C, Poaletti X, Bonnet D, Mvondo Mvondo D, et al. Determinants of immune reconstitution inflammatory syndrome in HIV type 1-infected patients with tuberculosis after initiation of antiretroviral therapy. Clin Infect Dis. 2004;39:1709-12.
89. Navas E, Martin-Davila P, Moreno L, et al. Paradoxical reactions of tuberculosis in patients with the acquired immunodeficiency syndrome who are treated with highly active antiretroviral therapy. Arch Intern Med. 2002;162(1):97-9.
90. Meybeck A, Just N, Nyunga M, Bourahla M, Wallaert B. Needle aspiration in paradoxical hypertrophy of tuberculous lymphadenitis. Rev Mal Respir. 2003;20:973-7.
91. Garcia Vidal C, Garau J. Systemic steroid treatment of paradoxical upgrading reaction in patients with lymph node tuberculosis. Clin Infect Dis. 2005;41:915-6; author reply 916-7.
92. Park KH, Cho OH, Chong YP, et al. Post-therapy paradoxical response in immunocompetent patients with lymph node tuberculosis. J Infect. 2010;61:430-4.
93. Afghani B, Lieberman JM. Paradoxical enlargement or development of intracranial tuberculomas during therapy: case report and review. Clin Infect Dis. 1994;19:1092-9.
94. Cho OH, Park KH, Kim T, et al. Paradoxical responses in non-HIV-infected patients with peripheral lymph node tuberculosis. J Infect. 2009;59:56-61.
95. Hawkey CR, Yap T, Pereira J, et al. Characterization and management of paradoxical upgrading reactions in HIV-uninfected patients with lymph node tuberculosis. Clin Infect Dis. 2005;40:1368-71.
96. Griffith DE, Aksamit T, Brown-Elliott BA, et al. An official ATS/IDSA statement: diagnosis, treatment, and prevention of nontuberculous mycobacterial diseases. Am J Respir Crit Care Med. 2007;175:367-416.
97. Wolinsky E. Mycobacterial lymphadenitis in children: a prospective study of 105 nontuberculous cases with long-term follow-up. Clin Infect Dis. 1995;20:954-63.
98. Diagnosis and treatment of disease caused by nontuberculous mycobacteria. This official statement of the American Thoracic Society was approved by the Board of Directors, March 1997. Medical Section of the American Lung Association. Am J Respir Crit Care Med. 1997;156:S1-25.
99. Campbell IA. The treatment of superficial tuberculous lymphadenitis. Tubercle. 1990;71:1-3.

CHAPTER 6

Conventional and Interventional Bronchoscopy in Tuberculosis

Semra Bilaçeroğlu, Atul C Mehta

INTRODUCTION

Owing to increasing immigrations, foreign travels, and human immunodeficiency virus (HIV) epidemic, tuberculosis (TB) remains one of the deadliest communicable diseases in the world. In 2013, it was estimated that 9.0 million people developed TB, 1.5 million died from the disease, and 360,000 were HIV-positive. Consistent with the slow annual decline of TB, it is estimated that 37 million lives were saved between 2000 and 2013 by effective diagnosis and treatment. However, as most TB deaths are preventable, the death toll from this disease is still unacceptably high.

Detecting cases with active pulmonary TB is crucial in TB control since appropriate treatment makes these cases noninfectious and prevents transmission of the disease. The diagnosis of pulmonary TB is mainly based on examination of the sputum smear and sputum microscopy is highly specific, low-cost, and essential for the Directly Observed Treatment, Short Course (DOTS) strategy of the World Health Organization which aims at a case detection rate of at least 70%.[1,2]

However, sputum smears do not reveal acid-fast bacilli (AFB) in all patients with suspected pulmonary TB and "smear-negative, culture-positive" state is observed in 22–61%. Furthermore, mycobacterial cultures take 6–8 weeks to confirm the diagnosis. Even with the DOTS approach providing access to standardized microscopy, sputum smear-negative pulmonary TB is still a common problem particularly in children and patients immunosuppressed with HIV infection or acquired immunodeficiency syndrome (AIDS). Thus, various bronchoscopic and nonbronchoscopic methods (Box 1) have been used to confirm active TB in these patients with suspected sputum smear-negative pulmonary TB.[2-5]

BOX 1	Methods for microbiological and/or histopathological diagnosis of tuberculosis in cases with sputum smear negativity or inadequate sputum
<ul><li>Nonbronchoscopic methods<ul><li>Sputum induction using hypertonic saline</li><li>Gastric lavage</li><li>Image-guided transthoracic needle aspiration</li><li>Postbronchoscopy sputum</li><li>Serological and molecular blood tests</li></ul></li></ul>	<ul><li>Rigid bronchoscopy</li><li>Flexible bronchoscopy<ul><li>Bronchial aspirate/washings</li><li>Brushing</li><li>Bronchoalveolar lavage</li><li>Transbronchial needle aspiration</li><li>Endobronchial biopsy</li><li>Transbronchial biopsy</li></ul></li></ul>

SPUTUM SMEAR NEGATIVITY: IMPORTANCE AND CAUSES

The number of bacilli in the sputum is proportional to the microscopic results of the properly prepared and examined sputum smear. For 10,000 bacilli per milliliter of sputum, there will be 100 bacilli in the sputum smear and one AFB will be seen per 100 oil immersion fields. About 100 viable bacteria per milliliter of the sputum are required to have the conventional mycobacterial culture of the sputum-positive on Löwenstein-Jensen medium.[6] "Sputum smear negativity" can be mentioned only if this result is obtained from a qualified and accredited laboratory. In developing countries, inspite of the widespread availability and accessibility to quality microscopy, commercial laboratories with varying standards still provide sputum examination with varying quality. Poor quality of the sputum sample (submitting saliva as sputum), improper preparation, staining, or examination of the sputum smear can cause false-negative results.[7]

Tuberculosis patients with severe immunosuppression such as late stage HIV disease (CD4+ ≤200/mm^3) tend to be sputum smear-negative. Moreover, some TB patients do not produce adequate sputum and some others producing adequate sputum are also smear-negative for unknown reasons although sputum collection, processing, and examination are properly performed.[2]

As shown by deoxyribonucleic acid finger printing studies, in areas of low TB transmission smear-negative, culture-positive index patients are responsible for 17% of the transmissions.[8] In areas of high transmission, the risk of infectivity of smear-negative TB particularly to young household is higher.[9] More than half of smear-negative patients will need chemotherapy by 12 months if not treated.[10] The mortality for smear-negative, culture-positive cases is 14.1% versus 34.7% in smear-positive patients at 18 months of follow-up.[11] Furthermore, treating smear-negative patients empirically with anti-TB therapy cannot be defended given the potential side effects of these drugs. As can be seen from the above data, early diagnosis of active smear-negative TB is crucial for the optimal management of the disease.

BRONCHOSCOPY

Bronchoscopic methods have been used solely or in combination to diagnose smear-negative TB (Box 1). Flexible bronchoscopy (FB) has been more frequently used to confirm the diagnosis of sputum smear-negative pulmonary TB whereas rigid bronchoscopy was used in the earlier days for preoperative evaluation and to check the results of drug therapy.[12-14]

Conventional Bronchoscopy

Among the patients suspicious for TB, diagnostic bronchoscopy is indicated in those with at least 2-3 AFB-negative sputum samples or who cannot expectorate sputum.[15,16] In those who cannot expectorate sputum, diagnostic yield of induced sputum (39-96%) has been found to be lower than that of FB (52-96%). Even the combination of three induced sputum and three gastric lavage samples can be diagnostic in only 43% of the cases.[17-20]

Clinical characteristics of those diagnosed by bronchoscopy are quite different than those diagnosed by sputum examination. Higher percentage of females and bedridden patients, absence of symptoms, atypical radiology (e.g., lower zone involvement, tuberculoma), shorter duration up to diagnosis, less nosocomial TB infection,[21] and higher yield for TB in malignancy (3-8%) are more frequently seen in bronchoscopically diagnosed TB patients.[18,22]

In nonendemic regions, routine mycobacterial examination of bronchoscopic specimens is unnecessary because of the low yield (0.8-2.9%). However, in moderately or highly endemic regions, it is necessary since the yield is higher (3.7-6.4%).[18,23-25] Inexperience of the bronchoscopist, using high-dose lidocaine (≥2 mL of 2% lidocaine) and low amount of bronchoalveolar lavage (BAL) fluid (<40 mL) decreases the diagnostic yield of bronchoscopy for TB. Wide ranges in diagnostic yields of bronchoscopy in TB can be ascribed to different geographic regions, prevalance of the disease, diagnostic methods, drugs used, and study design.[18,25,26]

Total yield of bronchoscopy in thoracic TB is 77% (11-96%). It can be exclusively diagnostic in 16-52% of the cases and can provide immediate diagnosis with microbiological smears and histological samples in 48% (9-79%). Cultures of bronchoscopic specimens, positive in 44-95% and exclusively positive in 20-47%, are more sensitive than cultures of prebronchoscopy sputum specimens (Table 1). In general, diagnostic yield of bronchoscopy is comparable in HIV-positive and HIV-negative cases with thoracic TB.[18,25-28] Through combination of histological specimens obtained by transbronchial biopsy (TBB) or endobronchial biopsy (EBB) and cultures of other bronchoscopic specimens, bronchoscopy can also be diagnostic in 47-95% of the cases with non-TB mycobacterial infections, particularly with *Mycobacterium avium-intracellulare*.[15-18,20,28]

Bronchoalveolar Lavage

Bronchoalveolar lavage smears and cultures provide a total diagnostic yield of 65% (34-93%) in pulmonary TB. Bronchoalveolar lavage is the sole and immediate means of diagnosis in 4-40% and 10-46%, respectively (Table 1). If enough lavage fluid is used and local anesthetics (e.g., lidocaine, tetracaine) that inhibit mycobacterial growth are limited or avoided before the procedure, BAL provides higher diagnostic yield than all other bronchoscopic methods. Mycobacterial cultures of BAL provide higher diagnostic yield than those of brushing or gastric lavage.[2,17-19,27]

Bronchial Lavage/Aspiration

The combined diagnostic yield of smears and cultures of bronchial lavage/aspiration specimens is 40% (19-95%) and higher than that of brushing. Cultures of bronchial aspirate can provide diagnosis exclusively in 4-47%. Immediate diagnosis can be obtained by smears in 4-30% (Table 1).[2,16,23,24]

Bronchial Brushing

In general, smears and cultures of brushing have low yields (0-73%) in pulmonary TB. Yield from brushing is usually lower than that of BAL or bronchial lavage/aspiration. Its additional contribution to the yields of other bronchoscopic methods is also not significant (0-10%). However, in endobronchial TB, brushing can be highly diagnostic (67-84%). Particularly, cultures from brushing are positive in 67-95% and can be the only means of diagnosis in 40-53% of these cases (Table 1).[2,18,29-31]

Transbronchial Needle Aspiration

In mediastinal TB lymphadenitis, 19-gauge transbronchial needle aspiration (TBNA), providing diagnosis in 85% (45-100%) of the cases, obviates mediastinoscopy or thoracotomy which are more invasive and costly. It is solely diagnostic in 68% (40-80%). Transbronchial needle aspiration; specimens can provide diagnosis by histology (65%), culture (60%), and smear (48%). Early diagnosis can be obtained by smears and histology in 78% (Table 1).[32-34]

TABLE 1	Diagnostic yields of bronchoscopic methods and pre- and postbronchoscopic sputum in sputum smear-negative thoracic tuberculosis						
Method	Overall	Exclusive	Immediate	Pathological	Smear	Culture
TBB	57–79%	12–20%	48%	68%	2%	2%
EBB	30–53%	<20%	<20%	–	very low	<20%
Brushing	0–73%	0–10%	–	–	–	–
TBNA	85% 45–100%	68% 40–80%	78%	65%	48%	60%
EBUS-TBNA	80–86%	53%	–	–	8–27%	8–47%
BAL	65% 34–93%	4–40%	10–46%	–	–	–
Bronchial lavage	40% 19–95%	4–47%	4–30%	–	–	–
PCR (BAL/EBUS-TBNA)	36–97%	–	59–91% PCR+TBB	–	–	–
Bronchoscopy (total)	77% 11–96%	16–52%	48% 9–79%	–	–	44–95%
Induced prebronchoscopic sputum	43% 39–96%	–	–	–	–	–
Postbronchoscopic sputum	–	Smear: 2–4% Culture: 0–10%	–	–	28% 6–76%	40% 4–79%

TBB, transbronchial biopsy; EBB, endobronchial biopsy; TBNA, transbronchial needle aspiration; EBUS-TBNA, endobronchial ultrasound-guided transbronchial needle aspiration; BAL, bronchoalveolar lavage; PCR, polymerase chain reaction.

Bronchial/Endobronchial Biopsy

The overall diagnostic yield of this method is 30–53% (Table 1). It can be immediately or exclusively diagnostic in less than 20%. Particularly in endobronchial TB, the yield is higher (40–84%). In endobronchial TB, AFB should also be sought for in the biopsy specimen during histological examination; however, the yield is low. Yield from the cultures of EBB specimen is less than 20%.[2,18,26,31]

Transbronchial Lung Biopsy

Overall diagnostic yield of TBB in pulmonary TB is 57–79% (Table 1). The cultures of TBB specimens have very low yield. Particularly in bronchogenic spread and miliary forms of TB, this method is diagnostic in 63–73% by histology (68%), smears (2%), and cultures (2%). Transbronchial biopsy is diagnostic immediately in 48% and exclusively in 12–20%.[2,30,31,35]

Postbronchoscopic Sputum

The overall and exclusive diagnostic yields of smears and cultures of postbronchoscopic sputum are 28% (6–76%) and 40% (4–79%) whereas the exclusive yields are 2–4% and 0–10%, respectively (Table 1). They do not significantly increase the yield over the combination of TBB and BAL.[2,30,31,36]

Interventional Bronchoscopy

Interventional bronchoscopy is an alternative strategy to surgery in the management of serious complications due to thoracic TB. The decision on whether a patient with TB complication is better suited for surgical or interventional bronchoscopic management is not straightforward. However, when indicated, surgery should be the treatment of choice in patients who can tolerate it.[37,38]

A variety of interventional bronchoscopic techniques can be performed using rigid or flexible bronchoscope in thoracic TB—endobronchial ultrasonography (EBUS), mechanical dilatation and reaming with rigid bronchoscope, balloon dilatation, stent placement, electrocautery, laser photoresection, argon plasma coagulation (APC), cryotherapy, fistula occlusion, and interventions for hemoptysis (Table 2). The main indication for interventional bronchoscopic procedures in thoracic TB is tracheobronchial stenosis.[37-41]

Tracheobronchial stenosis occurs in 15–18% of the cases with active pulmonary TB. Since it is usually underrecognized and misdiagnosed, the diagnosis is delayed. It usualy causes dyspnea, coughing, and obstructive pneumonia. Interventional bronchoscopic techniques are usually combined according to the indications (e.g., APC + balloon dilatation + stenting) in the management of tracheobronchial stenosis. Immediate relief of symptoms is achieved postintervention almost in all cases and about 50% of the cases stay asymptomatic for at least 2 years. Airway diameter can be increased from 4.5 mm to 11.9 mm in trachea, and from 2.6 mm to 8.3 mm in main stem bronchi. However, repeated sessions of interventions may be required in about 20% to maintain improvement.[37,38]

Other indications for interventional bronchoscopic procedures are mediastinal lymphadenopathy,[41] airway fistulas,[39] and hemoptysis.[40]

Endobronchial Ultrasound

Convex probe EBUS-or radial probe EBUS (RP-EBUS)-guided TBNA can be used for the diagnosis of hilar/mediastinal TB lymphadenopathy and parenchymal nodules adjacent to the airways.[41,42] Radial probe-EBUS is also useful in evaluating the individual layers of the

TABLE 2	Interventional bronchoscopic procedures used in the management of thoracic tuberculosis complications	
TB complication	**Interventional procedures**	**Efficacy**
Tracheobronchial stenosis	• Mechanical dilatation • Balloon dilatation • Hot treatments • Cryotherapy • Stenting • EBUS imaging	• Dilatation: 30–40% (high recurrence) • Combined: 50% (2 years)

Bronchopleural fistula	• Visualized fistula:
	  ○ Fibrin glue, hemoclipping, gelatinous sponge, cyanoacrylate
	• Distal fistula:
	  ○ Valves, spigots, stents, coils, atrial septostomy catheter
		• Valves, spigots: 70%

Bronchoesophageal fistula	• Fibrin glue, hemoclipping, gelatinous sponge, cyanoacrylate	–
Hemoptysis	• Iced saline, adrenaline electrocautery, argon plasma coagulation, Fogarty balloon catheter, double-lumen tube	–

TB, tuberculosis; EBUS, endobronchial ultrasonography.

bronchial wall. The images produced by RP-EBUS correlate well with histologic results and provide useful information for a planned bronchoscopic intervention, particularly for tracheobronchial stenosis by demonstrating the destruction of tracheobronchial cartilage or thickening of the airway wall (Table 2).[37]

Endobronchial ultrasound-guided transbronchial needle aspiration (EBUS-TBNA)[41-43] has comparable diagnostic performance to conventional TBNA[32-34] in hilar/mediastinal TB lymphadenitis and lesions adjacent to the airways (sensitivity: 65–94%, negative predictive value: 11–75%, accuracy: 80–85%). The overall diagnostic yield of EBUS-TBNA is 80–86% and 53% for pathologic and microbiologic specimens, respectively. Smears can be positive in 8–27%, cultures in 8–47%,[41-44] and polymerase chain reaction (PCR) test in 54%.[44] If pretest suspicion exists, EBUS-TBNA specimens should always be sent for dedicated microbiological analysis for TB (Table 1).

Combining EBUS-TBNA with conventional bronchoscopic methods (particularly conventional TBNA), preparing both smears and cell blocks, sampling more lymph node stations, and performing more needle passes can increase the diagnostic yield in TB lymphadenitis.[45,46]

Endobronchial ultrasound-guided TBNA can confirm granulomatous pathology. However, distinction of TB from sarcoidosis or another granulomatous disease depends upon correlating cytologic, microbiologic, radiologic, and clinical data in large series in TB endemic regions.[41-44,46]

Mechanical Dilatation and Debulking

Rigid bronchoscope itself can be used to dilate TB tracheobronchial stenosis. However, for very severe stenoses, balloon dilatation should be performed before mechanical dilatation (Table 2).

Firstly, the largest fitting rigid bronchoscope is inserted into the stenosed airway. Then, progressively larger-diameter rigid bronchoscopes are inserted until sufficient dilatation is achieved. Stenting may be required after mechanical dilatation in most of the cases.

To debulk the web-like scar tissue due to TB or the granulation tissue caused by the stent, the bevel of the rigid bronchoscope can also be used after APC, electrocautery, or laser treatments.[37,38]

Balloon Dilatation

This technique is minimally invasive, simple, and can be performed under local anesthesia. The expanding balloon dilates the stenosis radially (Fig. 1); thus, it is specifically suitable for treating annular cicatricial stenosis. Balloon dilatation should be the initial treatment for tracheobronchial stenosis. However, in most of the cases, early restenosis occurs. In noninflammatory bronchial stenosis, long-lasting clinical success with balloon dilatation is achieved in only 30–40% of the cases. Consequently, balloon dilatation alone is considered as an inadequate treatment for TB tracheobronchial stenosis and stenting is performed immediately afterward (Table 2).[37,38]

Stent Placement

Stenting is performed mainly to reestablish the patency of the central airways but also to support weakened cartilage in the presence of tracheobronchial malacia, and to seal the fistula due to TB erosion of the airway wall (Table 2). However, a stent should be placed only if the patient is definitely inoperable owing to long stenotic airway segments, severe stenosis at multiple levels, and/or compromised pulmonary reserve. Furthermore, if stent placement is decided on as management, then possible complications such as stent migration, granulation, retained secretions, and stent fracture must also be considered.[37,47]

Dumon silicone stent seems appropriate in TB airway stenosis (Figs 2A and B) since it is economical and can be removed or replaced easily when required. Ultraflex metallic stents should not be used as in all other benign stenoses because of difficulty in removal

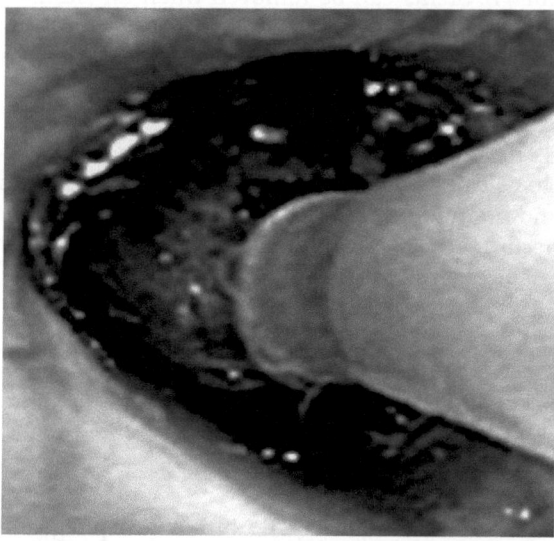

FIG. 1: Balloon dilatation of a bronchial stenosis due to endobronchial tuberculosis. *(For color version, see Plate 6)*

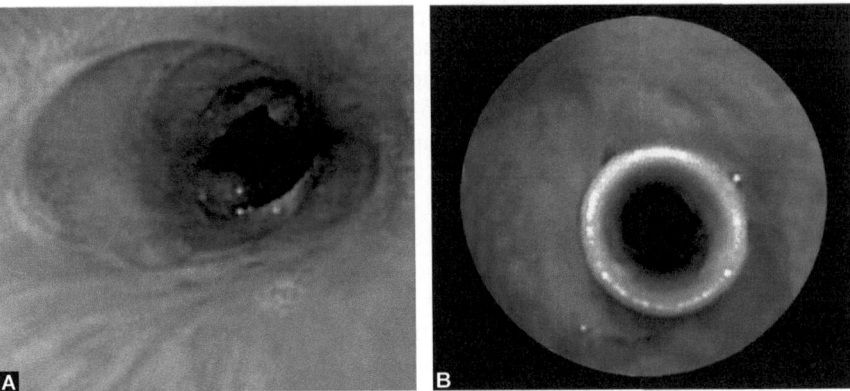

FIG. 2: A, Tracheal stenosis due to tuberculosis; **B,** A Dumon stent is placed and patency of trachea is reestablished. *(For color version, see Plate 6)*

and safety concerns in long term. Furthermore, metallic stents can cause problems related to formation of granulation tissue and stent deterioration due to metal fatigue.[37,38,47]

Dumon stents can migrate and cause granulation tissue but generally cause fewer complications than expandable metallic stents. These stent complications can be managed by stent removal or replacement, and application of APC, laser photoresection, or cryotherapy to the granulation tissue at the edges of the stent. For stenoses close to carina, Y-stent is well-suited and migrates less than straight stent.[37,47]

The nature of TB tracheobronchial stenosis (fixed narrowing or dynamic collapse) can be identified using serial flow-volume curves. In deciding whether or not a stent is needed, EBUS is useful to assess the condition of tracheobronchial wall regarding the presence of cartilaginous tracheobronchomalacia.[37]

In most of the cases with TB tracheobronchial stenosis, stent placement should be basically performed after balloon dilatation of the stenosed airway when the patients are smear-negative for TB. Stents can be removed when inflammation has diminished and severe malacia is absent. Removing the stent after 12 months or later can reduce restenosis in patients with incomplete stenosis.[37,38,47]

Hot Treatments

Electrocautery, APC, or laser [mostly neodymium-doped yttrium-aluminum-garnet (Nd:YAG)] (Figs. 3A to C) can be performed mainly to cut or resect endobronchial web-like fibrous bands and granulomas due to TB. After this procedure, dilatation and/or stenting is usually performed. Hot treatments are also useful to in ablating the stent-related granulation tissue obstructing the airway (Table 2).[37,38]

Cryotherapy

This cold method (Fig. 3D) can also be performed to ablate web-like scar tissue and granulomas due to TB and stent-related granulation tissue narrowing the airways (Table 2).[37]

Occlusion of Airway Fistulas

In HIV-negative patients with thoracic TB, bronchoesophageal fistula (BEF) and bronchopleural fistula (BPF) may rarely occur. However, there is increasing number of BEFs reported in HIV-infected TB patients owing to tendency for lymph node TB.[39,48]

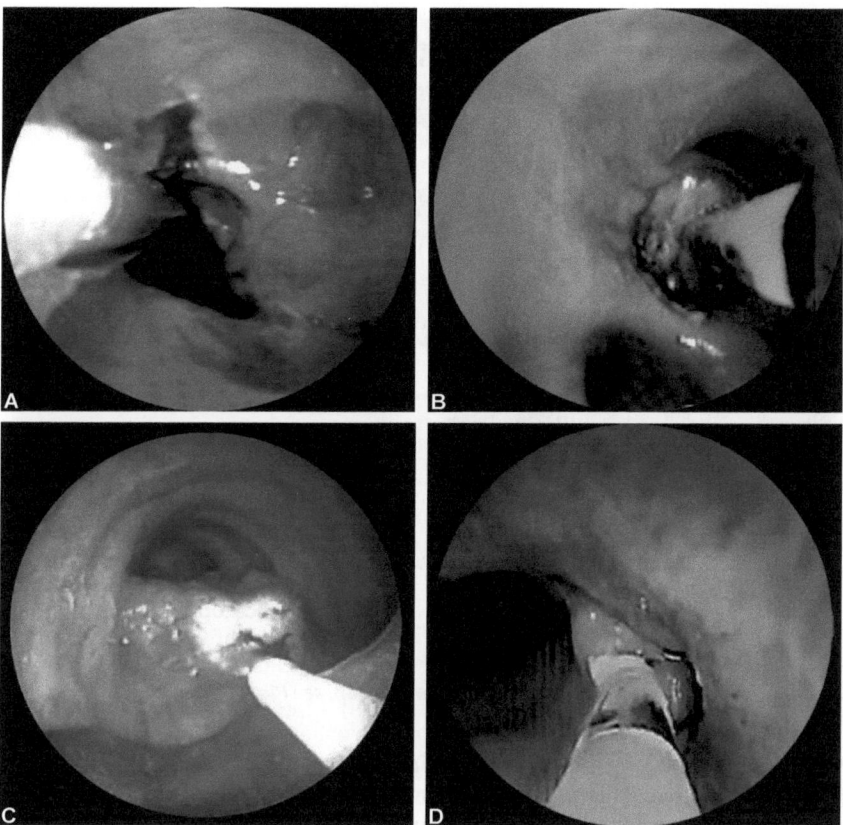

FIG. 3: Ablation of obstructing TB-related web-like and granulomatous tissues in the airways by **A,** electrocautery; **B,** argon plasma coagulation; **C,** laser; and **D,** cryotherapy. *(For color version, see Plate 7)*

If TB lymph nodes erode the adjacent bronchial or esophageal wall, a BEF, esophagomediastinal fistula or bronchomediastinal fistula may develop. Erosion of a bronchial TB ulcer into the esophagus, ulcerative esophageal TB perforating into the trachea or bronchus, or the development of traction diverticula between the respiratory tree and the esophagus may also lead to BEF.[48] Likewise, TB pyothorax/pyopneumothorax eroding into lung parenchyma and airways, or a large lung cavity eroding into pleural cavity may cause BPF.[39]

Bronchoesophageal fistulas and BPFs usually heal and close with anti-TB treatment. In simple BPFs, tube thoracostomy and pleurodesis are sufficient besides anti-TB treatment. However, fistulas that are large, chronic, or occurring after anti-TB treatment may be refractory. Surgical repair is the traditional treatment for all benign airway fistulas.[48]

In inoperable cases, fibrin glue, hemoclipping, gelatinous sponge, and cyanoacrylate have been used to repair visualized BEFs (Fig. 4) and BPFs endoscopically but the outcomes depend on the dimensions of the fistula.[39,48] For distal BPFs, reduction of leakage should be confirmed by balloon occlusion before Watanabe spigots,[49] endobronchial valves,[50] or tracheobronchial stents are placed. Watanabe spigots[49] and valves[50] have been shown to be successful (70%) in stopping leaks with sufficient experience. However, experience with coils, calf bones, and atrial septostomy catheters as sealants are limited (Table 2).[39,51]

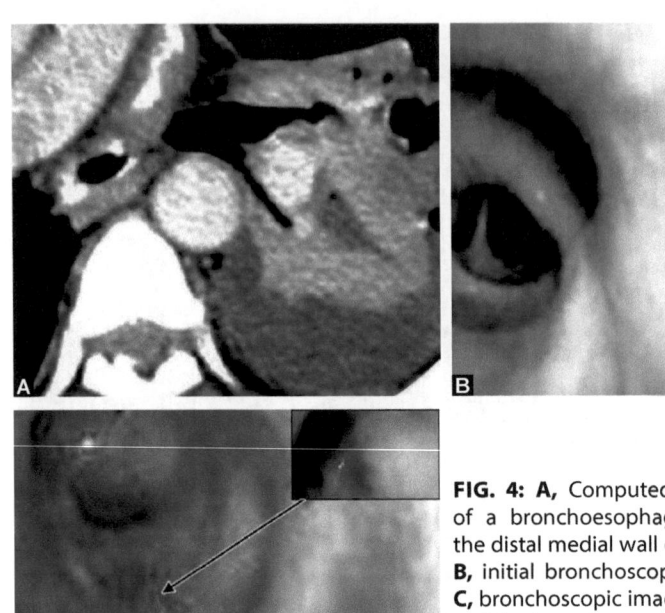

FIG. 4: A, Computed tomography image of a bronchoesophageal fistula (BEF) on the distal medial wall of left main bronchus; **B,** initial bronchoscopic image of the BEF; **C,** bronchoscopic image after closure of the BEF by bronchoscopic injection of cyanoacrylate glue (right upper corner: close-up image of BEF sealed with glue). *(For color version, see Plate 8)*

Bronchoscopic Interventions for Hemoptysis

Hemoptysis frequently occurs in both old or active pulmonary TB owing to bronchiectasis, fungus ball, broncholithiasis, destroyed lung, or erosion of bronchial or pulmonary arteries by cavitary infiltration. Chest computerized tomography and bronchoscopy are requisites for determining the site and origin of bleeding. The obvious cause of hemoptysis should be treated with specific measures. However, if the bleeding is life-threatening (massive and/or continuous), endobronchial interventions should be considered. Rigid bronchoscopy is preferred over fiberoptic bronchoscopy because of better ventilation and suctioning. Instillation of iced isotonic saline lavage, adrenaline, or thrombin-fibrinogen compounds to the bleeding site may be effective. Electrocautery or APC can also be applied if the bleeding site is endobronchially visible. Inserting and inflating of a Fogarty balloon catheter to tamponade over the bleeding area is another method to stop bleeding. In case all of the above interventions fail, intubation using a double-lumen tube can stabilize the bleeding until the definitive surgical treatment (Table 3).

Bronchial artery embolization can be beneficial in some cases; however, the recurrence rate is higher in TB. Surgical management, particularly lobectomy, is life-saving but should be performed very selectively to avoid postoperative morbidity and mortality.[40]

Bronchoscopic Methods and Forms of Intrathoracic Tuberculosis

Miliary Tuberculosis

Diagnosis of miliary TB can be a challenge since diagnosis is difficult and delay in diagnosis is associated with high mortality. Smears and cultures of sputum, gastric fluid, bone marrow aspiration/biopsy, or urine generally produce positive yields in less than half of the patients (14–67%) even if these methods are combined. Liver

| TABLE 3 | Diagnostic yields of bronchoscopic methods by forms of thoracic tuberculosis ||||||||
Form of TB	TBB (%)	EBB (%)	TBNA (%)	EBUS-TBNA (%)	Brushing (%)	BAL (%)	Bronchial lavage (%)	Total (%)
Miliary	73–88	–	–	–	25–57	25–64	15–45	73–86
Bronchogenic spread	30–50	–	–	–	30–50	30–90	35–40	60–90
Endobronchial	–	84	19	–	–	10	–	38–84
Lymphadenitis	–	9–75	75–100	80–86	9–75	–	–	75–100
Tuberculoma	40	–	–	–	<10	<10	–	50

TBB, transbronchial biopsy; EBB, endobronchial biopsy; TBNA, transbronchial needle aspiration; EBUS-TBNA, endobronchial ultrasound-guided transbronchial needle aspiration; BAL, bronchoalveolar lavage.

biopsy may show granulomas in the liver but noncaseating granulomas, found in about 25% of cases with miliary TB, are not specific for TB and can also be seen in other granulomatous disease such as sarcoidosis, berylliosis, mycosis, brucellosis and syphilis. Thus, liver biopsy can be diagnostic only if *Mycobacterium tuberculosis* (MTB) can be demonstrated with the granulomas.[18,52]

Considering the above-mentioned diagnostic challenges, bronchoscopy in miliary TB seems highly efficient with an overall diagnostic yield of 73–86%. It can be exclusively diagnostic in about 25% and provide early diagnosis in 63–76% by AFB on smears of bronchial brushing, BAL, or bronchial lavage specimens or by presence of granulomas in TBB specimens. Bronchial brushing can be diagnostic in up to 57% (smear: 30%, culture: 27%) while TBB specimens are positive in about 73% with most of the yield coming from histological examination (smear and culture: 5%, histology: 68%) (Table 3).[18,53,54]

Endobronchial Tuberculosis

Erosion of the tracheobronchial wall by TB lymph nodes, or bronchogenic spread of AFB-positive secretions coming from cavities can cause endobronchial TB. Particularly in regions with diminishing incidence of TB, diagnosis is often delayed owing to low suspicion of endobronchial TB that can lead to bronchostenosis and other serious sequelae despite adequate treatment. Asthma and bronchogenic carcinoma are the frequent misdiagnoses in cases with endobronchial TB.[55]

Elevated levels of interferon-γ and transforming growth factor-β (TGF-β) in bronchial washing fluid and lowered initial and post-treatment levels of TGF-β in serum have been implicated in the pathogenesis of endobronchial TB and airway stenosis during the course of this disease.[56]

Endobronchial TB can be seen in 4–74% of the adults and 38–57% of the children with TB and undergoing bronchoscopy. Endobronchial biopsy can be highly diagnostic in this form of TB (up to 84%) whereas TBNA and BAL provide diagnosis in only 19% and 10%, respectively (Table 3)[18,57,58]

There are seven different types of endobronchial TB (Fig. 5):
- Actively caseating
- Tumorous
- Edematous-hyperemic
- Granular
- Ulcerative
- Nonspecific bronchitic
- Fibrostenotic.[55]

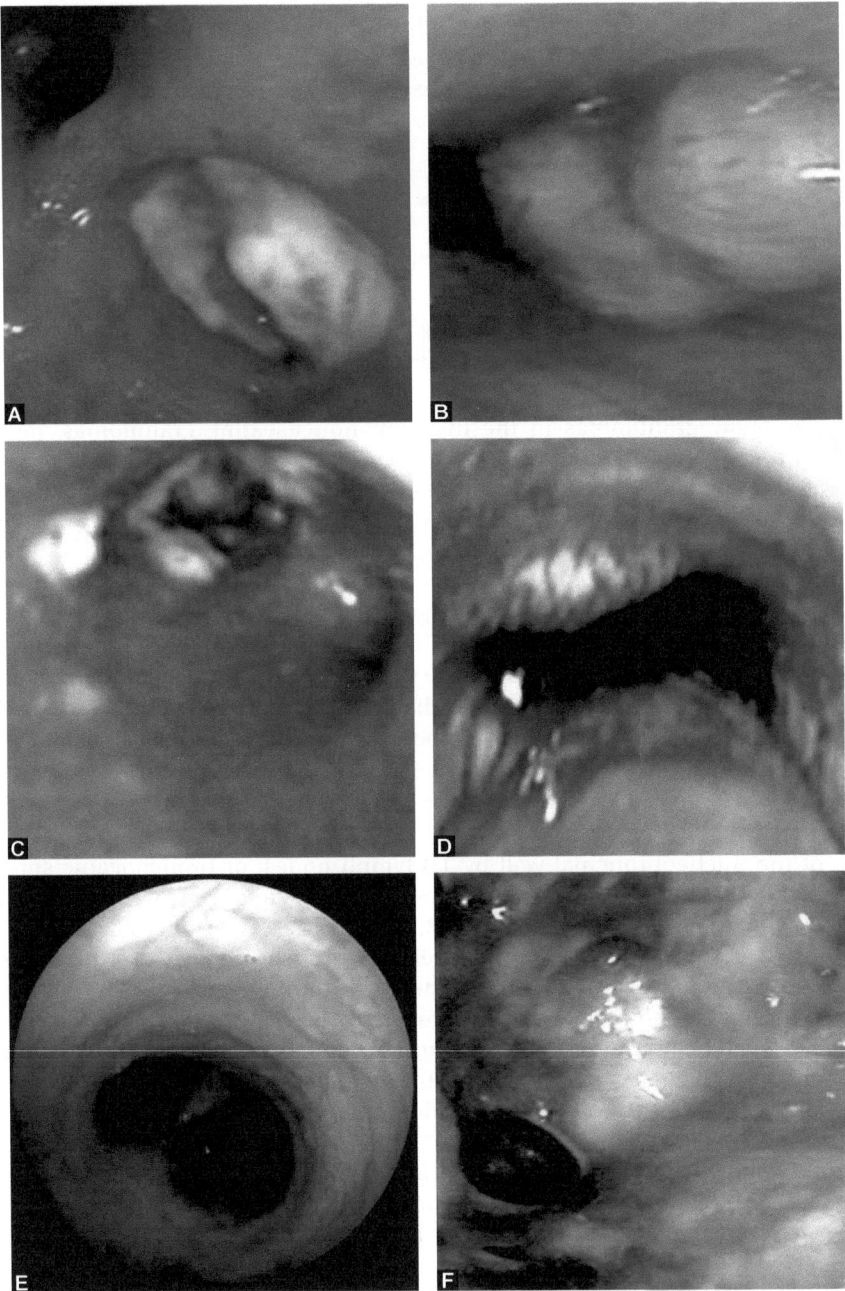

FIG. 5: Bronchoscopic images of different subtypes of endobronchial tuberculosis: **A,** actively caseating (with hyperhemia); **B,** tumorous; **C,** granular and edematous-hyperemic; **D,** ulcerating (with some stenosis); **E,** nonspecific bronchitic; **F,** fibrostenotic (with caseation and antracosis). *(For color version, see Plate 9)*

Of these, actively caseating, tumorous, and edematous-hyperemic varieties progress to fibrostenotic type more frequently (65–70%) than granular (18%), ulcerative, and nonspecific bronchitic varieties (0%) while fibrostenotic type does not show any improvement despite treatment. In tumorous type, new lesions may appear or initial lesions may increase in size. Bronchoscopy is useful in close follow-up of this complicated behavior of endobronchial lesions and progression to airway stenosis besides enabling visualization of the lesions and specimen collection from them.[55,58]

Tuberculoma (Solitary or Multiple Pulmonary Nodules)

In areas endemic for TB, radiologic pattern of solitary or multiple pulmonary nodules is not infrequent. However, importance of bronchoscopy in the diagnosis of tuberculoma(s) is not studied largely. Transbronchial biopsy and brushing guided by imaging methods (fluoroscopy, EBUS, or electromagnetic navigation) can be diagnostic in about half of the cases and provide rapid identification of TB in almost all of them. About 80% of immediate diagnoses are made by granulomas in TBB specimens (Table 3). Postbronchoscopic sputum is AFB-positive in only 5% of the cases with tuberculoma.[18,59]

Tuberculous Lymphadenopathy

In contrast to primary TB in childhood, TB lymphadenitis is an uncommon presentation in adults. Pulmonary infiltrates and hilar/mediastinal lymphadenopathy is the typical radiographic appearance in primary TB infection. However, involvement of only hilar/mediastinal lymph nodes with TB and absence of parenchymal lesions renders diagnosis complicated since sputum smear is usually negative and the differential diagnosis includes many diseases of granulomatous, infectious, and malignant etiology. Incidence of isolated involvement of intrathoracic lymph nodes by TB varies between 0.25 and 5.8%. In these cases with isolated lymphadenopathy, bronchoscopy is indicated to make a rapid diagnosis and to see whether there is any endobronchial TB.[32,60,61]

In intrathoracic TB lymphadenitis, the yield of bronchoscopy with only brushing and EBB varies between 9 and 75% depending on the presence of endobronchial lesion. When there is endobronchial involvement, the yield of bronchoscopy increases with brushing and EBB.[60,61] However, 19-gauge TBNA, independently of the endobronchial lesions, provides an overall diagnosis of 75–100%. Moreover, it is the only means of diagnosis in 80%. Thus, TBNA should be used routinely in diagnosing intrathoracic TB lymphadenitis.[32-34]

As mentioned earlier in the chapter, EBUS-TBNA[41-43] has an overall yield comparable to that of conventional TBNA[32-34] in this form of TB (Table 3). Thus, it appears to be rational and more cost-effective to use EBUS-TBNA to sample lymph nodes with smaller diameter (<1.5–2 cm) and/or at locations other than right lower paratracheal (4R) and subcarinal stations (7), or when conventional TBNA fails in patients with suspected TB lymphadenitis.[62-64]

Methods not in Routine Practice

Serodiagnostic Methods

Detection of MTB antigen and immunoglobulin G (IgG) antibody against MTB by radioimmunoassay or enzyme-linked immunosorbent assay in bronchial lavage/BAL fluid and serum in smear-negative TB has varying diagnostic performance (sensitivity: 70–72%, specificity: 82%, accuracy: 80%). Although serodiagnostic methods are found to be useful adjuncts to conventional tests, they are seldom used in routine clinical practice owing to their inconsistently reliable diagnostic performance.[2,65,66]

Estimation of Tuberculostearic Acid

Although not used and recommended in routine clinical practice, detection of tuberculostearic acid (TSA) in bronchial lavage and BAL specimens from sputum smear-negative patients can be a useful adjunct in early diagnosis of pulmonary TB. It has higher sensitivity than smears of bronchial lavage and BAL fluids. The sensitivity of TSA test is 40% in bronchial aspirate, 80% in BAL fluid, and 27% in TBB specimens while the combined sensitivity and specificity are 79–87% and 79%, respectively.[67,68]

Estimation of Adenosine Deaminase and Lysozyme

The diagnostic performance of adenosine deaminase (ADA) levels in bronchial aspirate and BAL fluid varies largely. Adenosine deaminase levels in BAL fluid greater than or equal to 2.5 IU/L have a sensitivity, specificity, and accuracy of 71–100%, 85–87%, and 81%, respectively. Since there is no significant difference in the mean bronchial aspirate/BAL fluid ADA levels between TB, malignancy and miscellaneous causes, their measurement is not recommended in the diagnosis of pulmonary TB.[69,70]

Given that lysozyme levels of bronchial aspirate/BAL fluid in pulmonary TB, infectious lung disease, or bronchogenic carcinoma are found to be comparable whereas BAL lysozyme levels are higher in interstitial lung diseases, this test is also not useful in diagnosing TB.[69]

Estimation of Lactate Dehydrogenase

The mean BAL fluid lactate dehydrogenase (LDH) level is significantly higher in pulmonary TB than controls. Very low levels of BAL fluid LDH levels (<60 mIU/mL), though not confirmatory, may occasionally be useful to exclude the diagnosis of active pulmonary TB. However, it cannot be advocated in routine use.[71]

Molecular Methods

Polymerase Chain Reaction

Overall, conventional or sequence capture PCR test on bronchial aspirate and BAL fluid has a sensitivity, specificity, positive and negative predictive values of 36–97, 73–96, 82–94, and 45–95%, respectively. However, it should be noted that there can be high false-positive results with PCR (4–26%). Bronchoalveolar lavage fluid/bronchial aspirate PCR examination can be a useful adjunct to TBB in the early diagnosis of sputum smear-negative pulmonary TB (59–91%) and can give reliable results even in culture-negative TB provided that there is appropriate clinical setting.[27,72-74]

Ligase Chain Reaction

The combined diagnostic yield of ligase chain reaction (LCR) and BACTEC 460 radiometric methods on BAL fluid has been found to be about 58% while that of sputum or bronchial aspirate culture is 42 and 47%, respectively. The negative predictive value of LCR method is low (52%). However, BAL fluid LCR test can be a rapid diagnostic tool in selected cases with sputum smear-negative pulmonary TB.[75]

Interferon-γ Release Assays

In sputum smear-negative patients, enzyme-linked immunospot assay with early antigenic target-6 and culture filtrate protein-10 peptides performed on mononuclear cells of BAL fluid and blood has shown that BAL fluid interferon-γ release assays (IGRAs) can be used selectively for the rapid diagnosis of TB.[76]

TRANSMISSION OF TUBERCULOSIS DURING BRONCHOSCOPY

Transmission by Bronchoscopy

Infectious transmission by bronchoscopy is a significant problem since there are large number of bronchoscopies performed in many institutions worldwide. Infectious complications due to bronchoscopy seem to be rare. However, most of them are possibly unreported or unrecognized since it may take months or years from MTB infection until clinical presentation. Furthermore, most MTB infections might not progress to active disease.

Although bronchoscope is disinfected, pseudoinfections may be seen if an organism contaminates bronchoscopic specimens from a patient with no sign of related disease. Unnecessary anxiety leads to further investigations and treatment for the isolate and also delay in diagnosis of actual disease. A pseudo-outbreak/pseudoepidemic is mentioned if bronchoscopic specimens of multiple patients are found to have AFB. However, only development of active disease after a bronchoscopic procedure with contaminated instruments can be named as true infection.[2,18,77] True infections are rare but cross-contamination of bronchial washings with MTB and transmission of MTB by FB have been reported.[78-80] All these cases with true infections result from lapses in standard infection control procedures and are preventable.

All bronchoscopes can be disinfected adequately in 2% alkaline glutaraldehyde at 20°C or peracetic acid for 20 minutes if thorough cleaning with detergent is performed before disinfection.[18,77]

Transmission to Staff and Bystanders

Increased coughing during diagnostic bronchoscopy causes spread of MTB by airborne route which may lead to TB outbreaks, particularly in units with highly susceptible patient populations.[81] Owing to bronchoscopy-related exposure to TB, skin test conversions in pulmonary fellows are higher than those of infectious disease fellows although TB exposure is comparable.[82] After a widespread nosocomial exposure, staff present during bronchoscopy have the highest skin test conversion rates.[83] However, despite all mentioned above, there have been no reliable reports and confirmed documents on development of active TB in healthcare staff after bronchoscopy.[18,77]

The Centers for Disease Control and Prevention (CDC) recommendations for preventing MTB transmission during bronchoscopy are as follows:[84]
- Bronchoscopy should be avoided in patients suspected of having infectious TB unless it is absolutely necessary and can be done with appropriate measures
- In patients with possibility of infectious TB, bronchoscopy should be performed using local exhaust ventilation devices (booths/special enclosures) or in a room with ventilation requirements for TB isolation
- Healthcare staff should wear respiratory protection in the rooms/enclosures where bronchoscopy is being performed on patients with possible infectious TB.

Precautions for infection (barrier clothing with gowns, gloves, mask and eye shields, needlestick precautions, and adequate ventilation) should be exercised fully in every procedure. There should be negative air pressure with engineering controls in the bronchoscopy area, 14 or more air changes per hour, and direct discharge of air to outside, or particulate air filtration before recirculation. If available, power air-purifying respirator hood that prevents MTB transmission should be used. Particulate respirator N95 is a minimally acceptable choice.[77,85]

REFERENCES

1. World Health Organization. (2014). Global tuberculosis report 2014. Executive summary, xi. [online] Available from: http://www.who.int/tb/publications/global_report/gtbr14_executive_summary.pdf?ua=1 [Accessed January, 2016].
2. Mohan A, Sharma SK. Fibreoptic bronchoscopy in the diagnosis of sputum smear-negative pulmonary tuberculosis: current status. Indian J Chest Dis Allied Sci. 2008;50:67-78.
3. Sputum-smear-negative pulmonary tuberculosis: controlled clinical trial of 3-month and 2-month regimens of chemotherapy. Lancet. 1979;1:1361-3.
4. Narain R, Rao MS, Chandrasekhar P, Pyarelal. Microscopy positive and microscopy negative cases of pulmonary tuberculosis. Am Rev Respir Dis. 1971;103:761-73.
5. Kim TC, Blackman RS, Heatwole KM, Kim TC, Rochester DF. Acid-fast bacilli in sputum smears of patients with pulmonary tuberculosis. Prevalence and significance of negative smears pretreatment and positive smears post-treatment. Am Rev Respir Dis. 1984;129:264-8.
6. Colebunders R, Bastian I. A review of the diagnosis and treatment of smear-negative pulmonary tuberculosis. Int J Tuberc Lung Dis. 2000;4:97-107.
7. Toman K. How many bacilli are present in a sputum specimen found positive by smear microscopy? In: Frieden T, editors. Toman's Tuberculosis: Case Detection, Treatment and Monitoring: Questions and Answers. 2nd ed. Geneva: World Health Organization; 2004. pp. 11-3.
8. Behr MA, Warren SA, Salamon H, et al. Transmission of Mycobacterium tuberculosis from patients smear-negative for acid-fast bacilli. Lancet. 1999;353:444-9.
9. Rouillon A, Perdrizet S, Parrot R. Transmission of tubercle bacilli: the effects of chemotherapy. Tubercle. 1976;57:275-99.
10. A study of the characteristics and course of sputum smear-negative pulmonary tuberculosis. Tubercle. 1981;62:155-67.
11. Narain R, Nair SS, Naganna K, Chandrasekhar P, Rao GR, Lal P. Problems in defining a "case" of pulmonary tuberculosis in prevalence surveys. Bull World Health Organ. 1968;39:701-29.
12. Kernan DJ. Bronchoscopy in pulmonary tuberculosis. Laryngoscope. 1937;47:777-91.
13. Shipman SJ. Diagnostic bronchoscopy in occult tuberculosis. Am Rev Tuberc. 1939;39:629-32.
14. Gronroos JA, Palva T, Saloheimo M. Bronchoscopic observations in pulmonary tuberculosis; with special reference to cytologic and bacterial findings. Acta Tuberc Scand. 1956;32:163-78.
15. Saglam L, Akgun M, Aktas E. Usefulness of induced sputum and fibreoptic bronchoscopy specimens in the diagnosis of pulmonary tuberculosis. J Int Med Res. 2005;33:260-5.
16. McWilliams T, Wells AU, Harrison AC, et al. Induced sputum and bronchoscopy in the diagnosis of pulmonary tuberculosis. Thorax. 2002;57:1010-4.
17. Conde MB, Soares SL, Mello FC, et al. Comparison of sputum induction with fiberoptic bronchoscopy in the diagnosis of tuberculosis: experience at an acquired immune deficiency syndrome reference center in Rio de Janeiro, Brazil. Am Respir Crit Care Med. 2000;162:2238-40.
18. Venkateshiah S, Mehta AC. Role of flexible bronchoscopy in the diagnosis of pulmonary tuberculosis in immunocompetent individuals. J Bronchol. 2003;10:300-8.
19. Brown M, Varia H, Bassett P, Davidson RN, Wall R, Pasvol G. Prospective study of sputum induction, gastric washing, and bronchoalveolar lavage for the diagnosis of pulmonary tuberculosis in patients who are unable to expectorate. Clin Infect Dis. 2007;44:1415-20.
20. Schoch OD, Rieder P, Tueller C, et al. Diagnostic yield of sputum, induced sputum, and bronchoscopy after radiologic tuberculosis screening. Am J Respir Crit Care Med. 2007;175:80-6.
21. Kobashi Y, Mouri K, Fukuda M, Yoshida K, Oka M. The usefulness of bronchoscopy for the diagnosis of pulmonary tuberculosis. J Bronchol. 2007;14:22-5.
22. Karnak D, Kayacan O, Beder S. Reactivation of pulmonary tuberculosis in malignancy. Tumori. 2002;88:251-4.
23. Yang CJ, Chen TC, Hung JY, et al. Routine culture for Mycobacterium tuberculosis from bronchoscopy in Taiwan. Respirology. 2007;12:412-5.
24. Kim MH, Suh GY, Chung MP, et al. The value of routinely culturing for tuberculosis during bronchoscopies in an intermediate tuberculosis-burden country. Yonsei Med J. 2007;48:969-72.

25. Shitrit D, Vertenshtein T, Shitrit AB, Shlomi D, Kramer MR. The role of routine culture for tuberculosis during bronchoscopy in a nonendemic area: analysis of 300 cases and review of the literature. Am J Infect Control. 2005;33:602-5.
26. Yuksekol I, Bal S, Ozkan M, et al. The value of fiberoptic bronchoscopy in diagnosis of smear negative pulmonary tuberculosis. Tuberk Toraks. 2003;51:405-9.
27. Tueller C, Chhajed PN, Buitrago-Tellez C, Frei R, Frey M, Tamm M. Value of smear and PCR in bronchoalveolar lavage fluid in culture positive pulmonary tuberculosis. Eur Respir J. 2005;26:767-72.
28. Tamura A, Muraki K, Shimada M, et al. Usefulness of bronchofiberscopy for the diagnosis of pulmonary non-tuberculous mycobacteriosis—an analysis mainly on pulmonary M. avium complex disease. Kekkaku. 2008;83:785-91.
29. Zainudin BM, Wahab Sufarlan A, Rassip CN, Ruzana MA, Tay AM. The role of diagnostic fiberoptic bronchoscopy for rapid diagnosis of pulmonary tuberculosis. Med J Malaysia. 1991;46:309-13.
30. Willcox PA, Benatar SR, Potgieter PD. Use of the flexible fibreoptic bronchoscope in diagnosis of sputum-negative pulmonary tuberculosis. Thorax. 1982;37:598-601.
31. Al-Kassimi FA, Azhar M, Al-Majed S, Al-Wazzan AD, Al-Hajjaj MS, Malibary T. Diagnostic role of fibreoptic bronchoscopy in tuberculosis in the presence of typical X-ray pictures and adequate sputum. Tubercle. 1991;72:145-8.
32. Bilaçeroğlu S, Günel O, Eriş N, Cağirici U, Mehta AC. Transbronchial needle aspiration in diagnosing intrathoracic tuberculous lymphadenitis. Chest. 2004;126:259-67.
33. Baran R, Tor M, Tahaoğlu K, et al. Intrathoracic tuberculous lymphadenopathy: clinical and bronchoscopic features in 17 adults without parenchymal lesions. Thorax. 1996;51:87-9.
34. Harkin TJ, Ciotoli C, Addrizzo-Harris DJ, Naidich DP, Jagirdar J, Rom WN. Transbronchial needle aspiration (TBNA) in patients infected with HIV. Am J Respir Crit Care Med. 1998;157(6 Pt 1):1913-8.
35. Wallace JM, Deutsch AL, Harrell JH, Moser KM. Bronchoscopy and transbronchial biopsy in evaluation of patients with suspected active tuberculosis. Am J Med. 1981:70:1189-94.
36. Chawla R, Pant K, Jaggi OP, Chandrashekhar S, Thukral SS. Fiberoptic bronchoscopy in smear-negative pulmonary tuberculosis. Eur Respir J. 1988;1:804-6.
37. Iwamoto Y, Miyazawa T, Kurimoto N, Miyazu Y, Ishida A, Matsuo K, et al. Interventional bronchoscopy in the management of airway stenosis due to tracheobronchial tuberculosis. Chest. 2004;126:1344-52.
38. Low SY, Hsu A, Eng P. Interventional bronchoscopy for tuberculous tracheobronchial stenosis. Eur Respir J. 2004;24:345-7.
39. Dalar L, Kosar F, Eryuksel E, Karasulu L, Altin S. Endobronchial Watanabe spigot embolisation in the treatment of bronchopleural fistula due to tuberculous empyema in intensive care unit. Ann Thorac Cardiovasc Surg. 2013;19:140-3.
40. Halezeroğlu S, Okur E. Thoracic surgery for haemoptysis in the context of tuberculosis: what is the best management approach? J Thorac Dis. 2014;6:182-5.
41. Navani N, Molyneaux PL, Breen RA, et al. Utility of endobronchial ultrasound-guided transbronchial needle aspiration in patients with tuberculous intrathoracic lymphadenopathy: a multicentre study. Thorax. 2011;66:889-93.
42. Sun J, Teng J, Yang H, et al. Endobronchial ultrasound-guided transbronchial needle aspiration in diagnosing intrathoracic tuberculosis. Ann Thorac Surg. 2013;96:2021-7.
43. Kuo CH, Lin SM, Lee KY, et al. Algorithmic approach by endobronchial ultrasound-guided transbronchial needle aspiration for isolated intrathoracic lymphadenopathy: A study in a tuberculosis-endemic country. J Formos Med Assoc. 2014;113:527-34.
44. Senturk A, Arguder E, Hezer H, et al. Rapid diagnosis of mediastinal tuberculosis with polymerase chain reaction evaluation of aspirated material taken by endobronchial ultrasound-guided transbronchial needle aspiration. J Investig Med. 2014;62:885-9.
45. van der Heijden EH, Casal RF, Trisolini R, et al. Guideline for the acquisition and preparation of conventional and endobronchial ultrasound-guided transbronchial needle aspiration specimens for the diagnosis and molecular testing of patients with known or suspected lung cancer. Respiration. 2014;88:500-17.
46. Çağlayan B, Salepçi B, Fidan A, et al. Sensitivity of convex probe endobronchial sonographically guided transbronchial needle aspiration in the diagnosis of granulomatous mediastinal lymphadenitis. J Ultrasound Med. 2011;30:1683-9.

47. Eom JS, Kim H, Park HY, et al. Timing of silicone stent removal in patients with post-tuberculosis bronchial stenosis. Ann Thorac Med. 2013;8:218-23.
48. Sasaki M, Mochizuki H, Takahashi H. A bronchoesophageal fistula that developed shortly after the initiation of antituberculous chemotherapy. Intern Med. 2013;52:795-9.
49. Watanabe Y, Matsuo K, Tamaoki A, Komoto R, Hiraki S. Bronchial occlusion with endobronchial Watanabe spigot. J Bronchol. 2003;10:264-7.
50. Toma TP, Kon OM, Oldfield W, et al. Reduction of persistent air leak with endoscopic valve implants. Thorax. 2007;62:830-3.
51. Yang L, Kong J, Tao W, et al. Tuberculosis bronchopleural fistula treated with atrial septal defect occluder. Ann Thorac Surg. 2013;96:e9-e11.
52. Sahn SA, Neff TA. Miliary tuberculosis. Am J Med. 1974;56:494-505.
53. Willcox PA, Potgieter PD, Bateman ED, Benatar SR. Rapid diagnosis of sputum negative miliary tuberculosis using the flexible fibreoptic bronchoscope. Thorax. 1986;41:681-4.
54. Maartens G, Willcox PA, Benatar SR. Miliary tuberculosis: rapid diagnosis, hematologic abnormalities, and outcome in 109 treated adults. Am J Med. 1990;89:291-6.
55. Chung HS, Lee JH. Bronchoscopic assessment of the evolution of endobronchial tuberculosis. Chest. 2000;117:385-92.
56. Kim Y, Kim K, Joe J, et al. Changes in the levels of interferon-gamma and transforming growth factor-beta influence bronchial stenosis during the treatment of endobronchial tuberculosis. Respiration. 2007;74:202-7.
57. Altin S, Cikrikcioğlu S, Morgül M, Koşar F, Ozyurt H. 50 endobronchial tuberculosis cases based on bronchoscopic diagnosis. Respiration. 1997;64:162-4.
58. Mariotta S, Masullo M, Guidi L, Aquilini M, Pabani R, Bisetti A. Tracheobronchial involvement in 84 cases of pulmonary tuberculosis. Monaldi Arch Chest Dis. 1995;50:356-9.
59. Lai RS, Lee SS, Ting YM, Wang HC, Lin CC, Lu JY. Diagnostic value of transbronchial lung biopsy under fluoroscopic guidance in solitary pulmonary nodule in an endemic area of tuberculosis. Respir Med. 1996;90:139-43.
60. Chang SC, Lee PY, Perng RP. Clinical role of bronchoscopy in adults with intrathoracic tuberculous lymphadenopathy. Chest. 1988;93:314-7.
61. Ayed AK, Behbehani NA. Diagnosis and treatment of isolated tuberculous mediastinal lymphadenopathy in adults. Eur J Surg. 2001;167:334-8.
62. Li K, Jiang S. A randomized controlled study of conventional TBNA versus EBUS-TBNA for diagnosis of suspected stage I and II sarcoidosis. Sarcoidosis Vasc Diffuse Lung Dis. 2014;31:211-8.
63. Bonifazi M, Zuccatosta L, Trisolini R, Moja L, Gasparini S. Transbronchial needle aspiration: a systematic review on predictors of a successful aspirate. Respiration. 2013;86:123-34.
64. Mehta AC, Wang KP. Teaching conventional transbronchial needle aspiration. A continuum. Ann Am Thorac Soc. 2013;10:685-9.
65. Udani PM, Samuel A, Kadiwal GV, et al. Diagnosis of intrathoracic tuberculosis by detection of tubercle and/or tubercular antigen (TB Ag) in bronchial aspirate. Indian J Pediatr. 1987;54:69-77.
66. Levy H, Wadee AA, Feldman C, Rabson AR. Enzyme-linked immunosorbent assay for the detection of antibodies against Mycobacterium tuberculosis in bronchial washings and serum. Chest. 1988;93:762-6.
67. Pang JA, Chan HS, Chan CY, Cheung SW, French GL. A tuberculostearic acid assay in the diagnosis of sputum smear-negative pulmonary tuberculosis. A prospective study of bronchoscopic aspirate and lavage specimens. Ann Intern Med. 1989;111:650-4.
68. Chan CH, Chan RC, Arnold M, Cheung H, Cheung SW, Cheng AF. Bronchoscopy and tuberculostearic acid assay in the diagnosis of sputum smear-negative pulmonary tuberculosis: a prospective study with the addition of transbronchial biopsy. Q J Med. 1992;82:15-23.
69. Orphanidou D, Stratakos G, Rasidakis A, et al. Adenosine deaminase activity and lysozyme levels in bronchoalveolar lavage fluid in patients with pulmonary tuberculosis. Int J Tuberc Lung Dis. 1998;2:147-52.
70. Reechaipichitkul W, Lulitanond V, Patjanasoontorn B, Boonsawat W, Phunmanee A. Diagnostic yield of adenosine deaminase in bronchoalveolar lavage. Southeast Asian J Trop Med Public Health. 2004;35:730-4.
71. Emad A, Rezaian GR. Lactate dehydrogenase in bronchoalveolar lavage fluid of patients with active pulmonary tuberculosis. Respiration. 1999;66:41-5.

72. Liam CK, Chen YC, Yap SF, Srinivas P, Poi PJ. Detection of Mycobacterium tuberculosis in bronchoalveolar lavage from patients with sputum smear-negative pulmonary tuberculosis using a polymerase chain reaction assay. Respirology. 1998;3:125-9.
73. Wong CF, Yew WW, Chan CY, Au LY, Cheung SW, Cheng AF. Rapid diagnosis of smear-negative pulmonary tuberculosis via fibreoptic bronchoscopy: utility of polymerase chain reaction in bronchial aspirates as an adjunct to transbronchial biopsies. Respir Med. 1998;92:815-9.
74. Chen NH, Liu YC, Tsao TC, et al. Combined bronchoalveolar lavage and polymerase chain reaction in the diagnosis of pulmonary tuberculosis in smear-negative patients. Int J Tuberc Lung Dis. 2002;6:350-5.
75. Kwiatkowska S, Marczak J, Zieba M, Nowak D. Clinical utility of a commercial ligase chain reaction kit for the diagnosis of smear-negative pulmonary tuberculosis. Int J Tuberc Lung Dis. 1999;3:421-5.
76. Jafari C, Ernst M, Kalsdorf B, et al. Rapid diagnosis of smear-negative tuberculosis by bronchoalveolar lavage enzyme-linked immunospot. Am J Respir Crit Care Med. 2006;174:1048-54.
77. Culver DA, Gordon SM, Mehta AC. Infection control in the bronchoscopy suite: a review of outbreaks and guidelines for prevention. Am J Respir Crit Care Med. 2003;167:1050-6.
78. Bryce EA, Walker M, Bevan C, Smith JA. Contamination of bronchoscopes with Mycobacterium tuberculosis. Can J Infect Control. 1993;8:35-6.
79. Prigogine T, Glupczynski Y, Van Molle P, Schmerber J. Mycobacterial cross-contamination of bronchoscopy specimens. J Hosp Infect. 1988;11:93-5.
80. Wheeler PW, Lancaster D, Kaiser AB. Bronchopulmonary cross-colonization and infection related to mycobacterial contamination of suction valves of bronchoscopes. J Infect Dis. 1989;159:954-8.
81. Jereb JA, Burwen DR, Dooley SW, et al. Nosocomial outbreak of tuberculosis in a renal transplant unit: application of a new technique for restriction fragment length polymorphism analysis of Mycobacterium tuberculosis isolates. J Infect Dis. 1993;168:1219-24.
82. Malasky C, Jordan T, Potulski F, Reichman LB. Occupational tuberculous infections among pulmonary physicians in training. Am Rev Respir Dis. 1990;142:505-7.
83. Catanzaro A. Nosocomial tuberculosis. Am Rev Respir Dis. 1982;125:559-62.
84. Guidelines for preventing the transmission of Mycobacterium tuberculosis in health-care facilities, 1994. Centers for Disease Control and Prevention. MMWR Recomm Rep. 1994;43(RR-13):1-132.
85. Fennelly KP. Personal respiratory protection against Mycobacterium tuberculosis. Clin Chest Med. 1997;18:1-17.

CHAPTER 7

Bronchogenic Tuberculosis

Dragana M Jovanovic, Atul C Mehta

INTRODUCTION

Exposure of *Mycobacterium tuberculosis* (Mtb)-naïve individuals to a pulmonary tuberculosis (TB) patient results in Mtb infection (30%) or primary TB and among infected ones, the lifetime risk of reactivation TB of 10%. Once TB develops, possible treatment outcomes include cure, treatment failure or death, but among presumably cured individuals TB relapses can occur. A previous history of TB does not confer immunity against all strains and re-exposure to another Mtb strain can lead to reinfection.

After primary infection, 10% of individuals develop a TB pneumonia with expansion of infiltrates, and may have hilar lymphadenopathy or present with disease at more distant sites, commonly with cervical lymph nodes, meningitis, pericarditis, or miliary dissemination. Progression to local disease or dissemination occurs more frequently in those with poor immune responses, such as human immunodeficiency virus (HIV), chronic kidney failure, poorly controlled diabetes mellitus (DM), and older adults.[1]

The lung is the most commonly affected organ in TB with more than 70% of the newly diagnosed cases of TB having lung involvement.[2] Although extrapulmonary involvement is common in persons with HIV infection, the rates of pulmonary involvement are 60–70%, in some series even up to 90%.[3]

Reactivation TB (postprimary disease, endogenous reinfection) represents 90% of adult cases among HIV-negative individuals, and results from reactivation of a previously dormant focus seeded at the time of the primary infection.

SYMPTOMS AND SIGNS

Given the wide spectrum of lung involvement in TB, from skin positivity with clear X-rays to advanced disease, a wide range of signs and symptoms can also be present. Symptoms are often divided into two categories:
1. Constitutional and
2. Pulmonary.[1,4]

The most frequently reported symptoms of active pulmonary TB include cough (23–47%), fever (18–79%), weight loss (7–24%), and hemoptysis (8–9%). The frequency of these symptoms differs significantly depending on whether the patient has primary TB or reactivation TB, all more common in the reactivation TB.

Reactivation TB may remain undiagnosed and potentially infectious for 2–3 years or longer, with development of symptoms only late in the course of the disease. Symptoms typically begin insidiously and are present for weeks or months before the diagnosis is made, usually with cough, weight loss, and fatigue developed in half to two-thirds of patients and fever and night sweats or night sweats alone in approximately one-half.

Cough, the most common symptom of pulmonary TB, may be nonproductive early in the course of the disease, but subsequently, as the infection progresses and the caseation necrosis and liquefaction occur, it becomes productive, often associated with mild hemoptysis. Chest pain may be localized and pleuritic. Spontaneous pneumothorax may also occur, often with chest pain and perhaps dyspnea. Dyspnea, shortness of breath typically is due to extensive parenchymal lung disease and may be associated with severe respiratory failure. Hemoptysis often occurs with more extensive disease but does not necessarily indicate an active TB. They may also result from bronchiectasis as a residual of healed TB; from rupture of a dilated vessel in the wall of an old cavity (Rasmussen's aneurysm); from bacterial or fungal infection [especially in the form of a fungus ball (aspergilloma or mycetoma)] in an old residual cavity or from erosion of calcified lesions into the lumen of an airway (broncholithiasis).

The systemic signs of TB include fever in approximately 35–80%[5,6] with often a classic fever pattern with a fever that develops in the late afternoon and typical "night sweats". Anorexia, wasting (consumption), and malaise are common features of advanced disease and may be the only presenting features in some patients.

Laboratory findings: Routine hematology and biochemistry analyses are frequently normal in the setting of pulmonary TB. The C-reactive protein can be elevated in upto 85% of patients.[7] Later in the course of disease, a variety of hematologic abnormalities, especially leukocytosis and anemia (usually normocytic)[8] can be registered. Metabolic disorders like hyponatremia[9,10] may be associated with the syndrome of inappropriate antidiuretic hormone secretion[11] or rarely with adrenal insufficiency. Hypoalbuminemia and hypergammaglobulinemia also may occur as late findings.

Physical findings are not particularly helpful. Crackles may be heard in the area of lung TB process, along with bronchial breath sounds when lung consolidation is close to the chest wall, occasionally amphoric breath sounds may be heard indicative of a cavity.

IMAGING

Radiography

Pulmonary TB nearly always causes detectable abnormalities on the chest X-ray, although in patients with HIV infection, a normal chest radiograph occurred in as many as 11% of patients with positive sputum cultures.[12]

Primary Tuberculosis

The most common radiographic appearance of primary TB is a normal radiograph. In primary TB, occurring as a result of recent infection, generally a middle or lower lung zone infiltrate is seen, often associated with ipsilateral hilar adenopathy (Fig. 1). Atelectasis usually results from compression of airways by enlarged lymph nodes. If the primary process persists beyond the time when specific cell-mediated immunity develops, cavitation may occur, i.e., progressive primary TB, particularly in malnourished or other immunocompromised patients (Fig. 2).

Typically, the TB infiltrates are small and subpleural in location, more commonly seen in adults, while hilar or paratracheal lymph node enlargement is a characteristic finding in primary TB most commonly seen in children (usually unilateral). Miliary involvement at the onset of disease is seen in less than 3% of cases, most commonly in children under 2–3 years of age, but can also be seen in adults. An isolated pleural effusion commonly of mild-to-moderate degree may be the only manifestation of primary TB as well.

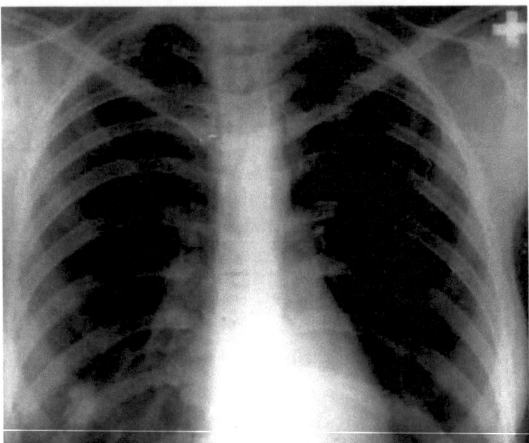

FIG. 1: Posteroanterior chest radiograph of a 21-year-old female patient who presented with a history of recent onset of coughing and night fever: a lower lung zone infiltrate associated with ipsilateral hilar adenopathy.

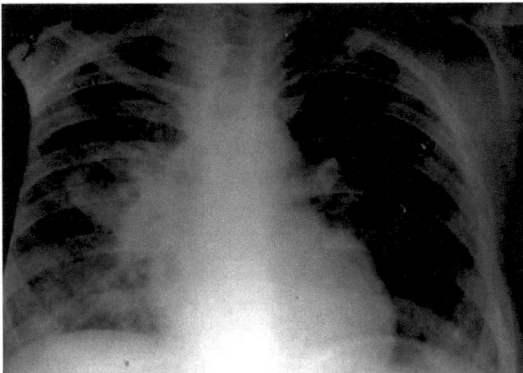

FIG. 2: Posteroanterior chest radiograph of a 27-year-old male patient who presented with night fever and hemoptysis: a primary tuberculosis cavity associated with ipsilateral hilar adenopathy.

Reactivation Tuberculosis

Most patients with reactivation TB have abnormalities on chest radiography, even in the absence of respiratory symptoms.[13-15] A normal chest radiograph is also possible even in active pulmonary TB in upto 10%.[16] Although, reactivation TB may involve any lung segment, the characteristic distribution suggesting the disease are the lesions in the apical posterior segments of the upper lobes (80–90% of patients) (Fig. 3) or the superior segment of the lower lobes and the anterior segment of the upper lobes.[17-19] This is the case in 95% of localized pulmonary TB, with the typical pattern of an airspace consolidation in a patchy or confluent nature and frequently increased linear densities to the ipsilateral hilum. As the lesions become more chronic, they become more sharply circumscribed and of irregular contour.

Cavitation is common noted in upto 40% of cases, with cavities associated with endobronchial spread of the disease; they typically have moderately thickened walls, while fewer than 10% of cases with air-fluid levels[19,20] (Figs. 4 to 6).

In the immunocompetent adult with TB, lymph node enlargement is rarely seen. When the disease progresses, infected material may be spread via the airways,

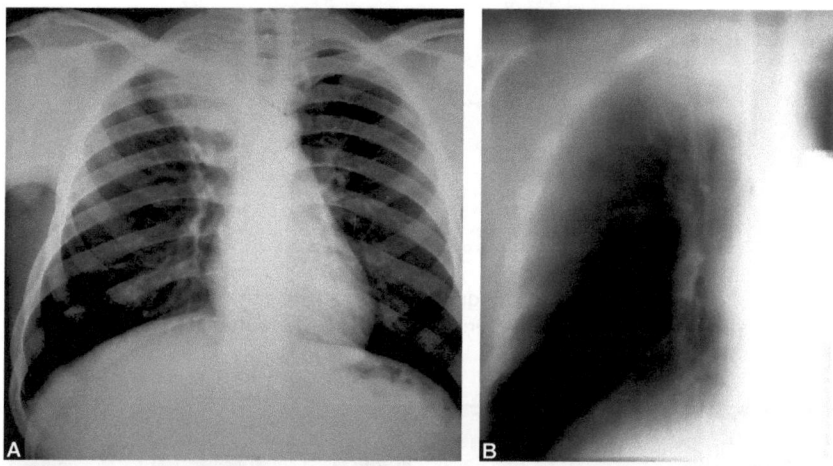

FIG. 3: Posteroanterior chest radiograph and the tomography from a 21-year-old male patient who presented with a history of recent onset of coughing and night sweats, showing tuberculosis lung lesion in the apical posterior segments of right upper lobe.

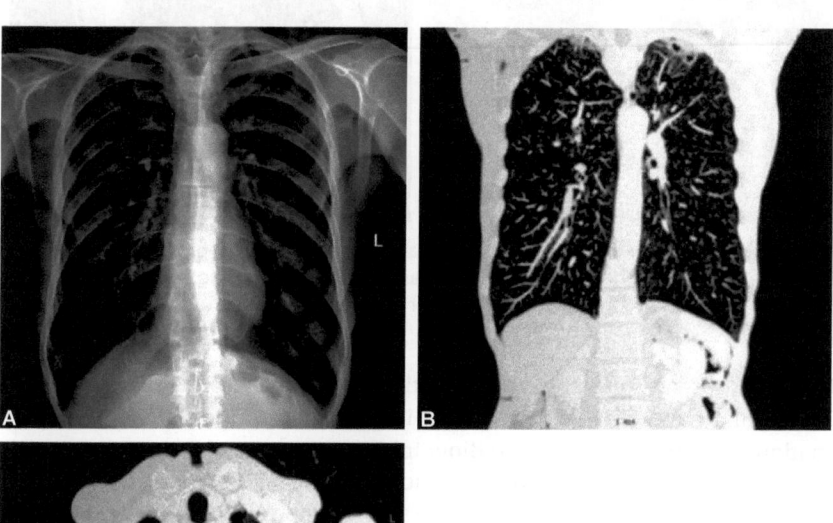

FIG. 4: Posteroanterior chest radiograph and the computed tomography scan from a 46-year-old male patient who presented with discrete hemoptysis: typical tuberculosis cavities in the apex of left upper lobe.

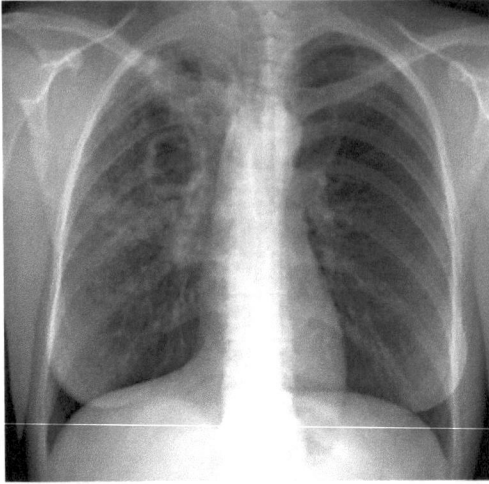

FIG. 5: Posteroanterior chest radiograph from a patient with the history of several months productive cough and fever: large tuberculosis cavities in the right lung.

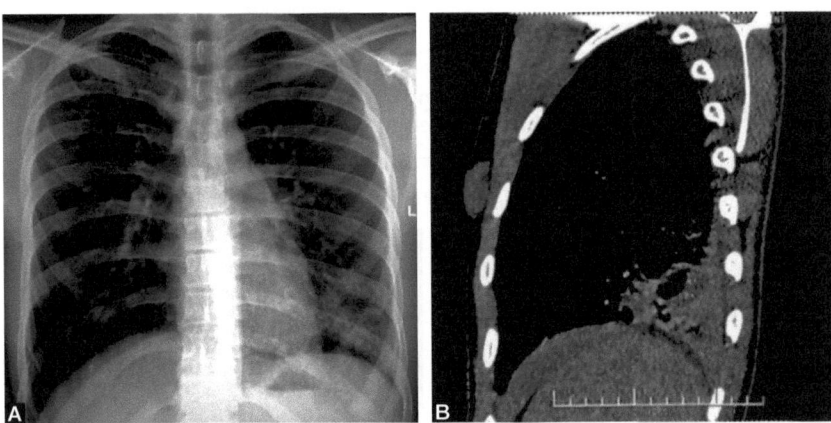

FIG. 6: Posteroanterior chest radiograph and computed tomography scan from a 22-year-old male patient with the history of asthma, often receiving corticosteroids and 3 months productive cough with fever: lower lobe cavitary tuberculosis in the left lung.

"bronchogenic" spread, into the lower portions of the involved lung or to the other lung. Erosion of a parenchymal focus of TB into a blood or lymph vessel may result in dissemination of the pathogen and a radiographic miliary pattern.

Lower lung field TB has the incidence in adults of 2–9%.[13,21] Elderly patients and those with HIV, diabetes, renal, or hepatic disease, those receiving corticosteroids, and those with underlying silicosis are at highest risk for lower lobe TB.[15,22] However, many patients with lower lobe TB have no underlying medical illnesses (Fig. 6).

In HIV-infected patients, radiographic findings are affected by the degree of immunosuppression; TB developing relatively early in the course of HIV infection tends to have typical radiographic findings with predominantly upper lobe infiltration and cavitation.[23] In more advanced HIV disease, the radiographic findings become more "atypical": lower lung zone or diffuse infiltrates and intrathoracic adenopathy are frequent while cavitation is uncommon. Surprisingly, at the end of the treatment for pulmonary TB, a substantial number of HIV-infected patients have normal radiographs.[24]

Healing of the tuberculous lesions usually results in development of a fibrotic scar with shrinkage of the lung parenchyma, volume loss, and often calcification. Upto 5% of patients with active TB present with upper lobe fibrocalcific changes thought to be indicative of healed primary TB. So, such patients with fibrocalcific changes should be evaluated for active TB in the setting of respiratory symptoms or absence of serial films documenting stability of the lesion.

Chest Computed Tomography

Computed tomography (CT) scans being more sensitive than plain chest radiography for diagnosis, particularly for smaller lesions located in the apex of the lung,[25] offer a more detailed examination than plain chest X-ray alone. In patients with primary TB, it typically demonstrates lobar consolidation in association with mediastinal or hilar adenopathy. The consolidation is usually well-defined, dense, homogeneous, and confined to a segment or lobe. CT may allow the visualization of tiny cavities as well as other parenchymal lesions that were not recognized on the plain chest X-ray.

Thus, approximately 20% of patients with tuberculous pleurisy have coexisting parenchymal disease on chest radiograph, but if chest CT scans are performed, more than 80% may have parenchymal abnormalities.[26]

High-resolution CT allows detection of early bronchogenic spread with the most common findings in reactivation TB of centrilobular nodules or branching linear structures (tree in bud) with or without bronchial wall thickening, lobular consolidation, cavity formation, bronchiectasis, and/or fibrotic changes (Figs. 7 and 8).

Some authors argue that CT findings such as the tree in bud and/or areas of centrilobular nodules are more consistent with active disease, but CT scans are not sufficiently reliable method to discriminate active TB from latent infection on each occasion.

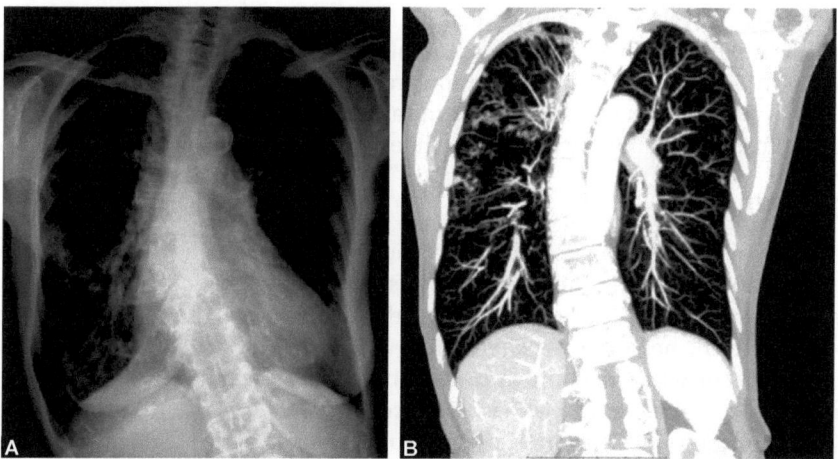

FIG. 7: Posteroanterior chest radiograph and computed tomography scan from a 57-year-old female patient with the history of several months dry cough and weight loss: reactivation tuberculosis of centrilobular nodules or branching linear structures (tree in bud).

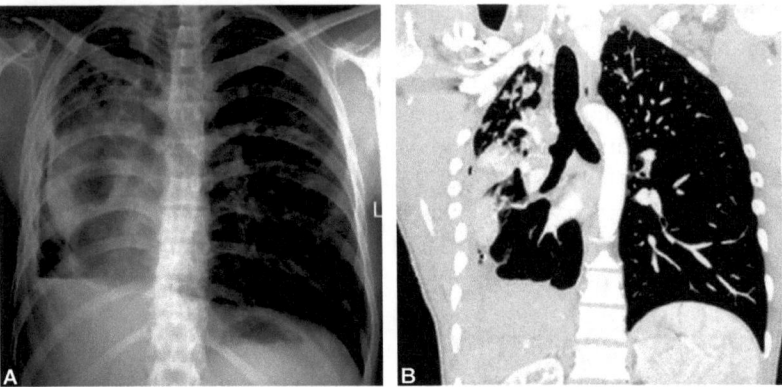

FIG. 8: Posteroanterior chest radiograph and computed tomography scan from a 26-year-old male patient with the history of tuberculosis relapse: massive bronchial wall thickening, cavities, bronchiectasis and fibrotic changes.

TUBERCULOSIS CHARACTERISTICS IN HUMAN IMMUNODEFICIENCY VIRUS-INFECTED PATIENTS

Some important differences are noticed regarding the clinical presentations of TB in patients with or without HIV infection. HIV-infected patients are more likely to present with disseminated disease and about 50% have extrapulmonary disease as compared to 20% of the general population. They tend to have an increased number and severity of symptoms and have a more rapid progression to death unless treatment is initiated. Surprisingly, at the end of the treatment for pulmonary TB, a substantial number of HIV-infected patients have normal radiographs.[24]

Radiographic findings of TB in HIV correlate with the degree of immunosuppression due to the CD4 cell depletion. Hilar and mediastinal lymphadenopathy are usually associated with lower CD4 counts (i.e., $<200/mm^3$), while cavitation is seen more commonly in patients with higher CD4 counts.

Tuberculosis developing relatively early in the course of HIV infection tends to have typical radiographic findings with predominantly upper lobe infiltration and cavitation.[23] In more advanced HIV disease, the radiographic findings become more "atypical": lower lung zone or diffuse infiltrates and intrathoracic adenopathy are frequent as well as pleural effusions and miliary infiltrates while cavitation is uncommon (Figs. 9 and 10).

DIAGNOSIS

For latent tuberculous infection (LTBI), tuberculin skin testing (TST) with purified protein derivative (PPD) is the current first step standard diagnostic test, interferon-gamma release assay (IGRA) following as the second step. tuberculin skin testing cannot distinguish, however, between latent and active infection. False-positive skin reaction can occur with infection with nontuberculous mycobacterial (NTM) infection or from Bacillus Calmette-Guérin (BCG) vaccination. False-negatives can occur with anergy due to immunocompromised states or recent or active infection, since it can take up to 10 weeks to develop a typical skin reaction. Guidelines for the use of PPD testing as a screening test for LTBI suggest that risk factor for tuberculous infection should affect the cutoff used to determine a positive result.[1,4,15]

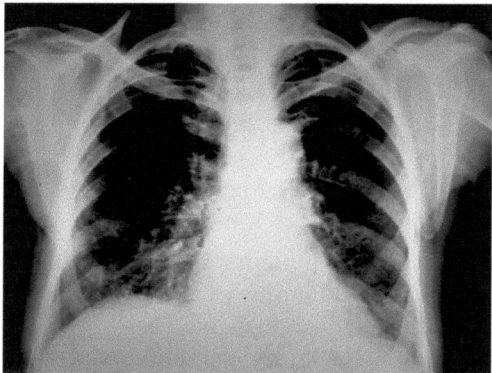

FIG. 9: Posteroanterior chest radiograph from a 60-year-old female Human immunodeficiency virus-positive patient with the tuberculosis lesions in lower lung lobes.

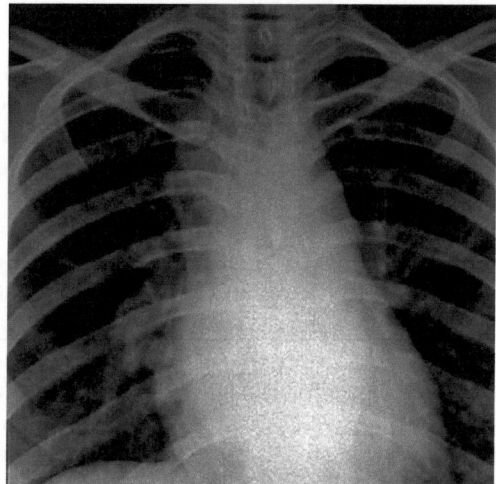

FIG. 10: Posteroanterior chest radiograph from a 37-year-old male Human immunodeficiency virus-positive patient with intrathoracic adenopathy bronchoscopically proven to be tuberculosis.

Newer technique for the diagnosis of latent infection, IGRA (the QuantiFERON-TB, QuantiFERON-TB Gold tests, the T-SPOT.TB test) is used increasingly to detect interferon-γ (IFN-γ) response to the Mtb-specific antigens, early secretory antigenic target-6 (ESAT-6), and culture filtrate protein-10.[27] Genes encoding these antigens are present in Mtb complex, but absent from BCG strain and most environmental NTM strains.[28,29]

The advantages of these tests include greater specificity (no cross reactivity with BCG and NTM) and improved sensitivity in immunosuppressed patients, and the lack of the need for follow-up in 48–72 hours. However, these tests are expensive and require some laboratory expertise, which limit their usefulness in the developing countries.[27,30,31]

The diagnosis of active TB often can be very difficult and it requires bacteriologic confirmation. Since a positive acid-fast smear is not specific for Mtb and other

TABLE 1	Sensitivity of sputum by smear and/or culture[32-35]		
Sputum sample	**By smear**	**By culture**	**By smear and/or culture**
Spontaneously produced	–	–	34–80%
Single sample	64%	70%	–
Induced sputum 3 samples	91%	99%	–

mycobacteria, both saprophytes and potential pathogens, that are usually acid-fast as well, can cause similar patterns of pulmonary disease. Thus, culture of Mtb is the only absolute way of confirming the diagnosis of active TB.

Freshly expectorated sputum is the best sample to stain and culture for Mtb. The sensitivity of expectorated sputum (by smear and/or culture) ranges from 34 to 80% in studies, and is highest in cavitary disease. If the patient is not spontaneously producing sputum, induced sputum is the next best specimen and a single induced sputum may have a yield of 64% for the diagnosis of TB by smear and 70% by culture. Increasing the number of induced sputum samples obtained to three increases the yield to 91% for smear and 99% for culture (Table 1).[32-35]

In some cases, bronchoscopy may be considered to obtain a sputum sample when none are expectorated or inducible. Since, irritation of the bronchial tree during the bronchoscopy procedure frequently leaves the patient with a productive cough, the collection of the postbronchoscopy sputum can be another valuable source of diagnostic material.[36-38]

Nucleic acid amplification (NAA) assays have become a useful adjunct in the diagnosis of TB. These assays amplify Mtb specific amino acid sequences using a probe. The advantage of these assays is that they require a much lower bacillus load to detect the presence of TB (10 bacillus vs 5,000–10,000 bacilli needed for smear-positivity and 10–100 organisms for positive culture). They are also very specific for Mtb and may not only detect Mtb, but also amplify sequences specific for isoniazid (INH) and rifampin resistance and thus may provide information on drug sensitivity as well. These sensitivity assays are not yet widely available for clinical practice; all are very expensive requiring a sophisticated laboratory as well. They are useful when attempting to confirm that a positive smear is indeed due to Mtb and may also be useful in cases with negative smears but a high clinical suspicion to suggest the diagnosis while awaiting the culture results.[39-43]

Still, in a significant number of cases, the diagnosis of TB had been made in the absence of bacteriologic confirmation, by a combination of a positive skin test, a compatible chest radiograph, and a therapeutic trial (clinical TB).

Bronchoscopy is essential diagnostic tool for endobronchial TB but also another possibility to obtain a specimen—not only a fiber aspirate but a biopsy sample to stain and culture for Mtb as well as to establish histologic diagnosis, in cases of suspected active pulmonary TB lesions in the absence of sputum bacteriologic confirmation.

The histological diagnosis of Mtb remains a diagnostic challenge despite different methods. There is evidence from recently published data that immunohistochemistry not only could confirm granulomatous tissue involvement but also can demonstrate Mtb antigen immunolocalization. It has been shown that positive immunohistochemical staining of TB granulomatous reactions not only highlights the presence of mycobacterial antigens for tissue diagnosis, but also morphologically localizes its distribution in different cells.[44]

In patients with HIV infection but without the manifestations of acquired immunodeficiency syndrome (AIDS), the TST is positive in 50–80% of patients with TB. Once an individual has developed AIDS, the TST is less likely to be positive, although reactivity may be seen in as many as 30–50% of patients. Active TB should be considered in any HIV-infected patient with a TST that has greater than 5 mm of induration. The proportion of positive sputum smears and cultures is similar for HIV-infected and uninfected patients. Therefore, the diagnostic algorithm of spontaneous or induced sputum followed by bronchoscopy with bronchoalveolar lavage (BAL) as for immunocompetent individuals should be followed. However, given the risk of rapid progression, the assumption must be that an acid-fast organism present in the sputum of a patient with HIV and pulmonary disease is Mtb, and treatment should be initiated while waiting for definitive identification of the organism.[1,15]

Specific Forms of Bronchogenic Tuberculosis

Tuberculoma usually manifests as a fairly discrete, sometimes with a spicular margin, nodule, or rounded mass lesion in the lungs. It can be a manifestation of primary infection or develop when a focus of reactivation TB becomes encapsulated,[45] cavitation is rare, and it represents the most common benign nodules representing up to 25% of all resected solitary pulmonary nodules.[46]

The differential diagnosis of pulmonary coin lesions is extensive, thus the diagnosis of tuberculoma can be difficult since sputum or fiber aspirate cultures are often negative. Differentiation between the active tuberculomas and malignant tumors is not easy, but cancer coexisting with tuberculoma may occur as well, mechanisms of this phenomenon remain unclear.[47,48] Invasive diagnostic procedures like fine needle aspiration or open lung biopsy are often necessary for diagnosis of tuberculoma.[49,50]

The benefits of surgical resection for pulmonary tuberculoma include the accurate diagnosis and differential diagnosis, determining future treatment strategies.[51] Limited pulmonary resection is required for patients with tuberculoma or most of other benign solitary pulmonary nodules,[52] preferably performed with the use of video-assisted thoracoscopic surgery, replacing traditional open thoracotomy (Fig. 11).[53-55]

Endobronchial tuberculosis (EBTB) is a chronic, progressive TB infection with bronchial and/or tracheal mucosal infiltration. It is characterized by hyperemia, edema,

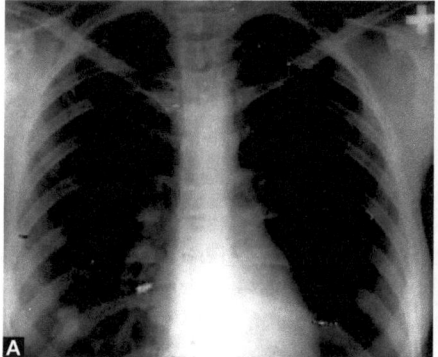 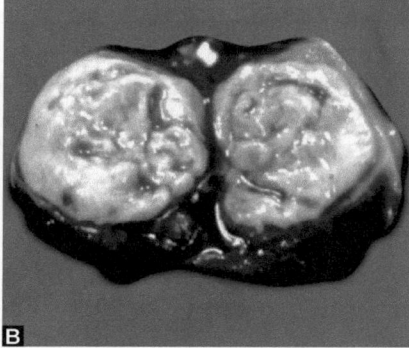

FIG. 11: Tumor-like lesion in the right lower lobe of a 46-year-old female patient with a long history of smoking who had surgery performed due to suspicion of lung cancer: histology finding of tuberculoma.

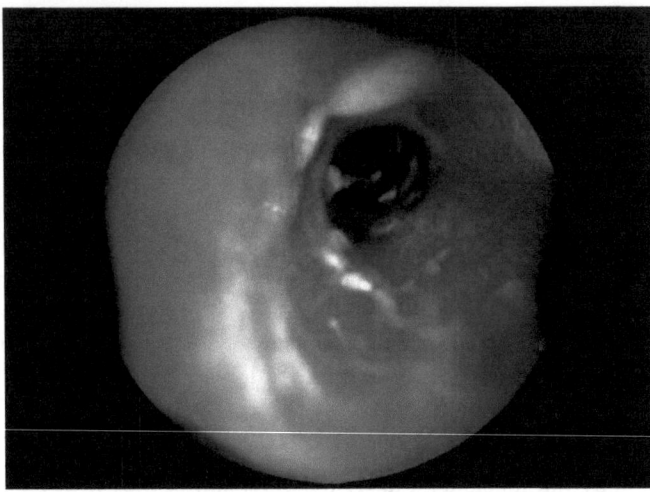

FIG. 12: Hyperemic, edematous mucosa of the trachea, covered with whitish (caseous) debris. Bronchoscopic biopsy revealed tuberculosis. A case of active-caseating form of endobronchial/tracheobronchial tuberculosis. *(For color version, see Plate 10)*

formation of granulation tissue, and sometimes with complicated clinical course, the occurrence of ulceration and bronchostenosis. This form of TB is often diagnosed with delay, until the onset of serious bronchial stenosis (Fig. 12).[56-58]

Endobronchial tuberculosis is noted in 10-40% of patients with active TB and often presents a diagnostic challenge because the clinical presentation varies, and positive rate of acid-fast bacillus (AFB) staining for sputum smears is low. Common chief complaints are often nondistinctive.

Although most EBTB patients have concurrent pulmonary lesions (often causing radiological findings to be misleading), some patients can have a normal chest radiography, even though the AFB positive sputum sample[56,59] and many published results evidenced normal chest radiographs in 10-20% of EBTB cases.[60,61] Normal chest radiography is one of major reasons the diagnosis of EBTB is often delayed.[62]

Bronchoscopy is essential diagnostic tool for EBTB. In patients investigated by bronchoscopy, the incidence of EBTB varies from 10 to 37%, often reported to be about 20%.[60]

Endobronchial tuberculosis occurs more commonly in young women, although a significant geriatric population is affected.[56,60]

Recently, the incidence of EBTB is shown to have two peaks with advancing age, thus also commonly observed in the old.[59] Possible reasons for that might be diminished immune function and comorbidities causing the reactivation of dormant bacilli, and the reinfection by exogenous bacilli.[63] Additionally, the extensive application of bronchoscopy due to suspicion of lung cancer also causes older patients with EBTB to be diagnosed. Racial and genetic differences might play an important role in the course and prognosis of EBTB. Published data on the detection rate of bacteriologic diagnostic methods of EBTB are rather controversial. Thus, some[58,64,65] confirm the assumption of high infectivity of patients with EBTB by the presence of simple sputum positive for AFB in 51.8-91% patients. In some other studies, significantly lower—9.1-17% smear sputum positive rate was observed.[56] Early EBTB diagnosis and early onset of therapy is of utmost importance to prevent the development of unwanted sequelae of bronchostenosis.

COMPLICATIONS

They include hemoptysis, bronchiectasis, extensive pulmonary destruction, pneumothorax, malignancy, and chronic pulmonary aspergillosis.

Hemoptysis

Hemoptysis occurs most frequently in the setting of active TB, but may also occur after completion of treatment.[66,67] Many patients with hemoptysis are AFB smear-positive and usually have cavitary disease. Mild hemoptysis is very frequent in acute infection while larger volume hemoptysis can occur later in the disease and may be due to rupture of a Rasmussen's aneurysm, still often fatal. Hemoptysis after the completion of therapy for TB only occasionally represents TB recurrence. In clinically healed TB patients, hemoptysis can occur due to the secondary development of an aspergilloma in residual cavities or due to exacerbations of bronchiectasis, rarely due to a carcinoma, or another infectious or inflammatory process. Patients with significant hemoptysis should undergo rapid evaluation to define the source of bleeding and enable immediate intervention and in some circumstances, conservative management is sufficient even for major or massive hemoptysis.[68,69] The exceptions are the cases of possible exsanguination, which require immediate surgical care.[70,71]

Bronchiectasis

Minor endobronchial disease of the distal bronchi is frequent finding in TB, but significant bronchial stenosis of major bronchi is rare. The same endobronchial processes may result in bronchiectasis due to destruction of the bronchial wall, usually involving the distal airways with a predilection for the upper lobes. Often this bronchiectasis is associated with little sputum production (dry bronchiectasis) and may manifest itself predominantly as low-grade hemoptysis. Infection with typical respiratory pathogens can convert "dry" to "wet" bronchiectasis, with frequent exacerbations of infection and occasionally hemoptysis.[1,4,15]

Extensive Pulmonary Destruction

Rarely, TB can cause progressive, extensive destruction of areas of one or both lungs.[72,73] In primary TB, occasionally lymph node obstruction of the bronchi together with distal collapse, necrosis, and bacterial superinfection can produce lung tissue destruction.[73] More commonly, destruction results from years of chronic reactivation TB, typically in the absence of effective chemotherapy leading to increased death risk of severe respiratory failure, superinfection, and massive hemoptysis. Radiographically, patients typically have large cavities and fibrosis of remaining lung (Fig. 13).[72,73]

Pneumothorax

Pneumothorax is a rare but serious complication of TB which is thought to occur from subpleural infection rupturing into the pleural space. This may lead to the spread of infection into the pleural space and, if left untreated, can lead to the development of an empyema with subsequent fibrothorax and associated trapped lung. A bronchopleural fistula may persist after a pneumothorax and, especially if untreated, may result in major problems from secondary or superimposed bacterial infection (mixed empyema) (Figs. 14 and 15).[74-76]

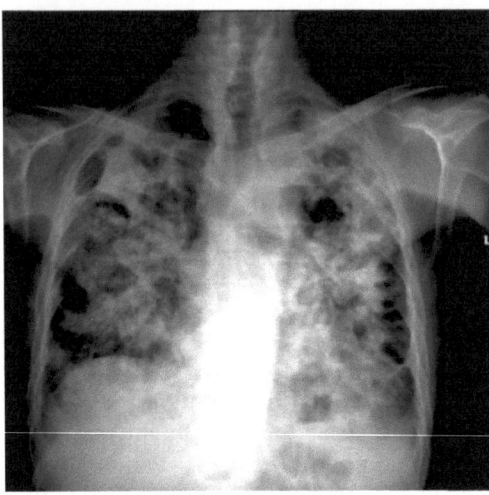

FIG. 13: Posteroanterior chest radiograph from a 62-year-old male, alcohol addicted, chronic bilateral multicavitary tuberculosis with extensive pulmonary destruction.

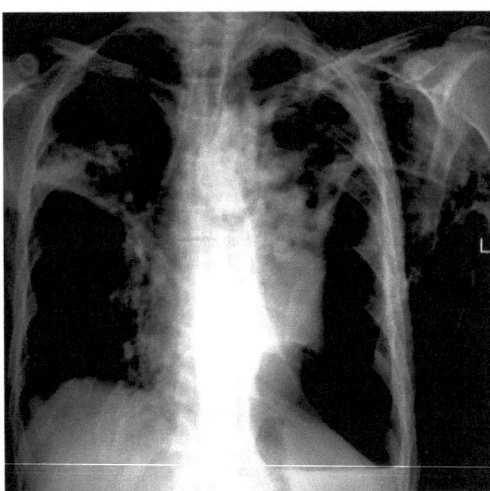

FIG. 14: Posteroanterior chest radiograph from a 32-year-old male with relapsed multicavitary tuberculosis and development of left-sided pneumothorax.

Chronic Pulmonary Aspergillosis

Even if TB is treated and cured, the destruction of lung parenchyma can lead to later complications as is colonization of cavities and areas of bronchiectasis that may occur with a variety of infectious agents. Aspergillus species may commonly colonize and/or infect areas of damaged lung. Chronic pulmonary aspergillosis as a sequela of pulmonary TB can further jeopardize patient's life due to its common complications, significant or massive hemoptysis (Fig. 16).[1,4,15,77,78]

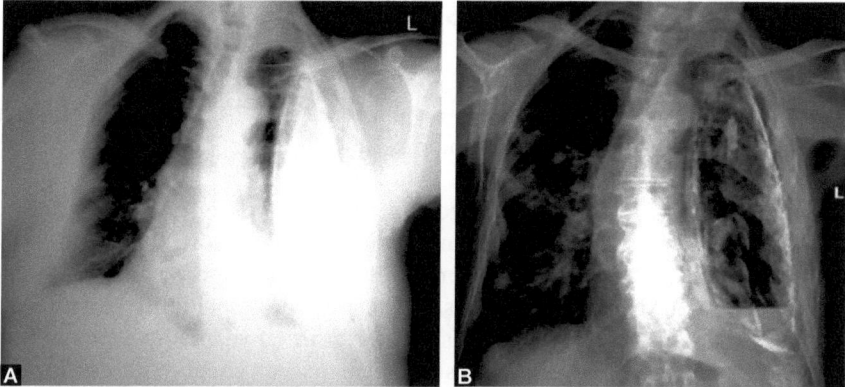

FIG. 15: Posteroanterior chest radiographs from an 82-year-old male with a history of treated pulmonary and pleural tuberculosis in his youth, massive sequela, developing pleural tuberculosis relapse with superimposed bacterial infection—proven mixed empyema: before and after evacuation of the empyema fluid, respectively.

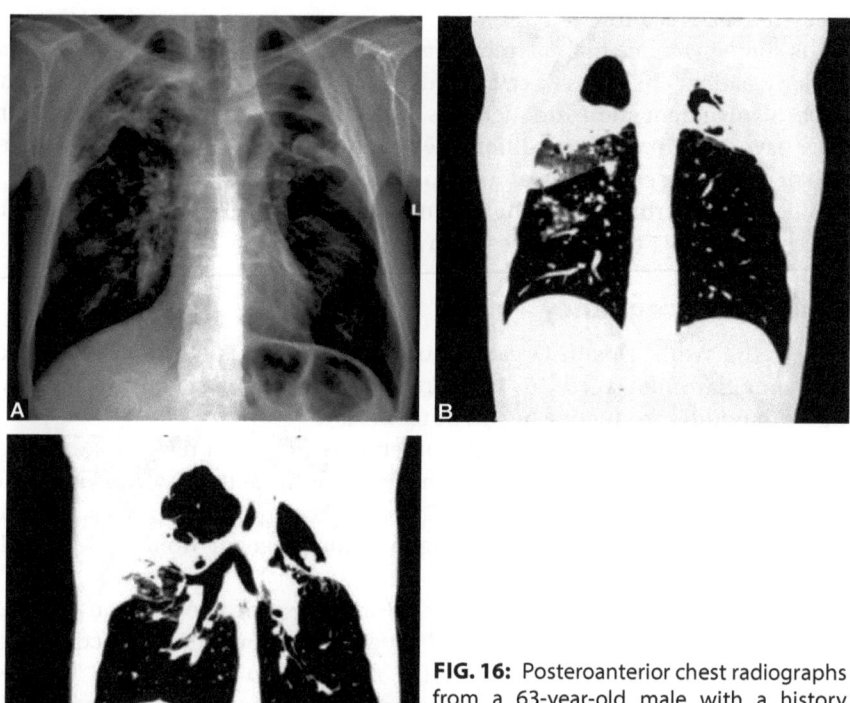

FIG. 16: Posteroanterior chest radiographs from a 63-year-old male with a history of treated bilateral cavitary pulmonary tuberculosis, presenting with massive hemoptysis due to development of chronic pulmonary aspergillosis as a sequela of pulmonary tuberculosis.

TUBERCULOSIS IN SPECIAL HOSTS

Tuberculosis in the Elderly

In nonendemic countries, the incidence of pulmonary TB is 2-3 times higher among older patients, especially those in old age homes, and the risk of death is higher compared with younger patients.[79,80]

Not only is increasing age a risk factor for the development of active TB, but the disease itself may present differently in the elderly, making it more difficult to recognize.

Comparative studies have suggested some differences in manifestations of pulmonary TB between elderly and younger patients. A meta-analysis including 12 studies noted no significant difference between patients greater than 60 years and patients less than 60 years with respect to time to diagnosis, prevalence of cough, sputum production, weight loss, or fatigue/malaise,[81] but less commonly observed findings among the elderly included fever, sweats, hemoptysis and a positive TST, and they were likely to present with the nonspecific symptoms of dyspnea, and fatigue. Findings noted more frequently among the elderly include anemia, elevated erythrocyte sedimentation rates, hyponatremia, hypoalbuminemia, leukopenia, and underlying disorders, comorbidities such as cardiovascular disease, chronic obstructive pulmonary disease (COPD), diabetes, malignancy, and gastrectomy.

There is some evidence that "atypical" radiographic findings are common in nearly half of elderly patients having TB: cavitary disease is less common and multilobar and lower lobe involvement more frequent, as well as a pleural reaction. However, not all studies have confirmed these differences, some of them pointing to an increased incidence of miliary disease in the older population.

It should be underlined that the diagnosis in older patients can be delayed or missed because of other comorbidities such as COPD.[82,83]

Tuberculosis in Pregnancy

According to the World Health Organization (WHO),[84] TB is the third leading cause of death among women aged 15-44 years. Tuberculosis can cause infertility and contributes to poor reproductive health outcomes.[85-88]

In resource-rich countries, pregnant women with high TB prevalence are migrants and people of foreign origin,[89-94] while in resource-limited countries, HIV-infected pregnant women are the group with high TB prevalence and mortality.[87,88,95-99]

The major problem concerning TB diagnosis for pregnant women is the delay in diagnosis.

Pregnancy itself is not a risk factor for TB and has not been shown to influence the pathogenesis of TB or the likelihood of progression from latent infection to active disease nor has it been shown to affect the response to treatment.[100-104] However, maternal infection can lead to congenital infection or neonatal infection. In addition, TB in pregnant women can present insidiously since symptoms of malaise and fatigue may be attributed to pregnancy rather than infection.[105]

Thus, TB in pregnant women is more difficult to diagnose because TB symptoms such as fatigue, shortness of breath, sweating, tiredness, cough, and mild fever are similar to physiological symptoms of pregnancy. Untreated TB or TB treated late may lead to severe consequences affecting both mother and child.[106,107] Without treatment, TB may lead to increased neonatal morbidity, low birth weight, prematurity, and increased pregnancy complications, including fourfold increases in maternal morbidity due to higher rates of abortion, postpartum hemorrhage, labor difficulties, and pre-eclampsia.[87,88,105]

Latent Tuberculosis

Screening for LTBI should be performed during pregnancy only for those women at high risk for progression from latent to active disease (e.g., women who have been infected recently and those who have HIV or are otherwise significantly immunocompromised).[87,88]

Tuberculin skin testing as a diagnostic tool for latent TB can be performed safely in pregnant women, and pregnancy does not alter the response to the TST.[90,108,109] However, its result can be affected by HIV infection or any situation that severely weakens the immune system (such as disseminated TB), as these could lead to false-negative results.[94,110,111] Bacillus Calmette–Guérin vaccination can also lead to TST-positive results in healthy women.[89,93] In a high HIV prevalence setting, other tests and clinical symptoms should therefore be taken into account in diagnosing TB[99] and the TST and anergy skin tests are recommended as a TB screening method in the prenatal care procedures.[112] In populations in which the majority of people are BCG vaccinated or their vaccination status is uncertain, TST is discouraged and IGRA is recommended for TB screening and diagnosis.[89,93] Interferon-gamma release assays are also safe in pregnancy and likely as effective for diagnosis of LTBI in pregnancy as in other circumstances.[89,113-115] The advantage of the IGRA test over TST is evident in TB screening and diagnosis for HIV-positive pregnant women, since its sensitivity is not affected by HIV infection.[110] Patients with positive LTBI screening results must undergo clinical evaluation to rule out active TB as in nonpregnant individuals, including radiographic examination of the chest (with appropriate shielding).[87,88]

Tuberculosis prevention includes BCG vaccination in childhood and INH prophylaxis for LTBI-positive pregnant women. A low completion rate of INH therapy was noted and a high risk of INH toxic hepatitis, with pregnant women having a 2.5-fold greater risk of INH hepatitis than nonpregnant women.

Active Tuberculosis

Active maternal infection may lead to congenital infection by hematogenous dissemination via the placenta, although congenital infection is very rare.

Pregnant patients with pulmonary TB typically have the same clinical manifestations as nonpregnant patients, although TB in pregnant women can present insidiously, since malaise and fatigue may be attributed to pregnancy rather than disease[91] and it can be difficult to recognize weight loss.[87,88]

The procedures for TB diagnosis for pregnant women include the sputum test (AFB) and the shielded chest X-ray.[90-92,111,116] The AFB smear test appears to have low sensitivity in pregnant women,[90,111,116] but is still used in low-resource settings as part of the procedure for diagnosing active TB due to its low cost and simple technique.[109,111] Acid-fast bacillus culture is used as a confirmation of diagnosis, but is time consuming and not available in low-resource settings.[91,109] Fluorescence microscopy is recommended as a substitute for AFB culture because it is cheaper;[109] but this procedure is for pulmonary TB cases only and cannot identify extrapulmonary TB without additional tests.

Treatment of TB in the setting of pregnancy should be initiated if the suspicion of active disease is moderate to high (such as a persistent upper lobe infiltrate and cough in a high-risk individual, and/or a positive AFB smear or NAA test), since untreated disease represents a greater hazard to the mother and fetus than anti-TB therapy. The principles in HIV-seronegative pregnant patients are the same as for nonpregnant patients, except for the exclusion of certain medications.[87,88] Regarding effectiveness and safety of anti-TB drugs, no significant association was noted between child abnormality and mother's exposure to anti-TB drugs, both for first- and second-line anti-TB drugs (including drugs of the aminoglycosides group, fluoroquinolone, thioamides, cycloserines, and terizidones) during pregnancy.[117-122]

Treatment outcome is generally positive. It has been shown that with an attentive follow-up and appropriate therapy, multidrug-resistant (MDR)-TB pregnant women can be cured and have a positive maternal outcome, and should therefore be given the option to continue with a pregnancy.[119,121,122] There is evidence that a delay in, or default, MDR treatment are the main causes of mortality and morbidity for mothers and babies.[87,88,120-122]

Tuberculosis in Diabetes Mellitus Patients

The association between DM and TB has been well recognized. Tuberculosis has increasingly become a problem in low-income countries, particularly those with HIV epidemics, and noninsulin-dependent DM a growing worldwide chronic disease, as a consequence of increases in obesity, changing patterns of diet and physical activity, and aging populations.[123-125]

The effect of diabetes on the development and severity of TB, and the complex interrelations between nutrition, obesity, diabetes, and TB represent a significant health problem particularly in the setting of the increasing overlap of populations at risk for both diseases.[126-128] Coaffliction with TB and DM is common, both in low-income and high-income countries.[124,129-131]

The higher risk of DM patients to TB is the most solid and clinically important finding, and hence, the best characterized aspect of the association between TB and DM.

Diabetes mellitus being an important risk factor for TB[132,133] has an impact at every stage of the natural history of TB with proven association between dysfunctional immunity and clinical characteristics of TB (Fig. 17). Current evidence is that the dysfunctional immune response of the DM host to Mtb antigens is likely to influence the development, clinical presentation, and outcomes of TB but the mechanisms involved are poorly understood.

Dysfunctional Innate and Adaptive Immunity to Mycobacterium Tuberculosis in Diabetes Mellitus Patients

Innate immunity to Mtb in the DM host: Diabetic monocytes significantly reduce binding and phagocytosis of Mtb most probably due to alterations in the diabetic monocyte as well as in serum opsonins for Mtb, particularly the C3 component of complement which mediates Mtb phagocytosis.[134,135]

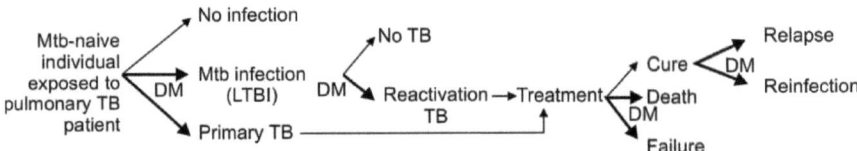

Mtb, *Mycobacterium tuberculosis*; DM, diabetes mellitus; LTBI, latent tuberculous infection.

FIG. 17: Impact of diabetes on the natural history of tuberculosis.

There is a reduced uptake of Mtb by alveolar macrophages within 2 weeks of infection,[136] as well as a delayed innate immunity to Mtb due to late delivery of Mtb bearing antigen-presenting cells to the lung draining lymph nodes.[137] These delays likely contribute to the higher risk of DM patients for Mtb infection and persistence.

Innate and adaptive immunity to Mtb in the DM host with LTBI and TB: There is no data on the type of immunity to Mtb that facilitates the progression from LTBI to TB in individuals with underlying DM (versus no DM), but an increasing number of studies in DM patients that developed TB indicate a paradoxical hyperinflammatory response.

Stimulation of peripheral white blood cells with mycobacterial antigens results in higher Th1 and Th17 responses, including higher IFN-γ and interleukin (IL)-17 secretion,[138-140] as well as other cytokines promoting immunity in TB-DM versus TB-no DM, such as IL-2 and granulocyte-macrophage colony-stimulating factor (GM-CSF).[138,139] Tuberculosis-DM cases also have a higher frequency of cytokine producing CD4+ Th1 cells in response to Mtb antigens (for IFN-γ, TNF-α, or IL-2).[139] These hyperactive responses in peripheral blood contrast with the results from few studies conducted at the site of infection (in BAL) where TB-DM patients appear to have reduced activation of immunity; one reported a lower proportion of activated alveolar macrophages, and another higher IL-10 (which is anti-inflammatory) and lower IFN-γ.[141] The impact of the host compartment (peripheral blood versus lung) requires further study (Table 2).

Impact of DM on the natural history of TB—risk of Mtb infection, persistence, and LTBI: The detection of a delayed and defective innate immune response to Mtb in DM provides indirect support for the higher risk of LTBI among contacts with DM. However, the relative risk of LTBI among contacts of TB patients with DM (vs no DM) has not been systematically measured in contemporary epidemiological studies, but preliminary findings suggest that DM patients may be more likely to become infected with Mtb.

The incidence of TB in patients with diabetes is evidently high.[123] Diabetes mellitus patients generally have a three-fold higher risk of developing TB. Most subsequent studies have confirmed that there is a significant TB risk in DM patients, but with variable effect sizes and even with some not showing a significant risk.[142-144] Several case-control studies have shown that the relative odds of developing TB in diabetic patients ranges from 2.44 to 8.33 compared with nondiabetic patients[145-148] and a number of large-scale longitudinal cohort studies have shown similar findings.[129,143,149,150]

This variation of studies data is likely the result of interaction or additive effects between the relatively "mild" contribution of DM to immune dysfunction and a variety

TABLE 2	Defective immune response to mycobacterium tuberculosis in diabetes mellitus host
Immunity to Mtb in Mtb-naïve hosts with DM (vs no DM)	**Immunity to Mtb in TB-DM hosts (vs. TB-no DM)**
Delayed T-cell priming	↑Th1 and Th17 cell-mediated response specific to Mtb antigens
↓IFN-γ	↓T-regulatory lymphocytes
↓Phagocytosis	↑IL-10 (anti-inflammatory)

Mtb, Mycobacterium tuberculosis; DM, diabetes mellitus; Th, helper T-cell; IFN, interferon; IL, interleukin; TB, tuberculosis.

of additional host factors that also depress immunity, vary across study populations, and are not always taken into account. In epidemiological studies, the most notable are poor glucose control and older age.[143,151,152]

Thus, TB develops most frequently in patients with poor diabetic control. It has been shown that diabetic patients who needed more than 40 units of insulin per day were twice as likely to develop TB as those using lower doses, thus linking severity of DM with risk of TB.[123]

Among studies with convincing data that DM is a moderate-to-strong risk factor for the development of active TB,[123,129,143,145-150] several studies provide evidence that insulin dependence, as a marker for severity of disease, predicts increased TB risk as well as does a poor glycemic control.[143,153,154]

The relationship between DM and other cofactors that enhance TB risk is emerging, particularly between DM and smoking.[155]

Radiographic Findings in Tuberculous Diabetic Patients

Pulmonary TB accounts for 70-80% of the cases, and it is generally accepted that compromised immunity facilitates early and late hematogenous dissemination of Mtb, predisposing to extrapulmonary TB. Current findings in DM patients consistently show lower extrapulmonary TB.[143,131,156-158] This may be due to a hyper-reactive cell-mediated immune response to Mtb in DM patients that may be suboptimal for containing Mtb growth within the lung, but effective for preventing its dissemination and reactivation elsewhere.[138,140,159]

The radiographic presentation of TB depends on many factors, including duration of illness and host immune status. It was widely believed that pulmonary TB in diabetic patients presented with an atypical radiographic pattern and distribution, particularly lower lung involvement which might be misdiagnosed as community-acquired pneumonia or cancer. Importantly, patients with pulmonary TB that do not have upper lobe involvement are less likely to have positive sputum smears and cultures.[160] In most series, multilobar disease or the presence of multiple cavities is more common in diabetic patients, but lower lung disease was rarely more common in diabetic patients than in controls, except, perhaps, in patients aged over 40 years.[161-165] Results vary substantially between studies and the frequency of unusual radiographic findings in diabetic patients has probably been overstated. The fact that TB-DM patients are more likely than TB-no DM to present with cavitary TB, particularly those with poor glycemic control, is in accordance with their robust cell-mediated immunity to Mtb antigens and their subsequent strong cell-mediated immune response.[166-168] Cavitary TB is accompanied by higher bacillary burden in the sputa of TB-DM patients.[131,158]

The higher frequency of pulmonary TB versus extrapulmonary TB, cavitary TB, and smear-positive TB would predict that TB-DM patients are more infectious than TB-no DM.[169] This is further supported by data indicating delays in their conversion to smear-negative or for prolonged culture-positivity during the course of treatment, having a significant public health impact.

In studies assessing time to sputum-culture conversion, diabetic patients seem to take longer to achieve culture negativity.[170,171] Together, these data suggest that although bacillary burden might be higher at presentation in diabetic patients, leading to modestly longer times to sputum-culture conversion, rates of sputum-culture conversion are similar to those of nondiabetic patients by 2-3 months of treatment.

However, there is growing evidence from observational studies that this TB-DM comorbidity is associated with not only delays in Mtb clearance during treatment, but treatment failures, death, relapse, and reinfection.[151,172,173]

Diabetes mellitus is most often associated with delayed mycobacterial clearance from sputum during the course of treatment,[172,174] why TB-DM versus TB-no DM patients have a higher proportion of smear-positives after completion of the intensive phase of treatment, or longer median days to mycobacterial clearance from sputum. These outcomes are early predictors of treatment failure (sputum smear or culture positivity at 5 months or later during treatment), which is also more likely in TB-DM versus TB-no DM.[173,175,176]

Nevertheless, in a systematic review and meta-analysis of contemporary literature, the risk of death in 23 unadjusted studies was nearly twofold, and this increased to 4.95 in four studies that adjusted for age and potential confounders.[176]

Although studies suggest that treatment failure and death are more frequent in diabetic patients whether aggressive management of DM would improve treatment, response remains unclear. Furthermore, because causes of death are not reported in most studies, it is not known whether excess mortality can be explained by increased severity of TB in diabetic patients or by the existence of comorbidities attributable to DM especially in more advanced age.

Tuberculosis-DM patients also appears to have a higher risk of relapse. The systematic review and meta-analysis reported a nearly fourfold risk of relapse in TB-DM versus TB-no DM.[176] A more recent prospective study further distinguished between relapses and reinfections and found higher adjusted odds of both in DM versus no DM (OR = 1.8 for both recurrence and relapse).[173] The higher frequency of adverse outcomes in DM patients suggests that the hyperreactive immune response to mycobacterial antigens in TB-DM patients is not effective for Mtb killing with possible explanations that higher Th1 and Th17 response is only present in the peripheral blood of TB-DM patients, while an anti-inflammatory response that facilitates Mtb growth is located at the site of infection, the lungs, and furthermore, this hyperreaction to Mtb antigens may contribute to lung tissue damage and hence, to the higher frequency of death in these patients.

The characteristics of TB in DM patients have been shown in box 1.

BOX 1 | Characteristics of tuberculosis in diabetes mellitus patients

- Coaffliction with tuberculosis (TB) and diabetes mellitus (DM) common[124,129-131]
- Delayed and defective innate immune response to *Mycobacterium tuberculosis* (Mtb) in DM and paradoxical hyperinflammatory cell-mediated immune response
- Diabetes mellitus an important risk factor for TB, a threefold higher risk of developing TB[132,133]
- Relative odds of developing TB in DM 2.44–8.33 compared with non-DM[129,143,145-150]
- Insulin dependence and poor glycemic control predict increased TB risk[143,153,154]
- Higher frequency of pulmonary TB (70–80% of the cases) versus extrapulmonary TB
- Multilobar disease or cavitary TB and smear-positive TB more common[161-165]
- Delays in conversion to smear-negative/prolonged culture-positivity during the course of treatment, treatment failure also more likely in TB-DM versus TB-no DM[173,175,176]
- The risk of death nearly twofold increased to 4.95 if adjusted for age and potential confounders[176]
- Higher risk of relapse, nearly fourfold risk of relapse in TB-DM versus TB-no DM[176]

Pulmonary Tuberculosis in Dialysis Patients

Dialysis patients are immunocompromised, having impaired cellular immunity, and at higher risk for TB. Diagnosis is difficult and often delayed due to extrapulmonary involvement and nonspecific symptoms. The incidence of extrapulmonary TB varies from 15.7 to 83.8% while in the general population, extrapulmonary TB accounts for 15–20%.[177-182] The common sites of involvement are lung, lymph node, pleura, and peritoneum.[183,184]

Several studies[185-193] have found a high incidence of TB during the first year after initiation of dialysis, attributed to the poor general health and reduced immunity at that stage.

As the incidence of TB is high in hemodialysis patients, with the predominance of extrapulmonary involvement, they should be evaluated periodically to exclude insidious infection and reduce morbidity and mortality. Physicians must be alert to unusual presentations and localizations of the disease; TB should be strongly suspected in endemic regions.[177,184]

Active Tuberculosis

Published data in 1980s strongly suggested that the incidence of active TB was much higher in dialysis patients than in the general population[185,194-196] with often atypical clinical presentation. Pulmonary disease is less common (<25% of cases) than in the general population. Fever, weight loss and anorexia in the context of pleural effusions, lymphadenopathy, ascites, and hepatomegaly being atypical presentation often led to delayed diagnosis.[177,184]

Active pulmonary TB should be suspected in cases of cough of greater than 2–3 weeks duration with fever, night sweats, weight loss, or hemoptysis; any patient at high risk for TB who has pneumonia that does not respond to conventional antibiotics (including HIV-positive, patients from endemic areas, or on immunosuppressive therapy); and asymptomatic patients with chest X-ray abnormalities suggestive of TB. Extrapulmonary TB should be considered in any unexplained illness manifested by some combination of prolonged fever, weight loss, lymphadenopathy, ascites, hepatomegaly, and pleural effusion.

For suspected active pulmonary TB, chest X-ray and sputum analysis are key analyses. Typical chest X-ray findings include focal upper lobe infiltrates, cavitation, and hilar adenopathy and fibrosis. Atypical findings include lower lobe or more extensive infiltrates, pleural effusions, and miliary TB. Clinically, suspicious features for active disease and no positive diagnostic test (detection of organisms by smear and/or culture, or positive findings of more sensitive and specific nucleic acid detection techniques) are not uncommon. The finding of caseating granulomas is suggestive, but not diagnostic of mycobacterial infection. Up to 20% of patients with a clinical diagnosis of TB never have positive bacterial confirmation. Therefore, nephrologists must have a high index of suspicion for the disease.[177,184]

Latent Tuberculosis

According to a number of studies using different diagnostic approaches, the prevalence of LTBI in chronic dialysis patients was high, ranging between 20 and 70%.[197-200] Dialysis patients have a much higher incidence of reactivation of latent TB, roughly tenfold higher risk than the general population, not only because of their immunosuppressed state but due to several other factors as well: immigrant populations from areas of endemic TB have a higher prevalence of end-stage kidney disease than residents of North America and Europe; highly likely transmission in a case of active TB patient in a hemodialysis unit, often atypical clinical manifestations of active TB more frequently involving organs other than the lungs, making quick diagnosis challenging. Latent TB must be diagnosed and treated before kidney transplantation, but the ability to diagnose latent TB has some limitations. However, other dialysis patients whose life expectancy is more than 10 years, but who are not transplant candidates must be screened and treated if they have evidence for latent TB as well. The underlying risk of having latent TB can be clinically assessed before deciding to screen for latent TB. Such is a case of immigrants from countries where TB is endemic, who are at considerably higher risk, and cases with typical abnormalities on routine chest X-ray that increase the probability of latent TB. Two tests currently available to detect latent TB are the same as for other population, the TST and IGRAs. Kidney failure induces some degree of immunosuppression that can result in a negative TST despite the presence of latent TB. The second problem with the TST is false-positives from exposure to atypical mycobacterial infections or to BCG vaccination, which is a common practice in much of the world outside of North America and parts of Europe. Thus in hemodialysis patients, TST is an insensitive test for the diagnosis of latent TB, missing about 80% of patients who probably have the disease. The advantage of the IGRA tests is that they have fewer false-negative results and greater sensitivity (of about 75%) in dialysis patients.[201] Given the expense of IGRA testing, a TST followed by an IGRA is the most cost-effective approach. Nevertheless, as even the combination of both tests will leave some false-negative results, clinical judgment still plays an important role. So, testing for latent TB should include also a clinical risk evaluation based on country of origin, prior Mtb exposure plus chest X-ray.[184]

Preventive therapy may not be useful in patients with short life expectancies which is the case in majority of patients on dialysis, additionally with the increased risk of adverse effects.

Short-course chemotherapy is effective, but, as adverse effects of anti-TB treatment are seen more frequently in these patients, they must be carefully observed during treatment.

High mortality of 17–75% in hemodialysis patients with TB is reported.[185,186,188,194,196,202-204] The delayed diagnosis and treatment played a major role in some instances while in other cases, the mortality was apparently caused by comorbid conditions. Reports of favorable outcome with no mortality are most likely due to early diagnosis and treatment.[187,189-191] A shorter duration of hemodialysis and being underweight were found to be significant risk-factors contributing to mortality.[205]

Tuberculosis in Solid Organ Transplant Recipients

Solid organ transplant (SOT) recipients are at risk for opportunistic infections including TB.

Tuberculosis in the allograft recipient is a common problem, particularly in developing countries where the TB incidence and prevalence in the general population is high.[206,207] The reported TB incidence in renal allograft recipients is 12.3%.[208,209]

The actual burden may be even much higher in the developing countries due to underreporting. The clinical presentation of TB differs in solid organ recipients and a high level of suspicion is important in diagnosing the problem.

Solid organ transplant recipients are at increased risk for opportunistic infections due to lifelong immunosuppression,[206] so other infections like cytomegalovirus downgrade host immunity and can activate occult TB infection as well. Also, the emergence of primary and secondary drug-resistant Mycobacterium may have a severe impact in the organ transplant setting.

The risk for active TB in SOT recipients is estimated to be 20–74 times higher than in the general population.[210] In addition to standard TB risk factors, there are several more: T-cell-depleting antibodies, higher intensity immunosuppression, liver disease, renal insufficiency and hemodialysis, DM and increased recipient age.[211-215] Particularly lung transplant recipients are at higher risk for TB.[206,212,216]

About 45–60% of TB occurs in the first year after transplantation. The median time for onset is at 9 months post transplantation.[217]

Reactivation from previously acquired infection is the predominant mode of developing TB in developing nations. Reinfection occurs only in a minority. This should especially be suspected in the presence of MDR organisms. The engrafted organ has also been shown to be the carrier in some rare cases.

The management of latent TB and active TB in the SOT population may differ by TB prevalence.

The frequency of active TB in SOT recipients in low-prevalence regions (<20 TB cases per 100,000 population) varies from 0.26 to 6.5%.[212,216,217] In addition to an increased risk for TB, TB-associated mortality is higher in SOT recipients (6–22%)[212,213,217,218] compared to other TB patients.[206]

In low-prevalence regions, extrapulmonary and disseminated TB is more common (45–67% of cases)[213,216,217] in SOT recipients, and it may occur in uncommon sites of TB involvement including kidneys, gastrointestinal tract, joints, and skin.

Symptoms may be nonspecific including fever, weight loss, and night sweats. Fever seen in most patients and TB should be considered in SOT recipients with fever of unknown origin.[206,217]

The lung is the major site of involvement followed by pyrexia of unknown origin as the other characteristic manifestation in high-prevalence regions. If there is no other conclusive evidence for other infections, empirical anti-TB therapy is usually justified.[219] The involvement of the liver, bone marrow, meninges, pericardial disease, or miliary disease is characteristic for disseminated disease, but lung involvement is universal in high-prevalence regions (noted in 85.2% of patients with disseminated disease).[220]

Chest imaging findings include focal infiltrates (40%), miliary pattern (22%), pleural effusions (13%), and nodules (5%) while cavities are unusual (4%).[206,217]

Fibrosis and regional adenopathy may be noted as well, the upper lobe is not often involved and the disease may be bilateral. Tuberculosis thus should be suspected in any patient with radiological evidence of pulmonary infiltrates. Occasionally, the diagnosis is made in asymptomatic patient who undergoes a chest X-ray for other reasons.

Time to diagnosis is often delayed due to extrapulmonary involvement, atypical presentations and imaging, and coinfections.[212,213,217,221] Lack of obvious TB risk factors may increase time to diagnosis as well.

There are difficulties in diagnosis, changes in the protocols of treatment as compared to the general population, the prognosis, risk factors for acquiring the disease.

Treatment of TB requires a multidrug regimen administered for appropriate duration in adequate doses. Compliance is equally important. Drug resistance and atypical mycobacterial infections are emerging problems and should be suspected in the nonresponding patients.

Overall mortality is approximately 30%. Higher mortality is due to immunosuppression and comorbidities.[217,222] Increased mortality is associated with delayed diagnosis, disseminated disease, prior organ rejection, and receipt of anti-T-cell antibodies.[206,217,222]

REFERENCES

1. Mason RJ, Broaddus VC, Martin TR, et al. Murray and Nadel's Textbook of Respiratory Medicine. 5th ed. Philadelphia: Saunders Elsevier; 2010.
2. Centers for Disease Control and Prevention (CDC). Trends in tuberculosis—United States, 2008. MMWR Morb Mortal Wkly Rep. 2009;58:249-53.
3. Small PM, Schecter GF, Goodman PC, Sande MA, Chaisson RE, Hopewell PC. Treatment of tuberculosis in patients with advanced human immunodeficiency virus infection. N Engl J Med. 1991;324:289-94.
4. Fishman A, Elias J, Fishman J, Grippi M, Senior RM, Pack AI. Fishman's Pulmonary Diseases and Disorders, 4th ed. New York: McGraw-Hill; 2008.
5. Kiblawi SS, Jay SJ, Stonehill RB, Norton J. Fever response of patients on therapy for pulmonary tuberculosis. Am Rev Respir Dis. 1981;123:20-4.
6. Arango L, Brewin AW, Murray JF. The spectrum of tuberculosis as currently seen in a metropolitan hospital. Am Rev Respir Dis. 1973;108:805-12.
7. Breen RA, Leonard O, Perrin FM, et al. How good are systemic symptoms and blood inflammatory markers at detecting individuals with tuberculosis? Int J Tuberc Lung Dis. 2008;12:44-9.
8. Cameron SJ. Tuberculosis and the blood—a special relationship? Tubercle. 1974;55:55-72.
9. Chung DK, Hubbard WW. Hyponatremia in untreated active pulmonary tuberculosis. Am Rev Respir Dis. 1969;99:595-7.
10. Vorherr H, Massry SG, Fallet R, Kaplan L, Kleeman CR. Antidiuretic principle in tuberculous lung tissue of a patient with pulmonary tuberculosis and hyponatremia. Ann Intern Med. 1970;72:383-7.
11. Lee P, Ho KK. Hyponatremia in pulmonary TB: evidence of ectopic antidiuretic hormone production. Chest. 2010;137:207-8.
12. Markowitz N, Hansen NI, Hopewell PC, et al. Incidence of tuberculosis in the United States among HIV-infected persons. The Pulmonary Complications of HIV Infection Study Group. Ann Intern Med. 1997;126:123-32.
13. Barnes PF, Verdegem TD, Vachon LA, Leedom JM, Overturf GD. Chest roentgenogram in pulmonary tuberculosis. New data on an old test. Chest. 1988;94:316-20.
14. Day JH, Charalambous S, Fielding KL, Hayes RJ, Churchyard GJ, Grant AD. Screening for tuberculosis prior to isoniazid preventive therapy among HIV-infected gold miners in South Africa. Int J Tuberc Lung Dis. 2006;10:523-9.
15. Pozniak A. (2016). Clinical manifestations and evaluation of pulmonary tuberculosis. [online] UpToDate website. Available from www.uptodate.com [Accessed January, 2016].
16. Marciniuk DD, McNab BD, Martin WT, Hoeppner VH. Detection of pulmonary tuberculosis in patients with a normal chest radiograph. Chest. 1999;115:445-52.
17. Lentino W, Jacobson HG, Poppel MH. Segmental localization of upper lobe tuberculosis; the rarity of anterior involvement. Am J Roentgenol Radium Ther Nucl Med. 1957;77:1042-7.
18. Woodring JH, Vandiviere HM, Fried AM, Dillon ML, Williams TD, Melvin IG. Update: the radiographic features of pulmonary tuberculosis. AJR Am J Roentgenol. 1986;146:497-506.
19. Poppius H, Thomander K. Segmentary distribution of cavities; a radiologic study of 500 consecutive cases of cavernous pulmonary tuberculosis. Ann Med Intern Fenn. 1957;46:113-9.
20. Farman DP, Speir WA. Initial roentgenographic manifestations of bacteriologically proven Mycobacterium tuberculosis. Typical or atypical? Chest. 1986;89:75-7.
21. Segarra F, Sherman DS, Rodriguez-Aguero J. Lower lung field tuberculosis. Am Rev Respir Dis. 1963;87:37-40.
22. Stead WW. Tuberculosis among elderly persons: an outbreak in a nursing home. Ann Intern Med. 1981;94:606-10.
23. Pitchenik AE, Rubinson HA. The radiographic appearance of tuberculosis in patients with the acquired immune deficiency syndrome (AIDS) and pre-AIDS. Am Rev Respir Dis. 1985;131:393-6.
24. Small PM, Hopewell PC, Schecter GF, Chaisson RE, Goodman PC. Evolution of chest radiographs in treated patients with pulmonary tuberculosis and HIV infection. J Thorac Imaging. 1994;9:74-7.

25. Im JG, Itoh H, Shim YS, et al. Pulmonary tuberculosis: CT findings—early active disease and sequential change with antituberculous therapy. Radiology. 1993;186:653-60.
26. Kim HJ, Lee HJ, Kwon SY, et al. The prevalence of pulmonary parenchymal tuberculosis in patients with tuberculous pleuritis. Chest. 2006;129:1253-8.
27. Sester M, Sotgiu G, Lange C, et al. Interferon-γ release assays for the diagnosis of active tuberculosis: a systematic review and meta-analysis. Eur Respir J. 2011;37:100-11.
28. Menzies D, Pai M, Comstock G. Meta-analysis: new tests for the diagnosis of latent tuberculosis infection: areas of uncertainty and recommendations for research. Ann Intern Med. 2007;146:340-54.
29. Liu F, Gao M, Zhang X, et al. Interferon-gamma release assay performance of pleural fluid and peripheral blood in pleural tuberculosis. PLoS One. 2013;8(12):e83857.
30. Pai M, Menzies D. Interferon-gamma release assays: what is their role in the diagnosis of active tuberculosis? Clin Infect Dis. 2007;44:74-7.
31. Dewan PK, Grinsdale J, Kawamura LM. Low sensitivity of a whole-blood interferon-gamma release assay for detection of active tuberculosis. Clin Infect Dis. 2007;44:69-73.
32. Nelson SM, Deike MA, Cartwright CP. Value of examining multiple sputum specimens in the diagnosis of pulmonary tuberculosis. J Clin Microbiol. 1998;36:467-9.
33. Craft DW, Jones MC, Blanchet CN, Hopfer RL. Value of examining three acid-fast bacillus sputum smears for removal of patients suspected of having tuberculosis from the "airborne precautions" category. J Clin Microbiol. 2000;38:4285-7.
34. Al Zahrani K, Al Jahdali H, Poirier L, René P, Menzies D. Yield of smear, culture and amplification tests from repeated sputum induction for the diagnosis of pulmonary tuberculosis. Int J Tuberc Lung Dis. 2001;5:855-60.
35. Davis JL, Cattamanchi A, Cuevas LE, Hopewell PC, Steingart KR. Diagnostic accuracy of same-day microscopy versus standard microscopy for pulmonary tuberculosis: a systematic review and meta-analysis. Lancet Infect Dis. 2013;13:147-54.
36. Anderson C, Inhaber N, Menzies D. Comparison of sputum induction with fiberoptic bronchoscopy in the diagnosis of tuberculosis. Am J Respir Crit Care Med. 1995;152:1570-4.
37. Conde MB, Soares SL, Mello FC, et al. Comparison of sputum induction with fiberoptic bronchoscopy in the diagnosis of tuberculosis: experience at an acquired immune deficiency syndrome reference center in Rio de Janeiro, Brazil. Am J Respir Crit Care Med. 2000;162:2238-40.
38. McWilliams T, Wells AU, Harrison AC, et al. Induced sputum and bronchoscopy in the diagnosis of pulmonary tuberculosis. Thorax. 2002;57:1010-4.
39. Cheng VC, Yew WW, Yuen KY. Molecular diagnostics in tuberculosis. Eur J Clin Microbiol Infect Dis. 2005;24:711-20.
40. Conaty SJ, Claxton AP, Enoch DA, Hayward AC, Lipman MC, Gillespie SH. The interpretation of nucleic acid amplification tests for tuberculosis: do rapid tests change treatment decisions? J Infect. 2005;50:187-92.
41. Lim TK, Mukhopadhyay A, Gough A, et al. Role of clinical judgment in the application of a nucleic acid amplification test for the rapid diagnosis of pulmonary tuberculosis. Chest. 2003;124:902-8.
42. Laraque F, Griggs A, Slopen M, Munsiff SS. Performance of nucleic acid amplification tests for diagnosis of tuberculosis in a large urban setting. Clin Infect Dis. 2009;49:46-54.
43. Campos M, Quartin A, Mendes E, et al. Feasibility of shortening respiratory isolation with a single sputum nucleic acid amplification test. Am J Respir Crit Care Med. 2008;178:300-5.
44. Karimi S, Shamaei M, Pourabdollah M, et al. Histopathological findings in immunohistological staining of the granulomatous tissue reaction associated with tuberculosis. Tuberc Res Treat. 2014;2014:858396.
45. Steele JD. The solitary pulmonary nodule. Report of a cooperative study of resected asymptomatic solitary pulmonary nodules in males. J Thorac Cardiovasc Surg. 1963;46:21-39.
46. Andreu J, Caceres J, Pallisa E, Martinez-Rodriguez M. Radiological manifestations of pulmonary tuberculosis. Eur J Radiol. 2004;51(2):139-49.
47. Ashizawa K, Matsuyama N, Okimoto T, et al. Coexistence of lung cancer and tuberculoma in the same lesion: demonstration by high resolution and contrast-enhanced dynamic CT. Br J Radiol. 2004;77(923):959-62.
48. Kim YI, Goo JM, Kim HY, Song JW, Im JG. Coexisting bronchogenic carcinoma and pulmonary tuberculosis in the same lobe: radiologic findings and clinical significance. Korean J Radiol. 2001;2(3):138-44.

49. Ishida T, Yokoyama H, Kaneko S, Sugio K, Sugimachi K, Hara N. Pulmonary tuberculoma and indications for surgery: radiographic and clinicopathological analysis. Respir Med. 1992;86(5):431-6.
50. Hsu K, Lee HC, Ou CC, Luh SP. Value of video-assisted thoracoscopic surgery in the diagnosis and treatment of pulmonary tuberculoma: 53 cases analysis and review of literature. J Zhejiang Univ Sci B. 2009;10(5):375-9.
51. Cherkasov VA, Stepanov SA, Rudoi EP. Immediate and late outcomes of surgical treatment in patients with tumor-simulating pulmonary tuberculosis. Probl Tuberk. 1997;(3):38-9.
52. Didenko GV. Results of surgical treatment in patients with pulmonary tuberculosis. Probl Tuberk Bolezn Legk. 2007;(11):26-8.
53. Congregado Loscertales M, Giron Arjona JC, Jimenez Merchan R, et al. Usefulness of video-assisted thoracoscopy for the diagnosis of solitary pulmonary nodules. Arch Bronconeumol. 2002;38(9):415-20.
54. Luh SP, Liu HP. Video-assisted thoracic surgery—the past, present status and the future. J Zhejiang Univ Sci B. 2006;7(2):118-28.
55. Prytz S, Hansen JL. Surgical treatment of "tuberculoma". A follow-up examination of patients with pulmonary tuberculosis resected on suspicion of tumour. Scand J Thorac Cardiovasc Surg. 1976;10(2):179-82.
56. Hoheisel G, Chan BK, Chan CH, Chan KS, Teschler H, Costabel U. Endobronchial tuberculosis: diagnostic features and therapeutic outcome. Respir Med. 1994;88(8):593-7.
57. Tetikkurt C. Current perspectives on endobronchial tuberculosis. Pneumon. 2008;21(3):239-5.
58. Chung HS, Lee JH. Bronchoscopic assessment of the evolution of endobronchial tuberculosis. Chest. 2000;117(2):385-92.
59. Kashyap S, Mohapatra PR, Saini V. Endobronchial tuberculosis. Indian J Chest Dis Allied Sci. 2003;45(4):247-56.
60. Ip MS, So SY, Lam WK, Mok CK. Endobronchial tuberculosis revisited. Chest. 1986;89(5):727-30.
61. Lee JH, Park SS, Lee DH, Shin DH, Yang SC, Yoo BM. Endobronchial tubeculosis. Clinical and bronchoscopic features in 121 cases. Chest. 1992;102(4):990-4.
62. Golshan M. Tuberculous bronchitis with normal chest X-ray among a large bronchoscopic population. Ann Saudi Med. 2002;22(1-2):98-101.
63. Kreisel D, Arora N, Weisenberg SA, et al. Tuberculosis presenting as an endobronchial mass. J Thorac Cardiovasc Surg. 2007;133(2):582-4.
64. Lee JH, Chung HS. Bronchoscopic, radiologic and pulmonary function evaluation of endobronchial tuberculosis. Respirology. 2000;5(4):411-7.
65. Kim HC, Kim HS, Lee SJ, et al. Endobronchial tuberculosis presenting as right middle lobe syndrome: clinical characteristics and bronchoscopic findings in 22 cases. Yonsei Med J. 2008;49(4):615-9.
66. Johnston H, Reisz G. Changing spectrum of hemoptysis. Underlying causes in 148 patients undergoing diagnostic flexible fiberoptic bronchoscopy. Arch Intern Med. 1989;149:1666-8.
67. Conlan AA, Hurwitz SS, Krige L, Nicolaou N, Pool R. Massive hemoptysis. Review of 123 cases. J Thorac Cardiovasc Surg. 1983;85:120-4.
68. Corey R, Hla KM. Major and massive hemoptysis: reassessment of conservative management. Am J Med Sci. 1987;294:301-9.
69. Muthuswamy PP, Akbik F, Franklin C, Spigos D, Barker WL. Management of major or massive hemoptysis in active pulmonary tuberculosis by bronchial arterial embolization. Chest. 1987;92:77-82.
70. Bobrowitz ID, Ramakrishna S, Shim YS. Comparison of medical v surgical treatment of major hemoptysis. Arch Intern Med. 1983;143:1343-6.
71. Uflacker R, Kaemmerer A, Picon PD, et al. Bronchial artery embolization in the management of hemoptysis: technical aspects and long-term results. Radiology. 1985;157:637-44.
72. Bobrowitz ID, Rodescu D, Marcus H, Abeles H. The destroyed tuberculous lung. Scand J Respir Dis. 1974;55:82-8.
73. Palmer PE. Pulmonary tuberculosis—usual and unusual radiographic presentations. Semin Roentgenol. 1979;14:204-43.
74. Ihm HJ, Hankins JR, Miller JE, McLaughlin JS. Pneumothorax associated with pulmonary tuberculosis. J Thorac Cardiovasc Surg. 1972;64:211-9.
75. Aktoğu S, Yorgancioglu A, Cirak K, Köse T, Dereli SM. Clinical spectrum of pulmonary and pleural tuberculosis: a report of 5,480 cases. Eur Respir J. 1996;9:2031-5.

76. Hussain SF, Aziz A, Fatima H. Pneumothorax: a review of 146 adult cases admitted at a university teaching hospital in Pakistan. J Pak Med Assoc. 1999;49:243-6.
77. Lorenz R, Kraman SS. Intracavitary mass in a patient with far-advanced tuberculosis. Chest. 1982;82:91-2.
78. van der Klooster JM, Bosman RJ, Oudemans-van Straaten HM, van der Spoel JI, Wester JP, Zandstra DF. Disseminated tuberculosis, pulmonary aspergillosis and cutaneous herpes simplex infection in a patient with infliximab and methotrexate. Intensive Care Med. 2003;29(12):2327-9.
79. Oursler KK, Moore RD, Bishai WR, Harrington SM, Pope DS, Chaisson RE. Survival of patients with pulmonary tuberculosis: clinical and molecular epidemiologic factors. Clin Infect Dis. 2002;34:752-9.
80. Wood R, Middelkoop K, Myer L, et al. Undiagnosed tuberculosis in a community with high HIV prevalence: implications for tuberculosis control. Am J Respir Crit Care Med. 2007;175:87-93.
81. Pérez-Guzmán C, Vargas MH, Torres-Cruz A, Villarreal-Velarde H. Does aging modify pulmonary tuberculosis? A meta-analytical review. Chest. 1999;116:961-7.
82. Mathur P, Sacks L, Auten G, Sall R, Levy C, Gordin F. Delayed diagnosis of pulmonary tuberculosis in city hospitals. Arch Intern Med. 1994;154:306-10.
83. Bobrowitz ID. Active tuberculosis undiagnosed until autopsy. Am J Med. 1982;72:650-8.
84. World Health Organization. (2016). Tuberculosis and gender. [online] Available from www.who.int/tb/challenges/gender/en/ [Accessed January, 2016].
85. TB alert. TB and women. [online] Available from: www.tbalert.org/about-tb/global-tb-challenges/tb-women/ [Accessed January, 2016].
86. World Health Organization. (2016). Women and tuberculosis. [online] Available from: www.who.int/tb/challenges/gender/women_and_tb/en/ [Accessed January, 2016].
87. Nguyen HT, Pandolfini C, Chiodini P, Bonati M. Tuberculosis care for pregnant women: a systematic review. BMC Infect Dis. 2014;14:617.
88. Friedman L, Tanoue L. (2014). Tuberculosis in pregnancy. [online] UpToDate website. Available from: www.uptodate.com. [Accessed January, 2016].
89. Worjoloh A, Kato-Maeda M, Osmond D, Freyre R, Aziz N, Cohan D. Interferon-gamma release assay compared with the tuberculin skin test for latent tuberculosis detection in pregnancy. Obstet Gynecol. 2011;118:1363-70.
90. Carter EJ, Mates S. Tuberculosis during pregnancy. The Rhode Island experience, 1987 to 1991. Chest. 1994;106:1466-70.
91. Knight M, Kurinczuk JJ, Nelson-Piercy C, Spark P, Brocklehurst P. Tuberculosis in pregnancy in the UK. BJOG. 2009;116:584-8.
92. Kothari A, Mahadevan N, Girling J. Tuberculosis and pregnancy—results of a study in a high prevalence area in London. Eur J Obstet Gynecol Reprod Biol. 2006;126:48-55.
93. Sepulveda RL, Gonzalez B, Gerszencveig R, Ferrer X, Martinez B, Sorensen RU. The influence of BCG immunization on tuberculin reactivity in healthy Chilean women in the third trimester of pregnancy. Tuber Lung Dis. 1995;76:28-34.
94. Llewelyn M, Cropley I, Wilkinson RJ, Davidson RN. Tuberculosis diagnosed during pregnancy: a prospective study from London. Thorax. 2000;55:129-32.
95. Gounder CR, Wada NI, Kensler C, et al. Active tuberculosis case-finding among pregnant women presenting to antenatal clinics in Soweto, South Africa. J Acquir Immune Defic Syndr. 2011;57:e77-84.
96. Khan M, Pillay T, Moodley JM, Connolly CA. Maternal mortality associated with tuberculosis-HIV-1 co-infection in Durban, South Africa. AIDS. 2001;15:1857-63.
97. Kali PB, Gray GE, Violari A, Chaisson RE, McIntyre JA, Martinson NA. Combining PMTCT with active case finding for tuberculosis. J Acquir Immune Defic Syndr. 2006;42:379-81.
98. Pillay T, Khan M, Moodley J, et al. The increasing burden of tuberculosis in pregnant women, newborns and infants under 6 months of age in Durban, KwaZulu-Natal. S Afr Med J. 2001;91:983-7.
99. Gupta A, Chandrasekhar A, Gupte N, et al. Symptom screening among HIV-infected pregnant women is acceptable and has high negative predictive value for active tuberculosis. Clin Infect Dis. 2011;53:1015-8.
100. Snider D. Pregnancy and tuberculosis. Chest. 1984;86:10S-13S.
101. Hamadeh MA, Glassroth J. Tuberculosis and pregnancy. Chest. 1992;101:1114-20.
102. Schaefer G, Zervoudakis IA, Fuchs FF, David S. Pregnancy and pulmonary tuberculosis. Obstet Gynecol. 1975;46:706-15.

103. Starke JR. Tuberculosis in childhood and pregnancy. In: Friedman LN (Ed). Tuberculosis: Current Concepts and Treatment. 2nd ed. Boca Raton: CRC Press; 2000. p. 191.
104. Davidson PT. Managing tuberculosis during pregnancy. Lancet. 1995;346:199-200.
105. Ormerod P. Tuberculosis in pregnancy and the puerperium. Thorax. 2001;56:494-9.
106. Bergeron KG, Bonebrake RG, Allen C, Gray CJ. Latent tuberculosis in pregnancy: screening and treatment. Curr Womens Health Rep. 2003;3:303-8.
107. Nhan-Chang CL, Jones TB. Tuberculosis in pregnancy. Clin Obstet Gynecol. 2010;53:311-21.
108. Targeted tuberculin testing and treatment of latent tuberculosis infection. American Thoracic Society. MMWR Recomm Rep. 2000;49:1-51.
109. Present PA, Comstock GW. Tuberculin sensitivity in pregnancy. Am Rev Respir Dis. 1975;112:413-6.
110. Jonnalagadda S, Payne BL, Brown E, et al. Latent tuberculosis detection by interferon-gamma release assay during pregnancy predicts active tuberculosis and mortality in human immunodeficiency virus type 1-infected women and their children. J Infect Dis. 2010;202:1826-35.
111. Sheriff FG, Manji KP, Manji MP, et al. Latent tuberculosis among pregnant mothers in a resource poor setting in Northern Tanzania: a cross-sectional study. BMC Infect Dis. 2010;10:52.
112. Mofenson LM, Rodriguez EM, Hershow R, et al. Mycobacterium tuberculosis infection in pregnant and nonpregnant women infected with HIV in the women and infants transmission study. Arch Intern Med. 1995;155:1066-72.
113. Mazurek GH, Jereb J, Lobue P, et al. Guidelines for using the QuantiFERON-TB Gold test for detecting Mycobacterium tuberculosis infection, United States. MMWR Recomm Rep. 2005;54:49-55.
114. Centers for Disease Control and Prevention. Tuberculosis (TB). (2016). [online] Available from: www.cdc.gov/tb/pubs/tbfactsheets/pregnancy.htm [Accessed January, 2016].
115. Lighter-Fisher J, Surette AM. Performance of an interferon-gamma release assay to diagnose latent tuberculosis infection during pregnancy. Obstet Gynecol. 2012;119:1088-95.
116. Doveren RF, Block R. Tuberculosis and pregnancy—a provincial study (1990-1996). Neth J Med. 1998;52:100-6.
117. Czeizel AE, Rockenbauer M, Olsen J, Sorensen HT. A population-based case-control study of the safety of oral anti-tuberculosis drug treatment during pregnancy. Int J Tuberc Lung Dis. 2001;5:564-8.
118. Tripathy SN, Tripathy SN. Tuberculosis and pregnancy. Int J Gynecol Obstet. 2003;80:247-53.
119. Tabarsi P, Moradi A, Baghaei P, et al. Standardised second-line treatment of multidrug-resistant tuberculosis during pregnancy. Int J Tuberc Lung Dis. 2011;15:547-50.
120. Oliveira HB, Mateus SH. Characterization of multidrug-resistant tuberculosis during pregnancy in Campinas, State of Sao Paulo, Brazil, from 1995 to 2007. Rev Soc Bras Med Trop. 2011;44:627-30.
121. Khan M, Pillay T, Moodley J, Ramjee A, Padayatchi N. Pregnancies complicated by multidrug-resistant tuberculosis and HIV co-infection in Durban, South Africa. Int J Tuberc Lung Dis. 2007;11:706-8.
122. Palacios E, Dallman R, Muñoz M, et al. Drug-resistant tuberculosis and pregnancy: treatment outcomes of 38 cases in Lima, Peru. Clin Infect Dis. 2009;48:1413-9.
123. Dooley KE, Chaisson RE. Tuberculosis and diabetes mellitus: convergence of two epidemics. Lancet Infect Dis. 2009;9:737-46.
124. Restrepo BI, Schlesinger LS. Impact of diabetes on the natural history of tuberculosis. Diabetes Res Clin Pract. 2014;106(2):191-9.
125. Mozaffarian D, Kamineni A, Carnethon M, Djousse L, Mukamal KJ, Siscovick D. Lifestyle risk factors and new-onset diabetes mellitus in older adults: the cardiovascular health study. Arch Intern Med. 2009;169:798-807.
126. Stevenson CR, Critchley JA, Forouhi NG, et al. Diabetes and the risk of tuberculosis: a neglected threat to public health? Chronic Illn. 2007;3:228-45.
127. Harries AD, Billo N, Kapur A. Links between diabetes mellitus and tuberculosis: should we integrate screening and care? Trans R Soc Trop Med Hyg. 2009;103:1-2.
128. Leung CC, Lam TH, Chan WM, et al. Lower risk of tuberculosis in obesity. Arch Intern Med. 2007;167:1297-304.
129. Stevenson CR, Forouhi NG, Roglic G, et al. Diabetes and tuberculosis: the impact of the diabetes epidemic on tuberculosis incidence. BMC Public Health. 2007;7:234.
130. Dooley KE, Tang T, Golub JE, Dorman SE, Cronin W. Impact of diabetes mellitus on treatment outcomes of patients with active tuberculosis. Am J Trop Med Hyg. 2009;80:634-9.

131. Restrepo BI, Fisher-Hoch SP, Crespo JG, et al. Type 2 diabetes and tuberculosis in a dynamic binational border population. Epidemiol Infect. 2007;135:483-91.
132. Jeon CY, Harries AD, Baker MA, et al. Bi-directional screening for tuberculosis and diabetes: a systematic review. Trop Med Int Health. 2010;15(11):1300-14.
133. Ottmani SE, Murray MB, Jeon CY, et al. Consultation meeting on tuberculosis and diabetes mellitus: meeting summary and recommendations. Int J Tuberc Lung Dis. 2010;14(12):1513-7.
134. Gomez DI, Twahirwa M, Schlesinger LS, Restrepo BI. Reduced Mycobacterium tuberculosis association with monocytes from diabetes patients that have poor glucose control. Tuberculosis. 2013;93(2):192-7.
135. Restrepo BI, Twahirwa M, Rahbar MH, Schlesinger LS. Phagocytosis via complement or Fc-gamma receptors is compromised in monocytes from type 2 diabetes patients with chronic hyperglycemia. PLoS One. 2014;9(3):e92977.
136. Martinez N, Kornfeld H. Diabetes and immunity to tuberculosis. Eur J Immunol. 2014;44(3):617-26.
137. Vallerskog T, Martens GW, Kornfeld H. Diabetic mice display a delayed adaptive immune response to Mycobacterium tuberculosis. J Immunol. 2010;184(11):6275-82.
138. Restrepo BI, Fisher-Hoch S, Pino PA, Salinas A, Rahbar MH, Mora F, et al. Tuberculosis in poorly controlled type 2 diabetes: altered cytokine expression in peripheral white blood cells. Clin Infect Dis. 2008;47:634-41.
139. Kumar NP, Sridhar R, Banurekha VV, Jawahar MS, Nutman TB, Babu S. Expansion of pathogen-specific T-helper 1 and T-helper 17 cells in pulmonary tuberculosis with coincident type 2 diabetes mellitus. J Infect Dis. 2013;208(5):739-48.
140. Walsh MC, Camerlin AJ, Miles R, et al. The sensitivity of interferon-gamma release assays is not compromised in tuberculosis patients with diabetes. Int J Tuberc Lung Dis. 2011;15(2):179-84.
141. Sun Q, Zhang Q, Xiao H, Cui H, Su B. Significance of the frequency of CD4+CD25+C127- T-cells in patients with pulmonary tuberculosis and diabetes mellitus. Respirology. 2012;17(5):876-82.
142. Leegaard A, Riis A, Kornum JB, et al. Diabetes, glycemic control, and risk of tuberculosis: a population-based case-control study. Diabetes Care. 2011;34(12):2530-5.
143. Leung CC, Lam TH, Chan WM, et al. Diabetic control and risk of tuberculosis: a cohort study. Am J Epidemiol. 2008;167(12):1486-94.
144. Dobler CC, Flack JR, Marks GB. Risk of tuberculosis among people with diabetes mellitus: an Australian nationwide cohort study. BMJ Open. 2012;2(1):e000666.
145. Mboussa J, Monabeka H, Kombo M, Yokolo D, Yoka-Mbio A, Yala F. Course of pulmonary tuberculosis in diabetics. Rev Pneumol Clin. 2003;59:39-44.
146. Shetty N, Shemko M, Vaz M, D'Souza G. An epidemiological evaluation of risk factors for tuberculosis in South India: a matched case control study. Int J Tuberc Lung Dis. 2006;10:80-6.
147. Coker R, McKee M, Atun R, et al. Risk factors for pulmonary tuberculosis in Russia: case-control study. BMJ. 2006;332:85-7.
148. Jabbar A, Hussain SF, Khan AA. Clinical characteristics of pulmonary tuberculosis in adult Pakistani patients with co-existing diabetes mellitus. East Mediterr Health J. 2006;12:522-7.
149. Kim SJ, Hong YP, Lew WJ, Yang SC, Lee EG. Incidence of pulmonary tuberculosis among diabetics. Tuber Lung Dis. 1995;76:529-33.
150. Shah BR, Hux JE. Quantifying the risk of infectious diseases for people with diabetes. Diabetes Care. 2003;26:510-3.
151. Baker MA, Lin HH, Chang HY, Murray MB. The risk of tuberculosis disease among persons with diabetes mellitus: a prospective cohort study. Clin Infect Dis. 2012;54(6):818-25.
152. Restrepo BI, Camerlin AJ, Rahbar MH, et al. Cross-sectional assessment reveals high diabetes prevalence among newly-diagnosed tuberculosis cases. Bull World Health Organ. 2011;89:352-9.
153. Olmos P, Donoso J, Rojas N, et al. Tuberculosis and diabetes mellitus: a longitudinal-retrospective study in a teaching hospital. Rev Med Chil. 1989;117:979-83.
154. Swai AB, McLarty DG, Mugusi F. Tuberculosis in diabetic patients in Tanzania. Trop Doct. 1990;20:147-50.
155. Reed GW, Choi H, Lee SY, et al. Impact of diabetes and smoking on mortality in tuberculosis. PLoS One. 2013;8(2):e58044.
156. Reis-Santos B, Locatelli R, Horta BL, et al. Socio-demographic and clinical differences in subjects with tuberculosis with and without diabetes mellitus in Brazil—a multivariate analysis. PLoS One. 2013;8(4):e62604.

157. Lin JN, Lai CH, Chen YH, et al. Risk factors for extra-pulmonary tuberculosis compared to pulmonary tuberculosis. Int J Tuberc Lung Dis. 2009;13(5):620-5.
158. Viswanathan V, Kumpatla S, Aravindalochanan V, et al. Prevalence of diabetes and pre-diabetes and associated risk factors among tuberculosis patients in India. PLoS One. 2012;7(7):e41367.
159. Kumar NP, Nutman T, Babu S. Expansion of pathogen-specific T-helper 1 and T-helper 17 cells in pulmonary tuberculosis with coincident type 2 diabetes mellitus. J Infect Dis. 2013;208:739-48.
160. Al-Tawfiq JA, Saadeh BM. Radiographic manifestations of culture-positive pulmonary tuberculosis: cavitary or non-cavitary? Int J Tuberc Lung Dis. 2009;13:367-70.
161. Ikezoe J, Takeuchi N, Johkoh T, et al. CT appearance of pulmonary tuberculosis in diabetic and immunocompromised patients: comparison with patients who had no underlying disease. AJR Am J Roentgenol. 1992;159:1175-9.
162. Morris JT, Seaworth BJ, McAllister CK. Pulmonary tuberculosis in diabetics. Chest. 1992;102:539-41.
163. Bacakoglu F, Basoglu OK, Cok G, Sayiner A, Ates M. Pulmonary tuberculosis in patients with diabetes mellitus. Respiration. 2001;68:595-600.
164. Perez-Guzman C, Torres-Cruz A, Villarreal-Velarde H, Salazar-Lezama MA, Vargas MH. Atypical radiological images of pulmonary tuberculosis in 192 diabetic patients: a comparative study. Int J Tuberc Lung Dis. 2001;5:455-61.
165. Shaikh MA, Singla R, Khan NB, Sharif NS, Saigh MO. Does diabetes alter the radiological presentation of pulmonary tuberculosis. Saudi Med J. 2003;24:278-81.
166. Perez-Guzman C, Torres-Cruz A, Villarreal-Velarde H, Vargas MH. Progressive age-related changes in pulmonary tuberculosis images and the effect of diabetes. Am J Respir Crit Care Med. 2000;162(5):1738-40.
167. Moran A, Harbour DV, Teeter LD, Musser JM, Graviss EA. Is alcohol use associated with cavitary disease in tuberculosis? Alcohol Clin Exp Res. 2007;31(1):33-8.
168. Chiang CY, Lee JJ, Chien ST, et al. Glycemic control and radiographic manifestations of tuberculosis in diabetic patients. PLoS One. 2014;9(4):e93397.
169. Behr MA, Warren SA, Salamon H, et al. Transmission of Mycobacterium tuberculosis from patients smear-negative for acid-fast bacilli. Lancet. 1999;353(9151):444-9.
170. Guler M, Unsal E, Dursun B, Aydln O, Capan N. Factors influencing sputum smear and culture conversion time among patients with new case pulmonary tuberculosis. Int J Clin Pract. 2007;61:231-5.
171. Restrepo BI, Fisher-Hoch SP, Smith B, et al. Mycobacterial clearance from sputum is delayed during the first phase of treatment in patients with diabetes. Am J Trop Med Hyg. 2008;79:541-4.
172. Jeon CY, Murray MB, Baker MA. Managing tuberculosis in patients with diabetes mellitus: why we care and what we know. Expert Rev Anti Infect Ther. 2012;10(8):863-8.
173. Jimenez-Corona ME, Cruz-Hervert LP, Garcia-Garcia L, et al. Association of diabetes and tuberculosis: impact on treatment and post-treatment outcomes. Thorax. 2013;68(3):214-20.
174. Jorgensen ME, Faurholt-Jepsen D. Is there an effect of glucose lowering treatment on incidence and prognosis of tuberculosis? A systematic review. Curr Diab Rep. 2014;14(7):505.
175. Viswanathan V, Vigneswari A, Selvan K, Satyavani K, Rajeswari R, Kapur A. Effect of diabetes on treatment outcome of smear-positive pulmonary tuberculosis—a report from South India. J Diabetes Complications. 2014;28(2):162-5.
176. Baker MA, Harries AD, Jeon CY, et al. The impact of diabetes on tuberculosis treatment outcomes: a systematic review. BMC Med. 2011;9:81.
177. Chaisson RE, Nachega JB. Tuberculosis. In: Warrel DA, Cox TM, Firth JD (Eds). Oxford Textbook of Medicine. 5th ed. Oxford: Oxford University Press; 2010. pp. 810-31.
178. Ates G, Yildiz T, Danis R, et al. Incidence of tuberculosis disease and latent tuberculosis infection in patients with end stage renal disease in an endemic region. Ren Fail. 2010;32(1):91-5.
179. Erkoc R, Dogan E, Sayarlioglu H, et al. Tuberculosis in dialysis patients, single centre experience from an endemic area. Int J Clin Pract. 2004;58(12):1115-7.
180. Malik GH, Al-Harbi AS, Al-Mohaya S, et al. Eleven years of experience with dialysis associated tuberculosis. Clin Nephrol. 2002;58(5):356-62.
181. Rao TM, Ram R, Swarnalatha G, et al. Tuberculosis in haemodialysis patients: a single centre experience. Indian J Nephrol. 2013;23(5):340-5.
182. Sen N, Turunc T, Karatasli M, Sezer S, Demiroglu YZ, Oner Eyuboglu F. Tuberculosis in patients with end-stage renal disease undergoing dialysis in an endemic region of Turkey. Transplant Proc. 2008;40(1):81-4.

183. Rutkowski B, Gillow AS, Kustosz J, Liberek T, Zdrojewski Z. Increasing incidence of tuberculosis in hemodialysis patients. Dial Transplant. 1997;26:21-5.
184. Richardson RM. The diagnosis of tuberculosis in dialysis patients. Semin Dial. 2012;25(4):419-22.
185. Lundin AP, Adler AJ, Berlyne GM, Friedman EA. Tuberculosis in patients undergoing maintenance hemodialysis. Am J Med. 1979;67:597-602.
186. Sasaki S, Akiba T, Suenaga M, et al. Ten years' survey of dialysis-associated tuberculosis. Nephron. 1979;24:141-5.
187. Shohaib SA, Scrimgeour EM, Shaerya F. Tuberculosis in active dialysis patients in Jeddah. Am J Nephrol. 1999;19:34-7.
188. Vartian CV. Tuberculosis in dialysis patients: an old association revisited. Infect Dis Clin Pract. 1997;6:247-9.
189. Al-Homrany M. Successful therapy of tuberculosis in hemodialysis patients. Am J Nephrol. 1997;17:32-5.
190. Cengiz K. Increased incidence of tuberculosis in patients undergoing hemodialysis. Nephron. 1996;73:421-4.
191. Hussein MM, Bakir N, Roujouleh H. Tuberculosis in patients undergoing maintenance dialysis. Nephrol Dial Transplant. 1990;5:584-7.
192. Mitwalli A. Tuberculosis in patients on maintenance dialysis. Am J Kidney Dis. 1991;18:579-82.
193. Moreiras-Plaza M, Pazos B, Courel MA, et al. Tuberculosis in dialysis patients. Nefrologia. 1995;15:581-6.
194. Malhotra KK, Parashar MK, Sharma RK, et al. Tuberculosis in maintenance haemodialysis patients. Study from an endemic area. Postgrad Med J. 1981;57:492-8.
195. Andrew OT, Schoenfeld PY, Hopewell PC, Humphreys AH. Tuberculosis in patients with end-stage renal disease. Am J Med. 1980;68:59-65.
196. Pradhan RP, Katz LA, Nidus BD, Matalon R, Eisinger RP. Tuberculosis in dialyzed patients. JAMA. 1974;229:798-800.
197. Habesoglu MA, Torun D, Demiroglu YZ, et al. Value of the tuberculin skin test in screening for tuberculosis in dialysis patients. Transplant Proc. 2007;39:883-6.
198. Lee SS, Chou KJ, Su IJ, et al. High prevalence of latent tuberculosis infection in patients in end-stage renal disease on hemodialysis: comparison of QuantiFERON-TB GOLD, ELISPOT, and tuberculin skin test. Infection. 2009;37:96-102.
199. Triverio PA, Bridevaux PO, Roux-Lombard P, et al. Interferon-gamma release assays versus tuberculin skin testing for detection of latent tuberculosis in chronic haemodialysis patients. Nephrol Dial Transplant. 2009;24:1952-6.
200. Passalent L, Khan K, Richardson R, Wang J, Dedier H, Gardam M. Detecting latent tuberculosis infection in hemodialysis patients: a head-to-head comparison of the T-SPOT.TB test, tuberculin skin test, and an expert physician panel. Clin J Am Soc Nephrol. 2007;2:68-73.
201. Segall L, Covic A. Diagnosis of tuberculosis in dialysis patients: current strategy. Clin J Am Soc Nephrol. 2010;5:1114-22.
202. Taskapan H, Utas C, Oymak FS, Gülmez I, Ozesmi M. The outcome of tuberculosis in patients on chronic hemodialysis. Clin Nephrol. 2000;54:134-7.
203. Chou KJ, Fang HC, Bai KJ, Hwang SJ, Yang WC, Chung HM. Tuberculosis in maintenance dialysis patients. Nephron. 2001;88:138-43.
204. Rutsky EA, Rostand SG. Mycobacteriosis in patients with chronic renal failure. Arch Intern Med. 1980;140:57-61.
205. Nakamura H, Tateyama M, Tasato D, et al. Active tuberculosis in patients undergoing hemodialysis for end-stage renal disease: a 9-year retrospective analysis in a single center. Intern Med. 2009;48:2061-7.
206. Horne DJ, Narita M, Spitters CL, Parimi S, Dodson S, Limaye AP. Challenging issues in tuberculosis in solid organ transplantation. Clin Infect Dis. 2013;57(10):1473-82.
207. Sundaram M, Adhikary SD, John GT, Kekre NS. Tuberculosis in renal transplant recipients. Indian J Urol. 2008;24(3):396-400.
208. John GT. Infections after renal transplantation in India. Indian J Nephrol. 2003;13:14-9.
209. Sakhuja V, Jha V, Varma PP, Joshi K, Chugh KS. The high incidence of tuberculosis among renal transplant recipients in India. Transplantation. 1996;61:211-5.

210. Munoz P, Rodriguez C, Bouza E. Mycobacterium tuberculosis infection in recipients of solid organ transplants. Clin Infect Dis. 2005;40:581-7.
211. Aguado JM, Torre-Cisneros J, Fortun J, et al. Tuberculosis in solid-organ transplant recipients: consensus statement of the group for the study of infection in transplant recipients (GESITRA) of the Spanish Society of Infectious Diseases and Clinical Microbiology. Clin Infect Dis. 2009;48:1276-84.
212. Torre-Cisneros J, Doblas A, Aguado JM, et al. Tuberculosis after solid-organ transplant: incidence, risk factors, and clinical characteristics in the RESITRA (Spanish Network of Infection in Transplantation) cohort. Clin Infect Dis. 2009;48:1657-65.
213. Canet E, Dantal J, Blancho G, Hourmant M, Coupel S. Tuberculosis following kidney transplantation: clinical features and outcome. A French multicentre experience in the last 20 years. Nephrol Dial Transplant. 2011;26:3773-8.
214. Ha YE, Joo EJ, Park SY, et al. Tacrolimus as a risk factor for tuberculosis and outcome of treatment with rifampicin in solid organ transplant recipients. Transpl Infect Dis. 2012;14:626-34.
215. Vandermarliere A, Van Audenhove A, Peetermans WE, Vanrenterghem Y, Maes B. Mycobacterial infection after renal transplantation in a Western population. Transpl Infect Dis. 2003;5:9-15.
216. Lopez de Castilla D, Schluger NW. Tuberculosis following solid organ transplantation. Transpl Infect Dis. 2010;12:106-12.
217. Singh N, Paterson DL. Mycobacterium tuberculosis infection in solid-organ transplant recipients: impact and implications for management. Clin Infect Dis. 1998;27:1266-77.
218. Klote MM, Agodoa LY, Abbott K. Mycobacterium tuberculosis infection incidence in hospitalized renal transplant patients in the United States, 1998-2000. Am J Transplant. 2004;4:1523-8.
219. John GT, Shankar V, Abraham AM, Mukundan U, Thomas PP, Jacob CK. Risk factors for post-transplant tuberculosis. Kidney Int. 2001;60:1148-53.
220. John GT, Shankar V. Mycobacterial infections in organ transplant recipients. Semin Respir Infect. 2002;17:274-83.
221. Aguado JM, Herrero JA, Gavalda J, et al. Clinical presentation and outcome of tuberculosis in kidney, liver, and heart transplant recipients in Spain. Spanish Transplantation Infection Study Group, GESITRA. Transplantation. 1997;63:1278-86.
222. Holty JE, Gould MK, Meinke L, Keeffe EB, Ruoss SJ. Tuberculosis in liver transplant recipients: a systematic review and meta-analysis of individual patient data. Liver Transpl. 2009;15:894-906.

CHAPTER 8

Miliary Tuberculosis

Ashok Shah, Shekhar Kunal

INTRODUCTION

Miliary tuberculosis is the most dreaded form of tuberculosis as it disseminates rapidly through the hematogenous system and often has a cryptic presentation. Thus, it frequently ensues in fatality if not detected on time. In a high tuberculous prevalence country like India, a patient presenting with miliary mottling on chest radiograph is assumed to be miliary tuberculosis until proved otherwise. This dangerous form of tuberculosis tends to have a nonspecific presentation and as such a high index of suspicion is required for prompt diagnosis. To compound the problem, the advent of human immunodeficiency virus (HIV)-acquired immunodeficiency syndrome (AIDS) has resulted in miliary tuberculosis reinventing itself and emerging in a drug-resistant form.

HISTORICAL PERSPECTIVE

"The captain of all these men of death that came against him to take him away, was the consumption, for it was that brought him down to the grave."

—John Bunyan, 1680

Tuberculosis "the white plague" has been described since ancient times. Ancient Indian scriptures like the Vedas do give a description of tuberculosis or "Yakshma" and so do the Chinese and Arabic texts.[1] It was Hippocrates who in 460 BC first gave an accurate description of this disease and coined the term "phthisis" the literal meaning of which was "wasting away".[2] He also gave the description of the disease in the *Book 1 "Of the Epidemics"*.[3] In 1689, Richard Morton in his book entitled *"Phthisiologia: or a Treatise of Consumptions"* gave a clear pathological description of tuberculosis by detailing the occurrence of tubercles on surface of the lungs.[4] Benjamin Marten in 1790 proposed the theory that tuberculosis is caused by some form of *animacula* or microorganism.[4] The word "tuberculosis" per se was coined by JL Schonlein, a German doctor in 1839.[5]

The term miliary is derived from the Latin word "miliarius" meaning resemblance to millet seeds. Miliary tuberculosis was first described in a postmortem study of a patient of tuberculosis by Theophilus Bonetus in 1679.[6] He had described a lung "seeded with minute tubercles" in his postmortem catalog *"Sepulcretum sive anatomia practica"*. The term "miliary" was first used in medical terminology in 1685 by Robert Boyle in his description of the skin lesions as "minute or miliary glandules of the skin".[6] The term "miliary tuberculosis" was coined by a Genevan physician, John Jacobus Manget. While republishing the works of Theophilus Bonetus, he also described the gross pathological picture and stated that the appearance was similar to that of multiple millet seeds. This led to the emergence of the term *"miliary"*.[6] Gaspard-Laurent Bayle (1774–1816) in his treatise

Recherches sur lephthisie pulmonaire (1810) while emphasizing that the tubercle was the essential feature of pulmonary phthisis, stated that miliary and caseous tuberculosis were two different entities. However, his pupil Rene-Theophile Hyacinthe Laënnec (1781-1826) proposed that miliary tuberculosis was related to caseating form of tuberculosis.[4] This theory was further confirmed by Buhl who stated that resorption of "the specific substance" from caseous foci led to miliary tuberculosis.[7] Weigert proposed the theory of vascular foci ("Weigert" tubercle) eroding into the vessels and leading to miliary tuberculosis. Jean-Antonie Villemin convincingly demonstrated disseminated tuberculosis in rabbits being caused by injection of caseous material from a tuberculous cavity.[3]

It was Hermann Heinrich Robert Koch, whose works especially in the field of infectious diseases, laid down the foundations of modern microbiology. On 24th March 1882, in his address "Über Tuberculose" during the monthly evening meeting of the Berlin Physiological Society, Koch announced the discovery of *Mycobacterium tuberculosis*. Using material from the grayish tubercles from the lungs of the dead patients, Koch with his own staining techniques (methylene blue and caustic potash) demonstrated the presence of beautifully stained bluish colored tubercular bacilli. Later on, Koch was able to successfully isolate *M. tuberculosis* in culture on cattle-blood serum solid media. Two weeks later, he published his works as *Die Aetiologie der Tuberculose* unfolding the secrets of the disease which had been a bane of mankind. In 1884, Robert Koch went on to publish his famous Koch's postulates, the basis of study for all the infectious diseases. In 1890, Koch announced the discovery of tuberculin as a curative agent for tuberculosis, a false hope which soon ended in disillusion. However, this agent turned out to be a diagnostic test for tuberculous infection. In 1905, Robert Koch was conferred the Nobel Prize in physiology and medicine for the discovery of *M. tuberculosis*.[5]

EPIDEMIOLOGY OF MILIARY TUBERCULOSIS

In 2014, the World Health Organization (WHO) global report estimated that there were 9.0 million new tuberculosis patients and 1.5 million deaths due to tuberculosis globally in 2013.[8] Miliary tuberculosis accounts for around 1-2%[9,10] of all tuberculosis patients and around 20%[10] of all the extrapulmonary tuberculosis patients. In the prechemotherapeutic era, miliary tuberculosis was more commonly seen among young children as the immature immune system in children led to hematogenous spread.[11] With the introduction of the Bacillus Calmette-Guérin (BCG) vaccine and effective chemotherapeutic regimens, there is a perceptible decline. In contrast, there is increase in incidence in the elderly subset and this has been linked to the advent of the AIDS pandemic, declining immunity, and use of immunosuppressive agents. A biphasic peak has been observed in age distribution of miliary tuberculosis with a higher incidence among 5th and 6th decades with a male predominance.[9,12-14] In a series of 100 patients between 1983 and 1994 from India, the mean age was around 35 years with 51% of patients being males.[15] The mean age in several other studies was around 40-60 years.[9,13,14]

Various conditions predispose to miliary tuberculosis. In the earlier case series of miliary tuberculosis, childhood infections such as measles and whooping cough were the major predisposing factors.[11] Measles virus not only led to damage to thymus in these children but also had a direct effect on lymphocytic response leading to depressed cellular immune response.[11] Malnutrition and alcoholism have been indicted as independent risk factors for miliary tuberculosis.[13] Comorbid conditions like diabetes mellitus, chronic renal failure, connective tissue disorders have all been shown to increase the incidence of miliary tuberculosis.[9] Pregnancy has of late been described as a predisposing factor.[16] A study from South Africa reported that 42% of their 109 patients with miliary tuberculosis had predisposing conditions which included alcoholism (16%), pregnancy (8%), steroids (6%), and diabetes (4%).[13] Risk of miliary tuberculosis is also higher in patients with HIV/AIDS, those on long-term steroids,[13] with solid organ transplants.[17] and those on immunosuppressive agents. In addition, patients on immunosuppressive agents or on biological immunomodulators like anti-tumor necrosis factor-α (TNF-α) agents for rheumatoid arthritis too have an increased predisposition for miliary tuberculosis.[18] Silicosis has also been described as one of the predisposing conditions for miliary tuberculosis.[19] The mortality rate in miliary tuberculosis is rather high, ranging from 20 to 30% in various series.[9,10,13,14]

PATHOGENESIS

Miliary tuberculosis is caused by the lymphohematogenous dissemination of *M. tuberculosis* bacilli which may occur either during the course of primary infection with mycobacteria or when there is a reactivation of a latent infection.[20] In the vast majority, host immune responses are able to contain the primary infection and result in either complete healing or persistence in the form of latent infection. However, in 10% of patients, the immune response is unable to contain the primary infection resulting in dissemination (Flowchart 1). During the course of primary infection, hematogenous spread of a small number of bacilli can occur to distant organs with high oxygen tension like liver, spleen, and brain. Although in majority of patients healing occurs with granuloma formation but in a small subset these foci of infection fail to heal and gain access to the lymphohematogenous system leading to acute miliary tuberculosis.[11] This phenomenon was frequently seen in children in the prechemotherapy era because of the poor immune response.[21] Reactivation of the latent focus of infection may also lead to miliary tuberculosis due to immunosuppression or HIV infection and the manifestation may vary from an acute presentation to the chronic cryptic form which may be difficult to recognize. Caseation and erosion into the nearby vascular structures

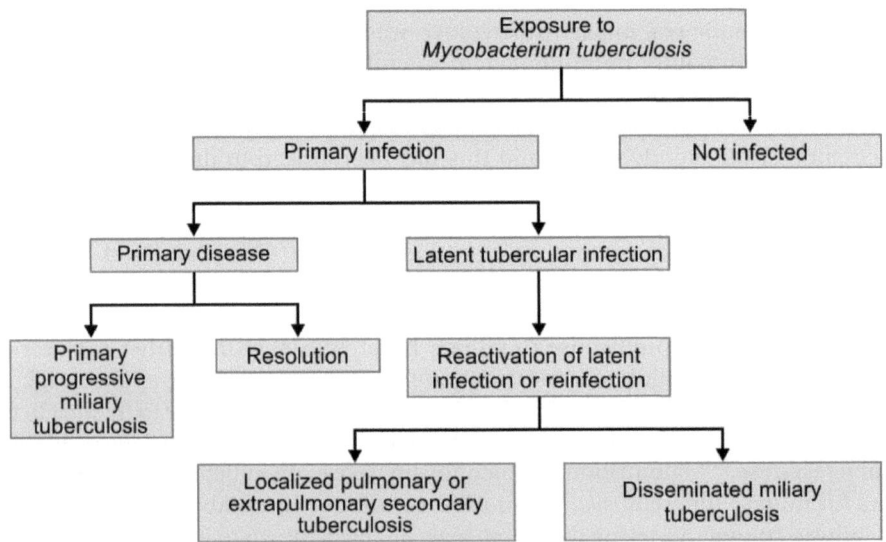

FLOWCHART 1: Pathogenesis of miliary tuberculosis.

results in spread to distant foci. Organ involvement varies depending on the site and the vascular structure affected. Whenever caseation of the mediastinal lymph node occurs, it leads to the involvement of thoracic duct culminating in dissemination in both the lungs. Dissemination to other organs commonly occurs whenever the pulmonary veins are affected.[11] When the main branch of pulmonary artery or its smaller branches are affected, the disease may occur in one lung or a portion of the lung.[22]

Millet seed-sized granulomatous foci remain the classical description of miliary tuberculosis. Grossly, these appear as small grayish-white pinhead sized lesions separated from the normal lung tissue.[22] These foci consist of epithelioid cells, macrophages, and Langhans giant cells. Depending on the presence or absence of caseous necrosis, miliary tubercles are further divided into "hard tubercles" and "soft tubercles", respectively.[22] Multiorgan spread along with pericardial, pleural effusion, or ascites may be seen due to serosal involvement.

IMMUNOLOGY

Immune response is predominantly cell mediated with pulmonary alveolar macrophages playing a central role in immunopathogenesis of tuberculosis. *Mycobacteria* phagocytosed by the macrophages and the dendritic cells are presented to the T cells. Two subsets of T cells, CD4+ T helper cells and CD8+ cytotoxic T cells form a part of the cell-mediated immunity.[23] The levels of CD4+ cells are decreased in patients with HIV resulting in an increased predisposition for miliary tuberculosis. The CD4+ T cells have two further subsets: (i) type 1 T helper (Th1) cells and (ii) type 2 T helper (Th2) cells. The Th1 cells produce tumor necrosis factor-α, interferon-γ, and interleukin-2 (IL-2).[23] These activate the macrophages and are responsible for killing of mycobacteria.[24] TNF-α plays a central role in the formation of a granuloma for the containment of tuberculous infection. Decreased TNF-α levels lead to failure in localizing the bacilli, thus predisposing to miliary tuberculosis. This has been frequently observed in patients on anti-TNF-α agents.[25] The Th2 cells produce IL-4, IL-5 which are chiefly responsible for activating B-lymphocytes and humoral immune system. The predominant type of immune response seen in miliary tuberculosis is the Th2 type which is unable to contain the bacilli leading to dissemination.[26] In patients with localized forms of pulmonary tuberculosis, there occurs a predominant Th1 response at the site of infection while in patients with miliary tuberculosis, a Th2 response is seen. This is evident from the increased IL-4 levels in the bronchoalveolar lavage (BAL) in patients with miliary tuberculosis.[27] Another subset of CD4+ cells, the regulatory T (Treg) cells have been identified of late. These cells produce tumor growth factor-β and IL-10. These cytokines lead to suppression of Th1-mediated cellular immune response. Originally studied in autoimmune diseases, the role of Treg cells has also been characterized in miliary tuberculosis. These Treg cells are CD4+, CD25+ but the characteristic marker of these cells is FoxP3+. Levels of these Treg cells are increased in miliary tuberculosis at the site of infection as evident by the raised FoxP3+ cells in BAL.[28] However, what controls this differential expression of various subsets of T cells needs to be elucidated.

CLINICAL FEATURES AND DIAGNOSTIC CRITERIA

The presentation of miliary tuberculosis has myriad forms ranging from an acute illness to a more chronic "cryptic" form. Multisystem involvement is a common feature with lungs being affected in a majority of patients. This is followed by liver, spleen, and the central nervous system (CNS).[9,12,14]

TABLE 1	Diagnostic criteria proposed for miliary tuberculosis[15]
S. No.	Diagnostic criteria
1	Clinical features suggesting a diagnosis of tuberculosis like fever with evening rise of temperature, loss of weight and appetite, tachycardia, and night sweats of >6 weeks duration and responding to antituberculous treatment
2	Characteristic miliary pattern on chest radiograph
3	Bilateral diffuse reticulonodular lung lesions on a background of miliary shadows demonstrable either on plain X-ray or high-resolution computerized tomography
4	Microbiological or histopathological features suggestive of tuberculosis

Constitutional symptoms are predominant with anorexia, weight loss, and fever being the common presentation. Fever, the most common symptom, seen in nearly 75-80% of patients[9,12-15] has a characteristic early morning spike. This is seen in two other conditions namely polyarteritis nodosa and enteric fever.[29] Fever with chills and rigors, frequently associated with bacterial or malarial infection has also been documented.[22] Gradual onset of symptoms of malaise and weight loss occurs in 60-65% of individuals with cough and breathlessness in 50% of cases.[9,12-15] Abdominal pain as a major symptom is seen in around 7-14% of patients with miliary tuberculosis.[30] The causes of abdominal pain in miliary tuberculosis include peritonitis, enteritis, retroperitoneal lymphadenitis, and rarely pancreatitis. Headache seen in 10-15% suggests meningeal involvement.[15] Other presenting complaints include hemoptysis, pleuritic chest pain, nausea, vomiting, and altered mental status. Clinical signs most consistent with miliary tuberculosis are pyrexia, hepatomegaly, and splenomegaly. Diffuse crepitations are audible on chest auscultation while neck stiffness points toward meningeal irritation.[9,12-15] Less common findings include impairment of consciousness, lymphadenopathy, and serositis.[9,12,14] Sharma et al.[15] proposed a diagnostic criteria for miliary tuberculosis which is depicted in a tabular form (Table 1).

ORGAN INVOLVEMENT IN MILIARY TUBERCULOSIS

Liver

Next to the lungs, the liver is second most common organ to be affected and is seen in 50-80% of patients.[9,12-15] Majority of patients present with hepatomegaly and asymptomatic elevation of liver enzymes. Munt[31] reported that of the 15 individuals with miliary tuberculosis, 14 had mild increase in levels of aspartate aminotransferase (AST) while 5 had increased alkaline phosphatase levels. Elevated serum bilirubin greater than 1 g% was seen in 24% but none had levels more than 2 g%. Fulminant hepatic failure, though rare, has also been reported.[32] Granulomas are commonly seen[33] but this histopathological finding is also observed in other conditions like sarcoidosis, brucellosis, histoplasmosis, and other granulomatous diseases.[32]

Spleen

Splenic involvement in tuberculosis occurs in two different forms, miliary due to lymphohematogenous dissemination which is the commoner form and the uncommon one as primary involvement of the spleen. Spleen is the third most common organ involved in miliary tuberculosis besides lung and liver. Left hypochondriac pain (dragging sensation) and fullness is the most common presenting symptom due to splenic involvement. Splenomegaly is a common clinical finding. In a series of 100 Indian patients of miliary tuberculosis, splenomegaly was found in 31% of them.[15] In various other case series, splenomegaly was found in around 30-40%.[12-14] Acute thrombocytopenic purpura associated with splenomegaly in miliary tuberculosis has been documented in literature.[34] Ultrasonography and computed tomography (CT) scan do form a good diagnostic modality for detection of splenic involvement in miliary tuberculosis.

Central Nervous System

Central nervous system involvement is seen in around 22% of patients with miliary tuberculosis.[35] Tuberculous meningitis (TBM) following miliary tuberculosis occurs frequently in the pediatric population. Dissemination of the tuberculous bacilli from the lungs to the meninges leads to the formation of small tuberculomas. These rupture into the subarachnoid space leading to TBM. In an Indian series of 60 patients with miliary tuberculosis and CNS involvement, most of them presented with fever, weight loss, headache, and/or vomiting. Tuberculous meningitis was a diagnosis in 35% of them while 45% patients were having TBM with tuberculomas.[35] Spinal cord involvement was seen in 15% of these patients. Imaging modality for diagnosis includes contrast-enhanced computed tomography brain and magnetic resonance imaging (MRI) brain with MRI being more sensitive than CT scan for tuberculomas.[36]

Skin

Skin lesions in miliary tuberculosis have been typically described as acute miliary tuberculosis of the skin (tuberculosis cutis miliaris acuta generalisata). Tuberculosis cutis miliaris acuta generalisata is a condition described in infants and young children with miliary tuberculosis.[37] Initially, lesions develop as pinhead sized papules evolving into vesicles and then forming a crust when vesicles rupture. This initial stage of papule formation characteristically appears as 2-3 mm dull-red flat-topped papule with a central crust. Healing occurs leaving behind a white scar surrounded by brownish pigmentation.[37,38] Biopsy from these reveals scanty, nonspecific, dermal infiltrate of lymphocytes, and plasma cells along with focal necrotic areas and abscess formation. True caseating granulomas are not present but tuberculous bacilli are abundantly seen along with vascular thrombi.[38] However, macules, large pustules, ulcers, purpuric lesions, and subcutaneous nodules can also be seen. Lesions are generally asymmetric in distribution with buttocks and thighs being commonly involved. These dermatological manifestations are frequently seen in immunocompromised patients and atypical lesions have also been described. These include metastatic subcutaneous abscesses, chronic skin ulcers, and erythematous, violaceous, infiltrated, dermohypodermal plaques.[39,40]

Ocular

Hematogenous dissemination often leads to ocular manifestations in the choroid which is the most vascular structure in the eye. Tubercles in the choroid are typically seen as grayish or yellowish lesions, one-fourth disc diameter (DD) in size, around one to two DD away from the optic disc, close to the posterior pole of the retina.[41] These choroidal tubercles when present are considered to be pathognomic of miliary tuberculosis. One of the earlier case series had reported that choroidal tubercles occurred in 38% of patients with miliary tuberculosis[41] while a recent study documented in 5%.[42] Choroidal tubercles can lead to visual loss due to macular involvement.[43] Other ocular manifestations in miliary tuberculosis include conjunctival ulcerations, uveitis, scleritis, retinal vasculitis, and retinal hemorrhages.[44]

Pyrexia of Unknown Origin

Miliary tuberculosis can masquerade as pyrexia of unknown origin (PUO) which is defined as a temperature greater than 38.3°C on multiple occasions. The fever lasts for more than 3 weeks and in spite of 1 week of inpatient investigation, a diagnosis has not been achieved. Cunha et al.[29] had described a patient of miliary tuberculosis presenting with PUO with characteristic early morning temperature spikes. In a series from Turkey, describing 117 patients of PUO, infections accounted for 36% with tuberculosis implicated in 70%. Of these, 50% were due to miliary tuberculosis which accounted for 12% of all patients with PUO.[45]

Hematological

A number of hematological abnormalities have been described in patients with miliary tuberculosis. Anemia, which is seen in 50% of the patients, is mainly normocytic normochromic type like anemia of chronic disease.[13] The degree of anemia correlates well with the duration of illness rather than its severity.[46] Other types of anemia include sideroblastic anemia and megaloblastic anemia. Megaloblastic anemia is usually due to folate deficiency as folate levels are frequently reduced, reflecting the poor physical condition, and decreased dietary intake of the patient.[46] In majority of patients, the total leukocytic count is either normal or shows slight leukocytosis with predominant polymorphonuclear cells.[47] Leukemoid reactions may also be seen and rarely when pancytopenia occurs, poor prognosis is usually the outcome but recovery had also been documented.[48] Hemophagocytosis which is histiocytic phagocytosis of the reticuloendothelial cells in the bone marrow has also been described in miliary tuberculosis and is not uncommon.[49] Disseminated intravascular coagulation too has also been reported and carries a bad prognosis.[48]

Kidneys

Renal involvement in miliary tuberculosis is not seen frequently. Hematogenous dissemination of bacilli into the glomerular arterioles leads to the formation of cortical microabscesses bilaterally. Majority of them heal spontaneously with only few of them progressing. Simon et al.[50] while describing renal involvement in 20 patients with miliary tuberculosis observed tuberculous bacilli in the urine of five patients. The presenting features include dysuria, hematuria, flank pain, and pyuria along with constitutional symptoms.

Acute Respiratory Distress Syndrome

Although acute respiratory distress syndrome (ARDS) is not commonly seen in miliary tuberculosis but when it occurs is usually associated with high mortality rates as compared to other causes of ARDS. Kim et al.[51] documented that ARDS developed in 8 of the 34 patients diagnosed with miliary tuberculosis (23.5%) over a 10-year period, 6 of whom died. It has been reported that certain factors like hypoalbuminemia, raised AST, alanine aminotransferase, and D-dimer are independent predictors of developing ARDS in patients with miliary tuberculosis.[52]

Other Uncommon Manifestations

Pregnancy and Puerperium

Hippocrates had postulated that pregnancy was beneficial in tuberculosis; however, currently it is thought to have a deleterious effect.[53] In pregnancy, miliary tuberculosis commonly presents with symptoms of shortness of breath, loss of appetite, weakness, and slight fever which may easily be mistaken for physiological manifestations of pregnancy. Henderson et al.[16] described two patients with miliary tuberculosis in 2nd and 3rd trimester of pregnancy, respectively. Both of them had constitutional symptoms, miliary shadows on chest radiograph and granulomatous lesions on lung biopsy which improved clinically and radiologically on appropriate antituberculous therapy. Postpartum placental examination showed necrotizing granulomas with acid-fast bacilli (AFB) stain positivity. Similarly, miliary tuberculosis presenting as PUO during puerperium has been documented in a 28-year-old female.[54]

Glandular Involvement in Miliary Tuberculosis

Miliary tuberculosis and Addison's disease: Primary adrenocortical failure was first described by Thomas Addison in a monograph in 1855. Armand Trousseau while confirming this clinical entity named it as Addison's disease. At that time, tuberculosis was thought to be responsible in 70–80% cases of the disease.[55] However, nowadays the association of tuberculosis with adrenal failure is not so common while miliary tuberculosis as a cause of Addison's disease is rather rare. Two patients of miliary tuberculosis associated with Addison's disease were described by Sadler et al.[56] Both of them had hypotension, hyperkalemia, hyponatremia, and constitutional symptoms as the presenting feature with miliary mottling seen on chest skiagram. One of them had choroidal tubercles, another pathognomic feature of miliary tuberculosis, on fundus examination. Subacute adrenal failure as an initial manifestation of miliary tuberculosis has been documented. A tuberculous mycotic aneurysm detected incidentally on autopsy was thought to be the source of tubercle bacilli.[57] More recently, Addison's disease caused by miliary tuberculosis and the administration of rifampicin has been documented from Japan. It was postulated that therapy with rifampicin precipitated an acute adrenal crisis as the drug affected cytochrome P-450 accelerating hepatic metabolism of corticosteroids. Besides serum levels of adrenocorticotropic hormone and cortisol, CT scan abdomen may demonstrate enlargement of adrenals, areas of necrosis as well as calcification in case of tuberculous involvement of the adrenal.[58]

Miliary tuberculosis and thyroid: Tuberculosis of thyroid was first described in 1862 by Lebert in a patient with disseminated tuberculosis.[59] The thyroid gland is affected in 7% of patients with miliary tuberculosis.[60]

Miliary tuberculosis and the pancreas: Tuberculosis rarely affects the pancreas as the pancreatic enzyme is not conducive for the seeding of the *Mycobacterium*. In 1944, in a large autopsy series of 1,656 tuberculosis patients, pancreatic involvement due to miliary tuberculosis was detected in 14 autopsies.[7] Since then sporadic case reports have documented the occurrence of pancreatic tuberculosis caused by miliary seeding. Patients usually present with nonspecific complaints such as vague abdominal pain, epigastric discomfort, back pain, and nausea and vomiting. Pancreatitis as an initial presentation of miliary tuberculosis has also been documented. The patient had presented with a 3-week history of abdominal pain followed by fever, malaise, and nausea and vomiting a week later. Serum amylase was raised and chest radiograph showed hilar and paratracheal involvement. Subsequently, ARDS resulted in mortality. Postmortem studies revealed miliary tuberculosis was present in the lungs along with caseous necrosis of the hilar nodes. Multiple microabscesses were present in the pancreas from where AFB were seen.[30] Similarly, a 31-year-old male with a normal X-ray chest with bilateral ground-glass opacities (GGOs) on chest CT presented with severe abdominal symptoms and open lung biopsy confirmed miliary tuberculosis. He was diagnosed as cryptic miliary tuberculosis presenting with pancreatitis. The patient had a favorable outcome with antituberculous therapy.[61]

Pleura in Miliary Tuberculosis

Miliary tuberculosis may lead to pneumothorax (Fig. 1), pleural effusions, and empyema.

In a series of 60 patients presenting with spontaneous pneumothorax, 57% of them had tuberculosis while miliary tuberculosis was seen in only 5%.[62] Unilateral, bilateral[63] as well as recurrent[64] cases of pneumothoraces have been described. Various possible hypotheses explaining the pathogenesis of pneumothorax include: (1) caseous necrosis and rupture of the confluent subpleural miliary nodules in the pleural space leading to pneumothorax (the most plausible explanation), (2) formation of subpleural blebs by the confluent subpleural nodules with subsequent rupture. This was demonstrated histopathologically as blebs with surrounding granulomatous inflammation and (3) interstitial emphysema as proposed by Peiken et al.[64] Pneumothorax may also occur during the course of treatment with antituberculous drugs and hence any patient presenting with increased dyspnea during course of treatment should be evaluated. Gupta et al.[65] reported an individual with a diagnosis of miliary tuberculosis presenting with recurrent pneumothorax during the course of treatment and managed by tube thoracostomy and pleurodesis.

Miliary tuberculosis may also present with pneumomediastinum and subcutaneous emphysema.[66] Excessive coughing in miliary tuberculosis results in a sudden increase in intra-alveolar pressure along with concomitant airway narrowing. This leads to the rupture of alveolar septa and air leaks into interstitial tissues of the lung. Through

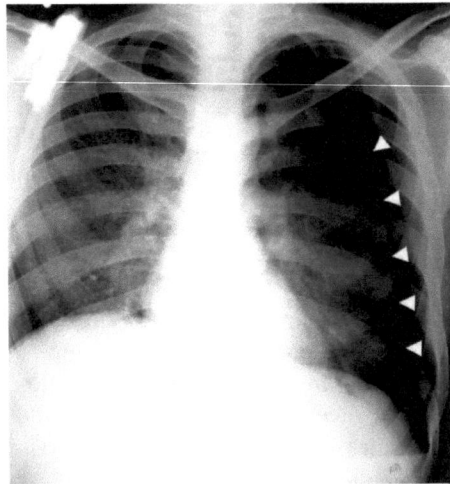

FIG. 1: Chest radiograph (posteroanterior view) showing the classical "miliary pattern" with left-sided pneumothorax (white arrow heads).

the peribronchial and perivascular spaces, air reaches the vascular adventitia of the hilum and into the mediastinum. The air then tracks along the fascial planes of the great vessels of the neck leading to subcutaneous emphysema. Management of pneumothorax includes tube thoracostomy with video-assisted thoracoscopic surgery and pleurodesis in recurrent cases.[64]

Polyserositis is not uncommon in patients with miliary tuberculosis. Pleural effusion in miliary tuberculosis is usually bilateral and tends to have a poor prognosis.[11]

Heart in Miliary Tuberculosis

Tuberculosis can affect the heart in 1-2% of the patients.[67] Tuberculous myocarditis, due to hematogenous spread of the bacilli, generally manifests as rhythm disturbances in the form of supraventricular tachycardias and atrioventricular blocks.[68] Other cardiac manifestations include native and prosthetic valve endocarditis, pericarditis, intracardiac mass, mycotic aneurysm, infection of a pacemaker pulse-generator pocket, and infection of ventriculoatrial shunt.[10]

COMPLICATIONS IN MILIARY TUBERCULOSIS

Complications are not uncommon in miliary tuberculosis and include "air-leak" syndromes such as unilateral/bilateral pneumothorax and pneumomediastinum.[62,63,66] Polyserositis, in the form of pleural and pericardial affection, is also known to complicate miliary tuberculosis. Pleural effusion in miliary tuberculosis usually tends to be bilateral as it is usually a polyserositis.[11] Electrolyte disturbances are also commonly seen in patients with miliary tuberculosis. Lymphadenopathy is a recognized complication of miliary tuberculosis.[11] Extensive lymphadenopathy involving the cervical, axillary, and inguinal regions with bilateral miliary mottling associated with pleural effusion, hepatomegaly, and ascites was documented.[69] Hyponatremia is the most common electrolyte disturbance and has been attributed to syndrome of inappropriate antidiuretic hormone secretion. Hypokalemia, another common electrolyte abnormality, frequently manifests as generalized weakness especially in the elderly.[11] Sepsis, septic shock, and ARDS are a few uncommon but grave complications (Table 2).

TABLE 2	Complications of miliary tuberculosis[1,10,12]
S. No.	Complications
1	"Air-leak" syndromes (pneumothorax, pneumomediastinum)
2	Sepsis, septic shock, disseminated intravascular coagulation
3	Acute respiratory distress syndrome
4	Adrenocortical insufficiency
5	Thyrotoxicosis
6	Pericarditis/pericardial effusion
7	Hyponatremia (due to syndrome of inappropriate antidiuretic hormone secretion), hypokalemia
8	Hematological abnormalities
9	Polyserositis
10	Lymphadenopathy

IMAGING IN MILIARY TUBERCULOSIS

Chest X-ray

Chest radiograph continues to remain the primary imaging diagnostic intervention in miliary tuberculosis but can also appear to be normal. Several case series have documented miliary lesions on chest radiograph in 30–93% of the patients.[12-14,70] In a radiological review of 71 patients with miliary tuberculosis, three observers detected miliary mottling on the chest radiograph in 59–69% with a good specificity but a poor sensitivity.[70] Many a times miliary mottlings may not be evident on initial presentation but develop in a week or two. Felson observed that miliary lesions are commonly seen around 2.5 weeks after an episode of hematogenous dissemination.[71] The usual description of these miliary shadows is "multiple well-defined nodules around 1–3 mm seen distributed well throughout the lung field predominantly in the lower lung fields".[71] Classically, these nodules are less than 3 mm in size; however, in 10% of the patients these nodules can be around 3–10 mm in size.[11] Initially, these nodules have a hazy appearance but sooner develop a sharper outline. Long et al.[72] documented that the number and size of miliary tubercles on chest radiograph are time dependent with majority of cases having 2.5–6 weeks gap between bacillemia and radiographic changes. The best way to identify these nodules is to scan the peripheral areas of the intercostal spaces in a well-penetrated film.[73] The caseous material and the collagen contribute to the appearance of the miliary shadows. Whenever these tubercles superimpose on each other, it gives the classic miliary appearance while if these nodules are not properly aligned along the plane of the film, a reticulonodular pattern is observed.[74] Sometimes due to the lymphatic involvement, a reticular pattern consisting of few thin dense lines may be seen, known as lymphangitis reticularis tuberculosa.[75] This is the lymphogenous form of miliary tuberculosis seen in chronic cases.[75]

Apart from the typical miliary pattern, other features seen on chest X-rays include areas of consolidation, GGOs, and lymphadenopathy. Pleural effusion is often seen (Fig. 2) and bilateral pleural effusion is not uncommon. Polyserositis is a well-known

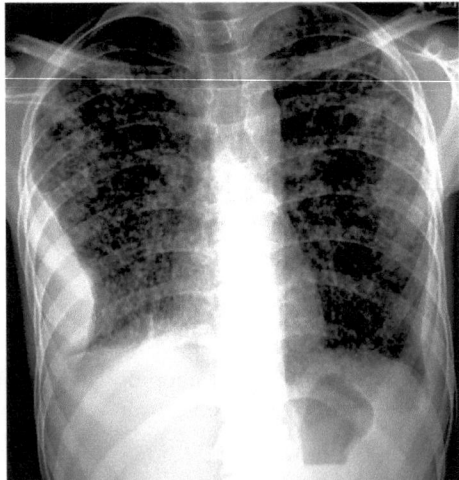

FIG. 2: Chest radiograph (posteroanterior view) showing miliary nodules in both the lung fields with bilateral pleural effusion (right to left).

BOX 1	Differential diagnosis of miliary mottlings[1,10,20]

- Infectious:
  - Mycobacterial:
    - *Mycobacterium tuberculosis*
    - Atypical mycobacterial infections
  - Viral:
    - Influenza
    - Measles
    - Varicella-zoster virus
    - Epstein-Barr virus
    - Cytomegalovirus
  - Bacterial:
    - *Staphylococcus aureus*
    - Pneumococcus
    - *Mycoplasma* infections
    - Brucellosis
    - Melioidosis
    - Tularemia
    - Psittacosis
  - Fungal:
    - Histoplasmosis
    - Blastomycosis
    - Coccidioidomycosis
    - Cryptococcosis
  - Parasitic:
    - Toxoplasmosis
    - Schistosomiasis
- Inflammatory causes:
  - Sarcoidosis
  - Hypersensitivity pneumonitis
  - Goodpasture syndrome
- Neoplastic:
  - Bronchoalveolar carcinoma
  - Lymphangitis carcinomatosis
  - Metastatic carcinoma
  - Lymphoma
- Other causes:
  - Tropical pulmonary eosinophilia
  - Hemosiderosis (mitral stenosis, heart failure)
  - Drug-induced (e.g., methotrexate, cyclophosphamide)
  - Pneumoconiosis

complication and includes pericardial effusion and ascites. Of the 71 patients with miliary tuberculosis, lymphadenopathy was identified on chest radiograph in 11 patients. Five of the patients had enlarged mediastinal nodes while one had enlarged hilar nodes and the rest five had both hilar and mediastinal lymphadenopathy. Pleural effusion was observed in 19 of the 71 patients with bilateral pleural effusion in five of them.[70]

The list for differential diagnosis of miliary opacities on chest radiograph has been detailed in box 1.

Computed Tomography Scan Chest

The advent of CT scan of the chest especially the high-resolution CT (HRCT) has emerged as a key diagnostic modality as on a conventional plain chest radiograph, the diagnosis can easily be missed. The HRCT findings include miliary nodules, GGOs, and reticular shadows. Miliary nodules, the commonest HRCT feature, are typically 1–2 mm in size, well defined, and are randomly distributed throughout the lung fields (Fig. 3).[76] A study from South Korea evaluated 25 patients with miliary tuberculosis and detected miliary nodules in 24 patients on HRCT.[76] These nodules are detected earlier on CT as compared to conventional radiograph. Miliary nodules, however, are a nonspecific finding on HRCT. High-resolution computed tomography done on 76 patients with miliary mottlings found that 54% patients had miliary tuberculosis while 26% of them had miliary metastasis, pneumoconiosis in 8%, and sarcoidosis in 5%.[77]

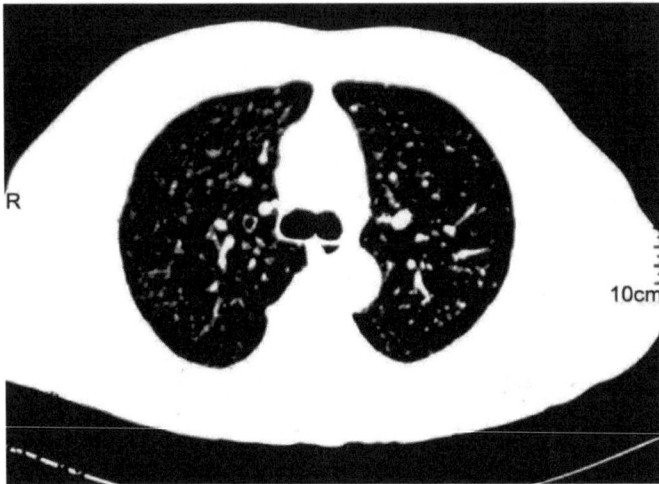

FIG. 3: Contrast-enhanced computed tomography chest (lung window) showing bilaterally randomly distributed miliary nodules.

Ground-glass opacities, the second most common HRCT finding, have been documented in 60–90% patients of miliary tuberculosis.[76,78,79] Ground-glass opacities represent tiny granulomas, focal areas of edema or alveolar wall thickening.[76] In patients with GGOs more than 50% present with dyspnea.[79] Transbronchial lung biopsy from these areas of focal ground-glassing had demonstrated multiple granulomas with AFB.[80]

Intralobular and interlobular septal thickening on HRCT occur due to the diffuse scattering of the granulomas along the pulmonary interstitium.[76] If present, pleural effusion can also be visualized (Fig. 4). In addition, pericardial effusions, mediastinal lymphadenopathy as well as calcifications may also be seen.

The findings on HRCT have a considerable difference among HIV-positive and HIV-negative patients with miliary tuberculosis. In a comparative study of the CT findings among HIV-positive and HIV-negative patients with miliary tuberculosis interlobular septal thickening, necrotic lymphadenitis and extrathoracic manifestations were more common in HIV-positive patients.[78]

Role of Ultrasound and Computed tomography Abdomen

Role of Ultrasonography primarily for diagnosis of miliary tuberculosis is limited. Ultrasonography is a useful adjunct in evaluation of liver and spleen and for documenting pleural effusion, ascites as well as intra-abdominal lymphadenopathy. Ultrasonography-guided hepatic or splenic biopsy may help in assessment of the granulomas of these organs. On Ultrasonography, the spleen when affected shows multiple small hypoechoic areas. However, CT scan of abdomen gives more detailed information. Computed tomography scan of the abdomen is more informative with tiny low-density foci seen when the liver and spleen are affected. These lesions are widely disseminated throughout this viscera.[81]

Role of Magnetic Resonance Imaging

Usefulness of MRI is restricted to the diagnosis of TBM following miliary tuberculosis where it is considered superior to CT scan. Lesions are generally found

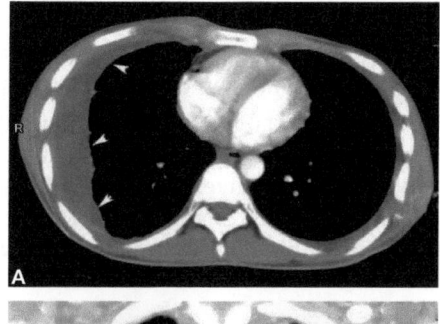
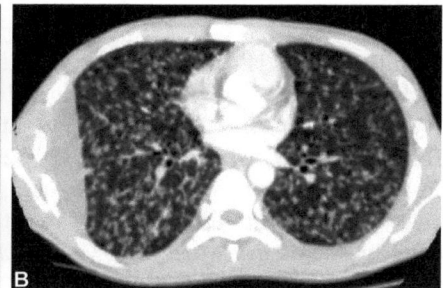
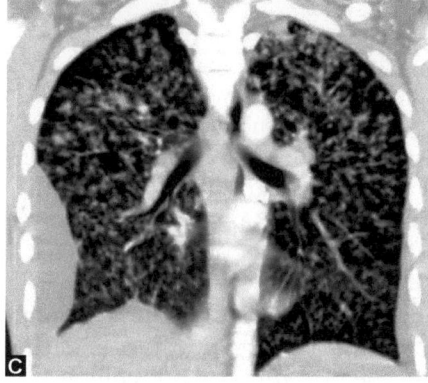

FIG. 4: A, Contrast-enhanced computed tomography (CECT) chest (mediastinal window) showing right-sided pleural effusion (white arrow heads); **B,** CECT chest (lung window) of the same patient showing randomly distributed miliary nodules bilaterally with right-sided pleural effusion; **C,** CECT chest (lung window coronal section) of the same patient showing randomly distributed miliary nodules bilaterally with right-sided pleural effusion.

at the corticomedullary junction in brain due to the hematogenous spread of the bacilli. These lesions are small in size (2–3 mm in diameter), diffusely scattered, and are hypointense on T2-weighted sequences. Postcontrast T1-weighted MR images show multiple, small, round, homogeneous, enhancing (usually ring enhancement) lesions.[82] Other findings on MRI include intracranial tuberculomas generally seen as low-intensity lesions with or without central hyperintensity (due to varying amount of caseous necrosis) and hypo- to isointense lesions on T1-weighted images.[83]

Nuclear Imaging Techniques

Initial studies regarding nuclear imaging modalities in miliary tuberculosis was through gallium 67 scans. Gallium 67 binds both to the inflammatory cells and the *Mycobacterium*. Gallium scintigraphy is thus a sensitive indicator for presence of active infection with *Mycobacterium*. It can also be used to identify the various sites of dissemination of the tuberculous bacilli.[84] In a series of 16 patients with miliary tuberculosis, gallium scan was positive in 13 patients with 10 of them having a diffuse uptake.[85] The drawback of gallium scintigraphy is the nonspecificity of this imaging modality. This nuclear imaging modality was superseded by the technetium-99m-methoxyisobutylisonitrile (MIBI) scintigraphy. Technetium-99m-MIBI scintigraphy was able to detect miliary tuberculosis with a sensitivity of nearly 100% with a poor specificity.[86] Newer nuclear imaging modalities like positron emission tomography-CT using 18-fluorodeoxyglucose have been used to assess activity of tuberculosis with further studies needed to define its diagnostic role in miliary tuberculosis.

TUBERCULIN SKIN TEST

Miliary tuberculosis is one of the few conditions where anergy occurs in the tuberculin test. Tuberculin test is generally positive during the early stages of dissemination. In a study by Sahn et al.,[47] 38% of the patients showed a positive tuberculin test with 1 tuberculin unit (TU) whereas with 5 TU, 52% had positive reaction. In a similar series by Mert et al.,[9] tuberculin positivity was 32% with 5 TU. Conversion from tuberculin negative to positive states occurs 2–4 months after initiation of treatment. Tuberculin positivity indicates infection with *Mycobacterium* and does not differentiate between active disease and latent infection.

ROLE OF INTERFERON-γ RELEASE ASSAYS

The newer diagnostic modality of interferon-γ release assay (IGRA) is superior as compared to tuberculin skin test for diagnosis of latent tuberculous infections. The sensitivity and specificity of IGRAs for pulmonary tuberculous infection is 86–89% and 94–98%, respectively.[87] Limited studies have been carried out in patients with miliary tuberculosis evaluating the performance of IGRAs. Two forms of IGRAs are commercially available: (1) QuantiFERON-TB Gold In-Tube assay which is an enzyme-linked immunosorbent assay and (2) T-SPOT.TB which is an enzyme-linked immunospot assay. These tests detect the interferon-γ released by the T-lymphocytes in response to stimulation by antigens, early secretory antigenic target-6 and culture filtrate protein-10 which are derived from the *M. tuberculosis* complex.[88] The sensitivity for QuantiFERON-TB Gold In-Tube assay was found out to be 63% in a study among 44 patients with miliary tuberculosis.[89] However, for the T-SPOT.TB test, the sensitivity was found out to be 93% in another series involving 43 patients with miliary tuberculosis.[88] A study comparing these two modalities demonstrated that sensitivity of QuantiFERON-TB Gold In-Tube was lower as compared to T-SPOT.TB test.[90] The authors suggested that this difference in results was due to the effect of immunosuppression on the sensitivity of QuantiFERON-TB Gold In-Tube test.[90]

Indeterminate results are quite common in miliary tuberculosis especially in patients with severe lymphocytopenia and extensive GGOs greater than 50%.[88] Lymphocytopenia leads to a decreased interferon release and thus indeterminate test results.[91]

ROLE OF SPUTUM SMEAR MICROSCOPY AND CULTURE

Sputum smear and culture has been the gold standard for diagnosis of tuberculosis. However, in cases of miliary tuberculosis, the yield is not so great. The overall outcome of sputum microscopy is 30–40% while positive culture is seen in 60% of patients.[9,13-15,31] Yield of AFB from other samples like gastric aspirates, bronchial washings is generally lower.

ROLE OF PULMONARY FUNCTION TESTS

The abnormalities seen in pulmonary function testing in miliary tuberculosis resemble that of an interstitial lung disease. The most consistent finding is impairment of diffusion capacity for carbon monoxide (DLCO). Spirometric abnormalities reported in 16 patients were a decreased forced vital capacity (FVC), forced expiratory volume in 1 second (FEV1), peak expiratory flow rate, and flow during the middle half of vital capacity [forced expiratory flow (FEF) 25–75] with increased FEV1/FVC (%), functional residual capacity, residual volume/total lung capacity (%). Diffusion capacity for carbon monoxide was low in these subjects.[92] Pipavath et al.[93] demonstrated a negative correlation between findings on HRCT and lung function and gas exchange parameters with worsening of parameters seen in severe disease.

Blood gas analysis reveals arterial hypoxemia with widening of alveolar-arterial oxygen gradient and hypocapnea due to hyperventilation in acute stages.[94]

ROLE OF BIOPSY

Biopsy has a varying yield depending on the tissue chosen. Biopsy finding includes the typical caseating granulomatous areas along with the AFB. Liver biopsy shows granulomatous inflammation in 90–95% in several case series[9,13-15,31] though culture positivity was rare from these samples. Similarly, other tissues like spleen, lymph node as well as bone marrow may be used with all of them having an average outcome. Kim et al.[95] evaluated 38 patients with miliary tuberculosis and reported the yield of biopsy from various tissue samples. The liver biopsy revealed granulomas in 11/12 (92%) biopsy specimens while granulomas on bone marrow biopsy were seen in 9/22 (41%) specimens. Only one-fourth of liver biopsy samples were culture-positive. Similarly, Mert et al.[9] reported granulomatous inflammation in biopsy samples from lungs in 11/13 patients (85%), in liver in 15/15 patients (100%), in bone marrow in 9/16 patients (56%).

ROLE OF FIBEROPTIC BRONCHOSCOPY IN MILIARY TUBERCULOSIS

Yield of sputum smear in case of miliary tuberculosis is quite low and hence for making a diagnosis fiberoptic bronchoscopy (FOB) and BAL play an important role. The first published report of FOB in the diagnosis of miliary tuberculosis was in 1975 by Sahn et al.[96] They reported a sputum smear-negative miliary tuberculosis patient diagnosed through transbronchial biopsy where the tissue specimen had numerous AFB with positive culture reports. Burk et al.[97] documented a 75% positive result among eight patients undergoing bronchoscopic biopsy. In a study of 41 patients with miliary tuberculosis, the diagnostic yield of FOB was 83% with rapid diagnostic techniques having a positive outcome in 79%.[98] In a similar study from our Institute, 73% of the sputum smear-negative miliary tuberculosis with miliary mottlings on chest X-ray were diagnosed with the help of FOB.[99] In a retrospective review[100] of bronchoscopic biopsies in 31 patients with miliary tuberculosis, caseating granulomas were found in 21 (67%). Since miliary tuberculosis involves the lung parenchyma diffusely, biopsy has a higher yield. It appears that FOB is one of the key diagnostic modality in the workup of patients with smear-negative miliary tuberculosis.

Analysis of the BAL fluid to determine its cellular composition in patients with miliary tuberculosis was first carried out by Sharma et al.[101] In comparison to the normal control subjects, patients with miliary tuberculosis had a higher total cellular and lymphocytic counts ($p < 0.01$) with significant decrease in alveolar macrophages ($p < 0.01$) in BAL fluid. Epithelioid cell granulomas were found in BAL fluid in two patients. However, smear for AFB and culture of the BAL fluid were negative in all cases.[101] A study from Japan analyzed the differential count of BAL fluid which showed that the total cellular count, neutrophils, and eosinophils, in BAL fluid of patients with miliary tuberculosis was not significantly different from controls ($p > 0.05$). Lymphocytic counts were increased in BAL fluid with peripheral lymphopenia. However, macrophages were lower in the BAL fluid with peripheral blood showing monocytosis. Analysis of the albumin content and immunoglobulin G levels in BAL fluid from these patients showed high values as compared to controls.[102] A study to analyze the lymphocytic subset in the BAL fluid in patients with miliary tuberculosis showed a lower percentage of CD4+ T-lymphocytes, a higher percentage of CD8+ T-lymphocytes, and a decreased CD4/CD8 ratio.[103]

DIAGNOSTIC UTILITY OF ADENOSINE DEAMINASE LEVELS

Adenosine deaminase (ADA) levels are increased in BAL fluid in miliary tuberculosis. Kubota et al.[104] measured the BAL fluid ADA activity in 65 subjects which included six patients with miliary tuberculosis who had a mean ADA activity of 5.02 ± 3.75 IU/L (mean ± SD). The levels were significantly increased and differed from other causes (p <0.01). Elevated ADA levels in BAL fluid may be an early diagnostic clue in miliary tuberculosis.

OTHER DIAGNOSTIC INVESTIGATIONS

In a study of 145 patients with miliary tuberculosis undergoing sternal marrow aspiration, tubercles were found in 16 of them.[105] Escobedo et al.[106] evaluated the role of polymerase chain reaction (PCR) for the diagnosis of miliary tuberculosis in 30 patients from bone marrow smears. Of the 30 patients, diagnosis was confirmed in 28 of them by routine microscopy and culture. Staining for AFB was positive in 13 respiratory specimens (sensitivity 43.3% and specificity 100%) and three in urine (sensitivity 10% and specificity 100%). Culture of sputum samples was positive in 14 of 30 patients (sensitivity 46.7% and specificity 100%), while in urine this was positive in five cases (sensitivity 16.7% and specificity 100%). Polymerase chain reaction was able to detect miliary tuberculosis in 21 patients with a sensitivity of 70% and specificity of 84.5%. The main drawback of PCR is the false-positive result occurring possibly due to contamination.[106]

MILIARY TUBERCULOSIS IN SPECIAL POPULATION

Pediatric Age Group

In the prechemotherapy era, miliary tuberculosis was predominantly seen in the pediatric age group. This was attributed to the poor cell-mediated immunity against the lymphohematogenous spread of the *Mycobacterium*. However, with the introduction of the BCG vaccine, incidence of miliary tuberculosis among children sharply declined. A comparative study of the necropsies performed in Belfast over two time periods, 1946-1949 and 1966-1969 reflected this changing pattern of miliary tuberculosis. During 1946-1949, miliary tuberculosis occurred in around 1.7% of all the autopsies with 54% of them being in the age group less than 20 years. However, in the 1966-1969 cohort, the incidence of miliary tuberculosis declined to 0.7% with majority of patients being adults.[107]

Natural History of Childhood Miliary Tuberculosis

Infection by *M. tuberculosis* may not herald into clinically manifest disease in all patients. Whenever infection occurs, within 3-8 weeks, there occurs the formation of Ghon focus and subsequently leading to the development of Ghon complex. During this stage, the child may develop fever, show tuberculin conversion, and primary complex may be evident on a chest radiograph. During the subsequent 1-3 months after primary infection, hematogenous dissemination of the tubercle bacilli and seeding into various organs occur. This is the period having maximum risk for development of miliary tuberculosis depending on the host immune response and virulence of the organism. Majority of patients develop an acute form of miliary tuberculosis; however, some children develop a chronic "cryptic" form.[108]

The single most important predictor for progression from infection to disease is age, the risk of disseminated infection being higher in infants and young children as compared to older children. The risk of miliary infection was shown to be 10–20% in the infants which decreased to 2–5% by second year of life and was 0.5% in the age group 10 years onward.[108]

Clinical Features

The most common presenting feature, fever, is seen in 60–80%.[109-111] Fever is typically high grade and persisting for weeks or months prior to diagnosis being established. The other symptoms include cough (60–70%),[109-111] weight loss and loss of appetite (40–50%),[110] vomiting, diarrhea, and night sweats. The most consistent clinical finding was hepatosplenomegaly seen in 60–70%.[109-111] Other findings included lymphadenopathy, pyrexia, and crepitations.[109-111]

Ocular examination tends to demonstrate choroidal tubercles, a feature considered to be pathognomic of miliary tuberculosis. In a series of 63 children, choroidal tubercles were detected in around 13%.[112] However, an earlier series documented choroidal tubercles in 113/170 (66%) patients with miliary tuberculosis.[113] Occurrence of choroidal tubercles was higher in patients with acute miliary tuberculosis than in subacute cases.[113] Tuberculin reactivity in several case series varied from 50 to 91%.[110-112] Miliary mottling was detected in chest radiograph in majority of children with miliary tuberculosis. In 1952, Debré[113] described three different forms of miliary mottling on chest X-ray in miliary tuberculosis. *"Granulie d'Empis"* is seen in acute form of miliary tuberculosis and consists of multiple tiny spots with no differences of size between them, is abundant and scattered throughout both the lung fields with no part of the lungs being clear of them. The other two forms are seen in subacute miliary tuberculosis where the spots are larger and unequal in size. These lesions heal spontaneously and have been termed as *"Granulie curable"*. They have a nonuniform distribution and appear denser near the hilum, where the lung is thicker and scarcer at the periphery. The other diagnostic modalities include sputum and gastric aspirates for AFB. The patients must also be evaluated for meningitis.

Complications

The single most important complication of miliary tuberculosis in children is TBM and a major cause of significant mortality and morbidity. Tuberculous meningitis is not uncommon in children with miliary tuberculosis and can occur in 20–40%. Of the 104 children with TBM, 32 (31%) children had miliary mottlings on chest radiograph. Cerebrospinal fluid findings included lymphocytosis with raised proteins and with a mortality rate of 16% in this particular study.[114] In a similar study among 84 children with miliary tuberculosis, TBM (28.5%) was the most frequent complication with mortality in 38%.[109]

Other complications include cervical lymphadenitis, renal tuberculosis, intestinal tuberculosis along with other nontuberculous complications like glomerulonephritis, osteomyelitis.[109]

Outcome

In the prechemotherapeutic era, outcome of acute miliary tuberculosis in the pediatric population was grim with high mortality rates. Mortality rates from several case series range from 7 to 18%.[109-112]

HUMAN IMMUNODEFICIENCY VIRUS AND MILIARY TUBERCULOSIS

With the spread of the HIV epidemic in the 1980s and 1990s, the incidence of miliary tuberculosis increased. Since cell-mediated immunity is responsible for containing infection in case of tuberculosis, a fall in CD4 count predisposes to disseminated tuberculosis. Clinical presentation in case of HIV-tuberculosis coinfection depends on the CD4 counts. Presentation in the form of miliary tuberculosis occurs in cases of advanced HIV infection with CD4 counts below 200/mm^3.[115]

Miliary tuberculosis in HIV patients may be due to reactivation of latent infection or due to secondary infection with the former being more common.[115] Miliary tuberculosis occurs in 10% of HIV-infected subjects and a high index of suspicion is needed for diagnosis due to nonspecific presentation.[116] A study in a tertiary care center in India among HIV-positive patients showed that 71% of the patients had pulmonary tuberculosis as an opportunistic infection out of which the rate of disseminated tuberculosis was found out to be 64%.[117] In another case series, the rate of miliary tuberculosis in HIV-tuberculosis coinfected individuals was determined to be 6.1%.[118] Majority of patients present with fever, cough, weight loss, and anorexia. Cutaneous lesions in miliary tuberculosis often seen in patients with HIV infection include tuberculosis cutis miliaris disseminata, lichen scrofulosorum, tuberculous ulcer, chancre, subcutaneous abscess, and a tuberculid-type of presentation.[119] A comparative study between miliary tuberculosis in HIV-positive and HIV-negative individuals showed that cutaneous involvement, lymphadenopathy, atypical presentation, and extrapulmonary involvement were more common in HIV-positive patients.[10] Tuberculin anergy is a common finding among HIV-infected patients with one series reporting the rates of tuberculin anergy to be 90% as compared to 40% in the non-HIV-infected patients.[115] In a series of 51 patients with miliary tuberculosis and HIV infection, miliary mottlings were seen in 22.[115] A comparison of the CT findings among HIV-seropositive and HIV-negative individuals showed that HIV-seropositive patients had significantly increased prevalence of interlobular septal thickening, necrotic lymph nodes, and greater extrathoracic involvement. The seropositive patients had a lower prevalence of large nodules. Computed tomography findings of patients with severe immunosuppression (CD4 count <50 cells/µL) were similar to those with a lower degree of immunosuppression (CD4 >50 cells/µL).[78]

Yield from sputum microscopy, culture as well as tissue biopsies are significantly higher in patients with miliary tuberculosis having HIV infection. This has been attributed to the fact that immunosuppressive state leads to a larger bacillary load. Histopathological studies have shown that HIV patients with miliary tuberculosis fail to develop a granuloma due to lack of adequate cellular immune response. The histopathological findings include acute granular necrosis containing nuclear debris and abundant AFB with very few epithelioid cells and lymphocytes. Granulomas are poorly defined or absent in a majority of patients.[115]

In a study to evaluate response to treatment in patients with miliary tuberculosis-HIV coinfection, the short-term outcome was favorable with 81% of the patients had significant clinical, bacteriological, and radiological improvement. The long-term outcome of these patients with advanced HIV disease was poor despite successful antituberculous therapy. The recurrence rate was high, with about a third of patients relapsing within 2 years of completing therapy.[120] Mortality rates ranged from 25 to 29% in patients with miliary tuberculosis and HIV coinfection.[115,120]

DRUG-RESISTANT MILIARY TUBERCULOSIS

Drug resistance especially, multidrug-resistance in tuberculosis (MDR-tuberculosis) is a global issue and is more frequently seen in developing countries. Inadequate dosing regimen, default on patient side, poor quality of drugs have all contributed in emergence of what could be a major challenge in treatment of tuberculosis. The WHO global report estimates that MDR-tuberculosis globally to be 3.5% in new cases and 20% in previously treated cases.[8] Globally, in 2013, there were an estimated 480,000 new cases of MDR-tuberculosis with approximately 210,000 deaths from MDR-tuberculosis.[8]

Drug-resistant Miliary Tuberculosis in Immunocompromised Hosts

The occurrence of drug-resistant miliary tuberculosis is common in immunocompromised patients as lowered immunity favors infection as well as dissemination of drug-resistant *Mycobacterium*. Daikos et al.[121] reported four patients with miliary tuberculosis and cutaneous spread of the tubercle bacilli. Of the four patients, three were diagnosed with drug-resistant miliary tuberculosis. Two of them were resistant to isoniazid, rifampicin, ethambutol, and ethionamide. Similarly, another case of rapidly progressive drug-resistant miliary tuberculosis in a 21-month-old HIV-positive girl was reported. Polymerase chain reaction was used for evaluation of drug resistance in this patient.[122]

Drug-resistant Miliary Tuberculosis in Immunocompetent Hosts

The description of MDR miliary tuberculosis in an immunocompetent host comes from India, in a 57-year-old, HIV-seronegative, nondiabetic patient having miliary tuberculosis coexistent with Pott's spine.[123] Bronchial aspirate was AFB-positive and culture reports showed *M. tuberculosis* resistant to rifampicin, isoniazid, streptomycin, kanamycin, and ethionamide but sensitive to fluoroquinolones, ethambutol, and para-aminosalicylic acid. Second line antituberculous treatment (ATT) led to marked clinicoradiological improvement within 10 weeks. A similar report from Germany documented drug-resistant miliary tuberculosis in a 27-year-old migrant worker resistant to all the first line antituberculous drugs.[124] The gold standard for diagnosis of drug-resistant tuberculosis is Mycobacterial culture and sensitivity studies. However, it takes around 8–12 weeks for a positive culture report with sometimes growth not being appreciable. Hence, newer molecular diagnostic tests like the line probe assay and cartridge-based nucleic acid amplification test (Xpert MTB/RIF) have been useful for early diagnosis. A recent case report from South Korea highlights the importance of these tests in establishing an early diagnosis of multidrug-resistant miliary tuberculosis.[125]

CHRONIC "CRYPTIC FORM"

The term "cryptic form" of miliary tuberculosis was first introduced by Proudfoot[126] when he described a series of patients with miliary tuberculosis presenting with nonspecific symptoms and lack of miliary mottling on chest radiograph. This obscure form of tuberculosis does not present with the classical clinical as well as radiological features. This leads to the diagnosis being delayed or completely missed and is often detected on autopsy. Due to this particular nature, this form of miliary tuberculosis warrants a high index of suspicion. This particular form is seen in a majority of older patients having a waning immune response to the tubercle bacilli. Yu et al.[127] proposed diagnostic criteria for cryptic form of miliary tuberculosis which includes presence of (i) nonspecific clinical and radiological features but positive bacteriological or histological findings of miliary tuberculosis either during life or at autopsy, (ii) nonspecific clinical and radiological features and negative bacteriological and histological findings but having a good response to antituberculous therapy. Majority of patients have an insidious presentation and are in an advanced stage of the disease. Comorbid conditions such as diabetes, malnutrition, and immunosuppression are a common association in these patients.[126]

EVOLUTION OF TREATMENT STRATEGIES

There has been a gradual evolution of the treatment strategies in case of miliary tuberculosis beginning from a single drug therapy to the current short-course combined chemotherapy. Current treatment strategy involves the use of short-course combined chemotherapy directly observed treatment short-course) in the treatment of miliary tuberculosis. The WHO treatment guidelines for tuberculosis classify miliary tuberculosis under "pulmonary tuberculosis".[128] As a result, all new cases of miliary tuberculosis should be treated using isoniazid, rifampicin, pyrazinamide, and ethambutol during the intensive phase for 2 months followed by isoniazid and rifampicin during the continuation phase for 4 months. Similarly, American Thoracic Society guidelines[129] and National Institute for Health and Care Excellence guidelines[130] also suggest a 6-month treatment of miliary tuberculosis. In patients with miliary tuberculosis and meningitis, treatment duration may be prolonged to 9-12 months.

Monitoring during the course of treatment is an important component of the treatment strategy. Since the antituberculous drugs are hepatotoxic, proper monitoring of the liver function tests should be done while on treatment. Since in patients with miliary tuberculosis asymptomatic increase of liver enzymes is quite common, ATT should not be stopped unless there has been a definite evidence of drug-induced hepatotoxicity.[1] Drug resistance is another issue that needs to be evaluated during the treatment of miliary tuberculosis. In suspected cases of drug resistance or failure to respond to treatment, culture and drug sensitivity should be done. Recently, the WHO has approved the use of GeneXpert in cases of diagnosis of drug resistance to rifampicin.[131]

In patients with HIV-miliary tuberculosis coinfection, antiretroviral therapy should be administered promptly along with ATT. Monitoring for drug interactions, management of immune reconstitution inflammatory syndrome (IRIS) following treatment and cotrimoxazole prophylaxis for *Pneumocystis jirovecii* (formerly *carinii*) pneumonia (PCP) form an integral part of treatment strategy.[1]

Role of Steroids

There have been limited data regarding the role of steroids in treatment of miliary tuberculosis. The only study which has described patient characteristics for comparison between corticosteroid and placebo-treated groups is from China. Of the 55 patients with miliary tuberculosis randomized into two groups, mortality rates were lower among the steroid-treated group (2 out of 27) as compared to the patients in the control group (5 out of 28). However, a similar study in the pediatric population failed to document any improvement following steroid treatment in miliary tuberculosis.[132]

Role of Bacillus Calmette–Guérin Vaccination

The protective efficacy of BCG vaccine varies in various forms of tuberculosis. Classically, the efficacy of BCG vaccine has been described ranging from 0 to 80%.[133] Higher protective effect was seen in disseminated and miliary forms of the disease as compared to the other forms of tuberculosis. In 1993, a meta-analysis consisting of 10 randomized controlled trials (RCTs) and eight case-control studies was conducted to determine the protective effect of BCG vaccine on miliary and meningeal forms of tuberculosis. The meta-analysis concluded that the protective effect of BCG vaccine was more homogenous and consistent in case of miliary tuberculosis as compared to other forms of tuberculosis. The overall protective effect of BCG vaccine in miliary tuberculosis was 86% in the RCTs and 75% in case of case-control studies.[133] Another meta-analysis regarding efficacy of BCG vaccination in miliary tuberculosis found out the protective efficacy to be 77%.[134]

PROGNOSTIC FACTORS IN MILIARY TUBERCULOSIS

Various factors determine outcome in patients with miliary tuberculosis. The factors commonly associated with poor prognosis include malnutrition, hypoalbuminemia, raised serum bilirubin levels, leukopenia, leukocytosis, lymphopenia, thrombocytopenia, and pleural, pericardial, or peritoneal involvement.[10,135] In a study to determine the predictors for the development of acute respiratory failure (ARF) and survival in patients with miliary tuberculosis, it was found out that ARF developed in 25% of patients (14 out of 56), with a 50% fatality rate. A high nutritional risk score (NRS) (≥3 points) was an independent risk factor for the development of ARF and fatality in these patients. A four-point NRS was defined according to the presence of four nutritional factors: (i) low body mass index (BMI) (<18.5 kg/m^2), (ii) hypoalbuminemia (<30.0 g/L), (iii) hypocholesterolemia (<2.33 mmol/L) and (iv) severe lymphocytopenia (<7 × 10^5 cells/L). Each risk factor was assigned a value of 1 if present or 0 if absent (with scores >3 were high risk scores). Acute respiratory failure, severe lymphocytopenia, hypocholesterolemia, low BMI, and higher NRS were risk factors for poor outcome in this study.[136]

CONCLUSION

Miliary tuberculosis can be a major diagnostic challenge. If not diagnosed on time and if left untreated it can spread rapidly and dreaded complications like TBM can occur. If detected on time, miliary tuberculosis responds well to appropriate therapy and the patient can be restored to good health.

REFERENCES

1. Mohan A, Sharma SK. History. In: Mohan A, Sharma SK (Eds). Tuberculosis. 2nd ed. New Delhi: Jaypee Brothers Medical Publishers (P) Ltd; 2009. pp. 10-1.
2. Ducati RG, Ruffino-Netto A, Basso LA, Santos DS. The resumption of consumption—a review on tuberculosis. Mem Inst Oswaldo Cruz. 2006;101:697-714.
3. Daniel TM. The history of tuberculosis. Respir Med. 2006;100:1862-70.
4. Breathnach CS. Richard Morton's Phthisiologia. J R Soc Med. 1998;91:551-2.
5. Sakula A. Robert Koch: centenary of the discovery of the tubercle bacillus, 1882. Thorax. 1982;37:246-51.
6. Klippe HJ, Kirsten D. Marcello Malpighi (1628-1694) and the terms miliary and tubercle. A completion of hitherto existing historical terminology. Pneumologie. 2011;65:432-5.

7. Auerbach O. Acute generalized miliary tuberculosis. Am J Pathol. 1944;20:121-36.
8. World Health Organization. (2014). Global tuberculosis report 2014. Geneva: WHO; [online] Available from www.who.int/tuberculosis/publications/global_report/en/ [Accessed January, 2014].
9. Mert A, Bilir M, Tabak F, et al. Miliary tuberculosis: clinical manifestations, diagnosis and outcome in 38 adults. Respirology. 2001;6:217-24.
10. Sharma SK, Mohan A, Sharma A. Challenges in the diagnosis and treatment of miliary tuberculosis. Indian J Med Res. 2012;135:703-30.
11. Crofton J. Miliary tuberculosis. In: Crofton J, Douglas A, editors. Respiratory Diseases. 2nd ed. Oxford: Blackwell Scientific Publications. 1975. pp. 224-31.
12. Campbell IG. Miliary tuberculosis in British Columbia. Can Med Assoc J. 1973;108:1517-9.
13. Maartens G, Willcox PA, Benatar SR. Miliary tuberculosis: rapid diagnosis, hematologic abnormalities, and outcome in 109 treated adults. Am J Med. 1990;89:291-6.
14. Al-Jahdali H, Al-Zahrani K, Amene P, et al. Clinical aspects of miliary tuberculosis in Saudi adults. Int J Tuberc Lung Dis. 2000;4:252-5.
15. Sharma SK, Mohan A, Pande JN, Prasad KL, Gupta AK, Khilnani GC. Clinical profile, laboratory characteristics and outcome in miliary tuberculosis. QJM. 1995;88:29-37.
16. Henderson CE, Turk R, Dobkin J, Comfort C, Divon MY. Miliary tuberculosis in pregnancy. J Natl Med Assoc. 1993;85:685-7.
17. Lian M, Chan W, Slavin M, Cohney S. Miliary tuberculosis in a Caucasian male transplant recipient and the role of intravenous immunoglobulin as an immunosuppressive sparing agent. Nephrology (Carlton). 2006;11:156-8.
18. Gin A, Dolianitis C. Multidrug resistant miliary tuberculosis during infliximab therapy despite tuberculosis screening. Australas J Dermatol. 2014;55:140-1.
19. Verma SK, Karmakar S. Pulmonary tuberculoma and miliary tuberculosis in silicosis. J Clin Diagn Res. 2013;7:361-3.
20. Baker SK, Glassroth J. Miliary tuberculosis. In: Rom WN, Garay SM, editors. Tuberculosis, 2nd ed. Philadelphia: Lippincott Williams and Wilkins; 2004. pp. 427-44.
21. Geppert EF, Leff A. The pathogenesis of pulmonary and miliary tuberculosis. Arch Intern Med. 1979;139:1381-3.
22. Rao KN. Pathology of pulmonary tuberculosis. In: Rao KN, editors. The Textbook of Tuberculosis. 2nd ed. New Delhi: Vikas Publishing House; 1981. pp. 171-2.
23. Mosmann TR, Sad S. The expanding universe of T-cell subsets: Th1, Th2 and more. Immunol Today.1996;17:138-46.
24. Cooper AM. Cell-mediated immune responses in tuberculosis. Annu Rev Immunol. 2009;27:393-422.
25. Tissot C, Couraud S, Meng L, Girard P, Avrillon V, Gérinière L, et al. Life-threatening disseminated tuberculosis as a complication of treatment by infliximab for Crohn's disease: report of two cases, including cerebral tuberculomas and miliary tuberculosis. J Crohns Colitis. 2012;6:946-9.
26. Kaufmann SH. Novel tuberculosis vaccination strategies based on understanding the immune response. J Intern Med. 2010;267:337-53.
27. Sharma SK, Mitra DK, Balamurugan A, Pandey RM, Mehra NK. Cytokine polarization in miliary and pleural tuberculosis. J Clin Immunol. 2002;22:345-52.
28. Sharma PK, Saha PK, Singh A, Sharma SK, Ghosh B, Mitra DK. FoxP3+ regulatory T cells suppress effector T-cell function at pathologic site in miliary tuberculosis. Am J Respir Crit Care Med. 2009;179:1061-70.
29. Cunha BA, Krakakis J, McDermott BP. Fever of unknown origin (FUO) caused by miliary tuberculosis: diagnostic significance of morning temperature spikes. Heart Lung. 2009;38:77-82.
30. Rushing JL, Hanna CJ, Selecky PA. Pancreatitis as the presenting manifestation of miliary tuberculosis. West J Med. 1978;129:432-6.
31. Munt PW. Miliary tuberculosis in the chemotherapy era: with a clinical review in 69 American adults. Medicine (Baltimore). 1972;51:139-55.
32. Godwin JE, Coleman AA, Sahn SA. Miliary tuberculosis presenting as hepatic and renal failure. Chest. 1991;99:752-4.
33. Cucin RL, Coleman M, Eckardt JJ, Silver RT. The diagnosis of miliary tuberculosis: utility of peripheral blood abnormalities, bone marrow and liver biopsy. J Chronic Dis. 1973;26:355-61.
34. Weiner JJ, Carter RF. Acute thrombocytopenic purpura hemorrhagica associated with tuberculosis (miliary) of the spleen: splenectomy-recovery. Ann Surg. 1941;113:57-61.

35. Garg RK, Sharma R, Kar AM, et al. Neurological complications of miliary tuberculosis. Clin Neurol Neurosurg. 2010;112:188-92.
36. Gee GT, Bazan C 3rd, Jinkins JR. Miliary tuberculosis involving the brain: MR findings. AJR Am J Roentgenol. 1992;159:1075-6.
37. Schermer DR, Simpson CG, Haserick JR, Van Ordstrand HS. Tuberculosis cutis miliaris acuta generalisata. Report of a case in an adult and review of the literature. Arch Dermatol. 1969;99:64-9.
38. Rietbroek RC, Dahlmans RP, Smedts F, Frantzen PJ, Koopman RJ, van der Meer JW. Tuberculosis cutis miliaris disseminata as a manifestation of miliary tuberculosis: literature review and report of a case of recurrent skin lesions. Rev Infect Dis. 1991;13:265-9.
39. del Giudice P, Bernard E, Perrin C, et al. Unusual cutaneous manifestations of miliary tuberculosis. Clin Infect Dis. 2000;30:201-4.
40. Rajpar S, Ladoyanni E, Abushaira H. A case of miliary tuberculosis presenting as metastatic subcutaneous abscesses and chronic skin ulcers. J Am Acad Dermatol. 2005;52:117.
41. Illingworth RS, Lorber J. Tubercles of the choroid. Arch Dis Child. 1956;31:467-9.
42. Baig MS, Masroor M, Burney JA. Frequency and visual outcome of choroidal tubercles with miliary tuberculosis. Pak J Ophthalmol. 2014;30:213-8.
43. Sharma PM, Singh RP, Kumar A, Prakash G, Mathur MB, Malik P. Choroidal tuberculoma in miliary tuberculosis. Retina. 2003;23:101-4.
44. Lamba PA, Srinivasan R. Conjunctival tuberculosis of endogenous origin associated with miliary tuberculosis. Indian J Ophthalmol. 1983;31:89-92.
45. Tabak F, Mert A, Celik AD, et al. Fever of unknown origin in Turkey. Infection. 2003;31:417-20.
46. Hunt BJ, Andrews V, Pettingale KW. The significance of pancytopenia in miliary tuberculosis. Postgrad Med J. 1987;63:801-4.
47 Sahn SA, Neff TA. Miliary tuberculosis. Am J Med. 1974;56:494-505.
48. Rosenberg MJ, Rumans LW. Survival of a patient with pancytopenia and disseminated coagulation with miliary tuberculosis. Chest. 1978;73:536-9.
49. Fujiki R, Shiraishi K, Noda K, et al. A case of hemophagocytic syndrome associated with miliary tuberculosis. Kekkaku. 2003;78:443-8.
50. Simon HB, Weinstein AJ, Pasternak MS, Swartz MN, Kunz LJ. Genitourinary tuberculosis. Clinical features in a general hospital population. Am J Med. 1977;63:410-20.
51. Kim JY, Park YB, Kim YS, et al. Miliary tuberculosis and acute respiratory distress syndrome. Int J Tuberc Lung Dis. 2003;7:359-64.
52. Deng W, Yu M, Ma H, et al. Predictors and outcome of patients with acute respiratory distress syndrome caused by miliary tuberculosis: a retrospective study in Chongqing, China. BMC Infect Dis. 2012;12:121.
53. Snider D. Pregnancy and tuberculosis. Chest. 1984;86:10S-13S.
54. Agarwal A. Miliary tuberculosis presenting as puerperial fever. Case Rep Infect Dis. 2011;2011:893515.
55. Pearce JM. Thomas Addison (1793-1860). J R Soc Med. 2004;97:297-300.
56. de Sadler MR, Beresford OD. Miliary tuberculosis associated with Addison's disease. Tubercle. 1971;52:298-300.
57. Braidy J, Pothel C, Amra S. Miliary tuberculosis presenting as adrenal failure. Can Med Assoc J. 1981;124:748-51.
58. Yokoyama T, Toda R, Kimura Y, Mikagi M, Aizawa H. Addison's disease induced by miliary tuberculosis and the administration of rifampicin. Intern Med. 2009;48:1297-300.
59. Terzidis K, Tourli P, Kiapekou E, Alevizaki M. Thyroid tuberculosis. Hormones (Athens). 2007;6:75-9.
60. Nieuwland Y, Tan KY, Elte JW. Miliary tuberculosis presenting with thyrotoxicosis. Postgrad Med J. 1992;68:677-9.
61. Hadjiangelis NP, Addrizzo-Harris DJ. Cryptic miliary tuberculosis with a clinical prodrome resembling pancreatitis. Respiratory Medicine Extra. 2006;2:95-7.
62. Agnihotri S, Sharma TN, Jain NK, Madan A, Mandhana RG, Saxena A. Spontaneous pneumothorax—a clinical study of eighty cases in Jaipur. Lung India. 1987;5:189-92.
63. Arya M, George J, Dixit R, Gupta RC, Gupta N. Bilateral spontaneous pneumothorax in miliary tuberculosis. Indian J Tuberc. 2011;58:125-8.
64. Liu WL, Wang HC, Luh KT, Yang PC. Recurrent bilateral pneumothoraces: a rare complication of miliary tuberculosis. J Formos Med Assoc. 2008;107:902-6.

65. Gupta PP, Mehta D, Agarwal D, Chand T. Recurrent pneumothorax developing during chemotherapy in a patient with miliary tuberculosis. Ann Thorac Med. 2007;2:173-5.
66. Narang RK, Kumar S, Gupta A. Pneumothorax and pneumomediastinum complicating acute miliary tuberculosis. Tubercle. 1977;58:79-82.
67. İrdem A, Başpınar O, Küçükosmanoğlu E. Dilated cardiomyopathy due to miliary tuberculosis. Anadolu Kardiyol Derg. 2013;13:499-500.
68. Agarwal MP, Avasthi R. Miliary tuberculosis presenting as myocarditis. Indian J Tuberc. 1994;41:171-2.
69. Köylü R, Tozkoparan E, Pabuşçu Y, Ciftçi F, Bilgiç H, Seber O. Unusual miliary tuberculosis presenting with generalized lymphadenopathy and abdominal involvement. Int J Tuberc Lung Dis. 1997;1:474-6.
70. Kwong JS, Carignan S, Kang EY, Müller NL, FitzGerald JM. Miliary tuberculosis. Diagnostic accuracy of chest radiography. Chest. 1996;110:339-42.
71. Felson B. Acute miliary diseases of the lung. Radiology. 1952;59:32-48.
72. Long R, O'Connor R, Palayew M, Hershfield E, Manfreda J. Disseminated tuberculosis with and without a miliary pattern on chest radiograph: a clinical-pathologic-radiologic correlation. Int J Tuberc Lung Dis. 1997;1:52-8.
73. Berger HW, Samortin TG. Miliary tuberculosis: diagnostic methods with emphasis on the chest roentgenogram. Chest. 1970;58:586-9.
74. Jamieson DH, Cremin BJ. High resolution CT of the lungs in acute disseminated tuberculosis and a paediatric radiology perspective of the term "miliary". Pediatr Radiol. 1993;23:380-3.
75. Price M. Lymphangitis reticularis tuberculosa. Tubercle. 1968;49:377-84.
76. Hong SH, Im JG, Lee JS, Song JW, Lee HJ, Yeon KM. High resolution CT findings of miliary tuberculosis. J Comput Assist Tomogr. 1998;22:220-4.
77. Jin SM, Lee HJ, Park EA, et al. Frequency and predictors of miliary tuberculosis in patients with miliary pulmonary nodules in South Korea: a retrospective cohort study. BMC Infect Dis. 2008;8:160.
78. Kim JY, Jeong YJ, Kim KI, et al. Miliary tuberculosis: a comparison of CT findings in HIV-seropositive and HIV-seronegative patients. Br J Radiol. 2010;83:206-11.
79. Lee J, Lim JK, Seo H, Lee SY, Choi KJ, Yoo SS, et al. Clinical relevance of ground glass opacity in 105 patients with miliary tuberculosis. Respir Med. 2014;108:924-30.
80. Oh YW, Kim YH, Lee NJ, et al. High-resolution CT appearance of miliary tuberculosis. J Comput Assist Tomogr. 1994;18:862-6.
81. Topal U, Savci G, Yurtkuran Sadikoglu M. Splenic involvement of tuberculosis: US and CT findings. Eur Radiol. 1994;4:577-9.
82. Sanei Taheri M, Karimi MA, Haghighatkhah H, Pourghorban R, Samadian M, Delavar Kasmaei H. Central nervous system tuberculosis: an imaging-focused review of a reemerging disease. Radiol Res Pract. 2015;2015:202806.
83. Park HS, Song YJ. Multiple tuberculoma involving the brain and spinal cord in a patient with miliary pulmonary tuberculosis. J Korean Neurosurg Soc. 2008;44:36-9.
84. Yang SO, Lee YI, Chung DH, et al. Detection of extrapulmonary tuberculosis with gallium-67 scan and computed tomography. J Nucl Med. 1992;33:2118-23.
85. Kao CH, Wang SJ, Liao SQ, Lin WY, Hsu CY. Usefulness of gallium-67-citrate scans in patients with acute disseminated tuberculosis and comparison with chest X-rays. J Nucl Med. 1993;34:1918-21.
86. Onsel C, Sönmezoglu K, Camsari G, et al. Technetium-99m-MIBI scintigraphy in pulmonary tuberculosis. J Nucl Med. 1996;37:233-8.
87. Tozlu M, Kalyoncu U, Alp S, Unal S, Calguneri M. Diagnostic accuracy of Quantiferon TB test for patients with SLE and miliary tuberculosis. Rheumatol Int. 2009;29:1395-6.
88. Lee YM, Park KH, Kim SM, et al. Diagnostic usefulness of a T-cell-based assay in patients with miliary tuberculosis compared with those with lymph node tuberculosis. Clin Infect Dis. 2013;56:e26-9.
89. Kim CH, Lim JK, Yoo SS, et al. Diagnostic performance of the QuantiFERON-TB Gold In-Tube assay and factors associated with nonpositive results in patients with miliary tuberculosis. Clin Infect Dis. 2014;58:986-9.
90. Hong SI, Lee YM, Park KH, Kim SH. Is the sensitivity of the QuantiFERON-TB gold in-tube test lower than that of T-SPOT.TB in patients with miliary tuberculosis? Clin Infect Dis. 2014;59:142.
91. Kobashi Y, Sugiu T, Mouri K, Obase Y, Miyashita N, Oka M. Indeterminate results of QuantiFERON TB-2G test performed in routine clinical practice. Eur Respir J. 2009;33:812-5.

92. Sharma SK, Mukhopadhyay S, Arora R, Varma K, Pande JN, Khilnani GC. Computed tomography in miliary tuberculosis: comparison with plain films, bronchoalveolar lavage, pulmonary functions and gas exchange. Australas Radiol. 1996;40:113-8.
93. Pipavath SN, Sharma SK, Sinha S, Mukhopadhyay S, Gulati MS. High-resolution CT (HRCT) in miliary tuberculosis (MTB) of the lung: correlation with pulmonary function tests and gas exchange parameters in north Indian patients. Indian J Med Res. 2007;126:193-8.
94. Sharma SK, Mohan A, Sharma A, Mitra DK. Miliary tuberculosis: new insights into an old disease. Lancet Infect Dis. 2005;5:415-30.
95. Kim JH, Langston AA, Gallis HA. Miliary tuberculosis: epidemiology, clinical manifestations, diagnosis, and outcome. Rev Infect Dis. 1990;12:583-90.
96. Sahn SA, Levin DC. Diagnosis of miliary tuberculosis by transbronchial lung biopsy. Br Med J. 1975;2:667-8.
97. Burk JR, Viroslav J, Bynum LJ. Miliary tuberculosis diagnosed by fibreoptic bronchoscopy and transbronchial biopsy. Tubercle. 1978;59:107-9.
98. Willcox PA, Potgieter PD, Bateman ED, Benatar SR. Rapid diagnosis of sputum negative miliary tuberculosis using the flexible fibreoptic bronchoscope. Thorax. 1986;41:681-4.
99. Pant K, Chawla R, Mann PS, Jaggi OP. Fiberbronchoscopy in smear-negative miliary tuberculosis. Chest. 1989;95:1151-2.
100. Aggarwal AN, Gupta D, Joshi K, Jindal SK. Bronchoscopic lung biopsy for diagnosis of miliary tuberculosis. Lung India. 2005;22:116-8.
101. Sharma SK, Pande JN, Verma K. Bronchoalveolar lavage (BAL) in miliary tuberculosis. Tubercle. 1988;69:175-8.
102. Ozaki T, Nakahira S, Tani K, Ogushi F, Yasuoka S, Ogura T. Differential cell analysis in bronchoalveolar lavage fluid from pulmonary lesions of patients with tuberculosis. Chest. 1992;102:54-9.
103. Kim JE, Seol HY, Cho WH, et al. Differential cell analysis and lymphocyte subset analysis in bronchoalveolar lavage fluid from patients with miliary tuberculosis. Tuberc Respir Dis. 2010;68:218-25.
104. Kubota M, Katagiri M, Yanase N, Soma K, Tomita T. Measurement of adenosine deaminase activity in bronchoalveolar lavage fluids as a tool for diagnosing miliary tuberculosis. Nihon Kyobu Shikkan Gakkai Zasshi. 1996;34:139-44.
105. Armstrong AR, Anderson W, Lee JH. Sternal marrow aspiration in miliary tuberculosis. Can Med Assoc J. 1951;65:468-9.
106. Escobedo-Jaimes L, Cicero-Sabido R, Criales-Cortez JL, et al. Evaluation of the polymerase chain reaction in the diagnosis of miliary tuberculosis in bone marrow smear. Int J Tuberc Lung Dis. 2003;7:580-6.
107. Jacques J, Sloan JM. The changing pattern of miliary tuberculosis. Thorax. 1970;25:237-40.
108. Marais BJ, Gie RP, Schaaf HS, et al. The natural history of childhood intra-thoracic tuberculosis: a critical review of literature from the pre-chemotherapy era. Int J Tuberc Lung Dis. 2004;8:392-402.
109. Kim PK, Lee JS, Yun DJ. Clinical review of miliary tuberculosis in Korean children. 84 cases and review of the literature. Yonsei Med J. 1969;10:146-52.
110. Hussey G, Chisholm T, Kibel M. Miliary tuberculosis in children: a review of 94 cases. Pediatr Infect Dis J. 1991;10:832-6.
111. Gurkan F, Bosnak M, Dikici B, et al. Miliary tuberculosis in children: a clinical review. Scand J Infect Dis. 1998;30:359-62.
112. Lincoln EM, Hould F. Results of specific treatment of miliary tuberculosis in children; a follow-up study of 63 patients treated with antimicrobial agents. N Engl J Med. 1959;261:113-20.
113. Debré R. Miliary tuberculosis in children. Lancet. 1952;260:545-9.
114. van den Bos F, Terken M, Ypma L, et al. Tuberculous meningitis and miliary tuberculosis in young children. Trop Med Int Health. 2004;9:309-13.
115. Hill AR, Premkumar S, Brustein S, et al. Disseminated tuberculosis in the acquired immunodeficiency syndrome era. Am Rev Respir Dis. 1991;144:1164-70.
116. Esteve E, Supervía A, Pallàs O, Martínez MT, Montero MM, Del Baño F. Miliary tuberculosis coinfection with human immunodeficiency virus. West J Emerg Med. 2010;11:405-7.
117. Sharma SK, Kadhiravan T, Banga A, Goyal T, Bhatia I, Saha PK. Spectrum of clinical disease in a cohort of 135 hospitalised HIV-infected patients from north India. BMC Infect Dis. 2004;4:52.

118. Deivanayagam CN, Rajasekaran S, Senthilnathan V, et al. Clinico-radiological spectrum of tuberculosis among HIV sero-positives: a Tambaram study. Indian J Tub. 2001;48:123-7.
119. Libraty DH, Byrd TF. Cutaneous miliary tuberculosis in the AIDS era: case report and review. Clin Infect Dis. 1996;23:706-10.
120. Swaminathan S, Padmapriyadarsini C, Ponnuraja C, et al. Miliary tuberculosis in human immunodeficiency virus infected patients not on antiretroviral therapy: clinical profile and response to short course chemotherapy. J Postgrad Med. 2007;53:228-31.
121. Daikos GL, Uttamchandani RB, Tuda C, et al. Disseminated miliary tuberculosis of the skin in patients with AIDS: report of four cases. Clin Infect Dis. 1998;27:205-8.
122. Innes S, Schaaf HS, Hoek KG, Rabie H, Cotton M. Unsuspected fatal drug-resistant tuberculosis in a closely monitored child: a plea for improved source-case tracing and drug susceptibility testing. South Afr J Epidemiol Infect. 2010;25:30-2.
123. Shah A, Panjabi C, Maurya V, Khanna P. Multidrug resistant miliary tuberculosis and Pott's disease in an immunocompetent patient. Saudi Med J. 2004;25:1468-70.
124. Sasse J, Teichmann D. Disseminated multiorgan MDR-TB resistant to virtually all first-line drugs. Eur Respir Rev. 2009;18:291-4.
125. Ko Y, Lee HY, Lee YS, et al. Multidrug-resistant tuberculosis presenting as miliary tuberculosis without immune suppression: a case diagnosed rapidly with the genotypic line probe assay method. Tuberc Respir Dis (Seoul). 2014;76:245-8.
126. Proudfoot AT, Akhtar AJ, Douglas AC, Horne NW. Miliary tuberculosis in adults. Br Med J. 1969;2:273-6.
127. Yu YL, Chow WH, Humphries MJ, Wong RW, Gabriel M. Cryptic miliary tuberculosis. Q J Med. 1986;59:421-8.
128. World Health Organization. Treatment of Tuberculosis: Guidelines, 4th edition. Geneva: WHO; 2009.
129. Blumberg HM, Burman WJ, Chaisson RE, Daley CL, Etkind SC, Friedman LN, et al. American Thoracic Society/Centers for Disease Control and Prevention/Infectious Diseases Society of America: treatment of tuberculosis. Am J Respir Crit Care Med. 2003;167:603-62.
130. National Institute for Health and Clinical Excellence, National Collaborating Centre for Chronic Conditions. Management of non-respiratory tuberculosis. Tuberculosis: Clinical Diagnosis and Management of Tuberculosis, and Measures for its Prevention and Control. London: Royal College of Physicians; 2006. pp. 63-76.
131. World Health Organization. Automated real-time nucleic acid amplification technology for rapid and simultaneous detection of tuberculosis and rifampicin resistance: Xpert MTB/RIF system for the diagnosis of pulmonary and extrapulmonary TB in adults and children: policy update (WHO/HTM/TB/2013.14). Geneva: World Health Organization; 2013.
132. Dooley DP, Carpenter JL, Rademacher S. Adjunctive corticosteroid therapy for tuberculosis: a critical reappraisal of the literature. Clin Infect Dis. 1997;25:872-87.
133. Rodrigues LC, Diwan VK, Wheeler JG. Protective effect of BCG against tuberculous meningitis and miliary tuberculosis: a meta-analysis. Int J Epidemiol. 1993;22:1154-8.
134. Trunz BB, Fine P, Dye C. Effect of BCG vaccination on childhood tuberculous meningitis and miliary tuberculosis worldwide: a meta-analysis and assessment of cost-effectiveness. Lancet. 2006;367:1173-80.
135. Wang JY, Hsueh PR, Wang SK, et al. Disseminated tuberculosis: a 10-year experience in a medical center. Medicine (Baltimore). 2007;86:39-46.
136. Kim DK, Kim HJ, Kwon SY, et al. Nutritional deficit as a negative prognostic factor in patients with miliary tuberculosis. Eur Respir J. 2008;32:1031-6.

CHAPTER 9
Tuberculosis Effusion and the Role of Closed Pleural Biopsy and Pleuroscopy

Dragana M Jovanovic, Violeta V Mihailovic Vucinic

INTRODUCTION

Tuberculosis (TB) is the leading cause of pleural effusions in some countries,[1] so the possibility of tuberculous pleuritis is considered in all patients with an undiagnosed pleural effusion. Extrapulmonary TB affecting mainly pleura and the lymph nodes represents the initial presentation in about 25% of adults with active TB disease. It is estimated that between 3 and 25% of patients with TB will have tuberculous pleuritis,[2] approximately 5% of human immunodeficiency virus (HIV)-negative patients, but the incidence of pleural TB is higher in patients who are HIV-positive. If the diagnosis is not made on time, usually the patient recovers, but with a high likelihood of subsequently developing pulmonary or extrapulmonary TB.

PATHOGENESIS

Tuberculous pleuritis is related to the rupture of a subpleural caseous focus in the lung into the pleural space[3,4] and it is thought to result from a delayed hypersensitivity reaction to mycobacteria and mycobacterial antigens in the pleural space.[2,5-7]

The key mechanisms include increased permeability of the pleural capillaries to protein caused by delayed hypersensitivity reaction resulting in higher rate of pleural fluid formation, while the lymphocytic pleuritis obstructs the lymphatics in the parietal pleura, leading to decreased pleural fluid removal from the pleural space. Thus in vast majority of cases, the bacillary burden in the pleural space is low. Although the development of pleural effusion occurs largely as a result of hypersensitivity reaction, still tuberculous pleurisy must be considered to be due to infection since culture of the fluid grows mycobacteria in some cases and culture of the pleural tissue usually grows mycobacteria. It may be the sequel to a primary infection 6–12 weeks previously or it may represent reactivation TB.[8]

In developed countries, it is considered that more pleural effusions are due to reactivation than follow a primary infection.[8,9]

INCIDENCE

The percentage of patients with TB who have pleural effusions varies markedly from country-to-country,[1,10-13] but generally between 3 and 25% of TB patients will have tuberculous pleuritis,[2] with the incidence of pleural TB higher in HIV-positive patients.

Immunocompromised patients in general, especially HIV-infected are more likely to develop TB than immunocompetent. In HIV-positive patients, the percentage of patients with tuberculous pleuritis is significantly higher than in immunocompetent patients as noted in reports from South Africa (38% vs. 20%),[11] Uganda (23% vs. 11%),[14] and

Zimbabwe (27% vs. 13%).[15] In other series of immunocompromised but HIV-negative hosts, the percentage of TB patients with pleural effusions has been less, occurring in only 11% patients with kidney transplants who developed TB,[16] and 10.4% patients who were on renal dialysis and developed TB.[17]

CLINICAL MANIFESTATIONS

Tuberculous pleuritis usually presents as an acute illness with fever, cough and pleuritic chest pain. The most frequent symptoms are cough (~70%), usually nonproductive, and pleuritic chest pain (~70%),[1,3,8] along with fever in approximately 85% of patients.[8]

Night sweats, chills, weakness, dyspnea, and weight loss can also occur. Patients with tuberculous pleural effusions (TPEs) may be dyspneic particularly if the effusion is large.

On occasions, the onset of tuberculous pleuritis is less acute with mild chest pain, low-grade fever, a nonproductive cough, weight loss, and fatigue.

Clinical manifestations in HIV-positive patients tend to be different with longer duration of illness and a lower incidence of chest pain.[18] Systemic signs and symptoms (night sweats, fatigue, diarrhea, hepatomegaly, splenomegaly, and lymphadenopathy) are more common in HIV-infected.[19]

Tuberculous pleuritis is usually unilateral and small-to-moderate in size, but can be of any size and it represents the third leading cause of massive pleural effusion registered in 12%, while malignancy in 55% and pneumonia in 22% of cases with massive pleural effusion (Fig. 1).[20]

Approximately 20% up to 50% of patients have coexisting parenchymal disease on chest radiograph,[21] but if chest computed tomography (CT) scans are performed, up to more than 80% have parenchymal lesions[22] which are almost always on the side of the pleural effusion and active. These lesions are located in the upper lobe in approximately three-fourths of HIV-negative cases, suggestive of reactivation TB (Fig. 2). Rarely, pleural TB can present with pleural-based nodules and thickening[1] (Fig. 3).

Natural history of untreated tuberculous pleuritis is that it usually resolves spontaneously, but the patient frequently develops active TB at a later date (approximately 2/3). The size of the original effusions and the presence or the absence of small radiological residual pleural disease do not correlate with the subsequent development of active TB.[23]

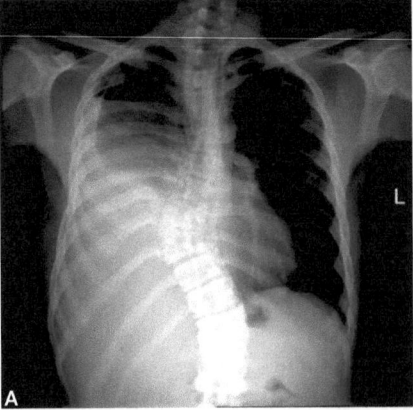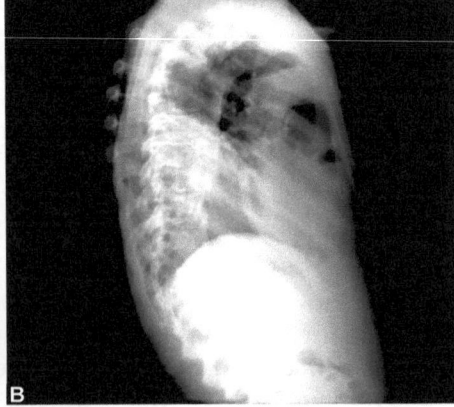

FIG. 1: Posteroanterior and profile chest radiograph of a 21-year-old male patient who presented with a history of recent onset of coughing, fatigue, and weight loss, showing right-sided massive pleural effusion which was proven by pleural biopsy to be TB effusion.

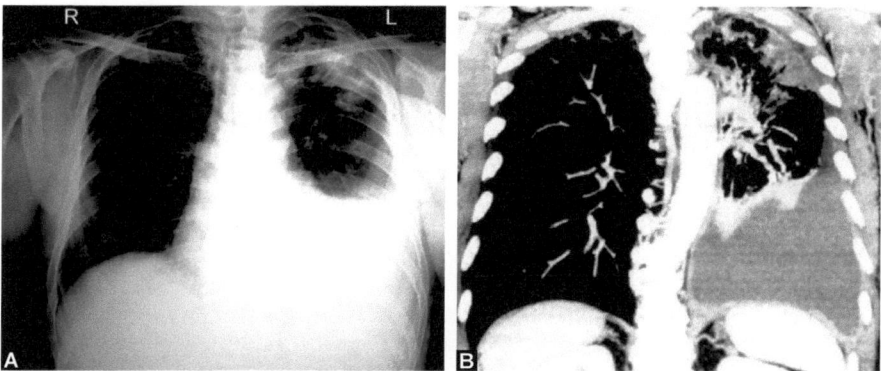

FIG. 2: A, Posteroanterior chest radiograph and; **B,** CT scan of a 58-year-old male patient who presented with a history of 4 months lasting dry cough, chest pain, and febrile episodes, showing left-sided massive pleural effusion with coexisting parenchymal disease.

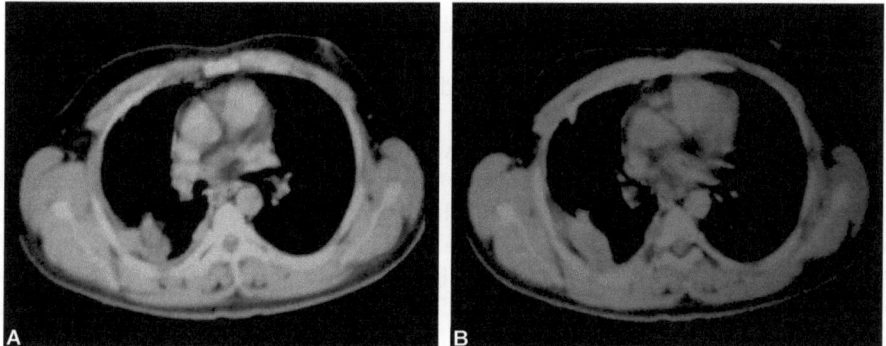

FIG. 3: Computed tomography scan of a 37-year-old male patient who presented with a history of recent chest pain and febrile episodes, showing pleural-based nodules and thickening.

DIAGNOSIS

Pleural fluid analysis and closed pleural biopsy are integral parts in the investigative workup of an exudative pleural effusion. Diagnostic evaluation of pleural effusion in the setting of suspected tuberculous begins with thoracentesis and pleural fluid routine studies. In cases of moderate-to-high suspicion for TB with nondiagnostic pleural fluid evaluation, pleural biopsy is warranted. In addition to pleural evaluation, routine laboratory diagnostic evaluation for TB is also necessary. Evaluation for concurrent HIV infection should be performed as well.

The definitive diagnosis of TPE depends on the demonstration of tubercle bacilli in the pleural fluid, sputum, or pleural biopsy specimen, and can also be established with reasonable certainty by demonstration of granuloma in the parietal pleura.

Microscopy of the pleural fluid for acid-fast bacilli (AFB) is positive in less than 5% of cases and mycobacterial culture of pleural fluid also has a low sensitivity of 35%.[21]

Diagnosis can be established by demonstrating granulomas or organisms on tissue specimens obtained via needle biopsy of the pleura or thoracoscopy. Closed pleural biopsy demonstrates granulomas in approximately 80% of cases, and its culture yields *Mycobacterium tuberculosis* in about 55%.

TABLE 1	Diagnostic yield of mycobacterial or/and histology analysis of pleural fluid or biopsy tissue sample			
Sample	Microscopy for AFB sensitivity	Mycobacterial culture sensitivity	Demonstrating granulomas or organisms on biopsy sample	Joint sensitivity of demonstrating granulomas or organisms and mycobacterial culture of biopsy tissue sample
Pleural fluid	<5%	35%	–	–
Closed pleural biopsy	–	About 55%	Approximately 80%	90%
Thoracoscopy biopsy	–	76%	Nearly 100%	–

Joint sensitivity of biopsy tissue samples is as high as 90%,[21] but closed pleural biopsy is a relatively invasive procedure and involves a long waiting time for mycobacteria culture results.

Thoracoscopy offers a nearly 100% positive diagnostic yield on histology and 76% positive on culture.[24,25]

Diagnostic yield of mycobacterial or/and histology analysis of pleural fluid or biopsy tissue sample has been shown in table 1.

The diagnosis can also be established with reasonable certainty by demonstrating elevated levels of adenosine deaminase (ADA) or γ-interferon in the pleural fluid.[26] Thus, the easiest and inexpensive way to establish the diagnosis of tuberculous pleuritis in a patient with a lymphocytic pleural exudate is to generally demonstrate a pleural fluid ADA level above 40 U/L. So, the first step is initial thoracentesis and the pleural fluid should be analyzed for the ADA level and differential cell count and the fluid should be cultured for mycobacteria.

Elevated pleural fluid levels of γ-interferon also are virtually diagnostic of tuberculous pleuritis in these patients.

Pleural Fluid Characteristics

The pleural fluid is an exudate that usually has predominantly lymphocytes and the pleural fluid protein level frequently exceeding 5 g/dL (50 g/L)—in 50–77% of cases, suggestive of tuberculous pleuritis.[1]

Most have more than 50% small lymphocytes but many have more than 90%.[3,1] However, it should be stressed that patients with symptoms lasting for less than 2 weeks are more likely to have predominantly polymorphonuclear leukocytes in tuberculous pleural exudates.[27]

If the pleural fluid contains more than 10% eosinophils, the diagnosis of tuberculous pleuritis is unlikely unless the patient has a pneumothorax or has had a previous thoracentesis.[1]

Low pH and low glucose concentration may be noted, these findings being more characteristic of chronic tuberculous empyema than TPE. The pleural fluid pH is usually above 7.30, but pH less than 7.30 is observed in about 20% of cases. Glucose level may be reduced but it usually is similar to the serum level. The pleural fluid glucose concentration is usually between 60 and 100 mg/dL (3.3 and 5.6 mmol/L), with glucose levels below 50 mg/dL (2.8 mmol/L) in 7–20% of tuberculous effusions, and occasionally extremely low glucose concentrations [<30 mg/dL (1.7 mmol/L)].

The pleural fluid lactate dehydrogenase (LDH) level is usually higher than the serum LDH level; it is elevated in approximately 75% of cases, with levels commonly exceeding 500 IU/L.

Pleural fluid in tuberculous pleuritis rarely has more than scattered mesothelial cells and it rarely contains more than 5% mesothelial cells,[1,28,29] with the exception of HIV-infected patients cases.

Mycobacterial Stain and Culture

Examination of the sputum for mycobacteria is frequently overlooked in the diagnostic workup of patients with an undiagnosed pleural effusion. Sputum examination is considered underutilized in the diagnosis of tuberculous pleuritis.[30] Routine smears of the pleural fluid for mycobacteria in immunocompetent individuals are not widely indicated because they are almost always negative unless the patient has a tuberculous empyema.[7,21] Nevertheless, smears should be obtained in immunocompromised hosts, smears being positive in approximately 20% of HIV-positive individuals.[18]

Pleural fluid cultures for mycobacteria should be obtained in any patient with an undiagnosed pleural effusion and in most series of immunocompetent patients with tuberculous pleuritis, the cultures are positive in less than 40%.[3,21]

The pleural fluid in HIV-positive patients is much more likely to be smear- and culture-positive for mycobacteria.[18,31] If the peripheral CD4 count is less than 100 cells/mm^3, approximately 50% of patients will have a positive smear for AFB on their pleural fluid.[18]

The use of a BACTEC system with bedside inoculation of the pleural fluid provides higher yields and faster results than do conventional methods, with positive cultures in 24% of HIV-negative patients and 75% of HIV-positive patients while the cultures are positive by the Lowenstein-Jensen medium in 12% of HIV-negative patients and 56% of HIV-positive patients. The additional advantage of the BACTEC system is that the mean time to a positive culture with the BACTEC system is 3.5 weeks compared with 4.7 weeks with the Löwenstein–Jensen medium.[31]

With the implementation of a liquid culture method, the diagnostic yield of pleural effusion mycobacterial culture is much higher than previously reported, 63% in a large series of 382 patients with tuberculous pleurisy from an endemic area, along with the diagnostic yields of 48% for sputum culture, 79% for the combination of effusion and sputum cultures, and 74% for histological examination of pleural biopsy specimens. The lymphocyte percentage was negatively associated with the probability of a positive effusion culture.[32]

Skin Tests

The tuberculin skin test is being utilized less and less in patients suspected of having tuberculous pleuritis, primarily because a negative test does not rule out the diagnosis of tuberculous pleuritis, so if the patient is markedly immunosuppressed with HIV infection or is severely malnourished, the skin test may remain negative.[21]

Adenosine Deaminase

The diagnosis can be established with reasonable certainty by demonstrating elevated levels of ADA or γ-interferon in the pleural fluid.[26]

Adenosine deaminase test is an easy, noninvasive, and inexpensive method for establishing the diagnosis of tuberculous pleuritis in high-incidence areas but the measurement of pleural fluid ADA levels could be used to rule out a tuberculous etiology of lymphocytic pleural effusions, regardless of the rate of TB prevalence as well.[1,33]

It is routinely used in high prevalence settings, whereas its value is questioned in areas with low prevalence.

Reported sensitivity and specificity of ADA in the diagnosis of pleural TB based on meta-analysis of 63 studies including 2,796 patients with tuberculous pleuritis and 5,297 with nontuberculous effusion were 92% and 90%, respectively.[34,35]

Three major meta-analyses, based on 75 studies including a total of 14,505 patients, performed over the last decade have demonstrated a uniformly high diagnostic performance of pleural ADA for TPE.[34-36]

Measurement of ADA level has thus become an important diagnostic tool in the evaluation of exudative pleural effusions because it is inexpensive, rapid, and has a high accuracy with sensitivity and specificity of up to 100% and 95%, respectively, for diagnosis of TPE.[37]

Adenosine deaminase levels in pleural fluid are also elevated in HIV patients even with very low CD4 cell counts[38,39] and also in renal transplant recipients with tuberculous pleurisy.[21,40]

The most widely accepted cutoff value for pleural fluid ADA is 40 U/L and the higher the level, the greater the chance is of the patient having TB.

However, roughly one-third of parapneumonic effusions and two-thirds of empyemas have ADA levels that exceed 40 U/L.[41] Elevated ADA levels in pleural fluid have also been reported in malignancies (5%, particularly lymphomas), infectious diseases (e.g., brucellosis, Q fever, mycoplasma, and chlamydia pneumonia) and connective tissue diseases such as rheumatoid arthritis,[2,42] which makes the test less useful in countries with a low prevalence of TB.[43,44]

Some studies have demonstrated correlation between pleural ADA level and CD4 lymphocyte counts[45] as well as lower mean ADA level in Japanese patients with TPE,[24] findings suggesting that patient immune status as well as demographic factors may affect pleural fluid ADA levels.[40,46] The combination of ADA and the pleural fluid lymphocyte proportion has been recognized as an excellent approach for increasing the specificity of ADA test[47] especially since it is routinely used in high prevalence settings most often related to limited health resources countries. Adenosine deaminase level of 40 U/L is considered a highly suitable cutoff level in patients younger than 40 years and it might constitute a virtual diagnosis of TPE when effusions are lymphocytic.[40,46] Pleural fluid ADA decreases with age and, therefore, increases the number of false-negative results for diagnosis of TPE when a fixed cutoff level is used in an older population compared to a younger population. Few studies were recently conducted in order to establish the optimal ADA levels for diagnosis of TPE for different age groups. There is evidence of a significant negative correlation between pleural fluid ADA and age, and for older patients, a lower ADA cutoff should be used to exclude TPE, pointing to ADA level for diagnosis of TPE according to different age groups: 72 IU/L in those less than or equal to 55 years and 26 IU/L in those greater than 55 years.

Two isoenzymes of ADA have been identified:
1. ADA-1
2. ADA-2

A number of studies have analyzed ADA and its isoenzymes in pleural effusions, and have found that ADA-2 isoenzyme is primarily responsible for the total ADA activity in tuberculous effusions, while ADA-1 is the major isoenzyme in parapneumonic effusions.[48,49]

As most of the ADA in TB pleural fluid is ADA-2, pleural levels of ADA-2 have the highest sensitivity among the different diagnostic parameters to distinguish pleural TB.[50]

Although a ratio of the ADA-1 to the total ADA of less than 0.42 would slightly increase the sensitivity and specificity of the ADA measurement in diagnosing tuberculous pleuritis, the separation of ADA into its isoenzymes is not necessary in the vast majority of cases and it would additionally increase costs.[51]

Summarizing Recommended Diagnostic Approach with ADA Testing: Since the first diagnostic step is initial thoracocentesis when the pleural fluid should be analyzed for the ADA level and differential cell count and the fluid should be cultured for mycobacteria, there are some recommended criteria for making diagnosis of pleural TB:

- If the fluid ADA is above 70 U/L and the pleural fluid has a lymphocyte-to-neutrophil ratio greater than 0.75, the diagnosis of tuberculous pleuritis is virtually established
- If the pleural fluid ADA is between 40 and 70 U/L and the patient has a lymphocyte-to-neutrophil ratio of more than 0.75, one can make a presumptive diagnosis of tuberculous pleuritis. If the patient's clinical picture is not typical for tuberculous pleuritis, consideration can be given to performing a needle biopsy of the pleura or thoracoscopy
- If the patient's pleural fluid ADA level is below 40 U/L, the diagnosis of TB is unlikely.

Nevertheless, if the patient has a clinical picture typical of tuberculous pleuritis and particularly, if the pleural fluid has a high percentage of lymphocytes, such cases should be further evaluated with needle biopsy of the pleura or thoracoscopy.[1]

Concern regarding the absence of culture and sensitivity data when the diagnosis relies primarily on the pleural fluid ADA value has been stated, and pleural biopsy is thereby advised mostly in high mycobacterial resistance scenarios.[2] On the other hand, the addition of a culture of the (closed) pleural biopsy to that of the pleural fluid increases the overall microbiological yield from 35 to 55%, and in some authors' opinion this invasive practice may be not justified in order to obtain such a diminished advantage of approximately 20%.[1,2,52]

Gamma-Interferon

The level of pleural fluid γ-interferon is also very efficient at distinguishing tuberculous from non-TPEs.

A meta-analysis of 22 studies that included 782 patients with TB and 1,319 patients with non-TPE showed that the mean sensitivity of the γ-interferon assay was 89%, the mean specificity was 97%, and the maximum joint sensitivity and specificity was 95%.[53]

It is impossible to establish a cutoff value overall as the units and the methods of measurement differ from study-to-study.[2]

A meta-analysis that reviewed 13 studies on γ-interferon and 31 on ADA, which included 1,189 patients concluded that both ADA and γ-interferon are accurate in diagnosing tuberculous pleuritis.[35]

Maximum joint sensitivity and specificity were 93% for ADA and 96% for γ-interferon.[35]

Similarly to the ADA levels, levels of γ-interferon are sometimes elevated with hematologic malignancies and empyemas.[54]

Nevertheless, the fact that measurement of ADA level is simpler and less expensive than the γ-interferon test makes it the preferred test.

Interferon-γ Release Assays

Interferon-γ release assays (IGRAs) measure γ-interferon release by sensitized T-cells from peripheral blood or pleural fluid in response to highly *M. tuberculosis*-specific antigens such as early secretory antigenic target-6 and culture filtrate protein-10.[2]

To date, IGRA is the best test for the diagnosis of latent TB infection (LTBI), especially in the Bacillus Calmette-Guérin-vaccinated populations.

QuantiFERON-TB Gold and T-SPOT.TB are most often used. These tests are good at identifying patients who have been infected with *M. tuberculosis*, however much less useful in identifying patients with pleural TB. A recent study aimed to examine the clinical accuracy of T-SPOT.TB on pleural fluid and peripheral blood for the diagnosis of pleural TB in high TB burden country has reported low diagnostic accuracy of peripheral blood T-SPOT.TB due to LTBI with the conclusion that pleural fluid T-SPOT.TB was a relatively useful and supplementary test to explore pleural TB in high TB burden countries, but its diagnostic accuracy needed to be validated in further large scale research.[55]

However, pleural fluid γ-interferon levels themselves are much superior to the IGRA in regards to both sensitivity and specificity,[56] so IGRAs are not recommended for diagnosis of tuberculous pleuritis.[25]

Since interferon-γ-induced protein-10 (IP-10) and its homologs involved in inflammatory lung injury are closely related to TB,[6,7] an increasing number of studies consider IP-10 to be a marker for the diagnosis of TB.[6-9] However, conflicting results have been reported and the exact role of IP-10 has remained unclear. Therefore, a very recent meta-analysis has been performed to establish the overall accuracy of IP-10 for diagnosing TB.[57] It comprised 14 studies based on 2,075 subjects and reported sensitivity 0.73, specificity 0.83, positive likelihood ratio 7.08, negative likelihood ratio 0.26, and diagnostic odds ratio 29.50. These findings suggest that IP-10 may improve the accuracy of TB diagnosis, but the results of IP-10 assays should be interpreted in parallel with conventional test results and other clinical findings.[57]

Nucleic Acid Amplification Tests

Nucleic acid amplification (NAA) assays amplify *M. tuberculosis*-specific nucleic acid sequences with a nucleic acid probe.[1,2]

Nucleic acid amplification tests enable direct detection of *M. tuberculosis* in clinical specimens such as pleural fluid within hours of their collection, and can also provide information regarding antimicrobial resistance.[2,52]

A pooled analysis of the data from 20 studies of pleural fluid NAA tests reported reasonably high specificity (97% for commercial and 91% for in-house tests), but generally poor and variable sensitivity (62% for commercial and 76.5% for in-house tests).[58]

However, although commercial tests have a reasonably high specificity of 98% in a systematic review and meta-analysis of 40 studies, they had a low and variable sensitivity of 62% for diagnosing TPE as well.[59]

New molecular and phenotyping tools offer the possibility of rapid diagnosis of active TB and enable prompt identification of drug-resistant strains.[60]

The performance of Xpert MTB/RIF, an automated molecular test for *M. tuberculosis* and resistance to rifampin (RIF), with a turnaround time of less than 2 hours, has been assessed.[60,61] Among culture-positive patients, a single, direct MTB/RIF test showed a sensitivity of 98.2% for smear-positive cases and 72.5% for smear-negative cases, while the specificity was as high as 99.2%. As compared with phenotypic drug susceptibility testing, MTB/RIF correctly identified 97.6% of RIF-resistant mycobacterial infections and 98.1% of RIF-sensitive mycobacterial infections.[60,61]

Another test, nested polymerase chain reaction (nPCR) assay targeting IS6110 gene sequence was investigated as a rapid diagnostic test for suspected tuberculous pleurisy. It has been shown that it can be a useful tool in the establishment of diagnosis of pleural TB where there is strong clinical suspicion and conventional techniques are negative. However, a combined analysis of nPCR, ADA activity, and other laboratory parameters can be helpful to achieve more rapid and accurate diagnosis.[62]

Pleural Biopsy

Blind needle biopsy of the pleura has been the most common way to make the diagnosis of tuberculous pleuritis over the past 50 years. Pleural tissue can also be obtained at thoracoscopy, but thoracoscopy is usually not necessary to make the diagnosis of tuberculous pleuritis.

The diagnostic yield of blind closed pleural biopsy is in the order of 80% for TB and less than 60% for pleural malignancy. Recent studies suggest that CT and/or ultrasound guidance may improve the yield. A second thoracocentesis combined with an image-assisted pleural biopsy with either an Abrams needle or cutting needle, depending on the setting, may therefore be an acceptable alternative to thoracoscopy. With such an approach, thoracoscopy may potentially be reserved for cases not diagnosed by means of closed pleural biopsy.[63]

Since tuberculous pleuritis generally represents more than 95% granulomatous pleuritis,[1] granuloma in the parietal pleura suggests tuberculous pleuritis; caseous necrosis and AFB need not be demonstrated.

Nevertheless, granulomatous pleuritis may be found in other diseases like fungal diseases, sarcoidosis, tularemia, and rheumatoid pleuritis.

Even if no granulomas are present on the biopsy, the biopsy specimen should be stained for AFB and cultured for *M. tuberculosis*.

In the study of 248 patients with tuberculous pleuritis, biopsy showed granulomas in 80%, the AFB stain of the biopsy was positive in 25.8% and the culture in 56%. At least one of the three tests was positive in 91%.[21]

Thoracoscopy

Thoracoscopy is usually not necessary to make the diagnosis of tuberculous pleuritis, but cases that remain undiagnosed warrant thoracoscopy. Many consider thoracoscopy the investigation of choice in exudative pleural effusions where a thoracocentesis was nondiagnostic and particularly when malignancy is suspected. It allows for the direct inspection of the pleura.[63]

Thoracoscopy is sometimes indicated when the clinical picture is confusing, and if the patient does have tuberculous pleuritis, thoracoscopy will establish the diagnosis in nearly 100% of cases.[25]

Thus, thoracoscopy has a diagnostic yield of 91–95% for malignant disease and as high as 100% for pleural TB.[63]

Sensitivity (%) of the different biopsy techniques in the diagnosis of TPEs with pleural fluid analysis (including ADA and differential cell counts) and histological results combined are presented in table 2.[25,63-66]

TABLE 2	Sensitivity of the different biopsy techniques in the diagnosis of tuberculous pleural effusions with pleural fluid analysis[25,64-66]		
Pleural fluid analysis	Image-assisted needle biopsy		Thoracoscopy
89	80		100
	93		–
–		100	
	100		

Source: Adapted and modified from Koegelenberg CF, Diacon AH. Pleural controversy: close needle pleural biopsy or thoracoscopy— which first? Respirology. 2011;16:738-46.

TREATMENT

Treatment of tuberculous pleuritis generally has three goals:
1. To prevent the subsequent development of active TB
2. To relieve the symptoms of the patient
3. To prevent the development of a fibrothorax.

Initial phase of a 6-month regimen generally consists of a 2-month period of isoniazid (INH), RIF, and pyrazinamide, and commonly ethambutol. Second phase of the treatment should be INH and RIF given for 4 months. Nine-month regimens using INH and RIF are reported to be also effective when the organisms are fully susceptible to the drug.[67,68]

Recently conducted study aimed to analyze the inhospital mortality rate of culture-confirmed tuberculous pleuritis with an emphasis on the clinical impact of pulmonary involvement has shown that in spite of adequate treatment in patients with pulmonary involvement a higher inhospital mortality rate was observed.[69]

Typical patient becomes afebrile within 2 weeks, but febrile episodes may persist as long as 2 months.[70]

If a therapeutic thoracentesis is performed at the same time that antituberculous therapy is initiated, most patients become afebrile within 5 days.[71,72]

The mean time for the complete resorption of pleural fluid is approximately 6 weeks, but it can be as long as 12 weeks.[70] Approximately, 50% of patients will have some residual pleural thickening 6–12 months after the initiation of antituberculous treatment (Fig. 4).[73] Occasionally, a fibrothorax is noted (Figs. 5 and 6).

Incidence of residual pleural thickening is slightly more common in patients with a low pleural fluid glucose, a high pleural fluid LDH level, and high pleural fluid cytokine levels.[73,74] It is more common if the pleural effusion is initially loculated as well.[75]

Complete removal of the pleural fluid does not appear to decrease the amount of residual pleural thickening,[76] while administration of a fibrinolytic may decrease the degree of residual pleural thickening in loculated TB pleural effusions.[77]

Paradoxical worsening of the pleural effusion after therapy started is confusing (17%),[78] it might be due to INH-induced lupus pleuritis.[79]

Occasionally, a peripheral lung nodule develops during treatment, which is almost always pulmonary TB and disappears during the continuation of antituberculous therapy.[80]

Some patients develop a pleural effusion while being treated for pulmonary TB as well.[81]

The role of corticosteroids in the treatment of tuberculous pleurisy is controversial, with no decrease of the degree of residual pleural thickening.[71,72,82]

Increased risk of Kaposi sarcoma in HIV-associated pleural TB is evidenced.[82,83]

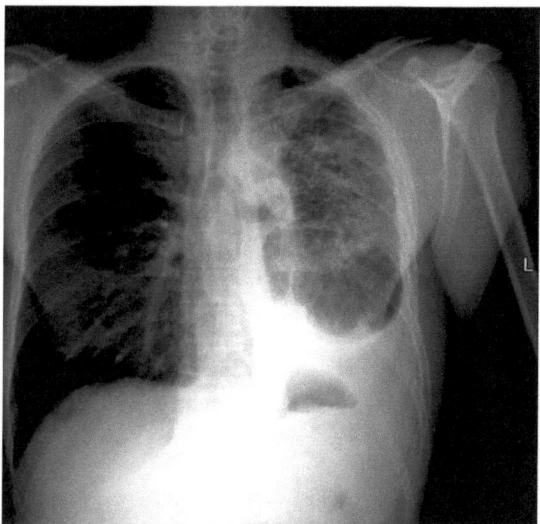

FIG. 4: Residual pleural thickening 8 months after the initiation of antituberculous treatment in a 32-year-old male patient.

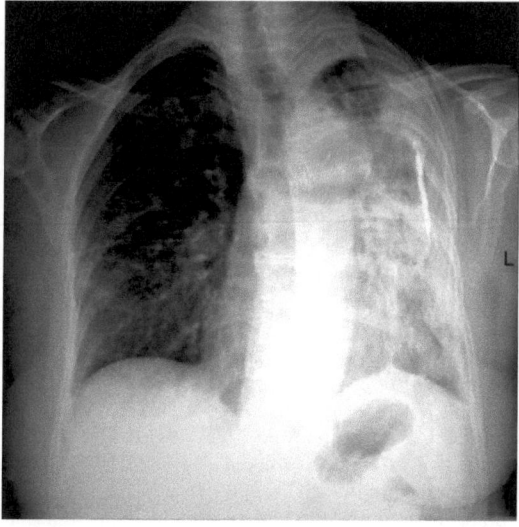

FIG. 5: Posteroanterior chest radiograph of a 70-year-old female patient who presented with a history of being treated for tuberculous pleural disease 30 years earlier, showing a left-sided fibrothorax with pleural calcification.

Based on Cochrane review, there are insufficient data to support evidence-based recommendations regarding the use of adjunctive corticosteroids in tuberculous pleurisy.[84]

Recommended approach is that if the patient is more than mildly symptomatic, a therapeutic thoracentesis is recommended, but if the patient continues to have severe systemic symptoms (fever, malaise, pleuritic chest pain) after the therapeutic thoracentesis, the administration of 80 mg of prednisone every other day until the acute symptoms have subsided is recommended. Thereafter, the corticosteroids are rapidly tapered.[1]

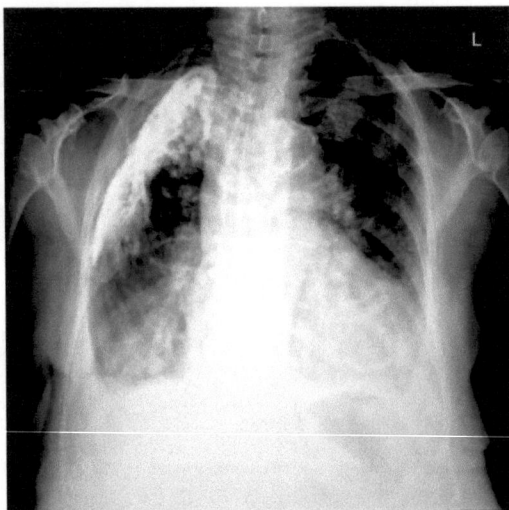

FIG. 6: Posteroanterior chest radiograph of a 78-year-old female patient who presented with a history of tuberculous pleural disease more than 45 years earlier, showing a right-sided fibrothorax with massive pleural calcification.

REFERENCES

1. Light RW. Pleural Diseases. 5th ed. Baltimore, MD: Lippincott Williams and Wilkins; 2007.
2. Porcel JM. Tuberculous pleural effusion. Lung. 2009;187:263-70.
3. Berger HW, Mejia E. Tuberculous pleurisy. Chest. 1973;63:88-92.
4. Stead WW, Eichenholz A, Stauss HK. Operative and pathologic findings in twenty-four patients with syndrome of idiopathic pleurisy with effusion, presumably tuberculous. Am Rev Tuberc. 1955;71:473-502.
5. Escudero BC, Garcia CM, Cuesta CB, et al. Cytologic and bacteriologic analysis of fluid and pleural biopsy specimens with Cope's needle. Study of 414 patients. Arch Intern Med. 1990;150:1190-4.
6. Ellner JJ, Barnes PF, Wallis RS, Modlin RL. The immunology of tuberculous pleurisy. Semin Respir Infect. 1988;3:335-42.
7. Frye MD, Sahn SA. (2014). Tuberculous pleural effusions in HIV-negative patients. [online] UpToDate website. Available from: www.uptodate.com [Accessed January, 2016].
8. Moudgil H, Sridhar G, Leitch AG. Reactivation disease: the commonest form of tuberculous pleural effusion in Edinburgh, 1980-1991. Respir Med. 1994;88:301-4.
9. Ong A, Creasman J, Hopewell PC, et al. A molecular epidemiological assessment of extrapulmonary tuberculosis in San Francisco. Clin Infect Dis. 2004;38:25-31.
10. Mlika-Cabanne N, Brauner M, Kamanfu G, et al. Radiographic abnormalities in tuberculosis and risk of coexisting human immunodeficiency virus infection. Methods and preliminary results from Bujumbura, Burundi. Am J Respir Crit Care Med. 1995;152:794-9.
11. Saks AM, Posner R. Tuberculosis in HIV positive patients in South Africa: a comparative radiological study with HIV negative patients. Clin Radiol. 1992;46:387-90.
12. Mehta JB, Dutt A, Harvill L, Mathews KM. Epidemiology of extrapulmonary tuberculosis. A comparative analysis with pre-AIDS era. Chest. 1991;99:1134-8.
13. Baumann MH, Nolan R, Petrini M, Lee YC, Light RW, Schneider E. Pleural tuberculosis in the United States: incidence and drug resistance. Chest. 2007;131:1125-32.
14. Awil PO, Bowlin SJ, Daniel TM. Radiology of pulmonary tuberculosis and human immunodeficiency virus infection in Gulu, Uganda. Eur Respir J. 1997;10:615-8.
15. Pozniak AL, MacLeod GA, Ndlovu D, Ross E, Mahari M, Weinberg J. Clinical and chest radiographic features of tuberculosis associated with human immunodeficiency virus in Zimbabwe. Am J Respir Crit Care Med. 1995;152:1558-61.

16. Queipo JA, Broseta E, Santos M, Sánchez-Plumed J, Budía A, Jiménez-Cruz F. Mycobacterial infection in a series of 1261 renal transplant recipients. Clin Microbiol Infect. 2003;9:518-25.
17. Malik GH, Al-Harbi AS, Al-Mohaya S, et al. Eleven years of experience with dialysis associated tuberculosis. Clin Nephrol. 2002;58:356-62.
18. Heyderman RS, Makunike R, Muza T, et al. Pleural tuberculosis in Harare, Zimbabwe: the relationship between human immunodeficiency virus, CD4 lymphocyte count, granuloma formation and disseminated disease. Trop Med Int Health. 1998;3:14-20.
19. Richter C, Perenboom R, Mtoni I, et al. Clinical features of HIV-seropositive and HIV-seronegative patients with tuberculous pleural effusion in Dar es Salaam, Tanzania. Chest. 1994;106:1471-5.
20. Porcel JM, Vives M. Etiology and pleural fluid characteristics of large and massive effusions. Chest. 2003;124:978-83.
21. Valdes L, Alvarez D, San Jose E, et al. Tuberculous pleurisy: a study of 254 patients. Arch Intern Med. 1998;158:2017-21.
22. Kim HJ, Lee HJ, Kwon SY, et al. The prevalence of pulmonary parenchymal tuberculosis in patients with tuberculous pleuritis. Chest. 2006;129:1253-8.
23. Sibley JC. A study of 200 cases of tuberculous pleurisy with effusion. Am Rev Tuberc. 1950;62:314-23.
24. Yeon KM, Kim CJ, Kim JS, Kim CH. Influence of age on the adenosine deaminase activity in patients with exudative pleural effusion. Tuberculosis Respir Dis. 2002;53:530-41.
25. Diacon AH, Van de Wal BW, Wyser C, et al. Diagnostic tools in tuberculous pleurisy: a direct comparative study. Eur Respir J. 2003;22:589-91.
26. Light RW. Establishing the diagnosis of tuberculous pleuritis. Arch Intern Med. 1998;158:1967-8.
27. Levine H, Szanto PB, Cugell DW. Tuberculous pleurisy. An acute illness. Arch Intern Med. 1968;122:329-32.
28. Light RW, Erozan YS, Ball WC Jr. Cells in pleural fluid. Their value in differential diagnosis. Arch Intern Med. 1973;132:854-60.
29. Hurwitz S, Leiman G, Shapiro C. Mesothelial cells in pleural fluid: TB or not TB? S Afr Med J. 1980;57:937-9.
30. Conde MB, Loivos AC, Rezende VM, et al. Yield of sputum induction in the diagnosis of pleural tuberculosis. Am J Respir Crit Care Med. 2003;167:723-5.
31. Luzze H, Elliott AM, Joloba ML, et al. Evaluation of suspected tuberculous pleurisy: clinical and diagnostic findings in HIV-1-positive and HIV-negative adults in Uganda. Int J Tuberc Lung Dis. 2001;5:746-53.
32. Ruan SY, Chuang YC, Wang JY, et al. Revisiting tuberculous pleurisy: pleural fluid characteristics and diagnostic yield of mycobacterial culture in an endemic area. Thorax. 2012;67:822-7.
33. Kelam MA, Ganie FA, Shah BA, et al. The diagnostic efficacy of adenosine deaminase in tubercular effusion. Oman Med J. 2013;28:417-21.
34. Liang QL, Shi HZ, Wang K, Qin SM, Qin XJ. Diagnostic accuracy of adenosine deaminase in tuberculous pleurisy: a meta-analysis. Respir Med. 2008;102:744-54.
35. Greco S, Girardi E, Masciangelo R, Capoccetta GB, Saltini C. Adenosine deaminase and interferon gamma measurements for the diagnosis of tuberculous pleurisy: a meta-analysis. Int J Tuberc Lung Dis. 2003;7(8):777-86.
36. Morisson P, Neves DD. Evaluation of adenosine deaminase in the diagnosis of pleural tuberculosis: a Brazilian meta-analysis. J Bras Pneumol. 2008;34(4):217-24.
37. Valdes L, San José E, Alvarez D, et al. Diagnosis of tuberculous pleurisy using the biologic parameters adenosine deaminase, lysozyme, and interferon gamma. Chest. 1993;103:458-65.
38. Riantawan P, Chaowalit P, Wongsangiem M, Rojanaraweewong P. Diagnostic value of pleural fluid adenosine deaminase in tuberculous pleuritis with reference to HIV coinfection and a Bayesian analysis. Chest. 1999;116:97-103.
39. Baba K, Hoosen AA, Langeland N, Dyrhol-Riise AM. Adenosine deaminase activity is a sensitive marker for the diagnosis of tuberculous pleuritis in patients with very low CD4 counts. PLoS One, 2008;3:e2788.
40. Tay TR, Tee A. Factors affecting pleural fluid adenosine deaminase level and the implication on the diagnosis of tuberculous pleural effusion: a retrospective cohort study. BMC Infect Dis. 2013;13:546.
41. Manuel Porcel J, Vives M, Esquerda A, Ruiz A. Usefulness of the British Thoracic Society and the American College of Chest Physicians guidelines in predicting pleural drainage of non-purulent parapneumonic effusions. Respir Med. 2006;100:933-7.

42. Gopi A, Madhavan SM, Sharma SK, Sahn SA. Diagnosis and treatment of tuberculous pleural effusion in 2006. Chest. 2007;131:880-9.
43. Maskell NA, Butland RJ. BTS guidelines for the investigation of a unilateral pleural effusion in adults. Thorax. 2003;58 Suppl 2:ii8-17.
44. Lee YC, Light RW. Adenosine deaminase for lymphocytic pleural effusions. International Pleural Newsletter. 2004;2:5-6.
45. Niwa Y, Kishimoto H, Shimokata K. Carcinomatous and tuberculous pleural effusions. Comparison of tumor markers. Chest. 1985;87:351-5.
46. Garcia-Zamalloa A, Taboada-Gomez J. Diagnostic accuracy of adenosine deaminase and lymphocyte proportion in pleural fluid for tuberculous pleurisy in different prevalence scenarios. PLoS One. 2012;7(6):e38729.
47. Burgess LJ, Maritz FJ, Le Roux I, Taljaard JJ. Combined use of pleural adenosine deaminase with lymphocyte/neutrophil ratio. Increased specificity for the diagnosis of tuberculous pleuritis. Chest. 1996;109:414-9.
48. Villegas MV, Labrada LA, Saravia NG. Evaluation of polymerase chain reaction, adenosine deaminase, and interferon-gamma in pleural fluid for the differential diagnosis of pleural tuberculosis. Chest. 2000;118:1355-64.
49. Pal S, Gupta S. Adenosine deaminase—the non-invasive marker of tuberculosis. J Indian Med Assoc. 2012;110(1):16-8.
50. Yurt S, Küçükergin C, Yigitbas BA, Seçkin S, Tigin HC, Koşar AF. Diagnostic utility of serum and pleural levels of adenosine deaminase 1–2, and interferon-γ in the diagnosis of pleural tuberculosis. Multidiscip Respir Med. 2014;9:12.
51. Perez-Rodriguez E, Castro DJ. The use of adenosine deaminase and adenosine deaminase isoenzymes in the diagnosis of tuberculous pleuritis. Curr Opin Pulm Med. 2000;6:259-66.
52. Light RW. Update on tuberculous pleural effusion. Respirology. 2010;15:451-8.
53. Jiang J, Shi HZ, Liang QL, Qin SM, Qin XJ. Diagnostic value of interferon-gamma in tuberculous pleurisy: a meta-analysis. Chest. 2007;131:1133-41.
54. Villena V, Lopez-Encuentra A, Pozo F, et al. Interferon gamma levels in pleural fluid for the diagnosis of tuberculosis. Am J Med. 2003;115:365-70.
55. Liu F, Gao M, Zhang X, et al. Interferon-gamma release assay performance of pleural fluid and peripheral blood in pleural tuberculosis. PLoS One. 2013;8(12):e83857.
56. Chegou NN, Walzl G, Bolliger CT, Diacon AH, van den Heuvel MM. Evaluation of adapted whole-blood interferon-gamma release assays for the diagnosis of pleural tuberculosis. Respiration. 2008;76:131-8.
57. Guo SJ, Jia LQ, Hu QJ, Long HY, Pang CS, Wen FQ. Diagnostic accuracy of interferon gamma-induced protein 10 for tuberculosis: a meta-analysis. Int J Clin Exp Med. 2014;7(1):93-100.
58. Dinnes J, Deeks J, Kunst H, et al. A systematic review of rapid diagnostic tests for the detection of tuberculosis infection. Health Technol Assess. 2007;11:1-196.
59. Pai M, Flores LL, Hubbard A, Riley LW, Colford JM Jr. Nucleic acid amplification tests in the diagnosis of tuberculous pleuritis: a systematic review and meta-analysis. BMC Infect Dis. 2004;4:6.
60. Leung CC, Feller-Kopman D, Niederman MS, Spiro SG. Year in review 2010: tuberculosis, pleural diseases, respiratory infections. Respirology. 2011;16:564-73.
61. Boehme CC, Nabeta P, Hillemann D, et al. Rapid molecular detection of tuberculosis and rifampin resistance. N Engl J Med. 2010;363:1005-15.
62. Gill MK, Kukreja S, Chhabra N. Evaluation of nested polymerase chain reaction for rapid diagnosis of clinically suspected tuberculous pleurisy. J Clin Diagn Res. 2013;7(11):2456-8.
63. Koegelenberg CF, Diacon AH. Pleural controversy: close needle pleural biopsy or thoracoscopy—which first? Respirology. 2011;16:738-46.
64. Hooper C, Lee YC, Maskell N. Investigation of a unilateral pleural effusion in adults: British Thoracic Society pleural disease guideline 2010. Thorax. 2010;65 Suppl 2:ii4-17.
65. Loddenkemper R, Boutin C. Thoracoscopy: present diagnostic and therapeutic indications. Eur Respir J. 1993;6:1544-55.
66. Koegelenberg CF, Bolliger CT, Theron J, et al. Direct comparison of the diagnostic yield of ultrasound-assisted Abrams and Tru-Cut needle biopsies for pleural tuberculosis. Thorax. 2010;65:857-62.
67. Small PM, Fujiwara PI. Management of tuberculosis in the United States. N Engl J Med. 2001;345:189-200.

68. Blumberg HM, Burman WJ, Chaisson RE, et al. American Thoracic Society/Centers for Disease Control and Prevention/Infectious Diseases Society of America: treatment of tuberculosis. Am J Respir Crit Care Med. 2003;167:603-62.
69. Shu CC, Wang JT, Wang JY, Lee LN, Yu CJ. In-hospital outcome of patients with culture-confirmed tuberculous pleurisy: clinical impact of pulmonary involvement. BMC Infect Dis. 2011;11:46.
70. Tani P, Poppius H, Maekipaja J. Cortisone therapy for exudative tuberculous pleurisy in the light of a follow-up study. Acta Tuberc Pneumol Scand. 1964;44:303-9.
71. Galarza I, Canete C, Granados A, Estopà R, Manresa F. Randomised trial of corticosteroids in the treatment of tuberculous pleurisy. Thorax. 1995;50:1305-7.
72. Wyser C, Walzl G, Smedema JP, Swart F, van Schalkwyk EM, van de Wal BW. Corticosteroids in the treatment of tuberculous pleurisy. A double-blind, placebo-controlled, randomized study. Chest. 1996;110:333-8.
73. Barbas CS, Cukier A, de Varvalho CR, Barbas Filho JV, Light RW. The relationship between pleural fluid findings and the development of pleural thickening in patients with pleural tuberculosis. Chest. 1991;100:1264-7.
74. Wong PC. Management of tuberculous pleuritis: can we do better? Respirology. 2005;10:144-8.
75. Han DH, Song JW, Chung HS, Lee JH. Resolution of residual pleural disease according to time course in tuberculous pleurisy during and after the termination of antituberculosis medication. Chest. 2005;128:3240-5.
76. Lai YF, Chao TY, Wang YH, Lin AS. Pigtail drainage in the treatment of tuberculous pleural effusions: a randomized study. Thorax. 2003;58:149-51.
77. Kwak SM, Park CS, Cho JH, et al. The effects of urokinase instillation therapy via percutaneous transthoracic catheter in loculated tuberculous pleural effusion: a randomized prospective study. Yonsei Med J. 2004;45:822-8.
78. Al-Majed SA. Study of paradoxical response to chemotherapy in tuberculous pleural effusion. Respir Med. 1996;90:211-4.
79. Hiraoka K, Nagata N, Kawajiri T, et al. Paradoxical pleural response to antituberculous chemotherapy and isoniazid-induced lupus. Review and report of two cases. Respiration. 1998;65:152-5.
80. Choi YW, Jeon SC, Seo HS, et al. Tuberculous pleural effusion: new pulmonary lesions during treatment. Radiology. 2002;224:493-502.
81. Gupta RC, Dixit R, Purohit SD, Saxena A. Development of pleural effusion in patients during antituberculous chemotherapy: analysis of twenty-nine cases with review of literature. Indian J Chest Dis Allied Sci. 2000;42:161-6.
82. Lee CH, Wang WJ, Lan RS, Tsai YH, Chiang YC. Corticosteroids in the treatment of tuberculous pleurisy: a double-blind, placebo-controlled, randomized study. Chest. 1988;94:1256-9.
83. Elliott AM, Luzze H, Quigley MA, et al. A randomized, double-blind, placebo-controlled trial of the use of prednisolone as an adjunct to treatment in HIV-1-associated pleural tuberculosis. J Infect Dis. 2004;190:869-78.
84. Engel ME, Matchaba PT, Volmink J. Corticosteroids for tuberculous pleurisy. Cochrane Database Syst Rev. 2007;(4):CD001876.

CHAPTER 10
Clinically Unrecognized Tuberculosis: Multidisciplinary Approach

Vesna Škodrić Trifunović

INTRODUCTION

Tuberculosis (TB) has existed for millennia and causes ill-health in millions of people each year. It is one of the top ten causes of death worldwide, ranking above human immunodeficiency virus (HIV)/acquired immune deficiency syndrome as one of the leading causes of death from an infectious disease. World Health Organization in 2013 reported 8.6 million newly diagnosed and 1.3 million deaths from TB.[1] Although, a declining trend in TB incidence and elimination of the disease at global level is still out of the reach. We have benefited from scientific and clinical progress, but at the same time there is a global increase of HIV infection, drug resistance in many countries, human migrations, etc. Also, there are many factors that facilitate transmission of disease, which include weakened immune system, overcrowding, malnutrition, smoking, and harmful use of alcohol. Tuberculosis primarily attacks the lungs but can affect any other organ as well. Despite the fact that TB is nowadays curable disease, cases of death caused by this disease are not rare. Tuberculosis therefore represents very significant health and social problem worldwide, but poses as the highest threat in developing countries.

In developed countries, TB is considered a rare disease which often leads to delayed or wrong diagnosis, especially when other organs are affected. Over 1 million people worldwide are misdiagnosed with TB. All these facts lead to the conclusion that there is a need for special caution (and increased suspicion of TB), because undiagnosed TB can easily result in complications and death.[2]

Identification of patients with active TB is important for both patients and society (as a whole). Early diagnosis and proper treatment will cure the sick and stop further spread of infection. It will also reduce nosocomial infections and professional risk of developing TB. Therefore, unrecognized TB can have clinical, epidemiological but also legal consequences.[3]

A BROAD SPECTRUM OF DIFFERENT DISEASES MAKES A PROBLEM IN DIAGNOSTICS

Most commonly affected organs are the lungs but any other organ can be affected by TB. Extrapulmonary forms of TB may be a complex diagnostic problem, depending on which organ is affected, which is the reason that the diagnosis may be delayed or wrong.[4,5] Abdominal TB is especially hard to recognize and in these cases, diagnosis is established by surgery or in the autopsy as unexpected TB.[6,7]

The differential diagnosis may include dozens of other diseases, and if TB is not considered, there is a great possibility of patient's death, especially in the elderly and immunocompromised.[2,4] Since clinical manifestations of TB in these patients are often nonspecific, the diagnosis of TB is sometimes very difficult. Atypical radiographic appearance, the existence of other comorbidities associated with TB may mask TB. Failing to suspect TB is the most common reason for late diagnosis.[4,5,8]

In the differential diagnosis of TB, physicians should think about the following diseases—flu, since early symptoms of TB are flu-like; upper respiratory infection; pneumonia; lung abscesses; respiratory fungal infections; lymphoma; silicosis; asbestosis, etc. In some cases, symptoms may suggest advanced lung malignancies.[2,4,9] In extrapulmonary forms, in addition to general symptoms, there are signs and symptoms of the affected organs.

DIAGNOSIS OF TUBERCULOSIS

Rapid diagnosis of TB is of crucial importance to control and reduce the spread of *Mycobacterium tuberculosis*.

The diagnosis of TB is based on clinical presentation, clinical examination, radiographic findings, and sputum smear and culturing. Despite the decades-long experience in diagnosing TB, many clinical studies have shown that errors in the diagnosis of TB are quite often.

The clinical history, in addition to the clinical presentation, is of great importance in establishing suspicion of TB. If the patient gives information of TB infection in the past or about the contact with TB patient in the last 2 years, physician should immediately take further diagnostic procedures. The first and most important step in the diagnosis of TB is to suspect on TB. For example, one study has shown that the time to diagnose TB was significantly shorter (8 days in average) when TB was mentioned as a differential diagnosis in chest X-ray (CXR) report comparing to when TB is not mentioned (20 days in average).[10]

Patients often complain of general symptoms such as adynamia, subfebrile temperatures, night sweating, loss of weight, but the most common and almost always present symptom is cough often followed by hemoptysis. Period from onset of symptoms to the initiation of therapy is very important for the outcome of the disease and the length of this period depends on the time when patient ask for the help and on the efficiency of healthcare system. The average period from onset of symptoms to the beginning of the treatment is 3 months, but can be much longer, which often results in a fatal outcome.[11] In patients with chronic diseases such as diabetes, chronic renal failure, or those on immunosuppressive therapy for various reasons, clinical presentation of TB can be significantly altered. Respiratory symptoms such as cough, coughing up, or hemoptysis may be absent or masked by general symptoms.[4,5,12] In these patients, they are often misdiagnosed as worsening of the underlying disease (worsening of glycemic control in diabetics or increase of blood urea nitrogen in patients with renal disease).

Chest Radiography

For early diagnosis of TB, it is the best to do CXR as soon as at the first visit, especially in all persons with symptoms of respiratory tract infections (productive cough) which are present for 3 or more weeks.

Chest X-ray findings in immunocompetent patients often include cavitations and infiltrates in the upper lobes. In contrast, radiological findings may be atypical for TB, may occur as a lung scattering in the lower lung fields, miliary scattering, etc. In persons with severe immunodeficiency, CXR findings resemble findings that are seen in primary TB of immunocompetent patients such as hilar adenopathy and pleural effusion. Normal chest radiographic findings do not exclude the diagnosis of pulmonary TB since radiographic signs may be well behind rapid evolution of active disease (the early onset of miliary TB) or in endobronchial forms of TB.[13,14]

Any patient with a history of TB infection or with an abnormal CXR consistent with past TB should be monitored on regular basis and referred to pulmonologist as needed. Routine screening of patients with comorbidity is not recommended but regular monitoring of these patients for early detection of TB can be helpful.

Sputum Smear and Culture

Although new molecular methods for the diagnosis of TB have been developed in the last two decades, acid-fast bacilli (AFB) smear microscopy and culture on Löwenstein–Jensen medium are still the "gold standards" for the diagnosis of active TB. However, in some cases, conventional microbiological methods for the detection of *M. tuberculosis* are often not quick enough since the treatment of active TB should start as soon as possible.

If there is a strong suspicion of TB and previous diagnostic tests (AFB) have failed to confirm the clinical diagnosis, it is essential to do histopathology examination. Rapid diagnostic tests are expensive and are used only when it is necessary to make an urgent decision on initiation of treatment.

Similarly, pathological and microbiological confirmation is necessary in the case of extrapulmonary TB. Type of specimen for diagnosis of extrapulmonary TB depends on which organ is affected. The most common patterns are tissue biopsy, aspirates, urine, pus, and normally sterile body fluids such as cerebrospinal fluid, synovial, pleural, pericardial, and peritoneal liquid. In the case of young children or adults who due to musculoskeletal illness or for any other reason are not able to cough up, gastric lavage is the preferable specimen. Diagnosis of peritoneal and pericardial TB is difficult and often requires invasive procedures. Adenosine deaminase activity is helpful in the diagnosis of tuberculous meningitis, tuberculous pleural effusion, and tuberculous peritonitis. Since these forms of TB are difficult to diagnose by only using classical methods, such as smear staining and culture, they often can remain undiagnosed.

FAILURE TO DIAGNOSE

Failure to recognize the symptoms of the disease can be made by general practitioners, internal medicine specialists, or even by a pulmonary medicine specialist. The diagnosis of active TB may be delayed or wrong due to the similarity of symptoms of TB and other respiratory diseases such as upper respiratory tract infections, cold, bronchitis, pneumonia, and flu. Chest X-ray findings may be similar to X-ray finding of the other lung diseases. These facts can affect the decision of clinicians in which direction to continue further diagnostics. According to published data, diagnosis of TB due to wrong medical decisions may be delayed 8–46 days.[15]

There are many factors associated with delay of diagnosis. Analyzing healthcare delays in relation to symptoms have shown that cough was strongly associated with shorter healthcare delays. If cough was longer present before patient visited physician, the period to make diagnosis of TB was much shorter. It was not proven that the presence of any other symptom or combination of symptoms could be a predictor of faster diagnosis.[10]

Current diagnostic algorithms require that if productive cough is present for 3 or more weeks, it is necessary to do chest radiography and sputum microbiological examination.

Analysis of respiratory symptoms typical for TB has shown that cough, hemoptysis, weight loss, fever, night sweats, and pain were omitted in 39–81% of cases. Analysis of the clinical examination showed that lung auscultation was omitted in 32–50%. Also, lymphadenopathy examination has been omitted in the 31–85% of patients. Retrograde analysis of the symptoms, physical signs, and CXR findings of the patients who died of unrecognized TB, indicates that they had symptoms, physical and radiographic findings for TB and other related diseases as well. These symptoms and signs were mostly fever, adynamia, and anorexia.[16]

Detailed analysis of clinical omissions have shown that if CXR, sputum specimen, and tuberculin skin test have not been done at the initial examination, the time to diagnose TB has been prolonged. Chest X-ray is not always reliable to indicate the possible TB and omission can happen in 38% of patients.[16] Based on CXR, TB can be wrongly diagnosed as a lung abscess, cancer, fungal infections, silicosis, berylliosis, or end-stage sarcoidosis.[2,4,5] Diagnosis of TB using CXR was significantly shorter if the first X-ray shows cavitations compared to those without visible cavitations. If there is no microbiological verification of TB, but X-ray shows cavitations in the lungs, it is necessary to do a bronchoscopy and histological diagnosis of TB.

Bronchoscopy has to be performed routinely in all patients with lung infiltrates suspected on TB, if there is no sputum smear nor culture verification. Endobronchial TB can mimic other diseases like lung cancer or asthma. If the patient has a history of asthma or chronic obstructive pulmonary disease, there is often diagnostic dilemma.[14]

Also, the time taken to diagnose TB depends on medical services where the patient initially asks for help. Most doctors in emergency rooms do not perform routine inspection of the lungs, but only when there are symptoms and signs of pulmonary disease. The time for detection of TB is shorter if patient comes with respiratory symptoms to the hospital first, because hospital doctors have a specialized education, and better access to diagnostic tools: CXR, sputum examination, computed tomography (CT), bronchoscopy, etc. but patients are often examined in emergency services due to nonrespiratory problems like gastrointestinal bleeding, abdominal pain, vertigo, tachycardia, petechial hemorrhages, etc. These patients are referred to other specialists and only if they develop prominent respiratory symptoms and signs, chest radiography is performed. Failures in these situations may arise from polymorphic clinical picture or urgency. Average number of days from first appearance to the diagnosis of TB was 10 days in a public health clinic, 18 days in hospital emergency rooms, and 51 days at private primary care physician office.[10] A special group of patients are immunocompromised patients, those who suffer from hematological, rheumatic, oncologic conditions, or conditions after organ transplantation. In this group, symptoms of the disease can be deceptive, and if a doctor does not routinely conduct periodic examination of the lung (CXR), the diagnosis of TB can be late resulting in death.

MISDIAGNOSIS OF TUBERCULOSIS LEADING TO DEATHS

Unrecognized TB represents great danger not only for the patient but also because of possibility of spread of the infection for the medical staff involved in the diagnosis and treatment, and can also be medicolegal problem.[3,17] Numerous cases of TB stay unrecognized until after the death.[2,7,18-20] It can be seen as a failure of the health system to timely recognize and treat potentially curable disease. These unrecognized cases of TB are also a source of further spread of the infection and poor epidemiological situation in the world today.[21]

Unrecognized TB is defined as clinically undiagnosed TB but later proven on autopsy. The most common errors in diagnosis of TB are happening in developed countries where there is low awareness due to low incidence of TB.[2,7]

Several studies from different parts of the world have indicated the problem of clinically unrecognized TB.[21] Thus, studies in the United States have shown that 3.9% and 5% of cases of active TB respectively were identified only after the death of the patient.[4,5,21] Many autopsy studies have suggested that the diagnosis of TB was omitted in a large number of patients during the life, even 18–54% of patients in whom later at autopsy was find pathological evidence of active TB.[7,20,22-30] In hospitals where autopsies are performed routinely, a diagnosis of active TB was omitted in 52%, and TB was wrongly declared as a cause of death in 16% of patients. It is important to note that in significant number of wrongly diagnosed TB cases, simple and basic diagnostic clinical actions were never documented.[16,22]

The reason why TB often stays unrecognized in human immunodeficiency virus (HIV)-infected are atypical clinical features, atypical CXR findings, extrapulmonary infection, and clinical picture that may be masked by underlying disease (HIV infection) or opportunistic infections.[27]

LENGTH OF HOSPITALIZATION

Length of hospitalization can be one of the factors for misdiagnosis of TB. It is considered that if patient was hospitalized for less than 48 hours, chances of misdiagnosing TB are higher. Such cases are often seen on autopsies, and reasons may be different.[28] For example, patients may come to a doctor in final stages of TB when it is already too late. Furthermore, miliary TB may be present as respiratory adult distress syndrome, and if not detected quickly lethal outcome is very likely.

Patients in which TB is not initially suspected length of hospitalization can be 2 or more weeks and death from TB can occur even before results of AFB smear or culture are obtained. Some studies point out that almost all cases of TB proven at autopsy in which the death occurred as a direct result of TB, major diagnostic omission was the lack of clinical suspicion of TB.[7,18,28]

CLINICOPATHOLOGICAL ANALYSIS OF DECEASED FROM TUBERCULOSIS

Diagnosis of TB at autopsy is a serious problem not only because the patient died of a potentially curable disease but also due to occupational exposure for pathologists as well as the risk of spreading nosocomial infection.[29,30]

Analysis of the reasons for nonrecognition of TB during life showed that 70% of patients had at least one more chronic disease; 64% had iatrogenic or other immunosuppressive condition caused by some chronic disease, 29% had a chronic lung disease, and other diseases such as diabetes, pulmonary fibrosis, and chronic renal disease were less often present.[2,31]

Studies that have been analyzing age in patients in whom TB was clinically unrecognized and later confirmed at autopsy showed that over 60% of cases were observed in the elderly.[30] In this group of patients, the symptoms were scarce, and the presence of other chronic diseases wrongly directed diagnosis.[2,4]

According to studies that were analyzing CXR findings in patients with TB, radiographic diagnosis was missed in 38% of cases.[16] Chest X-ray of these patients often shows radiological image of pneumonia or malignancy, or no abnormality is seen in case of intrabronchial form of TB.[2,14]

Miliary forms of TB are more frequently found at autopsy than diagnosed during the life of the patient. Miliary TB is the most common in the elderly and goes with the picture of chronic nonspecific process, subfebrile temperatures, and loss of weight. In these patients, TB is often not suspected or suspected too late, especially in countries where TB is rare. This finding in the elderly and risk factors (corticosteroids, other chronic diseases) should lead clinician to suspect TB. Negative tuberculin test does not exclude TB in these people.[4,13]

CASE STUDY 1

A female patient, 78 years old, was admitted to the emergency center, department of general surgery, because of melena. Starting from 2 weeks before the admission, apart from occasional black discoloration of the stool, she was febrile (up to 39°C), short of breath, lost appetite and weight, was sweating a lot, and felt malaise. She had no previous history of lung diseases, only of hypothyreosis for more than 10 years.

On admission, she appeared cachectic, subfebrile with impaired general condition. Gastroscopy was performed, with no signs of acute bleeding from stomach. Next morning, she was referred as outpatient to the examinations of the cardiologist and neurologist. Neurologist ordered brain computed tomography and cortical ischemic lesions were found. Cardiological examination was unremarkable. Seven days later, patient became tachypneic (25 breaths/minute), develops both central and peripheral cyanosis and she was urgently admitted in the clinic for pulmonary diseases and, for the first time, chest radiography was done (Fig. 1). Chest radiography could have been the key of diagnosis, if only was done earlier.

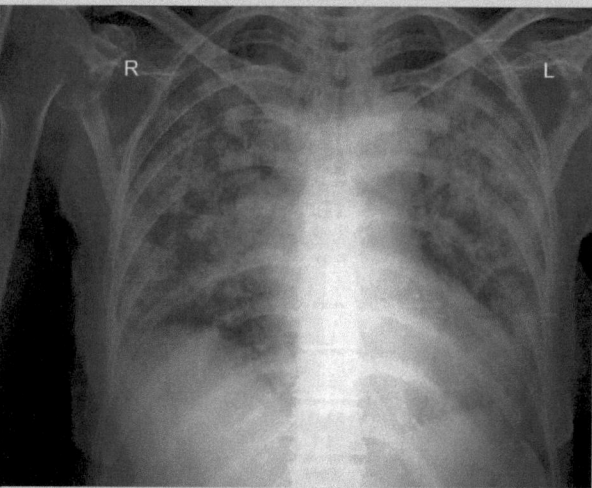

FIG. 1: Chest X-ray revealed both micronodular and confluent shadows with signs of excavation predominantly in left lower lobe.

Arterial blood gas analyses showed severe partial respiratory insufficiency (PaO$_2$ 4.4 kPa, PaCO$_2$ 4.0 kPa, pH 7.54, SaO$_2$ 71%), laboratory findings pointed to anemia, hepatorenal insufficiency, and inflammation with neutrophil predomination (93%). Sputum specimen was taken for acid-fast bacilli and antituberculous therapy immediately started. While waiting for the results of direct sputum microscopy, patient died with signs of cardiorespiratory insufficiency less than 24 hours after admission. Autopsy was done and it revealed miliary tuberculous granulomas in both lungs, along with generalized tuberculous granulomas in liver and kidney (Figs. 2 to 4).

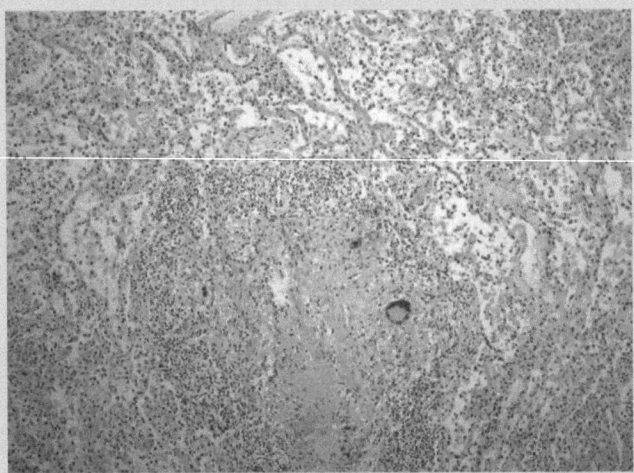

FIG. 2: Histopathology finding—lungs (HE, ×100): Areas of caseous necrosis, which are surrounded by rare epithelioid cells, giant multinucleated cells (Langhans cells), lymphocytes, and fibroblasts. *(For color version, see Plate 10)*

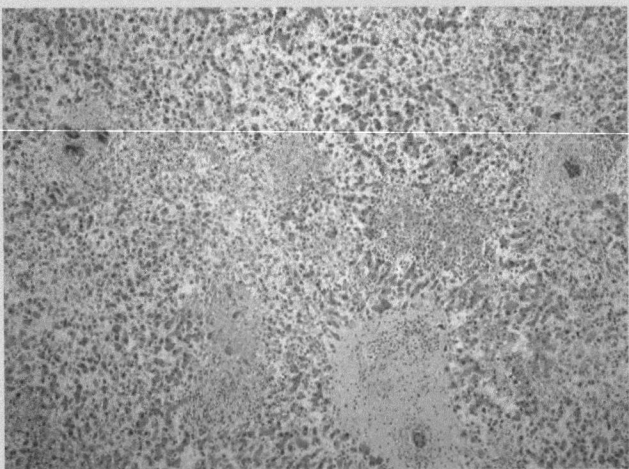

FIG. 3: Histopathology finding—liver (HE, ×100): Areas of caseous necrosis, which are surrounded by rare epithelioid cells, giant multinucleated cells (Langhans cells), and lymphocytes. *(For color version, see Plate 10)*

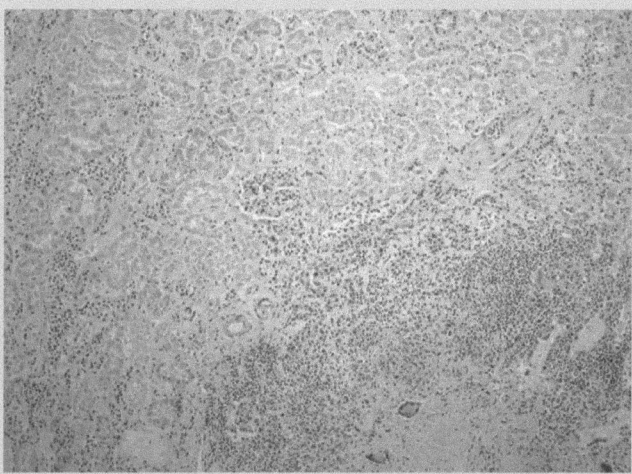

FIG. 4: Histopathology finding—kidney (HE, ×100): Small areas of caseous necrosis, which are surrounded by rare epithelioid cells, giant multinucleated cells (Langhans cells), and lymphocytes. *(For color version, see Plate 11)*

CASE STUDY 2

A female patient, 72 years old, was admitted to the gastroenterology department of the emergency center, because she thought that she vomited blood, although she was not sure if it was vomiting or coughing up blood (about 200 mL). Gastroscopy was performed and neither signs of bleeding from esophagus nor stomach were found, so she was referred to the pulmonologist and admitted in the clinic for pulmonary diseases because of hemoptysis.

Her medical history revealed bacterial meningitis 2 years ago and lung TB in her youth, but she was not able to give more details about it. On admission, laboratory results showed normal gas exchange, mild anemia, and slightly elevation of urea concentration in serum, but all other findings were normal.

Chest radiography and multislice computed tomography were performed (Figs. 5 and 6).

Upon arrival, urgent bronchoscopy was performed and a lot of fresh blood was seen in left and right bronchial tree. After aspiration, source of bleeding was observed in apical segment bronchus of the right upper lobe. The bronchus itself was narrowed with edematous, vulnerable mucosa. This finding is also compatible with edematous-hyperemic form of endobronchial TB, but suspicion of malignant disease was also raised (mediastinal lymphadenopathy, focal liver lesion). Hemoptysis was then stopped with conservative intrabronchial and systemic therapy.

Patient suddenly died on the third day of hospitalization with sudden onset of massive hemoptysis (more than 2L of blood in one episode), unresponsive to neither systemic nor bronchoscopic therapy.

Autopsy was done and it revealed miliary tuberculous granulomas in both lungs (Fig. 7) along with generalized tuberculous lymphadenitis (Fig. 8), and tuberculous granulomas in spleen and liver. One caseous lesion in right upper lobe invaded lobar bronchus and blood vessels (well-known mechanism of occurrence of endobronchial TB) and it was probable cause of massive hemoptysis. Focal lesion in the liver was calcified echinococcal cyst. As a cause of death was pronounced the generalized miliary TB.

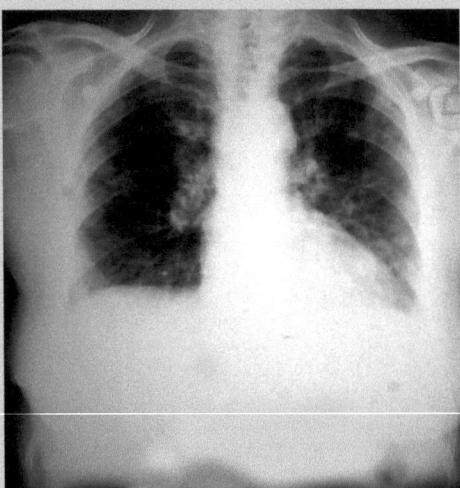

FIG. 5: Chest X-ray showing bilateral hilar adenopathy with calcifications was seen, also peribronchial and perivascular thickening and nodular shadows in both lungs. Scarring was also observed in both upper lobes.

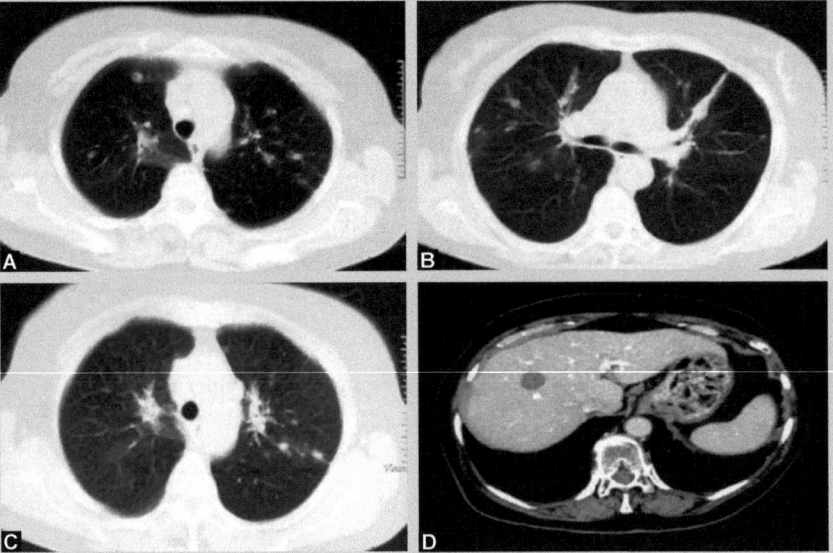

FIG. 6: A to **C,** Multislice computed tomography of the chest and upper abdomen revealed peribronchial thickenings and condensations in both lungs with predominantly calcified bihilar and mediastinal lymphadenopathy; **D,** Hypodense focal lesion was found in the liver.

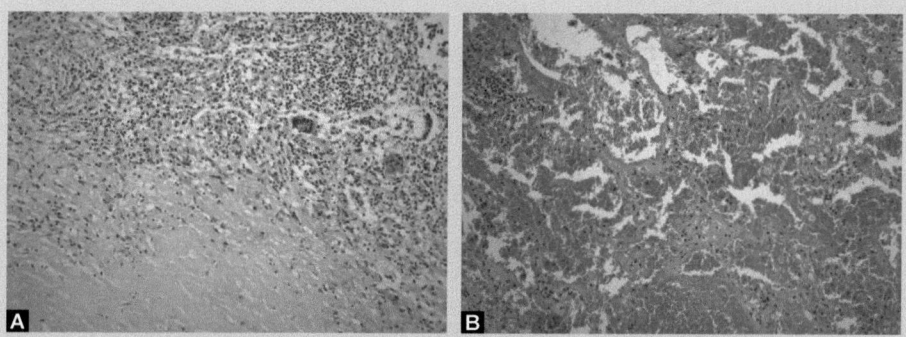

FIG. 7: Histopathology findings—lungs: **A,** Miliary tuberculous granulomas in both lungs are of different ages, primarily organized and calcified; **B,** Alveoli filled with erythrocytes. *(For color version, see Plate 11)*

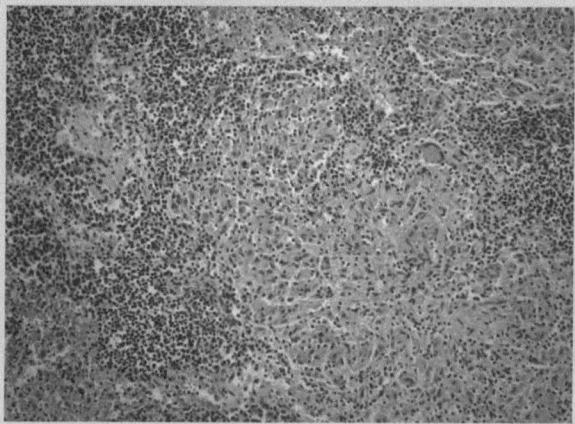

FIG. 8: Pulmonary hilar lymph nodes showed tuberculous granuloma with a field of caseous necrosis. *(For color version, see Plate 11)*

Courtesy: Pathologists, Institute of Pathology, Faculty of Medicine, University of Belgrade, Serbia.

CASE STUDY 3

A female patient, 68 years old, treated from asthma for 20 years and for 14 years from diabetes, on oral antidiabetics. She had weakness, fatigue, cough with whitish sputum expectoration, and wheezing starting 1 month prior to admission. She was treated with bronchodilators and antibiotics, but without improvement of her general condition and lung function tests. On chest radiography, a nodule in right upper lobe was seen (Fig. 9).

Due to failure to respond to the therapy, Multislice computed tomography of the chest was done and revealed pneumonic consolidation in apical segment of right upper lobe with slightly enlarged, reactive lymph nodes (11 mm in diameter) (Fig. 10)

On sputum microscopy, no acid-fast bacilli were observed and patient was referred to bronchoscopy on suspicion of intraluminal obstruction (lung cancer). On the bronchoscopic examination, mucosal swelling and hyperemia were found in tracheobronchial tree, biopsy results showed chronic bronchitis. Bronchial aspirate microscopy was negative, but the culture was positive (100 colonies) and *M. tuberculosis* was identified. Standard tuberculosis (TB) treatment was initiated.

In this case, there was no clinical suspicion on TB and the bronchoscopy was done on suspicion of lung cancer. Bacteriological confirmation of TB was unexpected.

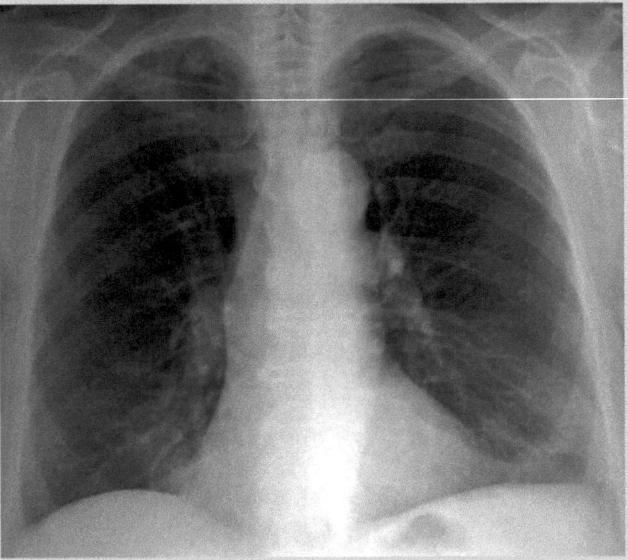

FIG. 9: Chest radiography showing nodular change in right upper lobe.

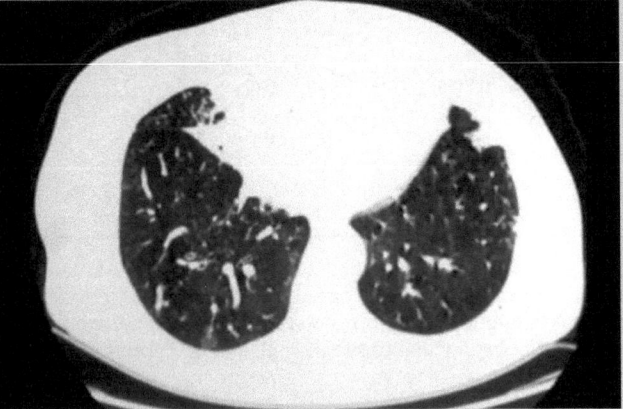

FIG. 10: Chest computed tomography showing suspected pneumonic consolidation in the right upper lobe.

CASE STUDY 4

A young man was referred to the abdominal surgeon because of abdominal pain in last 7 months, followed by malaise, weight loss, and jaundice. Laboratory findings showed high bilirubin (total and direct), transaminases, γ-glutamyl transferase (γ-GT), and alkaline phosphatases were moderately elevated. Tumor markers were all within normal range. Hepatitis markers were also negative [hepatitis B surface antigen (HBsAg), hepatitis C virus]. Ultrasonography revealed a solid hypoechogenic mass (40 mm) near the head of pancreas, and a few enlarged lymph nodes (Fig. 11). Computed tomography scan of the abdomen verified solid mass in the posterior of the head of the pancreas (Fig. 12).

The tumor in the pancreatic region was suspected and operation was performed. Intraoperative finding showed common bile duct stenosis caused by a mass in the posterior of the head of the pancreas. Lymph nodes were enlarged between 2 and 4 cm in diameter. Lymph nodes were removed and the bile duct repaired. Histology and polymerase chain reaction assay confirmed tuberculous lymphadenitis (Fig. 13). Patient received standard TB treatment and follow-up showed no signs of diseases relapse. Operative finding of tuberculous lymphadenitis as a cause of obstructive jaundice was unsuspected and operation was performed on suspicion of pancreatic tumor.

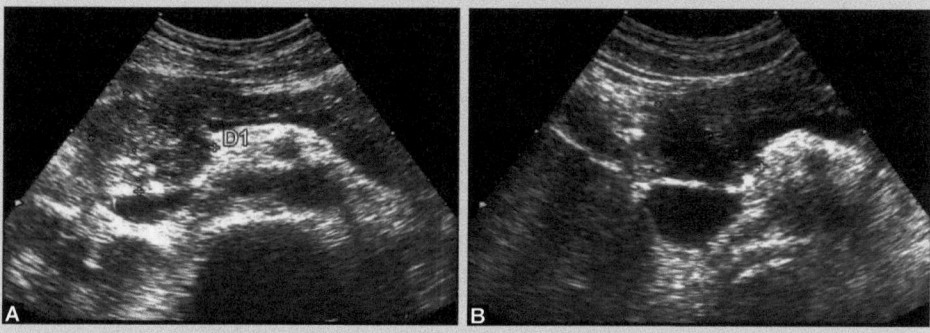

FIG. 11: Ultrasonography revealed a solid hypoechogenic mass (40 mm) near the head of pancreas and a few enlarged lymph nodes.
Courtesy: Dr Nikica Grubor, Clinic of Digestive Surgery, Clinical Center of Serbia, Belgrade, Serbia.

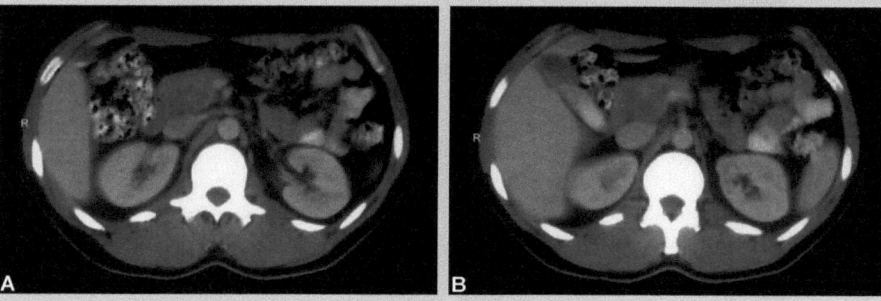

FIG. 12: Computed tomography scan of the abdomen verified solid mass in the posterior of the head of the pancreas.
Courtesy: Dr Nikica Grubor, Clinic of Digestive Surgery, Clinical Center of Serbia, Belgrade, Serbia.

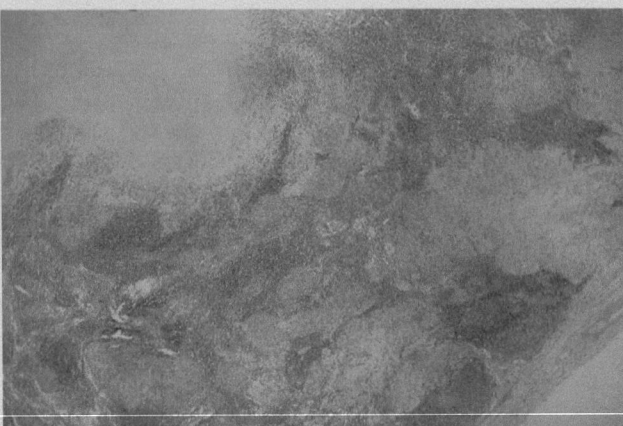

FIG. 13: Histopathology findings: Granulomatous lymphadenitis (HE, ×13).
(For color version, see Plate 12)

CASE STUDY 5

A male patient, 76 years old, with history of emphysema and frequent corticosteroid treatment was reported to the orthopedic surgeon because of constant swelling of the right wrist followed by moderate pain. Laboratory findings showed slightly elevated erythrocyte sedimentation rate (35 mm/1 h) and mild anemia. Chest radiography was done and it was normal. On the location of the swelling fistula was gradually formed, and from the smear *Staphylococcus aureus* was isolated. Patient started antibiotic treatment, according to antibiogram, but without success. Magnetic resonance imaging of the wrist revealed arthritis of small joints and flexor tenosynovitis.

Patient underwent operation and proliferation of the synovial membrane of radiocarpal joint was observed, together with a defects of distal parts of both ulna and radius, which were partially destroyed (Fig. 14). Also, effusions of the flexor tendons sheaths was identified. Histology report indicated toward tuberculous osteomyelitis and tenosynovitis. Patient was then referred to the pulmonologist and standard treatment for tuberculosis (TB) was started.

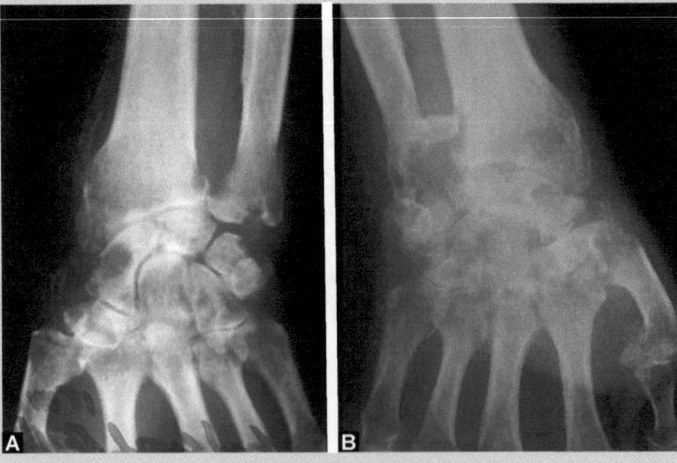

FIG. 14: Arthritis and destruction of distal parts of ulna and radius.

> Comment: The patient was immunodeficient due to frequent corticosteroid use during past years. In these rare cases of extrapulmonary TB, such as this one, with TB in the wrist joint, diagnosis is often established during operation because neither clinical picture nor other findings are specific. The main problem is that TB is not suspected at all, which inevitably leads to late diagnosis.
>
> This case demonstrates the different presentations and the diagnostic difficulties posed by atypical manifestations of TB. It also points out the value of maintaining a high degree of suspicion in endemic areas, even in the absence of microbiological evidence.

CONCLUSION

The fact is that people are still dying of clinically unrecognized TB both in developed and in developing countries. Possible reasons may be that in developed countries physicians often do not suspect TB since it is rare disease and in developing countries failures are most often due to lack of advanced diagnostic technologies. By increasing awareness of healthcare workers and doctors, unrecognized TB mortality can be significantly reduced. This is especially important since clinically unrecognized TB has negative consequences on both, sick individual and society and epidemiological situation in the region.[8,16,31]

REFERENCES

1. World Health Organization. (2010). Global tuberculosis control: WHO report 2010. [online] Available from www.who.int/tb/publications/global_report/2010/en/index.html. [Accessed January, 2016].
2. Katz I, Rosenthal T, Michaeli D. Undiagnosed tuberculosis in hospitalized patients. Chest. 1985;87:770-4.
3. Savić S, Savić B, Škodrić V. Undiagnosed tuberculosis as clinical, epidemiological and medicolegal problem: report of two cases. Srp Arh Celok Lek. 2006;134(11-12):541-5.
4. Rieder HL, Kelly GD, Bloch AB, Cauthen GM, Snider DE Jr. Tuberculosis diagnosed at death in the United States. Chest. 1991;100:678-81.
5. DeRiemer K, Rudoy I, Schecter GF, Hopewell PC, Daley CL. The epidemiology of tuberculosis diagnosed after death in San Francisco, 1986-1995. Int J Tuberc Lung Dis. 1999;3:488-93.
6. Čolović R, Grubor N, Jesic R, et al. Tuberculous lymphadenitis as a case of obstructive jaundice: a case report and literature review. World J Gastroenterol. 2008;14:3098-100.
7. Ashba JK, Boyce JM. Undiagnosed tuberculosis in a general hospital. Chest. 1972;61:447-51.
8. Ashkin D, Hollender ES, Narita M. "Won't get fooled again" (by tuberculosis). Chest. 1999;116:856-7.
9. Škodrić-Trifunović V. Risk factor for developing tuberculosis. Med Pregl. 2004;57(1):53-8.
10. Golub JE, Bur S, Cronin WA, et al. Patient and health care system delays in pulmonary tuberculosis diagnosis in a low-incidence state. Int J Tuberc Lung Dis. 2005;9:992-8.
11. Calder L, Gao W, Simmons G. Tuberculosis: reasons for diagnostic delay in Auckland. N Z Med J. 2000;113:483-5.
12. Škodrić-Trifunović V, Rašić T, Nagorni-Obradović L, Filipović S. Analysis of patients with tuberculosis and diabetes mellitus at the Institute of Pulmonary Diseases and Tuberculosis of the Clinical Center of Serbia (2000-2002). Med Pregl. 2004;57 Suppl 1:59-63.
13. Sharma SK, Mohan A, Sharma A, Mitra DK. Miliary tuberculosis: new insights into an old disease. Lancet Infect Dis. 2005;5(7):415-30.
14. Samardzić N, Jovanović D, Marković-Denić L, Roksandić-Milenković M, Popević S, Skodrić-Trifunović V. Clinical features of endobronchial tuberculosis. Vojnosanit Pregl. 2014;71(2):156-60.
15. Forssbohm M, Kropp R, Loytved G, et al. Death due to tuberculosis requiring treatment or an accompanying disease? A contribution to the lethality and mortality of tuberculosis in Germany. Pneumologie. 2011;65(10):607-14.
16. Field N, Murray J, Wong ML, et al. Missed opportunities in TB diagnosis: a TB process-based performance review tool to evaluate and improve clinical care. BMC Public Health. 2011;11:127.

17. Kantor HS, Poblete R, Pusateri SL. Nosocomial transmission of tuberculosis from unsuspected disease. Am J Med. 1988;84:833-8.
18. Bobrowitz ID. Active tuberculosis undiagnosed until autopsy. Am J Med. 1982;72:650-8.
19. Enarson DA, Grzybowski S, Dorken E. Failure of diagnosis as a factor in tuberculosis mortality. Can Med Assoc J. 1978;118:1520-2.
20. Edlin GP. Active tuberculosis unrecognized until necropsy. Lancet. 1978;1:650-2.
21. Mathur P, Sacks L, Auten G, Sall R, Levy C, Gordin F. Delayed diagnosis of pulmonary tuberculosis in city hospitals. Arch Intern Med. 1994;154:306-10.
22. Murray CJ, Wong ML. Processed-based performance review for the diagnosis of pulmonary tuberculosis. Mining Medical and Other Health Care Professionals Association of South Africa (MMOA); 2009. [online] Available from www.nioh.ac.za/?page=tb_tool&id=118. [Accessed January, 2016].
23. Rowinska-Zakrzewska E, Szopinski J, Remiszewski P, et al. Tuberculosis in the autopsy material: analysis of 1500 autopsies performed between 1972 and 1991 in the Institute of Tuberculosis and Chest Diseases, Warsaw, Poland. Tuber Lung Dis. 1995;76:349-54.
24. Lum D, Koelmeyer T. Tuberculosis in Auckland autopsies, revisited. N Z Med J. 2005;118:U1356.
25. Kircher T, Nelson J, Burdo H. The autopsy as a measure of accuracy of the death certificate. N Engl J Med. 1985;313:1263-9.
26. Linell F, Ostberg G. Tuberculosis in autopsy material, with special reference to cases not discovered until necropsy. Scand J Respir Dis. 1966;47:200-8.
27. Kramer F, Modilevsky T, Waliany AR, Leedom JM, Barnes PF. Delayed diagnosis of tuberculosis in patients with human immunodeficiency virus infection. Am J Med. 1990;89:451-6.
28. Pavić I, Radulović P, Bujas T, Perić Balja M, Ostojić J, Balicević D. Frequency of tuberculosis at autopsies in a large hospital in Zagreb, Croatia: a 10-year retrospective study. Croat Med J. 2012;53:48-52.
29. Flavin RJ, Gibbons N, O'Briain DS. Mycobacterium tuberculosis at autopsy—exposure and protection: an old adversary revisited. J Clin Pathol. 2007;60(5):487-91.
30. Chastonay P, Gardiol D. Extensive active tuberculosis at autopsy: retrospective study of a collection of adult autopsies (1961-1985). Schweiz Med Wochenschr. 1987;117(24):925-7.
31. Kattan JA, Sosa LE, Lobato MN. Tuberculosis mortality: death from a curable disease, Connecticut, 2007-2009. Int J Tuberc Lung Dis. 2012.

CHAPTER 11
Challenges in the Diagnosis and Treatment of MDR and XDR Tuberculosis

Müge Aydoğdu

INTRODUCTION

Tuberculosis (TB) is an infectious disease caused by the bacillus *Mycobacterium tuberculosis*. It typically affects the lungs (pulmonary TB) but can affect other sites as well (extrapulmonary TB). The disease spread in the air when sick people with pulmonary TB expel bacteria by coughing. Overall, a relatively small proportion (5-15%) of the estimated 2-3 billion people infected with *M. tuberculosis* will develop TB disease during their lifetime. However, the probability of developing TB is much higher among people infected with human immunodeficiency virus (HIV).[1,2]

Tuberculosis can usually be treated with a course of 6-month regimen of four standard, or first line, anti-TB drugs (isoniazid, rifampicin, ethambutol, and pyrazinamide/morphozinamide). If these drugs are misused or mismanaged, multidrug-resistant TB (MDR-TB), defined as resistance to isoniazid and rifampicin (the two most powerful anti-TB drugs), can develop. Multidrug-resistant TB takes longer to treat with second line drugs, which are more expensive and have more side effects. For most patients with MDR-TB, the current regimens recommended by the World Health Organization (WHO) last 20 months, and treatment success rates are much lower.[1-5]

Extensively drug-resistant TB (XDR-TB) can develop when these second line drugs are also misused or mismanaged, and therefore, also become ineffective. Because XDR-TB is resistant to first line and second line drugs, treatment options are seriously limited. It is therefore vital that TB control is managed properly.[1]

Antituberculosis drug resistance is a major public health problem that threatens progress made in TB care and control worldwide. Drug resistance arises due to improper use of antibiotics in chemotherapy of drug-susceptible TB patients. This improper use is a result of a number of actions including administration of improper treatment regimens and failure to ensure that patients complete the whole course of treatment. Essentially, drug resistance arises in areas with weak TB control programs. A patient who develops active disease with a drug-resistant TB strain can transmit this form of TB to other individuals.[1-5]

EPIDEMIOLOGY

Globally, 5% of TB cases were estimated to have had MDR-TB in 2014. Drug resistance surveillance data showed that an estimated 480,000 people developed MDR-TB in 2014 and 190,000 people died as a result of MDR-TB. Extensively drug-resistant TB has been reported by 105 countries in 2014. On average, an estimated 9.7% of people with MDR-TB have XDR-TB. If all notified TB patients (6.3 million) had been tested for drug resistance in 2014, an estimated 300,000 cases of MDR-TB would have been detected. In 2014, 123,000 patients with MDR-TB or rifampicin-resistant TB (RR-TB) were notified, of whom about 75% lived in the European region, India, South Africa, or China.[1]

Only 50% of the MDR-TB patients in the 2012 cohort of detected cases were successfully treated. Around 16% died, 24% did not have their treatment outcome documented or interrupted treatment, and in 10% the treatment failed. Only 26% of XDR-TB patients in the 2012 cohort had a successful outcome of treatment.[1]

DEFINITIONS

Resistance to anti-TB drugs is identified through laboratory tests. Both phenotypic methods that involve culturing of *M. tuberculosis* in the presence of anti-TB drugs and genotypic methods that identify specific mutations in the genome of the bacteria associated with resistance against individual drugs can be used. Tuberculosis drug resistance types are classified in table 1.[1,3-5] Recently, WHO revised the MDR/XDR-TB treatment outcome definitions (Table 2).[6]

TABLE 1	Definitions of tuberculosis drug resistance patterns
Drug resistance type	**Definition**
Monoresistance	Resistance to one first line anti-TB drug only
Polyresistance	Resistance to more than one first line anti-TB drug, other than both isoniazid and rifampicin
MDR	Resistance to at least both isoniazid and rifampicin
XDR	Resistance to isoniazid and rifampicin (i.e., MDR), any fluoroquinolone, and at least one of the three second line injectable drugs (capreomycin, kanamycin, and amikacin)
Rifampicin resistance	Resistance to rifampicin detected using phenotypic or genotypic methods, with or without resistance to other anti-TB drugs. It includes any resistance to rifampicin, in the form of monoresistance, polyresistance, MDR, or XDR

MDR, multidrug resistance; XDR, Extensive drug resistance; TB, tuberculosis.

TABLE 2	Treatment outcome categories and definitions for multidrug-resistant/extensively drug-resistant tuberculosis patients[6]
Treatment outcome category	**Definition**
Cured	Treatment completed as recommended by the national policy without evidence of failure and three or more consecutive cultures taken ≥ 30 days apart are negative after the intensive phase*
Treatment completed	Treatment completed as recommended by the national policy without evidence of failure, but no record that three or more consecutive cultures taken ≥ 30 days apart are negative after the intensive phase*
Treatment failed	Treatment terminated or need for permanent regimen change of at least two anti-TB drugs because of lack of conversion† by the end of the intensive phase or bacteriological reversion†† in the continuation phase after conversion to negative or evidence of additional acquires resistance to fluoroquinolones or second line injectable drugs or adverse drug reactions

Continued

Continued

TABLE 2	Treatment outcome categories and definitions for multidrug-resistant/extensively drug-resistant tuberculosis patients[6]
Treatment outcome category	**Definition**
Died	A person who dies for any reason during the course of treatment
Lost to follow-up	A patient whose treatment was interrupted for two consecutive months or more
Not evaluated	A patient for whom no treatment outcome is assigned (this includes cases "transferred out" to another treatment unit and whose treatment outcome is unknown)

*For regimens without a clear distinction between "intensive" and "continuation" phases, a cutoff 8 months after the start of treatment is suggested to determine when the criteria for "cured", "treatment completed" and "treatment failed" start to apply.

†Conversion (to negative); culture is considered to have converted to negative when two consecutive cultures, taken ≥ 30 days apart are found to be negative. In such cases, the specimen collection date of the first negative culture is used as the date of conversion.

††Reversion (to positive); culture is considered to have reverted to positive when, after an initial conversion, two consecutive cultures, taken ≥ 30 days apart, are found to be positive. For the purpose of defining "treatment failed" reversion is only considered when it occurs in the continuation phase.

CAUSES AND RISK FACTORS OF DRUG RESISTANT TUBERCULOSIS

There are two principal pathways leading to the development of active drug-resistant TB:[3]
1. Acquired (secondary) drug resistance: Acquired drug resistance is the result of inadequate, incomplete, or poor treatment quality that allows the selection of mutant resistant strains. If drug-susceptible TB is treated with a regimen exclusively based on a single effective TB medicine, there is a risk that bacteria with drug-resistant mutations will be selected and multiply further during the course of treatment, eventually becoming the dominant strain. If a person infected with a strain, initially resistant to a specific medicine is treated with that medicine plus a new additional medicine, then there is a risk of developing resistance to the additional medicine. Stepwise additions of drugs may eventually lead to more severe patterns of drug resistance and eventually to untreatable forms of TB[3]
2. Initial (primary) drug resistance: Primary or initial drug resistance means that a person has been infected with a drug-resistant TB strain. Transmission of drug-resistant TB occurs exactly in the same way as transmission of drug susceptible TB. High prevalence of drug-resistant TB in the community increases the risk of drug-resistant TB exposure in the community.[3]

Among the risk factors for MDR/XDR-TB, the most important one is prior TB treatment for greater than 1 month. This could particularly be the case if the treatment was inappropriate for the drug susceptibility of the strain. Other prominent risk factors include close contact to a patient with MDR-TB, migration, HIV infection, and young age. Environments favorable for TB transmission (such as crowding, poor ventilation, and poor infection control practices in health facilities), also contribute to transmission of drug-resistant TB. Patients with failure of retreatment regimens with first line anti-TB drugs (HRZES) have increased rates of MDR-TB, approaching to 90%. Besides patients who are on first line anti-TB treatment (HRZE) but still sputum smear-positive at month two or three of the treatment, and patients with relapse and return from loss to follow-up have increased risk of MDR-TB.[3]

All patients diagnosed with MDR-TB should preferably be tested also for XDR-TB. The two strongest risk factors for XDR-TB are:[3,7]

1. Failure of an MDR-TB treatment regimen, which contains second line drugs including an injectable agent and a fluoroquinolone
2. Close contact with an individual with documented XDR-TB or with an individual for whom treatment with a regimen including second line drugs is failing or has failed.

Similar to drug-susceptible TB, drug-resistant TB only progresses to active disease in a minority of those infected, and drug-resistant TB infection can remain latent for long periods of time. A poorly functioning immune system increases the risk of progression, and therefore, factors that can impair the immune system (e.g., HIV, under nutrition, diabetes, silicosis, smoking, alcohol abuse, a wide range of systemic diseases, and treatments with immunosuppressant) are also risk factors for developing drug-resistant TB disease.[3]

The WHO recommends five priority actions to address the global MDR-TB crisis and to prevent the development of drug resistant TB:[3,7]

1. Prevent the development of drug resistance through high quality treatment of drug susceptible TB—prevent development of MDR-TB as a first priority
2. Expand rapid testing and detection of drug-resistant TB cases
3. Provide immediate access to effective treatment and proper care
4. Prevent transmission through infection control—implement appropriate TB infection control measures and quickly enroll diagnosed patients on effective treatment to minimize the risk of disease transmission
5. Increase political commitment with financing—strengthen and sustain the MDR-TB response through high level political commitment, strong leadership across multiple governmental sectors, ever-broadening partnerships, and adequate financing for care and research.

DIAGNOSIS OF MULTIDRUG-RESISTANT/ EXTENSIVELY DRUG-RESISTANT TUBERCULOSIS[3,8-10]

Bacteriological examinations in patients with drug-resistant TB include sputum smear microscopy, culture and drug susceptibility testing (DST) as well as molecular techniques such as Xpert MTB/RIF and line-probe assay (LPA). Unfortunately, less than 25% of the estimated cases of MDR-TB are detected due to insufficient drug resistance testing. Microscopy and culture are still the basis of TB diagnostics.[3]

For a patient to be considered bacteriologically confirmed at the start of second-line treatment, the following criteria must be met:[3]

- At least one pretreatment specimen was positive on sputum smear microscopy, Xpert MTB/RIF or culture
- The collection date of the sample on which the laboratory examination was performed was less than 30 days before or 7 days after the initiation of second line treatment.

Examinations are required at the start of treatment to confirm the diagnosis of TB, and to determine the infectiousness of the patient. Patients with positive sputum smear are the most infectious. Both smear and culture should be used to monitor patients throughout the therapy. At least one sputum sample should always be cultured at the time of start of second line TB treatment. The monitoring of sputum culture is important for decisions on changes in treatment.[3]

Definitive diagnosis of drug-resistant TB requires that *M. tuberculosis* bacteria be detected and resistance to anti-TB drugs determined. This can be done by isolating the bacteria by culture, identifying it as belonging to the *M. tuberculosis* complex (MTBC), and conducting DST using solid or liquid media or by performing a WHO endorsed molecular test to detect TB DNA and mutations associated with resistance.[3]

Early detection of drug resistance allows the use of appropriate treatment regimens for patients, which has an important impact on improved TB control. The development of rapid methods for DST is crucial due to increasing rates of MDR-TB worldwide and the emergence of XDR-TB, with very high reported HIV-associated mortality. Spread of drug-resistant TB strains and the management of patients diagnosed with drug-resistant disease are among the most challenging difficulties faced by national TB control programs. This is compounded by a critical lack of appropriate diagnostic tools and vastly inadequate laboratory capacity.[3,8-10]

Conventional culture and DST methods require prolonged lengths of time to confirm mycobacterial growth and detect drug resistance, during which patients may be inappropriately treated, drug-resistant strains may continue to spread, and amplification of resistance may occur. Early and rapid diagnosis of TB and drug resistance will therefore have obvious benefits for patient and public health, including better prognosis, increased survival, prevention of acquisition of further drug resistance, and reduced spread of drug-resistant strains to vulnerable populations.

General Definitions for Drug Susceptibility Testing[3]

The following are definitions of the laboratory aspects:
- Phenotypic DST (conventional DST): Phenotypic testing determines if an isolate is resistant to an anti-TB drug by evaluating growth (or metabolic activity) in the presence of the drug
- Genotypic DST (molecular DST): Genotypic testing detects mutations in the TB genome associated with specific drug resistance. Note: Genotypic testing is also used to identify *M. tuberculosis* by detecting the presence of TB-specific mycobacterial DNA
- Direct testing: Direct testing refers to testing directly from a clinical sample (most commonly a sputum specimen). In direct DST, processed clinical samples are directly inoculated onto media with and without drugs, or processed for molecular testing
- Indirect testing: An indirect test requires the growth of a pure culture from the specimen; dilutions of the isolate are then inoculated into drug-containing and drug-free media. Indirect phenotypic tests have been extensively validated and are currently regarded as the reference standard. The most commonly used methods for solid media are the proportion, absolute concentration, and resistance ratio methods; and for liquid culture systems, the proportion method. Good concordance is seen between these methods for DST against first line anti-TB drugs. Several noncommercial culture and DST methods have been developed that are aimed for use in laboratories with limited resources as an interim solution pending capacity development for genotypic DST. Among these methods, microscopic observation of drug susceptibility, colorimetric redox indicator methods, and the nitrate reductase assays have shown to be inexpensive methods. These noncommercial methods have similar biosafety precautions to conventional culture and DST, and are therefore, only suitable for use at the central or regional level laboratories
- Critical drug concentration: This is the lowest concentration of a drug that inhibits growth of 95% of *M. tuberculosis* strains isolated from patients who have never been

treated with/exposed to that drug (i.e., presumably susceptible isolates), while at the same time not inhibiting growth of strains isolated from patients nonresponsive to therapy with that drug (i.e., presumably resistant to that drug). For some drugs, such as ethambutol, there is no optimal drug concentration that meets this definition. For such drugs, the concentration that shows the greatest difference between presumably susceptible and presumably resistant isolates is used in phenotypic DST. Typically, isolates of *M. tuberculosis* are tested against only the critical concentration of a drug.

Methods for Tuberculosis Diagnosis and Drug Susceptibility Testing[3,8-10]

- Microscopy: Smear microscopy is a low-cost and frontline tool for TB (but not drug-resistant TB) diagnosis. The introduction of light emitting diode fluorescence microscopy is recommended by the WHO and has increased test sensitivity without increasing overall costs; rather, it has reduced the turnaround time required allowing the screening of a larger number of slides at the peripheral level. The main purposes of microscopy for drug-resistant TB are to assess initial bacterial load, specimen triage to different diagnostic algorithms, monitor response to therapy, and to confirm the presence of acid-fast bacilli (AFB) rather than contaminants in the culture media, before proceeding to rapid identification tests. Microscopy for AFB cannot distinguish viable from nonviable organisms nor differentiate between drug-susceptible and drug-resistant *M. tuberculosis* bacteria, or between different species of mycobacteria. Its usefulness in drug-resistant TB treatment monitoring is therefore limited. Samples showing AFB by smear microscopy but negative to culture suggest that bacilli are not viable (caution is nonetheless warranted for these patients to be considered as possibly infectious); while samples showing AFB by smear microscopy but negative by molecular tests are likely to harbor nontuberculous mycobacteria (NTM)
- Culture of *M. tuberculosis*: Culture in liquid media is the current reference method for bacteriological confirmation of TB. However, good quality specimens, prompt transport to the laboratory, and quality of laboratory processing (appropriate digestion and decontamination, as well as good quality culture media and incubation conditions) are essential to optimize the yield of culture. Laboratory errors, such as mislabeling or cross-contamination between specimens during aerosol-producing procedures, may lead to false-negative or false-positive results. Therefore, laboratory findings should be always correlated with the patient's clinical condition and any diagnostic test should be repeated if necessary. In general, the recovery of tubercle bacilli is higher and the time to detection is shorter with liquid culture than with solid culture methods. However, liquid culture media being a more sensitive culture system has higher contamination rates than solid media. Nontuberculous mycobacteria are more frequently isolated with liquid media than with solid media. It is therefore essential to differentiate *M. tuberculosis* isolates from other mycobacteria
- Molecular testing:
  - Xpert MTB/RIF: In 2010, the WHO endorsed Xpert®MTB/RIF (Cephaid, Sunnyvale, USA), a PCR-based diagnostic tool. This tool detects both MTBC DNA and rifampicin resistance-associated mutations. The cartridge-based test has a turnaround time of approximately 2 hours and does not require a biosafety-level laboratory. The WHO recommends the use of the test as the initial diagnostic test rather than microscopy, culture, and DST in patients who are HIV-positive and in cases when resistance is suspected. It is also recommended in smear-negative cases in which suspicion of TB remains; but not recommended for

treatment monitoring. The simplicity of the test enables its use outside reference laboratories, improving patient access to TB diagnostics, and rapid DST. In a recent Cochrane meta-analysis, the test had a sensitivity of 88% and a specificity of 93% for diagnosing TB when used as an initial test, replacing microscopy. As an add-on test in cases with negative smear microscopy, the test yielded 67% sensitivity and 98% specificity. Rifampicin resistance was detected with 94% sensitivity and 98% specificity.[11] The major advantage of this test for TB control is the time required, less than 1 day, to detect *M. tuberculosis* and rifampicin resistance. By contrast, in the first multicenter implementation study, it took a median 20 days using LPAs (a DNA strip test that enables simultaneous molecular identification of TB and the most common genetic mutations causing resistance to rifampicin and isoniazid) and a median of 106 days using conventional DST to detect resistance.[12] In low-incidence countries, the positive predictive value of Xpert MTB/RIF is low, and therefore, the false-positive rate is higher. Thus, a confirmatory culture-based DST is always required.[13] Although Xpert MTB/RIF and LPAs are important steps, their accuracy, affordability, and simplicity still do not meet the criteria for a real point of care test. One key criterion for such a test is that it is able to deliver results during a single healthcare contact, i.e., within 3 hours. Providing accurate diagnosis and initiating treatment at the same health consultation would reduce the number of patients lost to follow-up. The desperate need for such a test, including resistance testing, is stressed by the fact that less than 25% of the estimated MDR-TB cases are currently detected

- o Line-probe assays: Molecular LPAs allow rapid detection of resistance to rifampicin (alone or in combination with isoniazid) and were endorsed by the WHO in 2008, with detailed policy guidance on their introduction at country level. With LPA technology, twelve specimens can be processed simultaneously and several batches of tests can be done per day. Hain Genotype® MTBDRplus (Hain, Nehren, Germany), a WHO endorsed test, can, in its latest version, detect resistance to rifampicin and isoniazid in both smear-positive and smear-negative (culture-positive) samples with high accuracy. An early evaluation study on smear-negative samples indicated 90.7% sensitivity and 96% specificity for rifampicin resistance and 93.5% sensitivity and 82.3% specificity for isoniazid resistance.[14] The use of the assay is technically more demanding and has a longer turnaround time compared with Xpert MTB/RIF, but it is a good alternative test for isoniazid and rifampicin resistance in reference laboratories. Line-probe assay provide the only currently available molecular routine test to detect resistance to fluoroquinolones, injectable drugs, and ethambutol (Genotype® MTBDRsl). This test has predominantly been evaluated in culture specimens. A new version of the test to be used directly with sputum samples is currently under evaluation. The test can currently only be recommended as a "rule-in" test for resistance to fluoroquinolones and injectables. A positive result should be confirmed by phenotypic DST. However, the test is not endorsed by the WHO and the results should be interpreted with caution
- Others: Other new diagnostic tests have become available but do not serve the goals outlined above. A urine dipstick test ((Determine® TB-LAM; Alere, Waltham, MA, USA)) checking for lipoarabinomannan (LAM) antigen to detect *M. tuberculosis*, only works well in patients with CD4 count below 50 cells/µL (with 66.7% sensitivity and >98% specificity).[15]

A summary of TB diagnostic methods and DST methods and turnaround times are provided in table 3.[3]

TABLE 3 Diagnostic methods and drug susceptibility test methods and turnaround times for multidrug-resistant tuberculosis and extensively drug-resistant tuberculosis[3]

Diagnostic method	Test name	Turnaround time	Description and comments
Smear microscopy	Conventional light microscopy—Ziehl-Neelsen	• 2 h	• Less sensitive than fluorescent/LED microscopy
	Conventional fluorescent microscopy	—	• Requires a quartz halogen or high pressure mercury vapor lamp • Sensitivity improved over light microscopy, observation time reduced • Expensive
	Light emitting diode (LED) fluorescence microscopy	—	• Improve sensitivity by 10% over conventional light microscopy • Observation time similar to conventional fluorescence microscopy • LED conversion kits for light microscopes are available
Solid culture	Löwenstein–Jensen	• 3 weeks smear positive • 4–8 weeks smear negative	• Egg-based medium, inexpensive
	Middlebrook and Cohn 7H10		• Agar-based medium. Less prone to contamination than Löwenstein–Jensen but more expensive
Automated liquid culture		• 8 days smear positive • 2–6 weeks smear negative	• Liquid culture systems • Fully automated systems that use either fluorimetric or colorimetric detection

Continued

Challenges in the Diagnosis and Treatment of MDR and XDR Tuberculosis

Continued

TABLE 3 Diagnostic methods and drug susceptibility test methods and turnaround times for multidrug-resistant tuberculosis and extensively drug-resistant tuberculosis[3]

Diagnostic method	Test name	Turnaround time	Description and comments
Noncommercial WHO endorsed culture and DST techniques	Media-based microscopic observation drug susceptibility (MODS)	• 2–21 days direct • 3–4 weeks indirect	• MODS is a manual liquid technique that uses basic laboratory equipment (including an inverted microscope) • Colonies are observed through the bottom of a sealed plastic container • Allows for H and R DST. MODS requires additional staff skills and a containment laboratory
	Nitrate reductase assay	• 6–9 days direct • 7–11 weeks indirect	• A colorimetric test using solid media • Allows for H and R DST • TB cells are cultured for 10 days and Griess reagent is added, which indicates the presence of growing cells
	Colorimetric redox indicator	• 3–5 weeks	• An indirect colorimetric test using liquid media. TB cells are cultured in the presence of a dye. Allows for H and R DST
Molecular testing	Line-probe assay (LPA)	• 1–2 days (direct on smear-positive specimen only)	• Two LPAs have been developed to detect M. tuberculosis resistant to R and H either directly or indirectly. Deoxyribonucleic acid targets are amplified by polymerase chain reaction (PCR) and hybridized to immobilized oligonucleotide targets. Results are visualized colorimetrically • If it is a smear-negative specimen, culture must be grown first
	Xpert MTB/RIF	• 2 h	• A fully automated test working in a dedicated platform performing detection of MTB and R resistance, using real-time PCR. Results are available in less than 2 h

DST, drug susceptibility testing; H, isoniazid; R, rifampicin.

Limitations of Drug Susceptibility Testing[3,8-10]

Molecular methods do not have perfect concordance with phenotypic culture-based DST methods and patient details such as treatment history and risk factors for drug-resistant TB should always be taken into account when interpreting laboratory results. All patients identified by molecular methods should be initiated on an appropriate WHO-recommended treatment regimen as soon as possible. Prompt treatment initiation will have a positive effect on patient outcomes, while the treatment regimen can be refined when additional testing results become available.

The reliability of DST (performed under optimal circumstances) varies with the drug tested:

- First line DST:
  - Most reliable for rifampicin and isoniazid
  - For rifampicin resistance, there is no complete concordance between phenotypic and genotypic detection methods. Emerging evidence suggests that DNA sequencing of the *rpoB* gene (the gold standard method for genotypic DST) may be a better although not perfect reference method than the phenotypic DST. The WHO continues to collect and evaluate emerging data on this issue and will formally review the accuracy of phenotypic resistance standards for DST once sufficient data becomes available. Given the resultant high sensitivity of molecular methods, a negative result generally excludes rifampicin resistance and no further testing to confirm negative results is required. In rare instances, when a patient is strongly presumed to have RR-TB even after a negative molecular test, follow-up testing using phenotypic culture-based DST may be used to test for rifampicin resistance resulting from a small number of mutations occurring outside the *rpoB* region
  - Less reliable and reproducible for streptomycin, ethambutol, and pyrazinamide (pyrazinamide testing can only be performed on liquid media after appropriate pH adjustment)
- Second line DST:
  - Has good reliability and reproducibility for second line injectable drugs (amikacin, kanamycin, capreomycin) and fluoroquinolones. According to current WHO policy guidance, routine DST for second line drugs should not be performed unless the required laboratory quality and biosafety standards are met, infrastructure and capacity have been established, rigorous quality assurance is in place, and sustainable high proficiency has been demonstrated for isoniazid and rifampicin testing. In order to retain proficiency and expertise, it is recommended that second line DST only be performed if at least 200 specimens are tested per year
  - At present, routine DST for group 4 drugs [ethionamide, prothionamide, cycloserine, terizidone, para-aminosalicylic acid (PAS)] and for group 5 drugs (bedaquiline, delamanid clofazimine, amoxicillin/clavulanate, clarithromycin, linezolid, imipenem, meropenem, thioacetazone) is not recommended as accuracy and reproducibility of laboratory testing cannot be guaranteed.

Presumptive Multidrug-resistant Tuberculosis when Rapid Genotypic Drug Susceptibility Testing is not Available[3]

When rapid DST is not available, there are selected groups of patients where the risk of MDR-TB is so high that a presumptive diagnosis of MDR-TB would apply and patients can

be directly enrolled on empiric MDR regimens. The MDR-TB regimen should be adjusted when conventional phenotypic DST results become available. The groups eligible for the presumptive diagnosis of MDR-TB and direct enrolment into an MDR regimen include:
- Failures of retreatment regimens with first line drugs: Patients in whom retreatment with first line drugs has failed in national TB control programs often have MDR-TB. If the quality of the drugs in the TB control program is uncertain or if the quality of directly observed therapy (DOT) is poor or unknown (i.e., if regular ingestion of medicines is uncertain), retreatment regimens may fail for reasons other than drug resistance
- Close contacts of drug-resistant TB cases that develop active TB disease. These patients can be enrolled for treatment with MDR regimens, pending DST results
- Failures of new regimens with first line anti-TB drugs in some settings. Since the prevalence of drug-resistant TB in this group of patients may vary greatly, the drug resistant TB rate in this group must be documented through appropriate testing and analysis before deciding whether empiric treatment for MDR-TB is justified and to determine which drugs should be included in empiric treatment.

TREATMENT OF MULTIDRUG-RESISTANT/ EXTENSIVELY DRUG-RESISTANT TUBERCULOSIS CASES

Definitions of Terms Used to Describe Treatment Strategies[3]

The following are definitions of terms often used to describe treatment strategies:
- Standardized treatment: Drug susceptibility data from representative patient populations are used as the basis for regimen design in the absence of individual DST. All patients in a defined group or category receive the same regimen. Suspected MDR-TB should be confirmed by DST whenever possible
- Individualized treatment: Each regimen is designed based on the patient's past history of TB treatment and individual DST results.

Tuberculosis programs often use a combination of standardized and individualized approaches. However, in situations where DST is unavailable or limited to only one or two first line drugs, programs will most commonly use a purely standardized approach.

The WHO-recommended grouping of anti-TB drugs has been shown in table 4.

TABLE 4	The World Health Organization-recommended grouping of antituberculosis drugs	
Group name	*Antituberculosis agent*	*Abbreviation*
Group 1: First line oral agents	• Isoniazid • Rifampicin • Ethambutol • Pyrazinamide • Rifabutine • Rifapentine	• H • R • E • Z • Rfb • Rpt
Group 2: Injectable anti-TB drugs	• Streptomycin • Kanamaycin • Amikacin • Capreomycin	• S • Km • Am • Cm

Continued

Continued

TABLE 4	The World Health Organization-recommended grouping of antituberculosis drugs	
Group name	**Antituberculosis agent**	**Abbreviation**
Group 3: Fluoroquinolones	• Levofloxacin • Moxifloxacin • Gatifloxacin	• Lfx • Mfx • Gfx
Group 4: Oral bacteriostatic second line anti-TB drugs	• Ethionamide • Prothionamide • Cycloserine • Terizidone • Paraaminosalicylic acid • Paraaminosalicylate sodium	• Eto • Pto • Cs • Trd • PAS • PAS-Na
Group 5: Anti-TB drugs with limited data on efficacy and/or long-term safety in the treatment of drug resistant TB (new anti-TB agents)	• Bedaquiline • Delamanid • Linezolid • Clofazimine • Amoxicillin/clavulanate • Imipenem/cilastatin • Meropenem • High dose isoniazid • Thiacetazone • Clarithromycin	• Bdq • Dlm • Lzd • Cfz • Amx/Clv • Ipm/Cln • Mpm • High dose H • T • Clr

TB, tuberculosis.

Designing and Administrating an Multidrug-resistant Tuberculosis Regimen

Early MDR-TB detection and the prompt initiation of an effective treatment are important factors in obtaining successful outcomes. The following are the basic principles involved in the treatment of MDR-TB (recommendations from the 2011 update of *Guidelines for the programmatic management of drug-resistant tuberculosis*):[16]

- The intensive phase of MDR-TB treatment should consist of at least four second line anti-TB drugs that are likely to be effective (including an injectable anti-TB drug), as well as pyrazinamide (conditional recommendation, very low quality evidence). Where there is unclear evidence about the effectiveness of a certain drug, this drug can still be part of the regimen; however, it should not be depended upon for success
- Multidrug-resistant regimens should include at least pyrazinamide, a fluoroquinolone, an injectable anti-TB drug, ethionamide (or prothionamide), and either cycloserine or PAS if cycloserine cannot be used (conditional recommendation, very low quality evidence)
- The drugs in the regimen should be judged to be "likely to be effective". An anti-TB drug is considered as such when:
  ○ The drug has not been used in a regimen that failed to cure the individual patent
  ○ Drug susceptibility testing performed indicates that it is susceptible to the drug (DST for isoniazid, rifampicin, groups 2 and 3 drugs is considered reliable; DST for all other drugs is considered not reliable enough for individual patient management)

- No known resistance to drugs with high cross-resistance
- No known close contacts with resistance to the drug
- Drug resistance surveys demonstrate that resistance to the drug is rare in patients with similar TB history

Note: It is not always possible that information of all five criteria can be ascertained. Therefore, clinical judgment is often necessary on whether to count a drug as "likely to be effective".

- There are conditions when more than five drugs are used. These conditions would be applicable when the effectiveness for a drug(s) is unlikely or questionable. One such relatively common condition is the treatment of XDR-TB
- Drugs that the patient is known to have a strong contraindication of usage due to drug-drug interactions, overlying toxicities, comorbidities, history of severe allergy or other adverse reactions, and/or pregnancy should not be used
- A fluoroquinolone should be used (strong recommendation, very low quality evidence). A later generation fluoroquinolone rather than an earlier generation fluoroquinolone should be used (conditional recommendation, very low quality evidence)
- In the treatment of patients with MDR-TB, ethionamide (or prothionamide) should be used (strong recommendation, very low quality evidence). This recommendation assumes the recommended drugs meet the criteria of "likely to be effective" and there are no contraindications to its use (such as severe adverse effects)
- The intensive phase (i.e., the initial part of treatment during which a group 2 injectable agent is used) lasts at least 8 months in total, but the duration can be modified according to the patient's response to treatment. The optimal duration of intensive phase following culture conversion, which is associated with treatment success, could not be inferred directly from the analysis used to revise the WHO programmatic management of drug-resistant TB guidelines in 2011. Some clinical experts may prefer that the intensive phase is continued for at least 4 months after culture conversion
- The total length of treatment is expected to be at least 20 months in most patients not previously treated for MDR-TB. Some clinical experts may prefer that total treatment be for at least 12 months past the point at which culture converts to negative, some others may prefer not to give less than 20 months in total
- Each dose is given under a patient-centered DOT throughout the treatment. A treatment card is marked for each observed dose. Directly observed therapy can be performed either at facility-based or community-based levels, keeping in mind that social support is an essential component of care and treatment delivery
- Any adverse effects of drugs should be managed immediately and adequately to relieve suffering, minimize the risk of treatment interruptions, and prevent morbidity and mortality due to serious adverse effects
- Antiretroviral therapy (ART) is recommended for all patients with HIV and drug-resistant TB, irrespective of CD4 cell count, as early as possible (within the first 8 weeks) following initiation of the anti-TB treatment (strong recommendation)
- The drug dosage is usually determined by age and weight
- Pyrazinamide, ethambutol, and fluoroquinolones should be given once a day. Depending on patient tolerance, once-a-day dosing is also used for oral second line anti-TB drugs from group 4; however, ethionamide/prothionamide, cycloserine, and PAS have traditionally been given in split doses during the day to reduce adverse effects
- All anti-TB drugs can be started at full dose. However, if tolerance is an issue, cycloserine, ethionamide, and PAS dosing can be increased gradually over a 2-week period[17]

- Injectable drugs can be given 5–7 days a week depending on the availability of a skilled medical person to give the intramuscular injections. Injectable anti-TB drugs should be given once daily, i.e., do not split the dose over the day. If adverse effects are problematic in a patient, the injectable agent may be given three times a week, preferably only after culture conversion[17]
- When possible, oral drugs are to be given 7 days a week under direct observation. Some programs suggest giving all drugs 6 days a week, but it is not known if this is equal to 7 days a week. Oral drugs should not be given 5 days a week (only the injectable agent is allowed to be on a 5 days a week schedule, see above)
- Pyrazinamide can be used for the entire treatment. Many drug-resistant TB patients have chronically inflamed lungs, which theoretically produce the acidic environment in which pyrazinamide is more effective. Alternatively, in patients doing well, pyrazinamide can be stopped with the injectable drug if the patient can continue with at least three likely effective drugs
- In MDR treatment strategies that initially enrol patients based on their strain being resistant to rifampicin alone, isoniazid may be included in the MDR regimen until DST to isoniazid can be done to determine if the isoniazid should be continued
- Patients with MDR-TB should be treated using mainly ambulatory care rather than models of care based principally on hospitalization (conditional recommendation, very low quality evidence).[16,18]

Table 5 describes the steps to build a regimen for drug-resistant TB treatment.[19]

TABLE 5	Steps to build a treatment regimen for drug-resistant tuberculosis	
Step 1	Choose an injectable (group 2): Choose a drug based on DST and treatment history. Streptomycin is generally not used because of high rates of resistance in patients with MDR-TB	• Kanamycin • Amikacin • Capreomycin
Step 2	Choose a higher generation fluoroquinolone (group 3): Use a later generation fluoroquinolone. If levofloxacin (or ofloxacin) resistance is documented, use moxifloxacin. Avoid moxifloxacin if possible when using bedaquiline or delamanid	• Levofloxacin • Moxifloxacin
Step 3	Add group 4 drugs: Add two or more group 4 drugs until there are at least four second line anti-TB drugs likely to be effective. Ethionamide/prothionamide is considered the most effective group 4 drugs. Consider treatment history, side effect profile, and cost. Drug susceptibility testing is not considered reliable for the drugs in this group	• Cycloserine/terizidone • Paraaminosalicylic acid (PAS) • Ethionamide/prothionamide
Step 4	Add group 1 drugs: Pyrazinamide is routinely added in most regimens; ethambutol can be added if the criteria for an effective drug are met. If isoniazid is unknown or pending, it can be added to the regimen until DST results become available	• Pyrazinamide • Ethambutol

Continued

Continued

TABLE 5	Steps to build a treatment regimen for drug-resistant tuberculosis	
Step 5	Add group 5 drugs: Consider adding group 5 drugs if four second line anti-TB drugs are not likely to be effective from groups 2–4. If drugs are needed from this group, it is recommended to add two or more. Drug susceptibility testing is not standardized for the drugs in this group. The drug-drug interactions betweem bedaquiline and delamanid have not been established and a recommendation about its combined use is not made in the WHO interim policy on these two drugs	• Bedaquiline • Delamanid • Linezolid • Clofazimine • Amoxicillin/clavulanate • Imipenem/cilastatin plus clavulanate • Meropenem plus clavulanate • High-dose isoniazid • Thiacetazone • Clarithromycin

Designing and Administrating an Extensively Drug-resistant Tuberculosis Regimen

There is very limited data on the different clinical approaches to XDR-TB and a recent review of treatment outcomes of XDR-TB patients could not find any associations between any specific drug or regimen and success; however, the analysis did indicate that success in XDR-TB patients was highest if at least six drugs were used in the intensive phase and four in the continuation phase.[20] A different meta-analysis provides empiric evidence that the use of later generation fluoroquinolones significantly improved treatment outcomes in patients with XDR-TB, even though DST demonstrated resistance to a representative fluoroquinolone.[21]

While data on efficacy and safety is limited, the incorporation of bedaquiline or delamanid into regimens designed to treat XDR-TB may be considered.[22,23] New anti-TB drugs are currently being developed and program managers should take care of WHO recommendations as they are released and updated though the website of the Task Force for New Drug Policy Development.[24] Box 1 summarizes the latest expert consensus on managing XDR-TB.[3]

Multidrug-resistant/Extensively Drug-resistant Tuberculosis in Patients Coinfected with Human Immunodeficiency Virus[5]

Extensively drug-resistant TB came to the attention of the world when extremely high mortality rates in patients coinfected with HIV were observed in South Africa.[25] All patients with MDR/XDR-TB need to be tested for HIV. If positive, ART should be started according to current guidelines.[16] Smear-negative TB is more common in patients who are HIV-positive.[26] Xpert MTB/RIF has a reasonable sensitivity in smear-negative cases.[11] To obtain a timely diagnosis of TB and rifampicin resistance, Xpert MTB/RIF is the recommended initial test for the diagnosis of TB in patients with HIV. Tuberculosis treatment should follow the guidelines for the management of MDR-TB. The WHO recommends starting ART within 8 weeks of starting MDR/XDR-TB treatment. Based on the evidence of drug-susceptible TB, it might be assumed that patients with advanced immunosuppression (CD4 count <50 cells/μL) should start ART within 2 weeks.[27-29]

> **BOX 1** — Treatment management for patients with documented or almost certain extensively drug-resistant tuberculosis
>
> - Use pyrazinamide and any other group 1 agent that may be effective
> - Use an injectable agent to which the strain is susceptible and consider an extended duration of use (12 months or possibly the whole treatment)
> - Use a higher generation fluoroquinolone such as moxifloxacin or gatifloxacin
> - Use all group 4 agents that have not been used extensively in a previous regimen or any that are likely to be effective
> - Add two or more group 5 drugs (consider adding bedaquiline or delamanid)
> - Consider adding a new investigational drug elligible for use under the compassionate use scheme if policy of the WHO endorses its use for XDR-TB
> - Consider high dose isoniazid treatment if low level resistance or absence of the kat G gene is documented
> - Consider adjuvant surgery if there is localized disease
> - Ensure rigorous respiratory infection control measures at the site where the patient is being treated
> - Consider the option of treatment in a hospital if the clinical condition of the patient is poor or major comorbidities coexist, or a shelter if the social condition of the patient prevents proper home care
> - Manage HIV coinfection
> - Provide comprehensive monitoring and full social support to enable adherence to treatment
> - Ensure that all patients have full acess to palliative and end of life care services with a patient centered approach to relief the suffering of the disease and its treatment

Treatment in Extrapulmonary and Central Nervous System Drug-resistant Tuberculosis[3]

Extrapulmonary drug-resistant TB is treated with the same strategy and duration as pulmonary drug-resistant TB; except the central nervous system (CNS) involvement. If the patient has symptoms suggestive of CNS involvement and is infected with drug-resistant TB, then the regimen should use drugs, which have adequate penetration into the CNS. Isoniazid, pyrazinamide, prothionamide/ethionamide, and cycloserine, all have good penetration into the cerebrospinal fluid, whereas kanamycin, amikacin, and streptomycin do so only in the presence of meningeal inflammation. Additionally, the penetration of capreomycin is less studied and not well determined. Paraaminosalicylic acid and ethambutol have poor or no penetration. The fluoroquinolones have variable cerebrospinal fluid penetration, with better penetration of moxifloxacin based on animal studies. There is no data on CNS penetration of clofazimine or clarithromycin. Linezolid is believed to penetrate the CNS, and has been used in meningitis treatment.[30] Imipenem has good CNS penetration, but children with meningitis treated with imipenem, had high rates of seizures (meropenem is preferred for meningitis cases and children).[31,32] No data is available regarding CNS penetration of bedaquiline or delamanid.

Surgery in Treatment of Drug-resistant Tuberculosis[3]

The most common surgical procedure in patients with pulmonary drug-resistant TB is resection surgery (taking out part or all of a lung). Large case series analysis has proven resection surgery to be effective and safe under appropriate surgical conditions.[33] It is considered an adjunct to chemotherapy and appears to be beneficial for patients when skilled thoracic surgeons and excellent postoperative care are available.[34] It is not indicated in patients with extensive bilateral disease. The case series that showed surgery to be effective may have a selection bias, as very sick patients with comorbidities, older patients, and those with extensive disease are often excluded from surgery.

The timing of surgery may be earlier in the course of the disease when the patient's risk of morbidity and mortality are lower, for example, when the disease is still localized to one lung or one lung lobe. Generally, at least 2 months of therapy should be given prior to resection surgery to decrease the bacterial infection in the surrounding lung tissue. Even with successful resection, the intensive phase and total treatment duration should also be given.

CHALLENGES IN TREATMENT OF MULTIDRUG-RESISTANT/EXTENSIVELY DRUG-RESISTANT TUBERCULOSIS CASES

Some points which are usully being discussed and need to be clarified in the treatment of MDR/XDR-TB are as follows:

- Some programs or clinicians may choose to use a shorter (e.g., 9–12 months) MDR-TB treatment regimen consisting of combinations of later generation fluoroquinolones (moxifloxacin or gatifloxacin), clofazimine, ethambutol, and pyrazinamide throughout the treatment period supplemented by prothionamide, kanamycin, and high dose isoniazid during an intensive phase. The evidence for these shorter regimens comes from limited observational studies. By May 2014, only one study of a patient series in Bangladesh using a short regimen had been published in a peer-reviewed journal.[35] An ongoing randomized clinical trial is evaluating the efficacy and safety of a shorter regimen to treat MDR-TB treatment and results should be available around 2017.[36] The combined off-label use of clofazimine and other drugs that prolong the QTc interval on the electrocardiography (ECG) (i.e., fluoroquinolones) in these regimens require active pharmacovigilance to enable proper surveillance management of safety issues. Those who choose to use shorter regimens should be aware that these regimens have not been evaluated in the treatment of XDR-TB, and are likely to acquire additional resistance in patients already harboring bacilli resistant to second line drugs. The longer treatment regimens for MDR-TB represent the standard of care that has been used more widely and for much longer;[37] they also have shown to bear good outcomes in a number of countries and the adverse drug reactions associated with them have been well documented[38]
- Increasing resistance to second line drugs poses additional challenges to diagnostics and treatment of drug-resistant TB. The Preserving Effective TB Treatment Study demonstrated resistance to at least one second line drug in 43.7% of 1,278 patients with MDR-TB from seven countries. Of these patients, 20.0% were resistant to at least one second line injectable drug and 12.9% to at least one fluoroquinolone.[39] Unpublished data from the author confirmed this trend in Europe. Given that resistance to these key drugs reduces further treatment success, such developments are relevant and worrying for the future management of drug-resistant TB[20]
- Rifampicin was licensed in 1964, but from then until December 2012, no new anti-TB drugs were registered worldwide. Then, bedaquiline, a diarylquinoline, was

approved under conditional licensing by the US Food and Drug Administration. The European Medicines Agency gave a conditional licensing recommendation for delamanid, a nitroimidazole, in November 2013, and to bedaquiline in December 2013. Even though both drugs received only conditional licensing, these are landmark events in the history of anti-TB drug development. Although licensing was based on phase IIb studies,[39-41] a phase III trial with delamanid is under way (clinical trials identifier: NCT01424670) and has completed recruitment, whereas a phase III trial with bedaquiline is pending (clinical trials identifier: NCT01600963). If adjustment is required in a drug-resistant TB regimen, at least two drugs should be changed simultaneously to avoid the development of immediate resistance to a single new drug added to a failing regimen. Unfortunately, there are no clinical data on the use of delamanid and bedaquiline together, and neither bedaquiline nor delamanid have been used in trials together with moxifloxacin,[41,42] the potentially most potent fluoroquinolone in TB treatment. Furthermore, although both these new drugs were generally tolerated well, cardiac toxicity and QT-interval prolongation remain a problem. The optimal use of these new drugs in MDR-TB regimens remains unclear. The WHO issued interim guidance, based on a low level of evidence. Bedaquiline should be used in cases when a regimen with four active drugs, excluding pyrazinamide, cannot be designed. Alternatively, the drug can be used in patients who have MDR-TB and additional resistance to any fluoroquinolone. It was stressed that bedaquiline should not be used for longer than 6 months and regular ECG testing is essential to detect pathological QT-interval prolongation[23]

- The potential to use high dose later generation fluoroquinolones (i.e., moxifloxacin 800 mg and levofloxacin 1,000 mg), which are more bactericidal and would potentially contribute to shortened treatment, is currently under discussion. However, there is a lack of safety data for long-term treatment and particular concerns about cardiac toxicity[43]
- Several recent studies confirmed the antimycobacterial activity of linezolid, which is currently the preferred class 5 drug.[4] A clinical trial in South Korea showed its beneficial effects in patients failing XDR-TB treatment.[44] A meta-analysis showed 93% culture conversion using individualized regimens with linezolid. Of the patients, 58.9% experienced adverse events and 68.4% had major adverse events. Neuropathies and cytopenias were the most frequent complications.[45] The optimal dosing is not yet known, although there is agreement on a maximum daily dose of 600 mg[4]
- Surgical treatment of MDR-TB might be an option and should be considered in selected cases with limited lesions and poor potential for cure otherwise.[46] However, no randomized data are available for guidance on patient selection and optimal timing for surgery.

REFERENCES

1. World Health Organization. Global tuberculosis report 2015. 20th ed. Geneva: WHO; 2015.
2. Tiemersma EW, van der Werf MJ, Borgdorff MW, Williams BG, Nagelkerke NJ. Natural history of tuberculosis: duration and fatality of untreated pulmonary tuberculosis in HIV negative patients. A systematic review. PLoS One. 2011;6(4):e17601.
3. Rich M, Jaramillo E. Companion handbook to the WHO guidelines for the programmatic management of drug-resistant tuberculosis. Geneva: WHO; 2014.
4. Lange C, Abubakar I, Alffenaar JW, et al. Management of patients with multidrug-resistant/extensively drug-resistant tuberculosis in Europe: a TBNET consensus statement. Eur Respir J. 2014;44:23-63.
5. Günther G. Multidrug-resistant and extensively drug-resistant tuberculosis: a review of current concepts and future challenges. Clin Med (Lond). 2014;14:279-85.

6. World Health Organization. (2013). Definitions and reporting framework for tuberculosis-2013 revision. [online] Available from: http://www.who.int/iris/bitstream/10665/79199/1/9789241505345-eng.pdf. [Accessed February, 2016].
7. WHO-Multidrug Resistant Tuberculosis (MDR-TB) Fact Sheet-2015 Update. [online] Available from: http://www.who.int/tb/challenges/mdr/mdr_tb_factsheet.pdf?ua=1. [Accessed February, 2016].
8. Migliori GB, Matteelli A, Cirillo D, Pai M. Diagnosis of multidrug-resistant tuberculosis and extensively drug-resistant tuberculosis: current standards and challenges. Can J Infect Dis Med Microbiol. 2008;19 (2):169-72.
9. Banerjee R, Schecter GF, Flood J, Porco TC. Extensively drug-resistant tuberculosis: new strains, new challenges. Expert Rev Anti Infect Ther. 2008;6(5):713-24.
10. Zumla A, Abubakar I, Raviglione M, et al. Drug-resistant tuberculosis: current dilemmas, unanswered questions, challenges, and priority needs. J Infect Dis. 2012;205 Suppl 2:S228-40.
11. Steingart KR, Sohn R, Schiller I, et al. Xpert® MTB/RIF assay for pulmonary tuberculosis and rifampicin resistance in adults. Cochrane Database Syst Rev. 2013;1:CD009593.
12. Boehme CC, Nicol MP, Nabeta P, et al. Feasibility, diagnostic accuracy, and effectiveness of decentralized use of the Xpert MTB/RIF test for diagnosis of tuberculosis and multidrug resistance: a multicenter implementation study. Lancet. 2011;377:1495-505.
13. Van Rie A, Mellet K, John MA, et al. False-positive rifampicin resistance on Xpert® MTB/RIF: case report and clinical implications. Int J Tuberc Lung Dis. 2012;16:206-8.
14. Crudu V, Stratan E, Romancenco E, Allerheiligen V, Hillemann A, Moraru N. First evaluation of an improved assay for molecular genetic detection of tuberculosis as well as rifampin and isoniazid resistances. J Clin Microbiol. 2012;50:1264-9.
15. Lawn SD, Kerkhoff AD, Vogt M, Wood R. Diagnostic accuracy of a low-cost, urine antigen, point-of-care screening assay for HIV-associated pulmonary tuberculosis before antiretroviral therapy: a descriptive study. Lancet Infect Dis. 2012;12:201-9.
16. World Health Organization. Guidelines for the programmatic management of drug-resistant tuberculosis. Geneva: World Health Organization; 2011. pp. 1-44. [online] Available from: http://www.who.int/tb/challenges/mdr/programmatic_guidelines_for_mdrtb/en/index.html. [Accessed February, 2016].
17. Curry International Tuberculosis Center, California Department of Health Sciences. (2008). Drug-resistant tuberculosis: a survival guide for clinicians. [online] Available from: http://www.currytbcenter.ucsf.edu/products/product_details.cfm?productID=WPT-11. [Accessed February, 2016].
18. Bassili A, Fitzpatrick C, Qadeer E, Fatima R, Floyd K, Jaramillo E. A systematic review of the effectiveness of hospital- and ambulatory-based management of multidrug-resistant tuberculosis. Am J Trop Med Hyg. 2013;89(2):271-80.
19. Varaine F, Rich M, editors. Tuberculosis: Practical Guide for Clinicians, Nurses, Laboratory Technicians and Medical Auxiliaries. Paris: Médecins San Frontières and Partners In Health; 2013. pp. 1-299.
20. Falzon D, Gandhi N, Migliori GB, et al. Resistance to fluoroquinolones and second-line injectable drugs: impact on multidrug-resistant TB outcomes. Eur Respir J. 2013;42:156-68.
21. Jacobson KR, Tierney DB, Jeon CY, Mitnick CD, Murray MB. Treatment outcomes among patients with extensively drug-resistant tuberculosis: systematic review and meta-analysis. Clin Infect Dis. 2010;51(1):6-14.
22. World Health Organization. The use of delamanid in the treatment of multidrug-resistant tuberculosis. Geneva: World Health Organization; 2014. pp. 1-47.
23. World Health Organization. The use of bedaquiline in the treatment of multidrug-resistant tuberculosis. Geneva: World Health Organization; 2013. pp. 1-64.
24. World Health Organization. (2016). Tuberculosis (TB) Task Force for New Drug Policy Development. [online] Available from: http://www.who.int/tb/advisory_bodies/newdrugs_taskforce/en/. [Accessed February, 2016].
25. Gandhi NR, Moll A, Sturm AW, et al. Extensively drug-resistant tuberculosis as a cause of death in patients co-infected with tuberculosis and HIV in a rural area of South Africa. Lancet. 2006;368:1575-80.
26. Chamie G, Luetkemeyer A, Walusimbi-Nanteza M, et al. Significant variation in presentation of pulmonary tuberculosis across a high resolution of CD4 strata. Int J Tuberc Lung Dis. 2010;14:1295-302.

27. Abdool Karim SS, Naidoo K, Grobler A, et al. Integration of antiretroviral therapy with tuberculosis treatment. N Engl J Med. 2011;365:1492-501.
28. Havlir DV, Kendall MA, Ive P, et al. Timing of antiretroviral therapy for HIV-1 infection and tuberculosis. N Engl J Med. 2011;365:1482-91.
29. Blanc FX, Sok T, Laureillard D, et al. Earlier versus later start of antiretroviral therapy in HIV-infected adults with tuberculosis. N Engl J Med. 2011;365:1471-81.
30. Tuberculosis Drug Information Guide. 2nd ed. California: Curry International Tuberculosis Center and California Department of Public Health; 2012.
31. Holdiness MR. Cerebrospinal fluid pharmacokinetics of the antituberculosis drugs. Clin Pharmacokinet. 1985;10:532-4.
32. Daley CL. Mycobacterium tuberculosis complex. In: Yu VL, Merigan TC Jr, Barriere SL (Eds). Antimicrobial Therapy and Vaccines. Philadelphia: Lippincott Williams & Wilkins; 1999. pp. 531-6.
33. Francis RS, Curwen MP. Major surgery for pulmonary tuberculosis: final report. Tubercle. 1964;45:5-79.
34. Centers for Disease Control and Prevention (CDC). Emergence of Mycobacterium tuberculosis with extensive resistance to second-line drugs—worldwide, 2000-2004. MMWR Morb Mortal Wkly Rep. 2006;55(11):301-5.
35. Van Deun A, Maug AK, Salim MA, et al. Short, highly effective, and inexpensive standardized treatment of multidrug-resistant tuberculosis. Am J Respir Crit Care Med. 2010;182(5):684-92.
36. STREAM to test a 9-month MDR-TB treatment regimen. (2014). [online] Available from: http://www.theunion.org/what-we-do/technical-assistance/tuberculosis-and-mdr-tb/treat-tb. [Accessed February, 2016].
37. Ahuja SD, Ashkin D, Avendano M, et al. Multidrug resistant pulmonary tuberculosis treatment regimens and patient outcomes: an individual patient data meta-analysis of 9,153 patients. PLoS Med. 2012;9(8):e1001300.
38. Bloss E, Kuksa L, Holtz TH, et al. Adverse events related to multidrug-resistant tuberculosis treatment, Latvia, 2000-2004. Intern J Tuberc Lung Dis. 2010;14(3):275-81.
39. Dalton T, Cegielski P, Akksilp S, et al. Prevalence of and risk factors for resistance to second-line drugs in people with multidrug-resistant tuberculosis in eight countries: a prospective cohort study. Lancet. 2012;380:1406-17.
40. Diacon AH, Donald PR, Pym A, et al. Randomized pilot trial of eight weeks of bedaquiline (TMC207) treatment for multidrug-resistant tuberculosis: long-term outcome, tolerability, and effect on emergence of drug resistance. Antimicrob Agents Chemother. 2012;56:3271-6.
41. Diacon AH, Pym A, Grobusch M, et al. The diarylquinoline TMC207 for multidrug-resistant tuberculosis. N Engl J Med. 2009;360:2397-405.
42. Gler MT, Skripconoka V, Sanchez-Garavito E, et al. Delamanid for multidrug-resistant pulmonary tuberculosis. N Engl J Med. 2012;366:2151-60.
43. Yew WW, Nuermberger E. High-dose fluoroquinolones in short-course regimens for treatment of MDR-TB: the way forward? Int J Tuberc Lung Dis. 2013;17:853-4.
44. Lee M, Lee J, Carroll MW, et al. Linezolid for treatment of chronic extensively drug-resistant tuberculosis. N Engl J Med. 2012;367:1508-18.
45. Sotgiu G, Centis R, D'Ambrosio L, et al. Efficacy, safety and tolerability of linezolid containing regimens in treating MDR-TB and XDR-TB: systematic review and meta-analysis. Eur Respir J. 2012;40:1430-42.
46. Marrone MT, Venkataramanan V, Goodman M, Hill AC, Jereb JA, Mase SR. Surgical interventions for drug-resistant tuberculosis: a systematic review and meta-analysis. Int J Tuberc Lung Dis. 2013;17:6-16.

CHAPTER 12
Childhood Tuberculosis

Varinder Singh, Kamal K Singhal

INTRODUCTION

Children with Tuberculosis (TB) are often at a disadvantage due to lack of simple diagnostic pathway. Most of TB control strategies focus on a bacteriological diagnosis, which was much harder to achieve in children due to difficulty in the access to specimen as well as due to paucibacillary primary disease. The current chapter details the pathogenesis of TB and describes the clinical features of various forms of TB in children. The chapter also discusses the utility and status of various available diagnostic tests in children with TB. The treatment of tuberculosis has undergone some changes in the recent times and we bring the up to date information on the drug combination and doses. The chapter also provides the information on monitoring of therapy and management of the adverse effects in detail. A brief on drug-resistant TB in children is also provided. Finally, it details about the preventive aspects of the disease too. The chapter thus covers all the important areas related to TB in children from epidemiology to clinical features, diagnosis, management and chemoprophylaxis in a succint fashion.

EPIDEMIOLOGY

Tuberculosis caused by *Mycobacterium tuberculosis*, is a major public health problem globally; mainly in the developing countries. In high-burden countries, children contribute an estimated 10–15% of the TB cases. In 2015, there were estimated to be 1,000,000 children living with TB. Children contribute to about 10% of the total TB cases but the exact burden of pediatric TB is not known due to difficulties in case ascertainment and inadequate surveillance. Furthermore, it is likely to be underdiagnosed in settings with diagnostic limitations (typically high burden resource limited communities) where case identification is based on smear positivity.[1] Pediatric TB is an indicator of inadequate TB control. Although young children are considered less infectious, due to paucibacillary nature of the disease and reduced tussive force: they do transmit the disease.

PATHOGENESIS

Entry and establishment of bacilli in human body constitutes infection. Infection is indicated by a positive tuberculin skin test (TST). The risk of developing disease after acquiring TB infection is dependent variably on age; nutritional and immune status of the child; genetic factors; virulence of the organism; load of infecting dose; and predisposing morbidities like measles, pertussis, and human immunodeficiency virus (HIV), etc. Primary infection before 2 years of age frequently progresses to serious disease within the first 12 months without significant prior symptoms. For young infants, this time span may be as short as 4–6 weeks.

CLINICAL FEATURES AND DIAGNOSIS

Incubation period is between 4 and 8 weeks. Although mostly subacute, the onset may sometimes be acute like in miliary TB. The mild subacute illness marking primary infection often goes unrecognized. Postmortem studies in high HIV burden African states have shown that about 10% of the deaths reported due to acute pneumonia are due to TB.[1] The clinical features of TB depend on the site of involvement.

Intrathoracic Tuberculosis

Primary Infection

It occurs when TB bacilli, inhaled via an aerosol droplet, reaches the terminal airway in a previously uninfected child. It leads to a localized pneumonic process (Ghon focus) at the site where these organisms settle. For the initial 4–6 weeks, multiplication of the bacilli occurs within this focus with the bacilli draining to the regional lymph nodes and beyond. During this early phase, when the cell-mediated immunity is not fully active, occult dissemination of the TB bacilli, in the absence of clinical disease, can occur. The Ghon complex constitutes the Ghon focus and the affected regional lymph nodes.

The symptoms and signs of primary pulmonary TB are variable and can sometimes be very subtle and it may be picked as a chance finding in chest skiagrams. Nonproductive cough and mild dyspnea are the most common symptoms. Almost half of the infants and children with radiographically moderate to severe pulmonary TB have no physical findings. Uncomplicated hilar or paratracheal lymphadenopathy remains the most common disease manifestation in most young children.

Progressive Primary Disease

The progression from primary complex to progressive primary disease is clinically indicated by onset of persistent, nonremitting clinical symptoms (mild fever, anorexia, weight loss, decreased activity). Cough with expectoration is more likely in advance disease. Clinical examination may show signs as per the pathology varying from scattered crackles to signs of consolidation or collapse. Cavitation is uncommon in immunocompetent children younger than 8–10 years age except in infancy. Endobronchial TB may present as persistent cough, wheeze, and respiratory distress mimicking asthma. Presence of fever and weight loss or inadequate weight gain and anorexia help differentiating it from asthma. Lymph nodes may lead to complete or partial collapse of the airway resulting in features suggestive of collapse or emphysema respectively.

Pleural Effusion

Tuberculous pleural effusion is uncommon in children less than 6 years of age and rare in children less than 2 years of age. Children usually have fever, anorexia, weight loss, and cough. Clinical presentation of pleural effusion depends on the amount of effusion. It is usually unilateral. Small to moderate effusions may present with pleuritic chest pain, decreased chest wall movement on the affected side, impaired note on percussion, and decreased air entry with pleural rub on auscultation. In larger effusions, pleurisy is replaced by discomfort and there is no pleural rub. There would be signs of mediastinal and tracheal shift to opposite side, with stony dullness on percussion. Tuberculosis usually involves pleural space as organisms from the subpleural pulmonary focus or caseating lymph node reach the pleural space, early in the course of a TB infection. The interaction of tubercular protein with the sensitized T-cells in the pleural space results in hypersensitivity reaction.

Less commonly, there can be tuberculous empyema which happens due to a large number of organisms spilling into the pleural space, usually from rupture of a cavity or an adjacent parenchymal focus into the pleura. A tuberculous empyema is usually associated with evident pulmonary parenchymal disease and pleural air on chest films.

Pleural aspiration for biochemical, cytological, and microbiological examination is needed for diagnosis. The pleural fluid is straw-colored exudate with protein levels between 2 and 4 g/dL; glucose between 20 and 40 mg/dL and several hundred to thousands of white blood cells, predominantly lymphocytes (polymorphs in early phase). Smear for acid-fast bacillus (AFB) is rarely positive but culture may be positive in less than 30% of cases. Adenosine deaminase (ADA) levels more than 40 IU/L may be suggestive of tuberculous pleural effusion but it is not diagnostic. Adenosine deaminase levels make poor distinction between TB effusion and partially treated bacterial effusions. Compared to pleural fluid, the pleural membrane is more likely to yield positive acid-fast stain, culture, or granuloma formation. The TST is positive in only 70–80% of cases. Cartridge based nucleic acid amplification tests (CBNAATs) like Xpert Rif do not perform well on pleural fluid though are fairly specific.

Reactivation Tuberculosis

It develops as a result of endogenous reactivation of primary infection, commonly in adolescents. The most frequent sites are the apical and posterior segments of the right and left upper lobe (Simon foci). Cavitation is common in reactivation TB. This form of disease usually remains localized to the lungs, because the established immune response prevents further extrapulmonary spread. Compared to children with primary pulmonary TB, older children and adolescents with reactivation TB are more likely to experience fever, anorexia, malaise, weight loss, night sweats, productive cough, hemoptysis, and chest pain. The physical examination findings on chest examination may suggest presence of cavity in the lung and crackles but the signs are often far less compared to the degree of parenchymal involvement.

Miliary Tuberculosis

It is a severe form of TB resulting from hematogenous spread of tuberculous bacilli throughout the body. Although occult dissemination is common following primary infections, it only progresses to disseminated disease in very young and immunocompromised children. In children younger than 2 years of age, primary infection may lead to severe disease within 12 months without any significant prior illness.[2] The onset of illness may be sudden with high-grade fever, weight loss, lymphadenopathy, cough, respiratory complaint, cyanosis, and even sensorial alteration. Examination may reveal fine creps and wheeze on auscultation, lymphadenopathy, and hepatosplenomegaly. Radiologically, it is seen as even sized miliary lesions (smaller than 2 mm), distributed bilaterally throughout the lungs. Half of the patients may reveal choroid tubercles and almost one-fourth may have associated meningitis.

Diagnosis of Pulmonary Tuberculosis

The diagnosis of pulmonary TB in children is challenging. In young children, the bacteriological diagnosis is difficult, due to the paucibacillary nature of the disease, nonspecific clinical presentation, and nonavailability of sputum. The diagnosis of TB in children is, therefore, mostly dependent on combination of clinical presentation (cough, fever, weight loss/no weight gain), history of contact with a known TB case, and result of TST and radiology. Also, a nonresponse of symptoms, particularly with persistence of the radiological shadows, to potent antibiotics is used as an additional ground for suspecting TB. In order to improve the predictive value of any test for TB, it is important that the suspects are identified using well-characterized clinical symptoms and have a high pretest probability to have TB. In high-burden countries like India, persistent cough with or without fever for more than 2 weeks duration is a common symptom complex used to identify those with presumptive TB (hitherto called as TB suspect). The Indian Academy of Pediatrics-Revised National Tuberculosis Control Program (IAP-RNTCP) guidelines for childhood TB in India specify that cases with fever persisting for more than 2 weeks without a known cause should be suspected and investigated for tuberculosis. It is important to document fever and not depend merely on impression. Fever can be of any type and the often-described evening rise of temperature is neither specific to this etiology nor commonly present. Likewise, a child with cough which is unremitting for the past 2 weeks should be considered as a TB suspect. Unexplained recent loss of weight (weight loss of >5% in past 3 months) may be more important pointer to TB than a static weight.

In individuals with presumptive TB, any of the available respiratory specimens [self-expectorated sputum/induced sputum (IS)/gastric lavage (GL)/bronchoalveolar lavage (BAL)] should be sent for workup. At least two specimens taken on two consecutive days be tested on smear for AFB. While GL is preferred in children who do not or cannot expectorate sputum, it requires overnight fasting and need for admission. Studies have reported that the collection can be done on ambulatory basis too, albeit with some loss of sensitivity.[3] Lately, a lot of interest has been generated around IS.[4,5] Induction of sputum is done by nebulizing with 3% saline (post priming with nebulized or inhaled β-2 agonist) and the secretions so induced are loosened by percussing the chest of the baby. These secretions are trapped from the nasopharynx by using a mucus trap attached to a wall or foot paddle suction. Induction of sputum can be easily performed in young children including infants with acceptable yield of the sample. Other specimens (tissue or fluid) depending on the site of tubercular involvement may include cerebrospinal fluid (CSF), pleural tap, ascitic tap, lymph node aspirate, joint fluid aspirate, abscesses, etc.

Studies comparing the yield of AFB (on both smear and culture) in IS versus GL have shown variable results; while some have shown the two techniques to be comparable but other studies show better yield with GL. Studies have also shown that the yield of two consecutive GL samples to be equivalent to one GL and IS taken on the same day.[4-6] Bronchoscopy and BAL is required in select cases of persistent pneumonia for diagnosis, or for children who are drug-resistant TB suspects as described later.

The bacteriological workup should include at least smear for AFB using either Ziehl-Neelsen (ZN) staining or fluorescent staining (like auramine or rhodamine), liquid culture (MGIT), and/or CBNAAT like Xpert Mtb/Rif™.

The sensitivity of ZN smear (about 0–15%) and culture (45–60%) is relatively poor in childhood TB. The smear examination using fluorescent light-emitting diode (LED) microscopy adds little (10% extra yield) to improve the diagnosis. With regards CBNAAT (Xpert Rif), there are three distinct advantages: firstly, rapid availability of result indicates presence or absence of TB within 2 hours; secondly, it also confirms presence or absence of resistance to rifampicin; thirdly, being cartridge-based, it has an inherent system of quality control, obviating risk of cross contamination. The World Health Organization (WHO) endorsed its use in adults in 2011 and later in children. Presently, it recommends its use in all children with pulmonary and/or extrapulmonary TB (EPTB) for respiratory (sputum, GL, and IS) and nonrespiratory (lymph node aspirates, CSF, pleural fluid, and other body fluids) specimens. In patients with associated HIV, suspected multidrug-resistant TB (MDR-TB), suspected TB meningitis (TBM), or with severe illness, it strongly recommends CBNAAT as the preferred initial test instead of conventional smear and culture. A negative CBNAAT result does not rule out TB.[7,8] Other in house nucleic acid amplification techniques, nonvalidated commercial polymerase chain reaction (PCR) tests and serology [immunoglobulin M (IgM), IgG, and IgA antibodies against *M. tuberculosis* antigens] are not recommended for use in pediatric TB.

The evidence among children, thus far, suggests that Xpert Rif performs somewhat poorly compared to culture but gives almost three times the sensitivity as compared to smear examination. On average about 40–50% of the cases of pediatric TB are likely to be missed by even the best of the methods available currently.[8] The bacteriological diagnosis can however be improved by accessing any additional specimens, e.g., about a fifth of the pulmonary cases may be confirmed through investigation of a concomitant peripheral lymphadenopathy.

The bacteriological diagnosis for TB is not simple and often not easily available or reliable in most resource-limited countries. However, efforts are being made to strengthen these globally, particularly, for the diagnosis of MDR-TB. In India, presently different tests are used for programmatic management of drug-resistant TB (PMDT) in India depending on the infrastructure available. This includes conventional solid Löwenstein–Jensen (LJ) media culture, the liquid culture (MGIT), and the rapid molecular assays such as line probe assay (LPA) and Xpert MTB/Rif.

Conventional drug susceptibility testing (DST), also known as phenotypic DST, evaluates growth of *M. tuberculosis* in the presence of drug-containing solid or liquid media. The molecular DST, also known as genotypic DST, evaluates for the presence of genetic mutations associated with phenotypic resistance. Conventional DST is available for more drugs, and is considered very reliable for isoniazid (INH), rifampicin (R), and streptomycin (S), but somewhat less reliable for other drugs such as ethambutol (E). Molecular DST, on the other hand, is highly reliable for rifampicin, but has less sensitive for detection of INH resistance. The time taken by the various tests to give drug sensitivity result is: 84 days by solid LJ media; 42 days by liquid culture (MGIT); around 72 hours by LPA (feasible only on smear-positive specimens); and around 2 hours by CBNAAT (Xpert MTB/Rif).

Radiology in Pulmonary Tuberculosis

Although certain radiological signs indicate a tubercular etiology, there are no pathognomic radiological signs of TB. Radiological signs strongly suggestive of TB are miliary (Fig. 1); paratracheal or hilar lymphadenopathy with or without parenchymal lung lesion (Fig. 2); and a chronic fibrocavitary lesion (Fig. 3). Enlarged hilar lymph node may lead to extraluminal or intraluminal compression/obstruction of airway leading to distal airway collapse or emphysema (Fig. 4). Adolescents may present with apical infiltrates with or without cavitation similar to adults.

Inhomogenous shadows or consolidations are also seen but are not as specific as the signs discussed above. Pleural effusion is seen due to rupture of a subpleural lesion into pleura (Fig. 5). Pneumothorax, due to rupture of bullous lesions, may occur uncommonly. A patchy or lobar air space opacity, which persists despite appropriate antibiotic therapy in a symptomatic case, should however merit workup for TB.

Ultrasonography, with the advantage of no radiation hazard, may be useful in assessing the pleural fluid for septae/fibrous strands to differentiate empyema

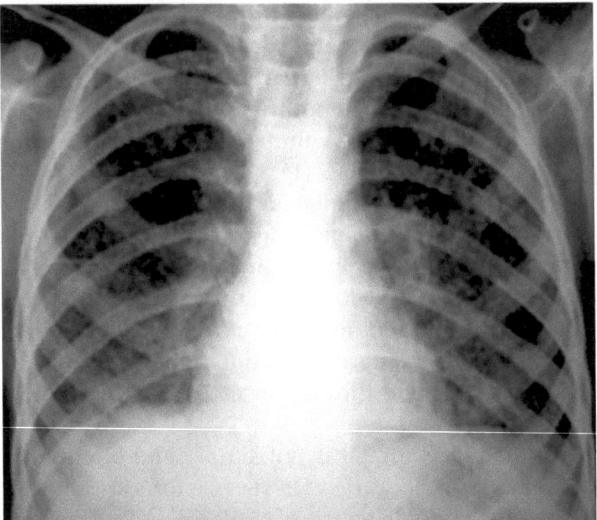

FIG. 1: Miliary tuberculosis.

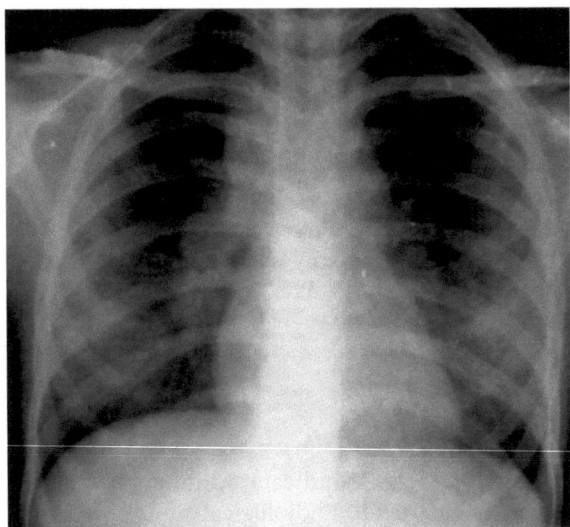

FIG. 2: Right hilar and paratracheal lymphadenopathy suggesting primary tuberculosis.

from tubercular effusion. The erect and lateral decubitus chest X-ray may also help differentiate loculated empyema from tubercular effusion. Contrast-enhanced computed tomography (CECT) chest can give more details but has high radiation cost than a digital chest X-ray (CXR). Given the high direct and indirect cost associated with CECT, it is considered to have limited utility in diagnosis of TB. However, CT is useful for guided tissue biopsy.

Tuberculin Skin Test
Tuberculin skin test is an immunological test which indicates present or past infection with *M. tuberculosis* but cannot help distinguish between latent infection and disease.

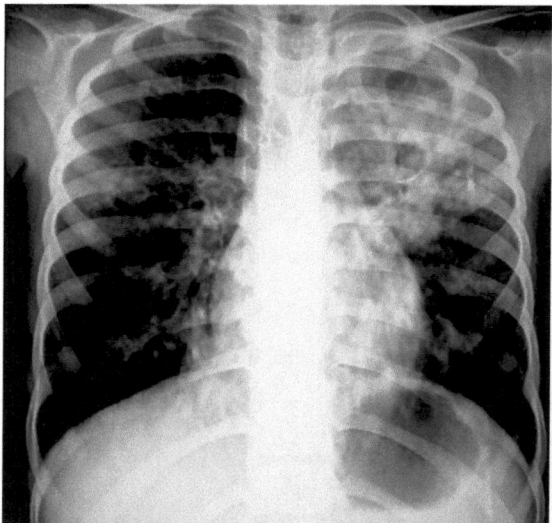

FIG. 3: Adult type fibrocavitary disease.

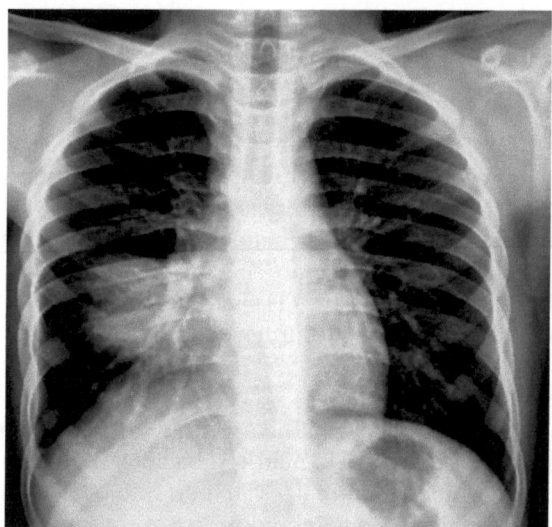

FIG. 4: Progressive primary tuberculosis with right middle lobe collapse with lower lobe pneumonia.

Of the number of skin tests available, Mantoux's method is recommended. It is used as an adjunct to other diagnostic tests in the diagnosis of TB in children. It is recommended to give 2 tuberculin units (TU) of PPD RT-23 (equivalent of 5 TU PPD-S) by intradermal injection on the volar surface of the forearm. It should form a wheal about 6 mm in size and the resulting induration is read after 48–72 hours. A positive Mantoux test is indicated by an induration of more than 10 mm. Degree of reaction or presence of necrosis and ulceration at the test site does not differentiate infection from disease. A positive result can still be read from 72 hours to 7th day. Repeat test may need to be given in the other forearm, if a patient reports 72 hours after injection with a negative result. Width of induration, not erythema, should be read horizontally using palpatory or ballpoint method. Previous

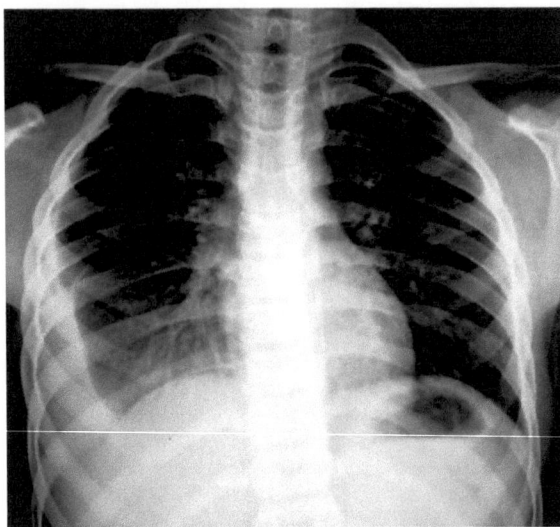

FIG. 5: Pleural effusion (right).

Bacillus Calmette–Guérin (BCG) vaccination has minimal influence on PPD reaction though can produce false-positive cross reaction in few.

Interferon-γ Release Assays

Interferon-γ release assays (IGRAs) measure *in vitro* response to antigens which are present only in *Mycobacterium tuberculosis* not in BCG vaccine strain and *Mycobacterium* other than tuberculosis. There are two advantages of IGRAs over TST:
1. It requires only one contact between the patients with the caregiver
2. It does not cross react with BCG so is more specific than TST.

Two commercially available IGRAs are: (1) Quantiferon Gold and (2) Tspot. The WHO does not recommend using IGRA in high-burden countries like India.[9]

Body Fluid Evaluation

Exudative (protein >3 g/dL) lymphocytic fluid aspirates from the pleura or peritoneal or pericardial effusions are suggestive of TB. Acid-fast bacillus staining of the aspirates may occasionally be positive for tuberculous bacteria. Xpert Mtb/Rif shows a better sensitivity than smear for CSF. The ascitic and pleural fluids do not show any significant yield with Xpert Mtb/Rif.

Histopathological Diagnosis

Depending on the organ involved tissue biopsy of pleura, lymph node, liver, bone marrow, transbronchial biopsy may show the presence of caseating granulomas. These can also be used for testing with Xpert Mtb/Rif.

The detailed recommendations by IAP-RNTCP for investigating a presumptive pulmonary TB case have been shown in flowchart 1.

The algorithm detailed in flowchart 1 is for new cases of pulmonary TB in children. While two consecutive specimens are tested for smear examination but usually a single specimen is subjected to MGIT culture or CBNAAT (Xpert Rif). Highly suggestive CXRs include either miliary, lymphadenopathy (hilar or mediastinal), or chronic fibrocavitary

Childhood Tuberculosis

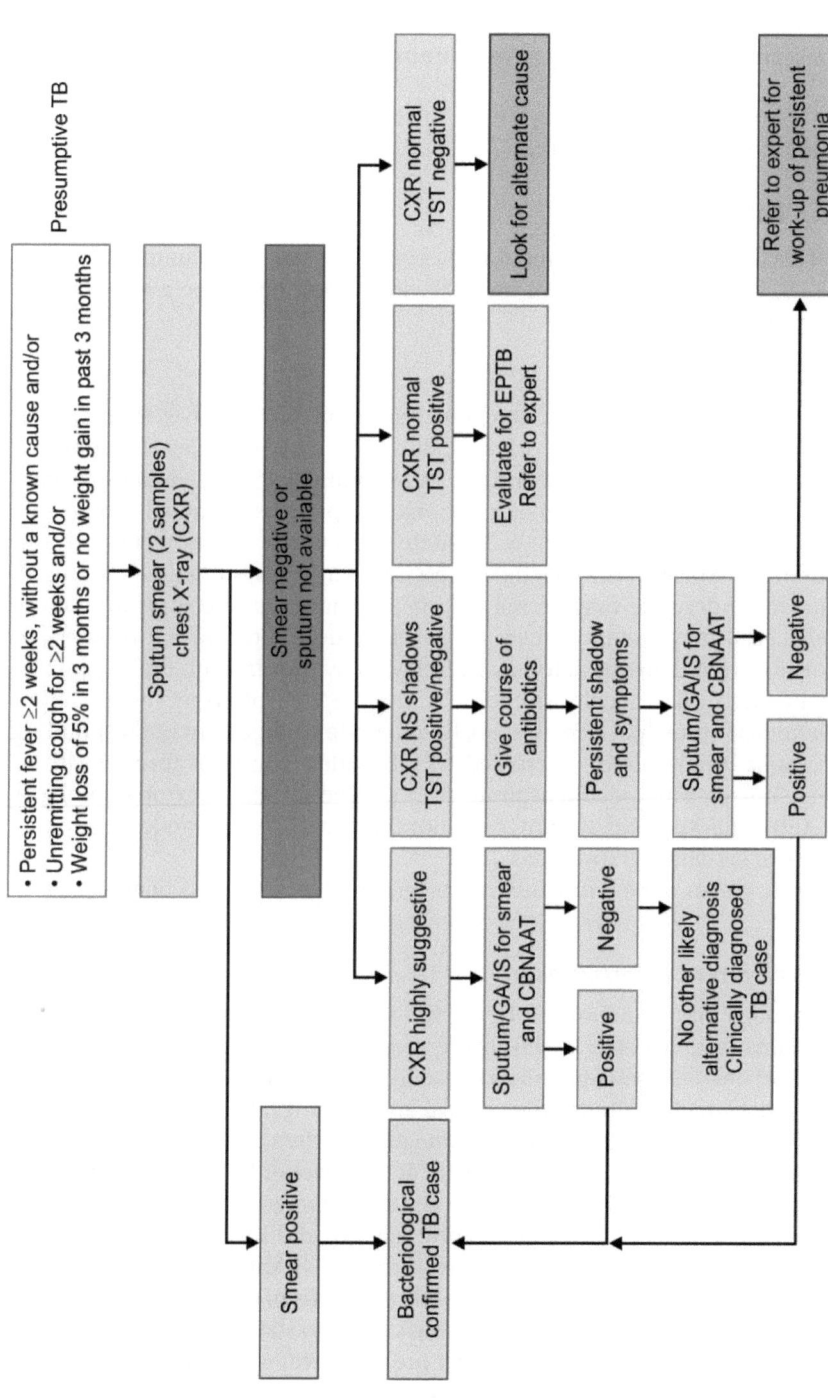

TB; tuberculosis; CBNAAT, cartridge based nucleic acid amplification test; GA, gastric aspirates; IS, induced sputum; EPTB, extrapulmonary tuberculosis.
FLOWCHART 1: Diagnostic algorithm for the diagnosis of pulmonary tuberculosis in children (Revised National Tuberculosis Control Program 2015).

lesions. As inadequately treated other pulmonary infections can mimic the symptoms and may not be distinguishable by radiology alone, a trial of antibiotics is often given as detailed in flowchart 1. Antibiotics like linezolid and fluoroquinolones should not be used for treating pulmonary infections as they have antitubercular activity which can confound the situation.

All TB cases should be offered testing for HIV. Therapeutic trial with anti-TB drugs is not recommended for establishing diagnosis.

Extrathoracic Tuberculosis

Lymph node tuberculosis (LNTB) and meningitis constitute the most common form of EPTB.[10,11] In EPTB, final diagnosis hinges on retrieving appropriate specimen (tissue or fluid aspirate) for workup.

Tuberculosis Lymphadenitis

Superficial lymphadenopathy is one of the most common forms (44-67%) of EPTB. Tuberculous lymphadenopathy may be primary, due to primary complex development in the cervical-pharyngeal lesion, or secondary. Tuberculous lymphadenopathy occurs 6-9 months after initial infection. Tubercular lymphadenopathy is a gradual progressive enlargement, over more than 2 weeks, and usually affects the anterior cervical and submandibular nodes. Typically, the affected lymph nodes are firm, sometimes fluctuant, with minimal or no tenderness; may be matted, or may have chronic sinus formation. If left untreated, LNTB may spontaneously resolve but more often would progress to caseation and necrosis (cold abscess). It may be followed by rupture with draining sinus. Diagnosis is established by fine needle aspiration cytology (FNAC) of suspect lymph nodes like large lymph nodes (more than 2 cm in size), lymph node enlargement not responding to a 1-2-week course of antibiotics, or matted lymph nodes with cold abscess with or without draining sinuses. Fine needle aspirate can be used for either cytopathology or demonstrating AFB or for Xpert Rif. If FNAC does not confirm TB, lymph node biopsy may show the presence of caseating granulomas.

Algorithm for diagnosis of pediatric tubercular lymphadenopathy has been shown in flowchart 2.

Central Nervous System Tuberculosis

Lymphohematogenous dissemination of the bacilli during the initial infection leads to formation of caseous lesions (Rich focus) in the meninges or the cerebral cortex. The caseous lesions (Rich focus) discharge tubercle bacilli in the subarachnoid space thereby producing an exudate which infiltrates the cortical and meningeal blood vessels leading to infarcts in the cerebral cortex. The thick exudate also hinders the normal flow of CSF in the ventricular system. Obstructed flow of CSF at the level of basal cisterns leads to communicating hydrocephalus. Thus, damage in central nervous system (CNS) TB is due to a combination of vasculitis, infarction, cerebral edema, and hydrocephalus. Central nervous system involvement is the most severe form of TB and commonly presents between 6 months and 4 years of age. The signs and symptoms of CNS TB can be divided into three stages. The illness usually progresses from stage 1 to stage 3 over several weeks, but in infants and young children, it may rapidly progress over days. Depending on the stage at which treatment is started, the prognosis progressively worsens from stage 1 to stage 3. Stage 1 typically lasts 1-2 weeks, characterized by nonspecific symptoms such as fever, headache, irritability, drowsiness, malaise, anorexia, inadequate weight gain or loss,

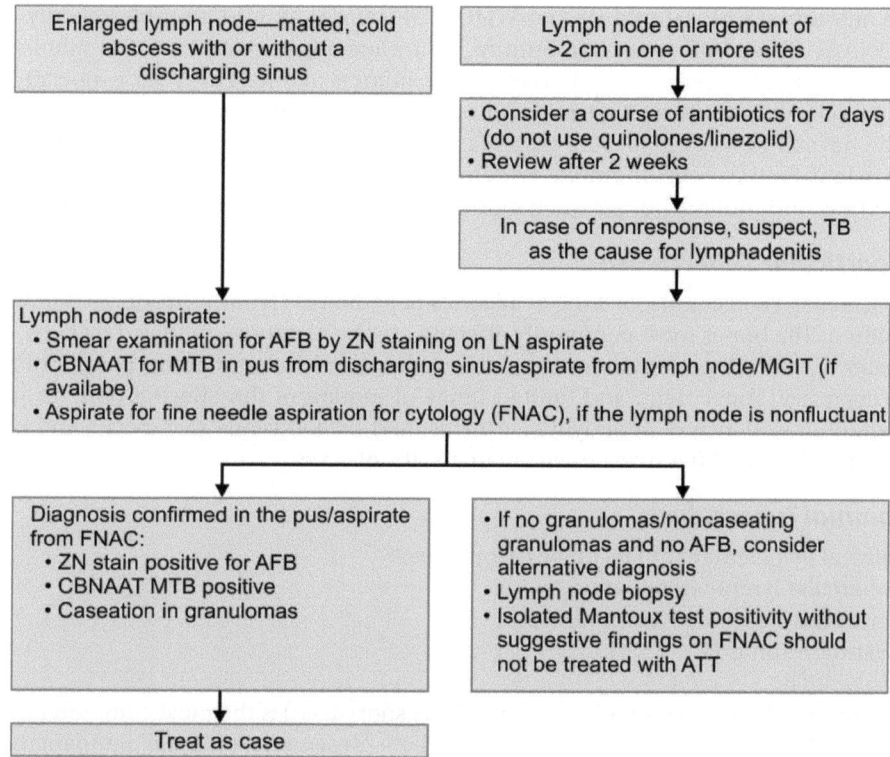

TB, tuberculosis; MTB, *Mycobacterium tuberculosis*; CBNAAT, cartridge based nucleic acid amplification test; ZN, Ziehl–Neelsen; AFB, acid-fast bacillus; ATT, antituberculosis treatment.

FLOWCHART 2: Algorithm for diagnosis of pediatric tubercular lymphadenopathy.

stagnation or regression of development milestones. Stage 2 begins abruptly with features indicative of increased intracranial pressure, meningeal irritability, and vasculitis. Clinical constellation in stage 2 includes lethargy, seizures, hypertonia, vomiting, cranial nerve palsies associated with basal meningitis, and other focal neurological deficits. Stage 3 is characterized by coma, hemiplegia or paraplegia, decerebrate posturing, deterioration in vital signs, and finally death.

Central nervous system TB can also present as an intracranial space-occupying lesion. Depending on the location, size, and perilesional edema, the manifestations of tuberculoma can be either of the following: seizures, headache, and neurological focal deficits. Paradoxical increase in size and even appearance of new tuberculomas are known to occur in patients of CNS TB, otherwise recovering on anti-TB treatment (ATT). It needs to be clinically differentiated from nonresponse to ATT. Severe clinical signs and symptoms of paradoxical response merit corticosteroids along with ATT. In TBM, the leukocyte count in CSF ranges from 10 to 500 cells/mm^3 but may occasionally be higher. Although majority of cells are lymphocytes, polymorphs may be seen in early illness. Cerebrospinal fluid biochemistry reveals glucose levels usually less than 40 mg/dL but rarely less than 20 mg/dL; and elevated protein levels as high as 400–5,000 mg/dL. High CSF ADA (various studies report cutoff between 7 and 11.3 IU/L) provides supportive evidence of TBM but poorly differentiates it from partially treated meningitis.[12] The microbiological yield on AFB smear and mycobacterial culture is directly proportionate to the amount of CSF sample. As per WHO, CSF sample should be preferentially sent for CBNAAT instead of smear and culture. Neuroimaging may reveal basal meningeal enhancement; hydrocephalus; tuberculoma(s); infarcts in different areas, especially the basal ganglia; or may even be normal. Tuberculin skin test may be nonreactive and CXR may be normal in 50 and 20–50% patients respectively. Nevertheless, effort should be made to look for these corroborative evidences since many a time it is these concomitant lesions (e.g., pulmonary, peripheral lymph node) that clinch the diagnosis of TBM.

Osteoarticular Tuberculosis

Osteoarticular TB accounts for 1.4% of all cases of pediatric TB and 5.9% of cases of EPTB in children. The bones most commonly affected are the vertebrae, followed by knee, hip, and elbow. Clinical presentation may include localized inflammation, pain, swelling, fever, decreased movement, and limited range of motion of the affected bone or joint. Radiographic evidence of spondylitis, arthritis, and osteomyelitis may occur and chest radiograph abnormalities may be seen in up to 50% of cases.

Abdominal Tuberculosis

The clinical involvement of TB can be of four types:
1. Tubercular lymphadenopathy
2. Peritoneal TB
3. Gastrointestinal TB
4. Visceral TB.

Abdominal lymphadenopathy (>15 mm in its short axis)) is the most common form of abdominal TB. Nodes most commonly involved are mesenteric, omental, peripancreatic, located at porta hepatis, and along the celiac axis. Peritoneal TB can be of three types. The most common type is wet ascitic type with large amount of free or loculated ascitic fluid. Fixed fibrotic type has matted bowel loops on imaging with occasional loculated ascites. The third type, dry plastic type, has fibrous peritoneal reaction, peritoneal nodules, and adhesions. Usually, a combination of these three types is seen. Isolated abdominal visceral involvement is uncommon. The most common site of gastrointestinal TB is the ileocecal junction. The usual clinical features of small intestinal TB are colicky abdominal pain, borborygmi, vomiting, and altered bowel habits. Barium follow-through study may suggest intestinal disease but is not confirmatory.

Congenital Tuberculosis

True congenital TB is rare, with fewer than 400 cases reported in literature. Initial infection occurring in the mother during or just prior to the pregnancy is more likely to affect the fetus. Clinical signs may manifest shortly after birth but more commonly from second to fourth week of life. Clinical manifestations resemble neonatal sepsis or any other congenital infection; and are neither definitive nor specific for congenital TB. The most common signs and symptoms in order of frequency are respiratory distress, hepatomegaly or splenomegaly, fever, lymphadenopathy, poor feeding, lethargy or irritability, abdominal distention, failure to thrive, ear drainage, and skin rashes. Other less common features may be jaundice, seizures, bloody diarrhea, and ascites. Less than half of the affected infants have meningitis. The diagnosis of neonatal TB requires high index of suspicion. It should be suspected in infants with signs and symptoms of bacterial or congenital infection not responding to conventional antibiotic and supportive therapy, with corroborative evidence of TB in mother.

TREATMENT

Current Regimes

Antitubercular drugs may have several different activities. Some drugs are bactericidal while others are bacteriostatic. Their action on various subpopulations of bacilli also differs, thus accounting for differences in their sterilizing activity, bactericidal activity, and prevention of emergence of resistance. The two-phase treatment has an intensive initial phase designated to eliminate quickly many logs of tubercle bacilli in all different metabolic populations. Therefore, intensive phase prevents deterioration of clinical condition and death by early killing of tubercle bacilli; and, reduces infectivity. The number and inclusion of drugs in initial phase should take into account the prevalence of drug resistance in the infectious pool of the community. The initial drug resistance to INH alone and INH and rifampin combined is around 15% and less than 5%, respectively. Therefore, now it is recommended to use a four-drug daily regime (RHZE) in the intensive phase followed by a three-drug (RHE) continuation phase. Rifampin and pyrazinamide form the backbone of modern chemotherapy. Rifampin is particularly effective against mycobacteria in closed caseous lesions, which are active in intermittent short spurts of only a few hours. Pyrazinamide works only in the acidic environment, e.g., inside macrophages and thus is useful only in intensive phase where there is inflammation. It reduces the treatment duration to 6 months due to its early sterilizing affect. Addition of ethambutol is useful if initial drug resistance to INH is high. Risk of ethambutol toxicity is low in children of all ages when given in recommended doses. Continuation phase eliminates most residual bacilli thereby reducing failures and relapses and is usually given for duration of 4 months except for patients with meningeal, disseminated, or bone TB where longer continuation phase (10 months) is recommended. Daily observed or intermittent directly observed treatment should always be given. Adherence to therapy is the key to its success and helps to prevent any emergence of resistance.

Intermittent therapy scores over daily therapy in terms of lower cost and operational ease in directly observed treatment short-course (DOTS). The scientific basis of intermittent chemotherapy is the long generation time (18–21 h) of the tubercle bacilli and lag period of *M. tuberculosis* culture after exposure to ATT. When the anti-TB drug has washed out, the tubercular bacilli continue to fall for some time before they begin remultiplication. This period is called "lag phase". It is possible to prevent further growth of bacilli if the next dose is given before the end of the lag period. Most efficacious intermittent therapy is thrice a week regimen. Intermittent therapy is not safe without observation and there is no margin for missing doses. In the presence of INH resistance, intermittent regimens may be increased risk of amplification of resistance to rifampicin. Moreover, in high HIV prevalence settings or in cases of confirmed HIV infection intermittent regimens should not be used. Thus in the background of high INH resistance with or without HIV coinfection, there are higher treatment failure rates and relapse with intermittent dosing regimens. Intermittent therapy under RNTCP DOTS strategy has effectively treated millions of cases successfully and made an impact on TB control in the country (Table 1). Presently, there is insufficient evidence to support or refute the use of intermittent treatment regimens over daily treatment regimens in children with TB.[13] However, growing from strength to strength, the need has been identified to address the issue of likely amplification of resistance in the presence of high INH initial resistance. The Standards of TB Care in India have recommended switching to a daily regime with mechanism to ensure adherence.[14] The national program in India is currently in a

TABLE 1	List of drugs used in treatment of drug sensitive and resistant tuberculosis as per the Revised National Tuberculosis Control Program	
Groups	Description of the group	Drugs
1	First line oral drugs	Isoniazid (H), rifampicin (R), pyrazinamide (Z), ethambutol (E)
2	Injectable drugs	Streptomycin (S), kanamycin, amikacin, capreomycin, viomycin
3	Fluoroquinolones	Ciprofloxacin, ofloxacin, levofloxacin, moxifloxacin, gatifloxacin
4	Second line oral drugs	Ethionamide, prothionamide, cycloserine, terizidone, para-aminosalicylic acid
5	Drugs with unclear efficacy	Clofazimine, linezolid, amoxicillin-clavulanic acid, thioacetazone, imipenem-cilastatin, high-dose isoniazid, clarithromycin

TABLE 2	Antituberculous drugs, dosages, and major side effects			
Drug (symbol)	Daily dosages per mg/kg body weight	Thrice weekly doses in mg/kg weight	Maximum per day dose (daily regime)	Major side effects
Streptomycin (S)	20 (15–30)	15	1,000 mg	Tinnitus
Rifampin (R)	15 (10–20)	15 (12–17)	600 mg	Hepatotoxicity, gastritis, flu-like illness
Isoniazid (H)	10 (7–15)	15 (12–17)	300 mg	Peripheral neuropathy, hepatotoxicity
Pyrazinamide (Z)	35 (30–40)	35 (30–40)	2,000 mg	Arthralgia, hepatotoxicit
Ethambutol (E)	20 (15–25)	30 (25–30)	1,600 mg	Ocular toxicity

transition phase, wherein intermittent DOTS shall be gradually replaced by daily therapy in the country.

Treatment of Retreatment Cases

Defaulter or relapse cases requiring retreatment are likely to have drug resistance, so all efforts should be made to isolate the bacteria and tailor their therapy as per drug sensitivity to prevent further amplification of resistance. The WHO recommended rapid diagnostic tests based on molecular testing for *M. tuberculosis* drug resistance can be used in addition to the conventional culture techniques to determine drug sensitivity. Till, the drug sensitivity pattern is known, retreatment regime using all the first line drugs of the armamentarium is given (2SHRZE/1HRZE/5HRE) ensuring adherence to therapy. This regime which adds a single drug the failing initial regime can be associated with a very high risk of developing resistance and thus is used as a waiting period regime and should ideally be continued if only the sensitivity to first-line drugs is established.

The WHO has recently revised the dosage for children after pharmacokinetic studies in children and table 2 lists the essential anti-TB drugs and their recommended doses.[15]

Place of Fixed Drug Combinations

To further ensure all the desired drugs are taken together without error, fixed drug combination (FDC) of the anti-TB drugs is recommended. The advantages of FDC are: safety; simplified treatment; reduced errors of missing drugs; reduced risk of emergence of drug resistance strains; and ease of drug supply, shipment, and distribution, from programmatic point of view. The WHO and the International Union Against Tuberculosis and Lung Disease (IUATLD) recommend FDC for treatment of TB. Good quality control and to ensure appropriate bioavailability of individual drugs is indispensable for FDCs. Most of the existing FDCs for children are not in correct dose combinations and efforts are on globally to get the correct three-drug FDC (RHZ) combination ready for licensing and marketing. It is only recently that adult FDC pill containing RHZ in 150 mg/75 mg/4000 mg combination and pediatric FDC pill containing RHZ in 75 mg/50 mg/150 mg combination have been approved and a combination of these can be used to treat patients in various weight bands.[16]

Adjunctive Treatment

Role of Corticosteroids as Adjunctive Therapy in Tuberculosis

In acute overwhelming TB, there is significant host response associated with tissue inflammation and fibrous proliferation. This heightened host response can lead to a poor clinical outcome. Corticosteroids have been effectively shown to reduce morbidity and mortality in patients with CNS TB; tubercular pericarditis, and pericardial effusion. They are also used for miliary disease with alveolar-capillary block, endobronchial TB with attendant localized emphysema or collapse-consolidation lesions, severe paradoxical response to drugs, and occasionally peritonitis or massive pleural effusions but there is limited to no quality evidence to support this practice. Corticosteroids can also be used to suppress severe drug-related hypersensitivity reactions.

Corticosteroid agents reduce mortality rates and long-term neurologic sequelae in patients with TBM by reducing vasculitis, inflammation, and intracranial pressure. Thus all children with TBM should be treated with adjuvant steroids irrespective of disease severity (prednisolone 2 mg/kg/day, maximum 60 mg/day or dexamethasone 0.6 mg/kg/day for 4 weeks followed by reducing course over 4 weeks).[15]

Role of Pyridoxine

Peripheral neuritis is a rare event in children on INH therapy, therefore, routine supplementation with pyridoxine is not necessary. However, special consideration should be given to those who have one or more of the following conditions:
- HIV coinfection
- Severely malnourished
- Chronic renal or liver disease
- Pre-existing peripheral neuropathy
- Exclusively breast fed babies.

In such situations, pyridoxine (in a dose of 25–50 mg/day) is used to prevent and treat central and peripheral nervous system side effects of INH.

Monitoring of Treatment

Children on treatment for TB need to be monitored for assessing the response to treatment, adherence to therapy, adverse event monitoring, and management. In addition, the other comorbid conditions (HIV, malnutrition, etc.) also need to be managed concomitantly. An initial visit within 2 weeks of starting therapy is good to check that the patient is getting the prescribed medicines in correct dose and combination and is tolerating them. Children can often vomit out these drugs even in the absence of any side effect, as they do for many other medications due to their poor taste, etc. Subsequently, a visit at 30 days after start of therapy, end of intensive phase, thereafter monthly till completion of treatment is optimal for the aforementioned purposes. Follow-up should preferably be continued even after completion of treatment, every 3–6 months for next 2 years, particularly in children with serious disease such as congenital TB or meningitis, or those with extensive residual chest radiographic findings at the end of chemotherapy.

Response to Therapy

Response to therapy is best monitored by bacteriological tools but given their poor sensitivity in childhood TB, response to treatment in children is more often made on the basis of clinical and radiological parameters.

The clinical improvement in patient on anti-TB drugs is the mainstay of assessing the response to therapy in children. Symptomatic improvement should be assessed by judging the improvement of fever, decrease in cough, weight gain, improved appetite and subjective well-being, and decrease in lymph node size. Majority of the patients show clinical improvement in symptoms and signs within 4 weeks' time.

In addition, the patients are assessed for resolution of the radiological abnormalities at the end of initial phase. An earlier radiological testing may only be done if there is a clinical deterioration to look for complications. In patients, who show increase or little change in radiological shadows with inadequate clinical response at the end of 2 months treatment, intensive phase can be extended by 4 more weeks while the patient is investigated for drug resistance. Normal chest radiograph appearance is not a necessary criterion for discontinuation of therapy. After completion of therapy, hilar adenopathy or scarring/fibrosis or residual lesions may be present for months to years.

To establish treatment outcome, the WHO recommends that all patients with pulmonary TB should have repeat sputum/gastric aspirate smears performed at the end of initial phase of treatment to detect conversion to negative status among those who were initially positive and to detect early failures in those who were AFB negative. To verify treatment success, additional sputum examinations should be done at least once before stopping treatment. Molecular methods like Xpert Rif are not useful for assessing bacteriological conversion as the DNA from dead bacilli may be detected for a long time even in a responding case. Sensitivity tests for all available drugs if possible should be performed for a new patient whose sputum is still positive at the end of the intensive phase of treatment, and for any patient suspected to be at risk of being drug-resistant, e.g., retreatment case or a disease in a MDR contact.

Treatment Adherence

Treatment adherence must always be checked along with response to treatment. It could be undertaken by asking the patient directly, by a pill count or prescription check, and by asking for the color of the urine. Where feasible, the patients should be offered DOTS. Local arrangements for supervision must be arranged either at the nearby health facilities, family practitioner, or by a responsible person/relative. The patients not on DOT should be followed up diligently. The patient must be made aware of his follow-up appointments to ensure continuation of treatment to completion and cure. To strengthen patient adherence, the patient and the caregiver should be educated about the illness and treatment, and regularly motivated during the course of treatment. Efforts should be made for prompt defaulter tracing. Often the complete treatment of a patient may entail socioeconomic assistance and advice for the family.

Adverse Event Monitoring and Management

All patients should be monitored clinically for adverse reactions during the period of chemotherapy. They should be informed about symptoms of common adverse reactions to the medications they are receiving. Routine biochemical monitoring is not recommended. Laboratory investigations are triggered by the occurrence of clinical adverse effects. Treatment stoppage or modification is often not needed in children as they tolerate these drugs very well and usually have only minor side effects.

Minor side effects such as gastrointestinal intolerance, mild skin rash, pruritus, or flushing are best managed by reassurance and symptomatic treatment and the patient should be encouraged to continue ATT. Nonsteroidal anti-inflammatory drugs provide symptomatic relief for pyrazinamide-related arthralgia. Skin rashes can usually be managed by withholding the causative drug and if it is really necessary to reintroduce the drug, the patient should undergo desensitization.

Major side effects which always necessitate change in treatment plan are detailed below:
- Hepatitis: As the anti-TB drugs are hepatic enzyme inducers, asymptomatic biochemical derangement without increase in bilirubin level may be tolerated till the enzymes remain up to five times the normal range. However, if patient develops jaundice, it is prudent to stop ATT immediately; for other symptoms like vomiting, nausea, etc. the treatment is altered if only the transaminases are three times or more than normal. The drugs are withheld till the serum bilirubin becomes normal and the enzymes are less than twice the upper limits of normal. Most patients with drug-induced hepatotoxicity can be successfully restarted on treatment. The drugs should be reintroduced sequentially starting with rifampicin, followed by INH and then pyrazinamide. The drugs can be restarted in full doses every 3 days or so while checking that the transaminases remain normal.[17] In sick cases, a nonhepatotoxic alternative regime using a combination of streptomycin, ethambutol, and fluoroquinolones can be given during the time the other drugs are withdrawn or are being reintroduced. The duration of therapy for which the original regime could not be given (i.e., period form withdrawal of therapy to its complete reintroduction of all its complements) is not counted for the purpose of calculating the total duration of therapy. All patients who require alteration from the standard regimen should be referred to experienced physicians and this is best done in a place where liver function can be carefully monitored.
- Peripheral neuropathy: Clinically manifest neuritis in children very rare. If at all it occurs, it manifests as pins and needles sensation in hands and feet. It is treated with pyridoxine 25–50 mg/day.
- Ocular toxicity: It is negligible in children on appropriate doses of ethambutol.

The development of any of the following conditions namely Stevens-Johnson syndrome; thrombocytopenia, shock and/or renal failure due to rifampicin; visual impairment due to ethambutol; eighth nerve damage from streptomycin contraindicates further use of the offending drug.

Drug-resistant Tuberculosis

Tuberculosis in children is a sentinel event and drug resistance in children is also more often a marker of the ongoing transmission of the resistant strains in the community. Acquired drug resistance is much less common in children as they have low bacillary load; however, amplification of resistance is possible in adolescents treated with weak initial therapy. Increased use of new diagnostics is ensuring that significantly more TB patients are correctly diagnosed, but major treatment gaps remain and funding is insufficient. Globally, 3.5% of new and 20.5% of previously treated TB cases (about 0.48 million cases) were estimated to have had MDR-TB in 2015.[18] On average, an estimated 9.0% of patients with MDR-TB have extensively drug-resistant TB. Progress in the detection of drug-resistant TB has been facilitated by the use of new rapid diagnostics. Globally, the success rate of treatment was 52%.[18] Health system weaknesses, lack of effective regimens, and other treatment challenges are responsible for unacceptably low cure rates, and the MDR-TB response is seriously hampered by insufficient funding.[19] Comprehensive studies on resistance to anti-TB drugs in children are limited and the prevalence of drug-resistant TB in children is not well defined, given the difficulties of culture confirmation in this age group. But the pattern of drug resistance among children reflects that found among adults in the same population as most resistance in children is caused by primary transmission of a resistant organism. A recent study from India documented INH resistance in 12.6% and MDR-TB in 4% of culture-positive pediatric cases; similar to drug resistance rate in adult population in the area. Similar experience has been reported from Western Cape Province of South Africa as well as Peru.[19-22] Clinical management as well as outcome of treatment of MDR-TB in children is also not adequately documented.

The spectrum of disease or type of disease (pulmonary or extrapulmonary) caused by MDR bacilli is not any different from that caused by drug sensitive bacilli. Children and adolescents with drug-resistant TB tend to have features of primary TB as hilar and/or mediastinal lymphadenopathy, segmental lesions, or pleural involvement. Thus, it may not be possible to differentiate between the two on the basis of clinical and radiological features, though in three of these studies around one-third to one-half of patients had cavitary disease on CXR and a very high proportion were smear/culture positive (44–94%).[19-23] The authors had concluded that this was probably due to delay in starting appropriate treatment and advanced stage of disease. Furthermore, the patients who acquire MDR-TB due to noncompliance with anti-TB therapy often have cavitary consolidations (50%) and generally demonstrate a postprimary radiographic pattern. Nevertheless, approximately one-third of adult patients in one of the study did not show the "expected" radiographic pattern. The adult patients who developed primary MDR-TB during an outbreak showed noncavitary consolidations, pleural effusions, and a primary radiographic pattern (70%).[23]

A high index of suspicion is, therefore, required to diagnose drug-resistant TB early and the presence of risk factors as mentioned in the earlier section should be sought in every case, especially history of contact with a known case of MDR-TB. In such cases, the DSTs (rapid tests if possible) should be ordered and results obtained at the earliest for starting appropriate treatment thus avoiding delay and its serious consequences.

Regimen for MDR-TB comprises of six drugs, i.e., kanamycin, levofloxacin, ethionamide, pyrazinamide, ethambutol, and cycloserine for 6–9 months of the intensive phase and four drugs, i.e., levofloxacin, ethionamide, ethambutol, and cycloserine to cover 18 months of the continuation phase. Work is on to start a shorter regime which also in addition uses Clofazimine for MDRTB; based on the encouraging experience from Bangladesh. Three drugs viz. para-aminosalicylic acid (PAS), moxifloxacin, and capreomycin are used as reserve/substitute drugs in this regimen. It is important to state that all such cases should only be treated by those who have experience of managing such cases. A detailed discussion on the topic is beyond the scope of this chapter and the readers are referred to other resources for the same. The IUATLD, WHO, and some others have provided useful guidance easily accessible via internet.[24]

PREVENTION

The only available vaccine against TB presently is BCG. It is a live-attenuated vaccine. Despite the variable protective effect (0–80%) and little ultimate effect on global TB control, its effect in preventing severe forms of TB like miliary and meningitis makes this vaccine presently indispensable. At the community level, factors predisposing to TB are poverty, HIV, poor access to health facilities, and overcrowding.

CHEMOPROPHYLAXIS

Isoniazid, as single drug, is recommended for chemoprophylaxis in asymptomatic children in contact with cases of infectious pulmonary TB. The recommended dose of INH as per RNTCP is 10 mg/kg administered daily for 6 months. Before considering a patient for chemoprophylaxis, every effort should be made to rule out tubercular disease. There should not be any clinical manifestations of disease (fever, cough, weight loss, anorexia, hepatosplenomegaly, lymphadenopathy, or pulmonary signs). Radiology may be done in doubtful cases. The indications of chemoprophylaxis in asymptomatic children include the following:
- Children less than 6 years of age with a smear-positive contact
- HIV-infected children with exposure to an infectious tubercular case or a positive (≥5 mm) TST
- TST-positive children receiving immunosuppressive therapy (e.g., on daily steroids or chemotherapy, etc.)
- Children of mothers having TB during pregnancy after ruling out congenital TB.

Childhood TB has its own distinct features and diagnostic pathway which is at variance from adults and needs to be understood. The nuances in treatment of TB in children are also highlighted.

REFERENCES

1. Chintu C, Mudenda V, Lucas S, et al. Lung diseases at necropsy in African children dying from respiratory illnesses: a descriptive necropsy study. Lancet. 2002;360(9338):985-90.
2. Marais BJ, Gie RP, Schaaf HS, et al. The natural history of childhood intra-thoracic tuberculosis: a critical review of literature from the pre-chemotherapy era. Int J Tuberc Lung Dis. 2004;8(4):392-402.
3. Lobato MN, Loeffler AM, Furst K, Cole B, Hopewell PC. Detection of Mycobacterium tuberculosis in gastric aspirates collected from children: hospitalization is not necessary. Pediatrics. 1998;102(4):E40.
4. Zar HJ, Hanslo D, Apolles P, Swingler G, Hussey G. Induced sputum versus gastric lavage for microbiological confirmation of pulmonary tuberculosis in infants and young children: a prospective study. Lancet. 2005;365(9454):130-4.
5. Ruiz Jiménez M, Guillén Martín S, Prieto Tato LM, et al. Induced sputum versus gastric lavage for the diagnosis of pulmonary tuberculosis in children. BMC Infect Dis. 2013;13:222.
6. Mukherjee A, Singh S, Lodha R, et al. Ambulatory gastric lavages provide better yields of Mycobacterium tuberculosis than induced sputum in children with intrathoracic tuberculosis. Pediatr Infect Dis J. 2013;32(12):1313-7.

7. Nicol MP, Workman L, Isaacs W, et al. Accuracy of the Xpert MTB/RIF test for the diagnosis of pulmonary tuberculosis in children admitted to hospital in Cape Town, South Africa: a descriptive study. Lancet Infect Dis. 2011;11(11):819-24.
8. Zar HJ, Workman L, Isaacs W, Dheda K, Zemanay W, Nicol MP. Rapid diagnosis of pulmonary tuberculosis in African children in a primary care setting by use of Xpert MTB/RIF on respiratory specimens: a prospective study. Lancet Glob Health. 2013;1(2):e97-104.
9. World Health Organization. Use of tuberculosis interferon-gamma release assays (IGRAs) in low- and middle-income countries: policy statement. Geneva: World Health Organization; 2011.
10. Jain SK, Ordonez A, Kinikar A, et al. Pediatric tuberculosis in young children in India: a prospective study. Biomed Res Int. 2013;2013:783698.
11. Zenebe Y, Anagaw B, Tesfay W, Debebe T, Gelaw B. Smear positive extra pulmonary tuberculosis disease at University of Gondar Hospital, Northwest Ethiopia. BMC Res Notes. 2013;6:21.
12. Tuon FF, Higashino HR, Lopes MI, et al. Adenosine deaminase and tuberculous meningitis—a systematic review with meta-analysis. Scand J Infect Dis. 2010;42:198-207.
13. Bose A, Kalita S, Rose W, Tharyan P. Intermittent versus daily therapy for treating tuberculosis in children. Cochrane Database Syst Rev. 2014;1:CD007953.
14. Standards of Tuberculosis care in India WHO 2014. Available from: http://www.tbcindia.nic.in/showfile.php?lid=3061[Accessed July, 2017].
15. Rapid Advice Treatment of tuberculosis in children. WHO 2010. Available from: http://apps.who.int/ [Accessed July, 2017].
16. New fixed-dose combinations for the treatment of TB in children. Available from: www.who.int/tb/FDC_Factsheet.pdf?ua=1 [Accessed July, 2017].
17. Donald PR. Antituberculosis drug induced hepatotoxicity in children. Pediatr Rep. 2011;3(2):e-16.
18. World Health Organization. (2016). Global tuberculous report 2016. [online] Available from: http://www.who.int/tb/publications/global_report/gtbr2016_executive_summary.pdf [Accessed July, 2017].
19. Mukherjee JS, Joseph JK, Rich ML, et al. Clinical and programmatic considerations in the treatment of MDR-TB in children: a series of 16 patients from Lima, Peru. Int J Tuberc Lung Dis. 2003;7(7):637-44.
20. Schaaf HS, Shean K, Donald PR. Culture confirmed multidrug resistant tuberculosis: diagnostic delay, clinical features, and outcome. Arch Dis Child. 2003;88(12):1106-11.
21. Schaaf HS, Gie RP, Beyers N, Sirgel FA, de Klerk PJ, Donald PR. Primary drug-resistant tuberculosis in children. Int J Tuberc Lung Dis. 2000;4(12):1149-55.
22. Drobac PC, Mukherjee JS, Joseph JK, et al. Community-based therapy for children with multidrug-resistant tuberculosis. Pediatrics. 2006;117(6):2022-9.
23. Fishman JE, Sais GJ, Schwartz DS, Otten J. Radiographic findings and patterns in multidrug-resistant tuberculosis. J Thorac Imaging. 1998;13(1):65-71.
24. Curry International Tuberculosis Center. (2011). Drug-resistant tuberculosis: a survival guide for clinicians. [online] Available from: http://www.currytbcenter.ucsf.edu/sites/default/files/mdrtb_book_2011_1.pdf. [Accessed February, 2016].

CHAPTER 13
Tuberculosis in Immunocompromised

Vesna Škodrić Trifunović

INTRODUCTION

Tuberculosis (TB) is still, at the beginning of the 21st century, most widespread infectious disease. It is estimated that one-third of humanity is infected with *Mycobacterium tuberculosis*. Every year, 9 million, are newly infected and about 2 million people die.[1,2] The largest number of people infected live in poor parts of the world, sub-Saharan Africa, Southeast Asia, and Latin America.

In the modern world, there are many factors that impair the immune balance and thereby increase the risk of developing TB. Even despite prevention measures and implementation of powerful anti-TB drugs, TB still represents big social and health problem. Application of new developments in medicine, such as organ transplantation, long-term use of immunosuppressive therapy in the treatment of various diseases, dialysis, and successful treatment of malignant diseases, contributed to extension of life expectancy, but in the same time contributed to development of different, long-term secondary immunodeficient states. Besides this, there is a growing number of human immunodeficiency virus (HIV)-positive people, as well as an increasing number of diabetic patients with general decline in the resistance of the organism.[3] Algorithm of the clinical spectrum of immunodeficient condition is shown in flowchart 1.[3]

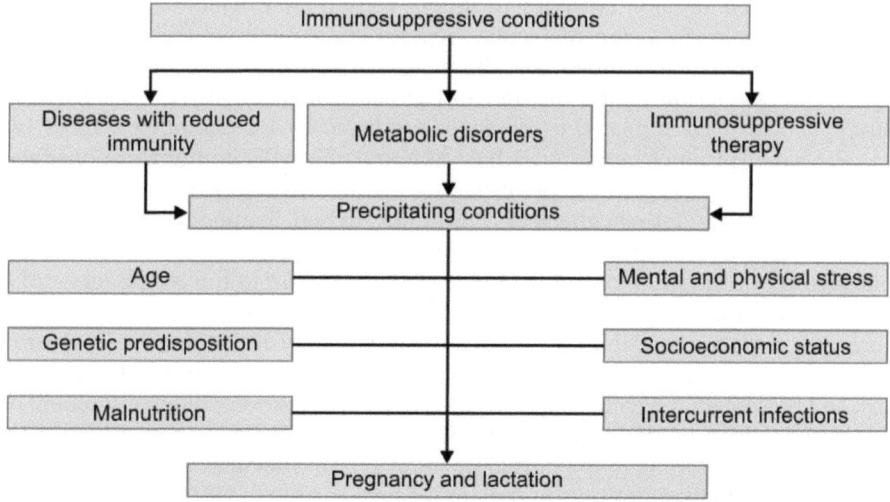

FLOWCHART 1: Algorithm of the clinical spectrum of immunodeficient states.

In immunocompetent persons, the greatest risk of progression of infection to active disease is during the first 2 years after the infection, and over time the risk is reduced in proportion to the time elapsed.[4] However, in people with compromised cellular immunity period from infection to the development of the disease is much shorter compared to people with intact immune system.[5]

The importance of recognizing TB in these immunodeficient states is that its clinical-radiological picture is uncharacteristic and often masked by symptoms and signs of underlying disease.[3] Therefore, immunocompromised people should be actively supervised by a doctor for early detection and commencement of treatment.

TUBERCULOSIS AND HUMAN IMMUNODEFICIENCY VIRUS INFECTION

Although the association between TB and acquired immunodeficiency syndrome (AIDS) was described early, soon after discovery of the first case of AIDS, this extremely important phenomenon has not received sufficient attention until the early 1990s of the 20th century.

Infection with HIV is the strongest known risk factor for progression of latent TB to active disease. Incidence of TB in people with AIDS is 20 times higher than in the general population. Clinical presentation of TB in HIV-infected person is dramatically different than in immunocompetent people. It is the most common disease associated with HIV in which the life of the patient is directly threatened and often it is the first clinical manifestation of AIDS.[2,6] In HIV-positive, TB usually occurs without pre-existing AIDS mainly because of the fact that *M. tuberculosis* is more virulent than other pathogens associated with HIV infection such as *Pneumocystis carinii* and *M. avium* complex. Mild immunosuppression (CD4 count between 250–500 cells/mm^3) allows the occurrence of TB, and therefore TB is considered for the first indication of HIV infection because it occurs before the awakening of opportunistic infections (*P. carinii*, *M. avium* complex, and cryptococcosis) which are characteristic of severe immunosuppression (CD4 50–125/mm^3).[7] Intensity and extent of symptoms of TB are more pronounced in HIV-positive than in HIV-negative and rapid fatal outcome is very likely if treatment is not started immediately.

People infected with HIV are at significantly higher risk of primary TB, the reactivation of latent TB or new episodes of illness caused by exogenous reinfection than HIV-negative people. By using molecular fingerprinting methods (restriction fragment length polymorphism), it is unequivocally demonstrated that exogenous reinfection is predominantly responsible for the recurrence of retreatment TB among HIV-positive people.[8]

Susceptibility to TB is related to cytokines produced by T lymphocytes. The T helper (Th)-1 cells, which produce interferon-γ, have a central role in the immune response against *Mycobacterium*. Unlike Th1 cells, Th2 cells produce interleukin (IL)-4 and IL-10 and do not contribute to the antimycobacterial immunity. When lymphocytes of HIV-infected individuals with TB are exposed to *M. tuberculosis in vitro*, they produced less amounts of γ-interferon but the same of IL-4 and IL-10 in comparison to the lymphocytes of HIV-negative patients suffering from TB. These data suggest the possibility that a reduced Th1 cells immune response contributes to increased susceptibility of HIV-positive people to TB.[7]

As HIV infection primarily damages the function of CD4+ T lymphocytes and macrophages, and preservation of cellular immunity is required to prevent the development of the clinical manifestation of TB, it is considered that the HIV infection is now the most potent of all known factors leading to the development of TB. On the other hand, active TB leads to stimulation of cellular immunity and therefore propagation of HIV infection and further deepening of immunosuppression, since HIV replicates mostly in activated lymphocytes.[2,9]

Clinical Forms: Pulmonary and Extrapulmonary

The HIV-infected pulmonary forms of TB significantly give way to extrapulmonary forms of the disease. Frequency of extrapulmonary TB ranges from 40 to 80% and increases with the severity of immunosuppression, compared with 10–20% of HIV-uninfected.[10] Disseminated disease and lymphadenitis are extremely rare in patients without HIV infection, and have been observed in 20–40% of TB and HIV-coinfected patients.[11]

Cervical, supraclavicular, and axillary lymph nodes are often the localization of peripheral lymphadenitis. Intrathoracic and intra-abdominal lymph nodes, which are otherwise rare place for TB in HIV-negative individuals, are often affected in HIV-positive with advanced immune deficiency. In HIV-positive, lymph nodes affected by tuberculous infection have an increased tendency for the formation of caseous necrosis, which leads to frequent abscess formation, fistula, and unusual localization of infection. Retroperitoneal lymph nodes may erode into the wall of the stomach or pancreatic cancer, mediastinal lymph glands in the esophagus, trachea or bronchus, and mesenteric lymph nodes in the lower intestine.[11]

Involvement of the central nervous system (CNS) occurs in 5–10% of HIV-positive patients with TB. The most common is meningitis but brain tuberculoma often occurs as well. Involvement of the pleura, pericardium, skin, and soft tissue (e.g., abscess of the breast, skin, liver, kidney, etc.) may occur as result of hematogenous dissemination of *Mycobacterium*. The bone marrow may also be affected, which should be considered especially when associated fever (above 39.5°C), chest X-ray, signs of miliary spread to the lungs and elevated serum alkaline phosphatase, and lactate dehydrogenase in serum.[11]

In general, those with higher count of CD4+ lymphocytes (>200/mL) often have classical clinical picture of TB, while those with lower CD4+ counts (<200/mL) are often atypical. In fact, some atypical presentations of TB in HIV-positive look like typical clinical presentation of the primary disease, very well known to pediatricians.[12]

Diagnosis of Tuberculosis in Human Immunodeficiency Virus-positive

Since manifestations of TB in HIV-positive are often nonspecific, the diagnosis of TB is sometimes very difficult. Decreased tuberculin skin sensitivity, atypical radiographic appearance, other infections associated with HIV, all together may mask TB. Mistake not to suspect TB is the most common reason for late diagnosis. Tuberculosis must be considered when a person infected with HIV has one or more of the following: fever, cough, pulmonary infiltrates, lymphadenopathy, meningitis, brain abscess, pericarditis, pleural effusion, or intra-abdominal, musculoskeletal, and skin abscesses. The probability of reactivation of TB is increased among HIV-positive patients who had previously suffered from TB, whose tuberculin skin test is positive, or who have emigrated from countries or belong to racial or ethnic group with a high prevalence of TB. A recent hospitalization in a hospital with nosocomial epidemic of TB, homelessness, intravenous drug abuse, alcoholism, and recent stay in prison, also have to be seriously considered as risk factors of TB reactivation.[13]

Chest radiographic findings correlate with the degree of immunosuppression caused by HIV infection. Among patients with relatively well-preserved immune system (CD4 >200/mL) with a positive tuberculin skin reaction and no other infections associated with HIV, X-ray findings are often identical to the ones in immunocompetent patients, including cavitations and infiltrates in the upper lobes. In contrast, in people with severe immunodeficiency, chest X-ray findings resemble findings seen in primary TB of immunocompetent patients, such as hilar adenopathy and pleural effusion or even signs or miliary scattering.[7,12] Normal chest radiographic findings do not exclude the diagnosis of pulmonary TB since radiographic signs may be well behind rapid evolution of active disease.[6]

In patients with intrathoracic lymphadenopathy, findings of computed tomography (CT) of the chest usually indicate packets of enlarged lymph glands often with central areas of low density corresponding to caseous necrosis. In patients with disseminated TB, CT scan of the abdomen shows intra-abdominal lymphadenopathy and focal lesions of the liver or spleen. In case of CNS involvement, findings are hypodense zones in brain mass.[12,14]

Sputum smear is positive in 30–70% of HIV-positive patients with TB. In patients with less advanced immunodeficiency, in whom radiographic findings correspond to changes in postprimary TB, smear sensitivity is similar to one in immunocompetent patients with postprimary TB. In HIV-positive patients with more advanced immunodeficiency, in whom radiographic changes are characteristic of primary or miliary TB, smear sensitivity for *Mycobacterium* is lower than in immunocompetent adults.[10,13]

Conventional microbiological methods for the detection of *M. tuberculosis* are often not fast enough, so, the treatment of active TB in HIV-infected should start as soon as possible. Polymerase chain reaction can detect *M. tuberculosis* in 6–8 hours, and even better, nucleic acid hybridization techniques can identify *Mycobacterium* complex after only 2 hours which make these two methods very helpful in early detection of *M. tuberculosis*.[13] Rapid diagnostic tests are expensive and are used only when it is necessary to make an urgent decision on initiation of treatment or use of other diagnostic procedures.

Treatment of Tuberculosis and Human Immunodeficiency Virus Together

In HIV-positive patients with TB, the priority is to treat TB, especially pulmonary TB with positive sputum smear due to the need to interrupt transmission of TB. However, patients with TB associated with HIV can be simultaneously treated with antiretroviral therapy and anti-TB drugs. Deciding when to begin antiretroviral therapy needs careful assessment. For example, in the case of a patient who is at high risk of dying during the treatment of TB (i.e., disseminated TB and/or CD4 count <200/mm^3), it may be necessary to simultaneously treat the patient with anti-TB and antiretroviral therapy.[15] On the other hand, for patients with pulmonary TB as the first manifestation of HIV infection, which does not seem to have a high risk of death, it can be safely to postpone beginning antiretroviral therapy while not completed the initial phase of the treatment of TB. This reduces the risk of immune reconstitution syndrome and avoids the drug interactions.[13,16]

Preventive therapy in HIV-positive individuals is of 12 months. The daily dose of isoniazid is 10 mg/kg for adults and 5 mg/kg for children. Alternatively, administration of isoniazid and rifampicin can be applied every 3 months.

TUBERCULOSIS AND MALIGNANCY

Advanced carcinomas are accompanied by immune system disorders. Moreover, the extent of malignant disease is closely related to the degree of immune dysfunction. Experimental data indicate defects in the function of T- and B-lymphocytes, as well as disorders of macrophages, in the etiology of reduced immune capacity in patients suffering from cancer. Additionally, chemotherapy and radiation primary damage proliferating cells, including mature lymphocytes and their precursors in the bone marrow, which cause long-term immunosuppression. Loss of immunity induced by either local or systemic effects of tumor and/or by applied radio and chemotherapy is important for the reactivation of TB, which significantly contributes to the mortality of cancer patients.[17,18]

Tuberculosis is most common in hematological malignancies, followed by lung cancer, breast cancer, and gastrointestinal tract cancers. It is not uncommon for lung tumors to destroy places of latent TB and induce reactivation of dormant *M. tuberculosis* in the field of secondary immunodeficiency caused by malignant disease.[18]

Coexistence of TB and lung cancer may lead to diagnostic dilemmas since symptoms and signs of both diseases are often similar. This may cause delays in making timely diagnosis and starting early treatment which might lead to poor prognosis.[18]

METABOLIC DISORDERS AS RISK FACTORS

There are many diseases and metabolic disorders that are considered for important risk factors for awakening latent foci of TB. Special significance, due to their frequency and their impact on immune system, have metabolic disorders that occur in diabetes mellitus (DM), chronic ethylisme, chronic renal failure, liver disease, hyperthyroidism, malnutrition, etc.

Tuberculosis and Diabetes Mellitus

It is well known that DM increases the risk of infections of different etiology. It is believed that with more pronounced glucose intolerance and complications in organs and blood vessels, there is a greater tendency to reactivation of TB. The disorder in the metabolism of carbohydrates leads to the development of ketosis, ketoacidosis, and shifts of acid-base status toward the acidic one, thus reducing the mobility of alveolar macrophages and their role in phagocytosis. On the other hand, infection, in this case of TB acts as a stress factor and activates the adrenal glands to secrete adrenaline and cortisol, which further worsens glycemic regulation. All this together, adversely affects the formation of antibodies, the function of polymorphonuclear cells, and macrophages.[18] Tuberculosis among people with DM is two to three times higher compared to those with no diabetes.[19,20]

In this group of patients, radiographic patterns might be altered. Thus, TB in diabetics often presents as a lower lung involvement on chest X-ray. This is important because atypical radiographic findings in these patients might be misdiagnosed as a lung cancer or community-acquired pneumonia which might further lead to initiation of wrong therapy and loss of precious time for these patients. Also, chest X-ray in diabetics can show multilobar disease and presence of multiple cavities.[21-23]

It is also important to mention that treatment failure and death are more frequent in diabetics, though it is not completely understood if it is because of increased severity of TB in these patients or because of comorbidities associated with DM.[24]

Growing number of diabetics that was estimated to be 285 million in 2010 and an expected increase to 439 million by 2030 does not indicate a good epidemiological situation in the future.[25] Experts are concerned about the growing epidemic of DM and TB, especially in poor and developing countries, where there is the fastest growing prevalence of DM but also the highest rate of TB incidence of the world.[26]

Tuberculosis in Patients with Chronic Renal Insufficiency

Nephropathy, dialysis, and kidney transplants are well known risk factors for awakening dormant forms of *M. tuberculosis* from latent foci. The incidence of TB in patients with chronic renal insufficiency is significantly higher than in the general population, which is especially important in regions where TB is endemic.[27]

Immunosuppression in this disease is caused not only by the underlying disease but also by toxic effects of nitrogen metabolites and application of immunosuppressive drugs (cyclosporine, azathioprine, corticosteroids).[18,28] Other conditions that can occur within the clinical picture of chronic renal failure and may contribute to lower immunity are malnutrition, vitamin D deficiency, and hyperparathyroidism.[27,29]

Difficulties in identifying TB in renal patients are due to atypical clinical pictures with few respiratory symptoms and mostly general signs and symptoms. Tuberculosis in these patients should be considered if they report fatigue, fever, anorexia, malaise, cough, weight loss, and if there is no positive therapeutic response to conventional antibiotics. Extrapulmonary TB is common in patients with terminal renal disease, and lymph nodes are the most common extrapulmonary localization. Radiological findings may be atypical for TB, may occur as a lung scattering in the lower lung fields, miliary scattering, or as extrapulmonary forms.[18]

Any patient with chronic kidney disease and a history of TB infection or with an abnormal chest X-ray consistent with past TB should be monitored on regular basis and referred to pulmonologist as needed. Using tuberculin skin test for routine screening of patients with chronic kidney disease or those on hemodialysis is not recommended but assessment of individual patient risk of developing active TB may be helpful.[27]

Recommended chemoprophylaxis in this group of patients is to use isoniazid 300 mg daily for 6 months or isoniazid plus rifampicin for 3 months or rifampicin alone for 4-6 months. Pyridoxine 10-25 mg daily should always be given with isoniazid in order to prevent neuropathy.[27]

TUBERCULOSIS AS A RESULT OF THE APPLICATION OF IMMUNOSUPPRESSIVE THERAPY

Immunosuppressive therapy used in management of many chronic and malignant diseases and conditions after organ transplantation significantly prolongs life of many patients, but in the same time creates iatrogenic immunodeficiency which contributes to the increased risk of developing TB. Drugs that are commonly used as immunosuppressive therapy are corticosteroids, methotrexate, cyclophosphamide, and inhibitors of TNF-α (infliximab, etanercept, and adalimumab).

Corticosteroids

Immunosuppressive effects of corticosteroids are the least selective, affecting the entire leukocyte cell lineage, including B and T lymphocytes, macrophages, granulocytes, and monocytes. In addition, glucocorticoids suppress the immune response by inhibiting release of vasoactive and chemotactic substances, as well as the ability of neutrophils to adhere to the endothelium and cause vasodilation and chemotaxis.[30] High doses of corticosteroids also reduce antigen-presenting cell function and thereby increase the risk of uncontrolled growth and spread of low virulent strains of bacteria, viruses, fungi, and mycobacteria, and lead to clinical presentation of infection without pronounced signs and symptoms of inflammation.[31]

The risk of developing TB is increased by about 12 times in patients receiving long-term corticosteroid therapy, and the risk begins increasing after only 1 month of corticosteroid therapy at a dose greater than 15 mg/day.[31]

Based on mentioned above, there is dilemma if patients on prolonged corticosteroid therapy should be given chemoprophylactic medications or it is sufficient just to increase observation of these patients. In areas with a high degree of multidrug-resistant TB, chemoprophylaxis would probably not yield the expected results so only regular monitoring of these patients for early detection of TB is recommended.[32]

Methotrexate

Methotrexate is used in the treatment of severe forms of psoriasis, rheumatoid arthritis, leukemia in children, non-Hodgkin's lymphoma, and a large number of solid tumors. The use of low-dose methotrexate, especially when used in combination with a corticosteroid, is an important risk factor for the reactivation of TB.[30] Due to the increasing use of low-dose methotrexate in the treatment of rheumatoid arthritis, as well as its combination with corticosteroids, it is necessary that doctors who follow these patients always have in mind the possibility of this complication.

Drugs Used in Treatment of Connective Tissue Diseases

Although systemic connective tissue diseases are commonly associated with mild and nonspecific infections, drugs used to control this group of diseases can lead to severe immunosuppression, and subsequent development of pulmonary and systemic infections. Traditional protocol for treatment of systemic collagen diseases includes corticosteroids, methotrexate, and cyclophosphamide. New drugs used for the treatment of collagen-vascular diseases are inhibitors of tumor necrosis factor-α (TNF-α). These drugs are very effective in reducing and slowing down degenerative changes in inflammatory arthritis as well as changes in granulomatous diseases. Several inhibitors of TNF-α so far approved and most widely and successfully employed are infliximab, etanercept, and adalimumab.[33,34]

The formation of granulomas is a common feature of many collagen-vascular diseases. The measure of effectiveness of TNF-α inhibitors is their ability to facilitate dissolution of granulomas.[35] However, TNF-α inhibitors are not able to differentiate between pathological granulomas in collagen-vascular diseases and granulomas created to control specific infectious diseases such as TB.[36] As a result of TNF-α inhibitors, there is dissolution of pathological and protective granulomas.

Tumor necrosis factor-α is an essential cytokine in the formation and maintenance of granulomas. Macrophages and T-lymphocytes produce TNF in response to an interaction with a number of pathogens, which further stimulates the production and release of IL-1 and other inflammatory cytokines, chemokines, and adhesion molecules which all together attract and activate cells necessary for formation of granulomas.[37] Blockade of TNF-α, either by switching off TNF receptors or administrating neutralizing TNF antibodies, leads to incomplete formation or degradation of previously formed granulomas. It is proved that TNF is necessary to maintain the integrity of the already formed granulomas in latent TB, and application of neutralizing antibodies against TNF leads to a rapid reactivation of TB infection.[38]

Most reported cases of infection (TB, histoplasmosis, aspergillosis, listeriosis, and cryptococcosis) were associated with infliximab. There are several possible reasons for this. Infliximab is a most potent inhibitor of TNF-α that acts by binding soluble and transmembrane forms of TNF-α, and thus prevents a remote interaction with the cellular receptors, the p55 and p75.[38] Also, infliximab is administered as a bolus injection leading to high-peak serum concentrations, which can temporarily shut down the cell-mediated immunity and allow the pathogen to escape immune sequestration. In contrast, adalimumab and etanercept are administered subcutaneously and thus achieve lower peak serum levels which are less likely to disrupt the immune system.[39]

The incidence of active TB after induction of anti-TNF therapy with infliximab is four to five times higher than in the general population.[40,41] The clinical picture of active TB after inducing infliximab develops rapidly, averagely in 12 weeks, and 98% of cases of active TB occur over a period of 6 months after the application of an inhibitor of TNF-α.[42] The incidence of serious, life-threatening TB, as well as disseminated forms of disease is greater than in patients not treated with anti-TNF agents. Exclusion of active TB and treatment of latent TB infection are the basis for the safe induction of anti-TNF therapy.[40]

The sensitivity of the tuberculin skin test used in diagnosis of latent TB infection is compromised in patients on immunosuppressive therapy and gives a large number of false-negative results. Since, most of the patients who are candidates for anti-TNF therapy are already on some kind of immunosuppressive therapy, tuberculin skin tests are not suitable for screening of latent TB infection in these patients. In the absence of screening tests for latent TB, which would represent the gold standard, before applying anti-TNF therapy it is necessary to assess the risk of latent TB activation. It can be done by checking the history of the previous active TB, assessing the risk of infection caused by contact with patients with active TB, or by chest radiography for the detection of residues of previous TB.[43]

TUBERCULOSIS AFTER ORGAN AND TISSUE TRANSPLANTATION

The total risk for the development of pulmonary infection in organ and tissue recipients depends on many factors including the degree of iatrogenic immunosuppression, type of transplant, type of immunosuppressive therapy, epidemiological situation of the region, and exposure to specific pathogens.[44] Majority of these patients also have additional health conditions, such as diabetes, renal insufficiency, malnutrition, and other diseases, which further increase the risk of infection. It has been shown that already existing virus infection, such as Epstein-Barr virus, cytomegalovirus, HIV, hepatitis C virus infection, increase the tendency of the recipient to bacterial and fungal infections.[45] There are other factors too, for example, in lung transplantation mucociliary clearance might be decreased due to bronchial constrictions at the site of anastomosis or denervation of the graft with decrease in cough reflex. Passive transmission of infection from donor to recipient is also possible.

Compared to other causes of post-transplantation pneumonia, a lung infection caused by *M. tuberculosis* and other atypical mycobacteria are rare, only 2% of all post-transplantation pneumonia. However, what gives the importance to this condition is that the risk of developing TB is almost 70 times higher among organ recipients than in the general population.[46,47]

Tuberculosis in organ recipients may develop due to reactivation of latent foci, nosocomial infection, or direct transmission from cadaveric or living donor infected with *M. tuberculosis*. Nosocomial infection and transmission from the donor can be proven by modern methods such as DNA fingerprinting. However, most cases of transplanted TB are result of awakening of latent form. Nearly 50% of organ recipients who are suffering from transplanted TB have pulmonary form of the disease, and about one-third develops disseminated TB.

All potential organ recipients should have tuberculin skin test done before organ transplantation. Although up to 70% of patients may be nonreactive, those with positive tests are considered to be at high risk.

Isoniazid prophylaxis should be considered in recipients with a positive tuberculin skin test (induration equal to or greater than 5 mm), radiology visible sequelae of an old active TB, inadequate data about treatment of previous TB in recipient or donor, data on close contact with infectious patient, or in newly infected (tuberculin skin test conversion to positive). Hepatotoxicity caused by isoniazid, a relatively rare development of TB in nonendemic areas and the existence of effective treatment of active TB are the most common arguments against routine chemoprophylaxis after organ transplantation.[48,49] On the other side, close to one-third of recipients with TB, die and roughly the same number experience allograft rejection. Although TB in these patients is curable when detected on time, unusual disease presentation often delays the diagnosis and large number of cases is discovered only at autopsy table. Therefore, chemoprophylaxis of TB after organ transplantation certainly should be considered in high-risk group. The current recommendation for prophylaxis is 9-month course of isoniazid.[50]

CASE STUDY 1

A 53-year-old female has been treated for systemic vasculitis with immunosuppressive therapy since 2001 (pulse doses of cyclophosphamide XII cycle, mycophenolate mofetil 750 mg for 4 years, prednisone 15 mg/day for several years). Dry cough, occasional fever, loss of appetite, and weight loss started 8 months before admission. The patient previously has been treated at a local hospital for suspected bilateral pneumonia. At the admission to the clinic in July 2012, she was in good general condition, without signs of respiratory insufficiency (spirometry detected mild airflow obstruction); the laboratory analysis showed mildly accelerated erythrocyte sedimentation rate (ESR), leukocytosis (13.3×10^9/L), and slightly elevated nitrogen materials.

Chest X-ray revealed inhomogeneous, poorly delineated, shadows in lower lung fields suggestive to bilateral pneumonia (Fig. 1). Bronchoscopy was preformed and signs of inflammation were seen. Sputum smear microscopy showed acid-fast bacilli (AFB); cultures of sputum were positive for *M. tuberculosis* (100 colonies). The treatment for TB was started.

Comment: In this case, TB was manifested with atypical radiographic picture, so the patient initially was treated as from pneumonia.

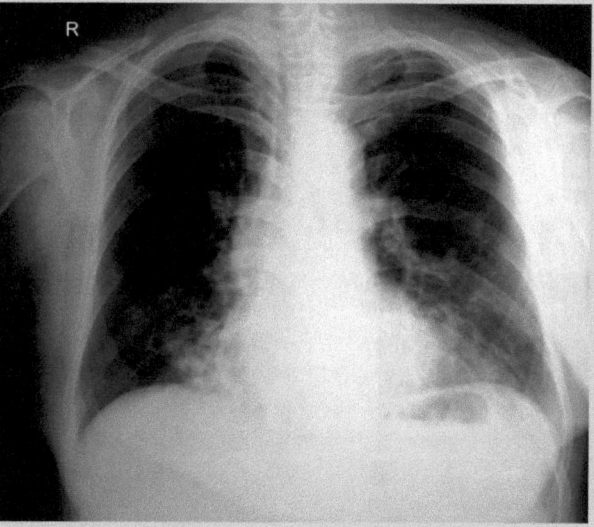

FIG. 1: Chest X-ray findings: Bilateral finely granular/miliary appearance; in lower lung fields hyperintensity and inhomogeneous shadowing.

CASE STUDY 2

A 48-year-old male became ill 10 days prior to admission to the hospital with fever (up to 39.7°C), dry cough, and weight loss of 5 kg. The patient had a history of alcohol consumption. At the admission to the hospital, the patient was confused, disoriented, dyspneic, tachypneic, cyanotic, no signs of heart failure, without peripheral lymphadenopathy, giving the impression of critically ill patient. Chest X-ray shows bilateral, symmetrical miliary shadows in lung's parenchyma and tomography revealed annular shadows in the right upper lobe (Figs. 2 and 3).

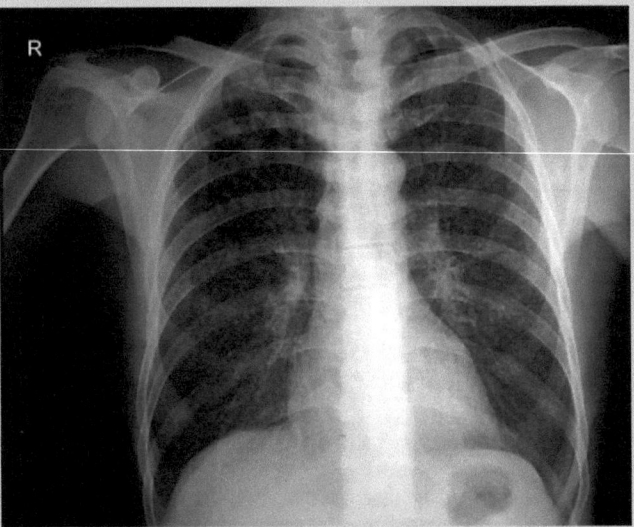

FIG. 2: Chest X-ray: Bilateral, symmetrical miliary shadows in lung's parenchyma.

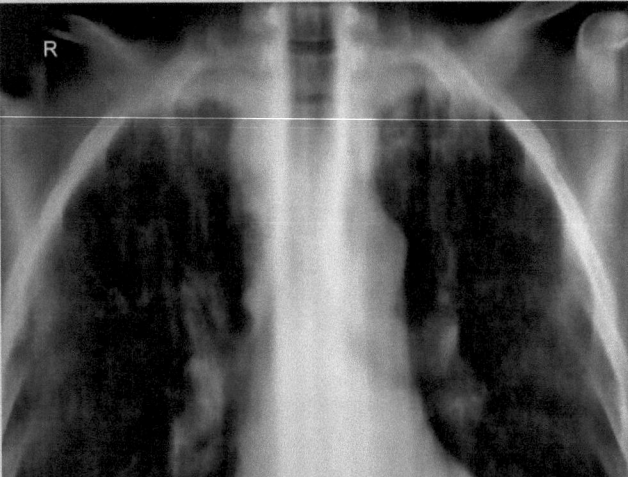

FIG. 3: Tomography: Annular shadows in the right upper lobe.

In laboratory results: Lymphopenia (9.8%; absolute number 0.8×10^9/L), mild anemia, (red blood cells: 3.53×10^{12}/L, hemoglobin 106 g/L, hematocrit: 0.313) and thrombocytopenia (132×10^9/L) were found. Elevated aspartate aminotransferase (164 U/L), alanine aminotransferase (108 U/L), alkaline phosphatase (161 U/L) and γ-glutamyl transferase (136 U/L) serum levels were detected. Ultrasound of the abdomen revealed slightly enlarged spleen, while the other findings were normal. Acid-fast bacilli were observed in the sputum, while urine and blood cultures were positive. Drug susceptibility testing showed *M. tuberculosis* sensitive to first-line TB drugs. Blood was taken for HIV testing and it gave positive results; further treatment of TB and HIV infection was continued in the center for HIV infection. Magnetic resonance imaging of the brain revealed multiple, focal lesions located supra- and infratentorial, cortical and subcortical; those lesions may be TB granulomas, which are common in miliary TB. The diagnosis was generalized miliary TB (Fig. 4). Conducted tests confirmed the presence of TB in the lungs, CNS, and kidneys.

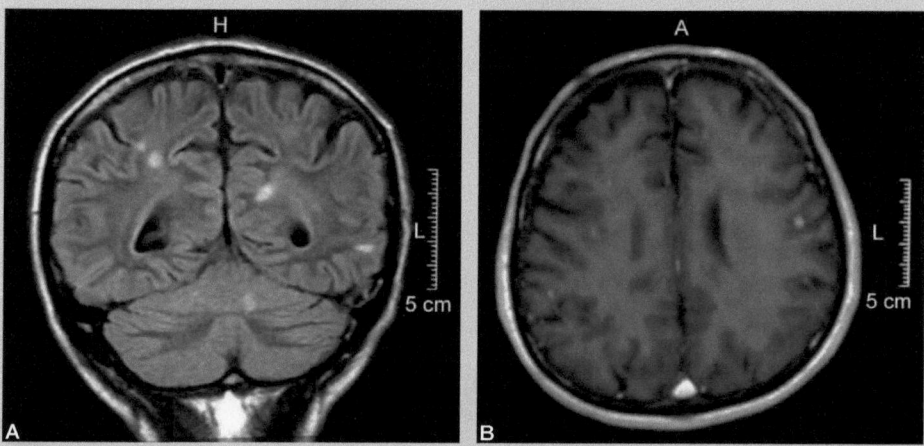

FIG. 4: A and **B,** Magnetic resonance imaging of the brain: Multiple, focal lesions located supra- and infratentorial, cortical and subcortical; those lesions may be tuberculosis granulomas, which are common in miliary tuberculosis.

CASE STUDY 3

A 62-year-old male has been treated for progressive systemic sclerosis (methotrexate 7.5 mg weekly) since 2006 and for hypothyroidism since 2008. Three months prior to admission, his main complains were dry cough, shortness of breath, and intensified fatigue on exertion. At the admission to the clinic (September 2013), the patient was in good general condition without signs of respiratory failure.

On chest X-ray, striped-patchy shadows in the right lower lung field can be seen (Fig. 5). Computed tomography of the chest revealed bilateral reticular changes in the lung parenchyma, mediastinal lymphadenopathy, and subcarinal lymph nodes enlargement (Fig. 6).

Biochemical analysis: Accelerated ESR (90/h), mild anemia, and hypoalbuminemia, while other results were in normal range. Spirometry results were normal and there was mild reduction in diffusion tests for carbon monoxide (DLCO 63%, KCO 83%). Sputum culture was positive. Genotyping showed that it was *M. tuberculosis*; drug susceptibility testing showed *M. tuberculosis* sensitive to first-line TB drugs. Standard TB treatment was applied.

Comment: In this case, pulmonary TB was a result of immunodeficiency due to long-term immunosuppressive therapy, but also because of progressive systemic sclerosis as well.

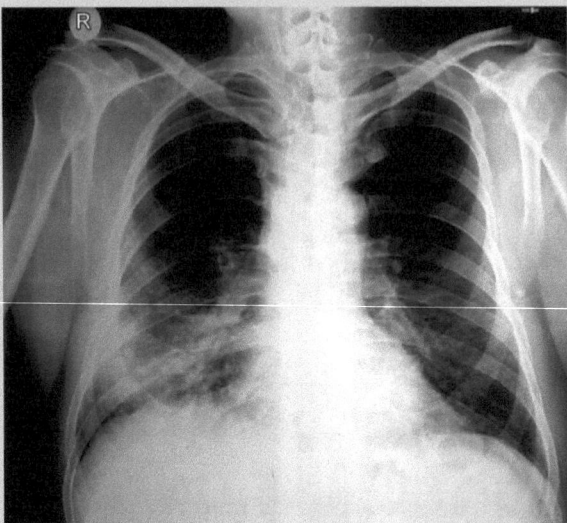

FIG. 5: Chest X-ray: Striped-patchy shadows in the right lower lung field.

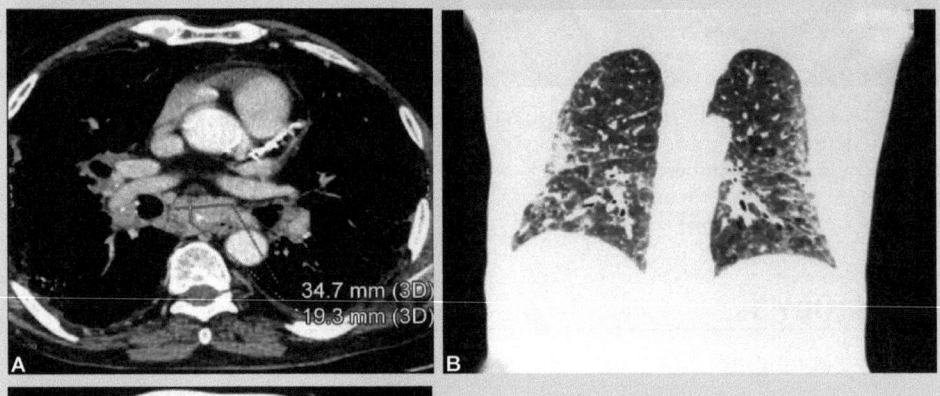

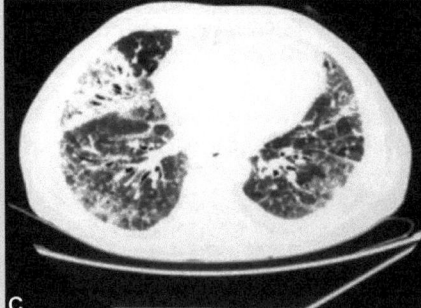

FIG. 6: A to **C,** Computed tomography of the chest: Bilateral reticular changes in the lung parenchyma with craniocaudal propagation; in the lower lobes more dense fibrotic changes with traction bronchiectasis and small zones of ground-glass opacities. In the left pleural space fluid collection about 15 mm thick, mediastinal lymphadenopathy with lymph nodes up to 20 mm in diameter, and conglomerate of subcarinal lymph nodes with dimensions of 35 × 20 mm.

CASE STUDY 4

A 60-year-old female diagnosed with Crohn's disease in 2000 and resection of the colon in the same year due to primary disease. After this the patient was on chronic immunosuppressive and anti-inflammatory therapy. Ten months prior to admission, she had symptoms such as shortness of breath, pain in the right half of the chest, cough with whitish sputum, and occasionally blood-stained content. She was admitted to the clinic in June 2013 to clarify nature of changes in the right lung suspected for tumor. At the admission, patient was in good general condition without signs of respiratory failure. Chest X-ray and CT scan revealed tumor-like infiltration in the upper right lung lobe with excavation (Figs. 7 and 8). Laboratory studies showed signs of inflammatory syndrome [C-reactive protein (CRP) 19.7, ESR 78/h].

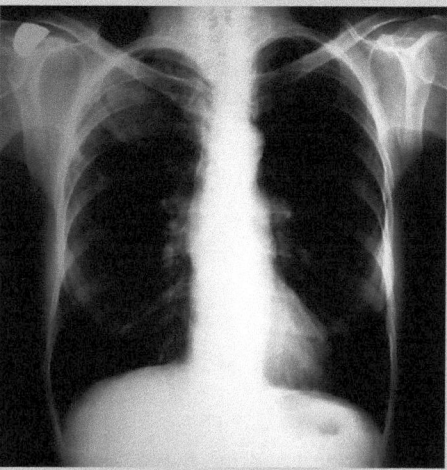

FIG. 7: Chest X-ray: Tumor-like infiltration in the upper right lung lobe with suspected excavation.

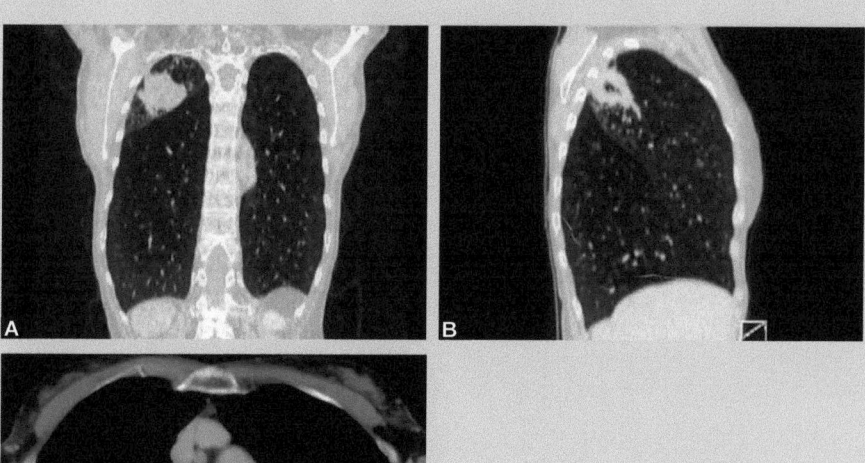

FIG. 8: A to **C,** Computed tomography of the chest: In posterior segment of the right lung, a mass was seen with central colliquation while in the lower left lobe was mass of 15 mm in diameter.

and mild anemia. Bronchoscopy was performed twice and results showed indirect signs of possibly neoplastic process, without histopathologic verification. Percutaneous biopsy of infiltration in the right lung was done, but histopathologic findings were still unreliable. It was decided to perform diagnostic-therapeutic surgical thoracotomy. The patient underwent right upper lobectomy and histopathologic findings showed: pulmonary caseous TB (Fig. 9), bronchiectasis (Fig. 10), granulomatous caseous lymphadenitis. Standard TB treatment was applied.

Comment: Both radiographic and bronchoscopic findings were highly suggestive of lung cancer, therefore patient underwent surgery. Histological findings were clinically unexpected.

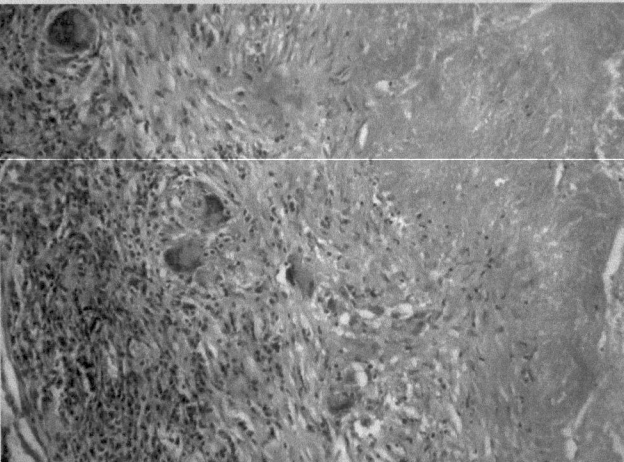

FIG. 9: Histopathology findings: Lung parenchyma (H ×20): Specific granuloma with predominant caseous necrosis surrounded by giant cells of Langhans type. *(For color version, see Plate 12)*

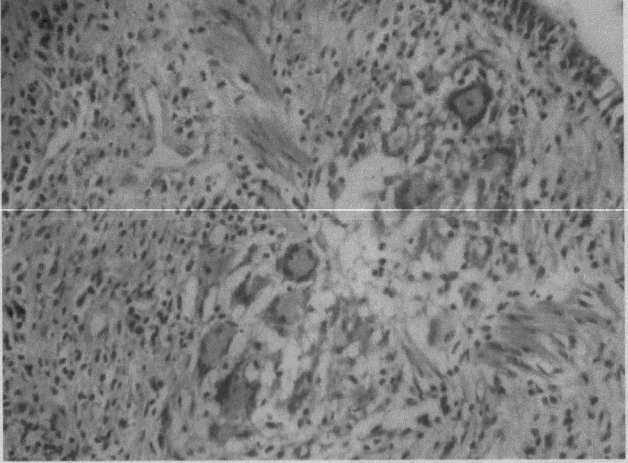

FIG. 10: Histopathology findings (H ×20): Specific bronchiectasis: In bronchial wall are present numerous productive granulomas consisted of epitheloid hystiocytes and giant cells of Langhans type. *(For color version, see Plate 12)*

Courtesy: Pathologist Jelena Stojsic, Department of pathology, Clinical Center of Serbia, Belgrade, Serbia.

CASE STUDY 5

A 47-year-old male was diagnosed with lung adenocarcinoma in 2010. It was treated surgically—lobectomy of the left upper lobe. Adjuvant chemotherapy was given (six cycles). In meantime, metastatic deposits in the CNS were diagnosed and treated with surgical resection. After brain surgery, patient got fever (up to 37.5°C), productive cough, and weight loss. At the admission in October 2013, patient was in good general condition without signs of respiratory failure. Chest X-ray: in the remaining part of the left lung diffuse blotchy partly confluent shadowing was noticed (Fig. 11). The CT of the chest: diffuse zones of consolidation, with excavations in the remaining part of the left lung. Laboratory studies: ESR accelerated, mild anemia. Direct microscopy of sputum samples showed AFB in large numbers. Standard TB treatment was initiated, but patient died few months later due to lung cancer progression.

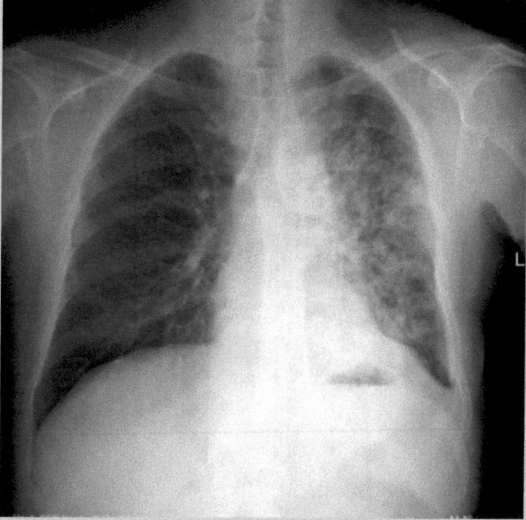

FIG. 11: Chest X-ray: In the remaining part of the left lung diffuse blotchy partly confluent shadowing was noticed.

CASE STUDY 6

A 42-year-old female has been treated for ulcerative colitis with immunosuppressant and anti-inflammatory therapy since 2002. She had been ill for 20 days before admission with fever (up to 37.3°C), cough, and occasionally coughing up blood-stained content. At the admission (August 2013), she was in good general condition, without signs of respiratory failure. Chest X-ray revealed linearly inhomogeneous hyperintensity shadows with excavation in the right upper lobe, CT scan of the chest were also performed (Figs. 12 and 13).

In laboratory studies, there were signs of inflammation (ESR 52/h, CRP 14.1). By direct microscopy of sputum AFB were not found, but cultures were positive and anti-TB treatment was started.

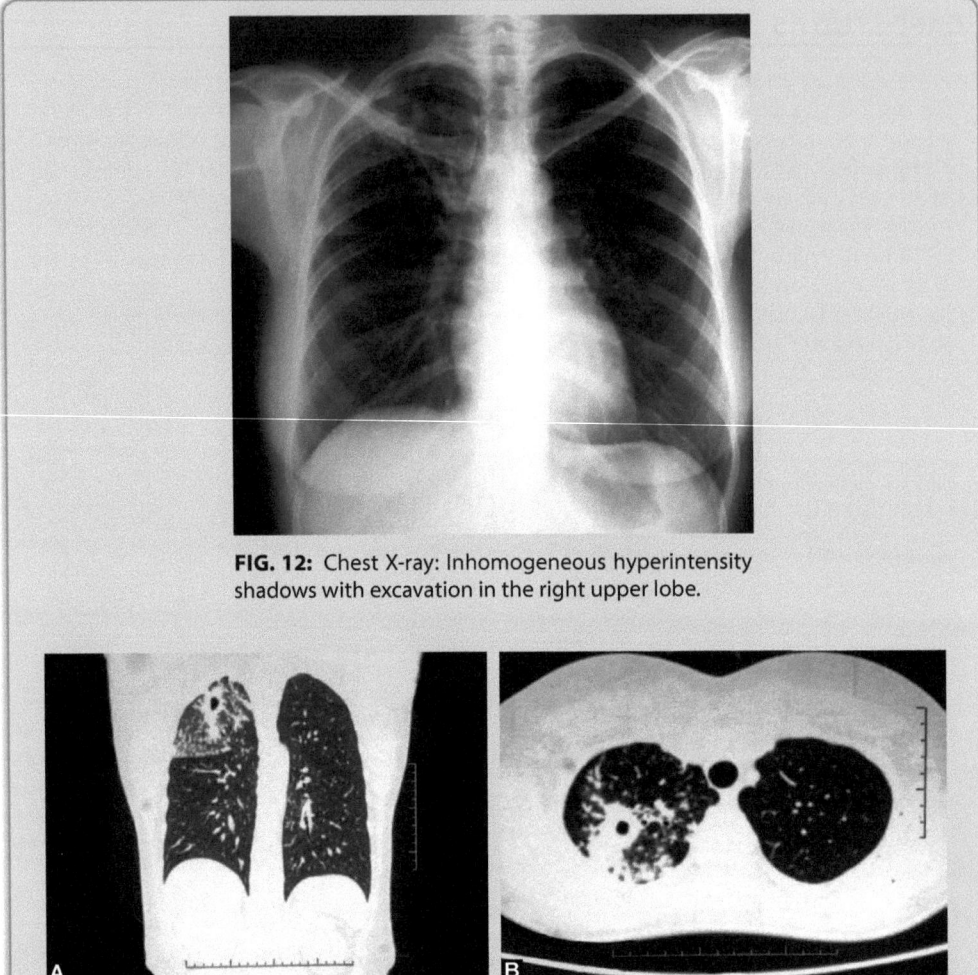

FIG. 12: Chest X-ray: Inhomogeneous hyperintensity shadows with excavation in the right upper lobe.

FIG. 13: A and **B,** Computed tomography scan of the chest: In the upper right lobe plenty of micronodular, excavated masses 27 mm in diameter and in the lower left lobe less numerous micronodular changes.

REFERENCES

1. World Health Organization. Global tuberculosis control: WHO report 2010. [online] Available from: http://www.who.int/tb/publications/global_report/2010/en/index.html. [Accessed February, 2016].
2. Pawlowski A, Jansson M, Sköld M, Rottenberg ME, Källenius G. Tuberculosis and HIV co-infection. PLoS Pathog. 2012;8(2):e1002464.
3. Škodrić V. Pulmonary tuberculosis in states of immunodeficiency. In: Djurić O. i sar. Tuberculosis. Belgrade: Savremena Administracija; 1996. pp. 515-33.
4. Andrews JR, Noubary F, Walensky RP, Cerda R, Losina E, Horsburgh CR. Risk of progression to active tuberculosis following reinfection with Mycobacterium tuberculosis. Clin Infect Dis. 2012;54(6):784-91.

5. Rieder HL. Tuberculosis. In: Rieder HL, editor. Epidemiologic Basis of Tuberculosis Control. 1st ed. Paris: IUATLD; 1999. pp. 63-121.
6. Sterling TR. Pham PA, Chaisson RE. HIV infection-related tuberculosis: clinical manifestations and treatment. Clin Infect Dis. 2010;50 Suppl 3:S223-30.
7. Havlir DV, Barnes PF. Tuberculosis in patients with human immunodeficiency virus infection. N Engl J Med. 1999;340:367-73.
8. Middelkoop K, Bekker LG, Shashkina E, Kreiswirth B, Wood R. Retreatment tuberculosis in a South African community: the role of re-infection, HIV and antiretroviral treatment. Int J Tuberc Lung Dis. 2012;16(11):1510-6.
9. Kwan CK, Ernst JD. HIV and tuberculosis: a deadly human syndemic. Clin Microbiol Rev. 2011;24(2):351-76.
10. Fischl MA, Daikos GL, Uttamchandani RB, et al. Clinical presentation and outcome of patients with HIV infection and tuberculosis caused by multiple-drug-resistant bacilli. Ann Intern Med. 1992;117:184-90.
11. Kaye K, Frieden TR. Tuberculosis control: the relevance of classic principles in an era of acquired immunodeficiency syndrome and multidrug resistance. Epidemiol Rev. 1996;18:52-63.
12. Shafer RW, Edlin BR. Tuberculosis in patients infected with human immunodeficiency virus: perspective on the past decade. Clin Infect Dis. 1996;22:683-704.
13. Pape JW. Tuberculosis and HIV in the Caribbean: approaches to diagnosis, treatment, and prophylaxis. Top HIV Med. 2004;12:144-9.
14. Ferreira M, Ferrazoli L, Palaci M, et al. Tuberculosis and HIV infection among female inmates in Sao Paulo, Brazil: a prospective cohort study. J Acquir Immune Defic Syndr Hum Retrovirol. 1996;13:177-83.
15. Török ME, Farrar JJ. When to start antiretroviral therapy in HIV-associated tuberculosis. N Engl J Med. 2011;365:1538-40.
16. Havlir DV, Kendall MA, Ive P, et al. Timing of antiretroviral therapy for HIV-1 infection and tuberculosis. N Engl J Med. 2011;365:1482-91.
17. Harikrishna J, Sukaveni V, Kumar DP, Mohan A. Cancer and tuberculosis. JIACM. 2012;13(2):142-4.
18. Škodrić-Trifunović V. Risk factor for developing tuberculosis. Med Pregl. 2004;57:53-8.
19. Škodrić-Trifunović V, Rašić T, Nagorni-Obradović LJ, Filipović S. Analysis of patients with tuberculosis and diabetes mellitus at the Institute of Pulmonary Diseases and Tuberculosis of the Clinical Center of Serbia (2000-2002). Med Pregl. 2004;57:59-63.
20. Li L, Lin Y, Mi F, et al. Screening of patients with tuberculosis for diabetes mellitus in China. Trop Med Int Health. 2012;17:1294-301.
21. Faurholt-Jepsen D, Range N, PrayGod G, et al. The role of diabetes on the clinical manifestations of pulmonary tuberculosis. Trop Med Int Health. 2012;17:877-83.
22. Hendy M, Stableforth D. The effect of established diabetes mellitus on the presentation of infiltrative pulmonary tuberculosis in the immigrant Asian community of an inner city area of the United Kingdom. Br J Dis Chest. 1983;77:87-90.
23. Wang CS, Yang CJ, Chen HC, et al. Impact of type 2 diabetes on manifestations and treatment outcome of pulmonary tuberculosis. Epidemiol Infect. 2009;137:203-10.
24. Dooley KE, Chaisson RE. Tuberculosis and diabetes mellitus: convergence of two epidemics. Lancet Infect Dis. 2009;9(12):737-46.
25. Chen L, Magliano DJ, Zimmet PZ. The worldwide epidemiology of type 2 diabetes mellitus—present and future perspectives. Nat Rev Endocrinol. 2012;8:228-36.
26. Wild S, Sicree R, Roglic G, King H, Green A. Global prevalence of diabetes: estimates for the year 2000 and projections for 2030. Diabetes Care. 2004;27:1047-53.
27. Milburn H, Ashman N, Davies P, et al. Guidelines for the prevention and management of Mycobacterium tuberculosis infection and disease in adult patients with chronic kidney disease. Thorax. 2010;65:557-70.
28. Lindenfeld J, Miller GG, Shakar SF, et al. Drug therapy in the heart transplant recipient: part I: cardiac rejection and immunosuppressive drugs. Circulation. 2004;110:3734-40.
29. Chan TY. Vitamin D deficiency and susceptibility to tuberculosis. Calcif Tissue Int. 2000;66:476-8.
30. di Girolamo C, Pappone N, Melillo E, Rengo C, Giuliano F, Melillo G. Cavitary lung tuberculosis in a rheumatoid arthritis patient treated with low-dose methotrexate and steroid pulse therapy. Br J Rheumatol. 1998;37:1136-7.

31. Hannaes OC, Bergmann A. Tuberculosis emerging in patients treated with corticosteroids. Eur J Respir Dis. 1983;64:294-7.
32. Pal D, Behera D, Gupta D, Aggarwal A. Tuberculosis in patients receiving prolonged treatment with oral corticosteroids for respiratory disorders. Ind J Tub. 2002;49:83-6.
33. Karampetsou MP, Liossis SN, Sfikakis PP. TNF-α antagonists beyond approved indications: stories of success and prospects for the future. QJM. 2010;103(12):917-28.
34. Galloway JB, Hyrich KL, Mercer LK, et al. Anti-TNF therapy is associated with an increased risk of serious infections in patients with rheumatoid arthritis especially in the first 6 months of treatment: updated results from the British Society for Rheumatology Biologics Register with special emphasis on risks in the elderly. Rheumatology. 2011;50(1):124-31.
35. Wallis RS, Broder M, Wong J, Lee A, Hoq L. Reactivation of latent granulomatous infections by infliximab. Clin Infect Dis. 2005;41:S194-8.
36. Rich EA, Torres M, Sada E, Finegan CK, Hamilton BD, Toossi Z. Mycobacterium tuberculosis (MTB)-stimulated production of nitric oxide by human alveolar macrophages and relationship of nitric oxide production to growth inhibition of MTB. Tuber Lung Dis. 1997;78:247-55.
37. Wallis RS, Amir-Tahmasseb M, Ellner JJ. Induction of interleukin 1 and tumor necrosis factor by mycobacterial proteins: the monocyte western blot. Proc Natl Acad Sci U S A. 1990;87:3348-52.
38. Dinarello CA. Differences between anti-tumor necrosis factor-alpha monoclonal antibodies and soluble TNF receptors in host defense impairment. J Rheumatol. 2005;74:40-7.
39. Ehlers S. Tumor necrosis factor and its blockade in granulomatous infections: differential modes of action of infliximab and etanercept? Clin Infect Dis. 2005;41:S199-203.
40. Jianfeng C, Qian C. P-030 infliximab and tuberculosis infection: a meta-analysis. Inflamm Bowel Dis. 2013;19:S37.
41. Wolfe F, Michaud K, Anderson J, Urbansky K. Tuberculosis infection in patients with rheumatoid arthritis and the effect of infliximab therapy. Arthritis Rheum. 2004;50:372-9.
42. Keane J, Gershon S, Wise RP, et al. Tuberculosis associated with infliximab, a tumor necrosis factor alpha-neutralizing agent. N Engl J Med. 2001;345:1098-104.
43. Ponce de Leon D, Acevedo-Vasquez E, Sanchez-Torres A, et al. Attenuated response to purified protein derivative in patients with rheumatoid arthritis: study in a population with a high prevalence of tuberculosis. Ann Rheum Dis. 2005;64:1360-1.
44. Fishman JA, Rubin RH. Infection in organ-transplant recipients. N Engl J Med. 1998;338:1741-51.
45. Snydman DR. Epidemiology of infections after solid-organ transplantation. Clin Infect Dis. 2001;33:S5-8.
46. Kotloff RM, Ahya VN, Crawford SW. Pulmonary complications of solid organ and hematopoietic stem cell transplantation. Am J Respir Crit Care Med. 2004;170:22-48.
47. Singh N, Paterson DL. Mycobacterium tuberculosis infection in solid-organ transplant recipients: impact and implications for management. Clin Infect Dis. 1998;27:1266-77.
48. Higgins RS, Kusne S, Reyes J. Mycobacterium tuberculosis after liver transplantation: management and guidelines for prevention. Clin Transplant. 1992;6:81-90.
49. Hussain Z, Naqvi R, Hashmi A, Hafiz S, Naqvi A, Rizvi A. Tuberculosis in renal allograft recipients. Transplant Proc. 1996;28:1516-7.
50. Currie AC, Knight SR, Morris PJ. Tuberculosis in renal transplant recipients: the evidence for prophylaxis. Transplantation. 2010;90(7):695-704.

CHAPTER 14
Smoking and Tuberculosis: A Pernicious Association

Ashok Shah, Shekhar Kunal, Kamal Gera

INTRODUCTION

Currently, it is estimated that tobacco usage annually is responsible for loss of 6 million lives worldwide. More than 5 million deaths are attributed to direct tobacco use while secondhand smoke contributes to around 0.6 million deaths. Amongst men, it accounts for 16% of deaths, and in women, 7% of deaths each year.[1,2] Tobacco usage thus is one of the major preventable cause of premature mortality and significant morbidity.

This enormous annual toll of mortality is expected to rise to more than 8 million by 2030 unless urgent corrective measures are taken. Globally, more than 20% of people older than 15 years smoke tobacco.[3] Low- and middle-income countries account for nearly 80% of world's 1 billion smokers. There is a distinct shift of tobacco epidemic from industrialized to developing countries with estimates showing that tobacco is likely to kill around 450 million people in the next 50 years.[4,5]

In 2012, more than 700 million people in developing countries consumed around 4,400 billion cigarettes with China and India having the dubious distinction of harboring the greatest number of smokers worldwide.[6,7] Global adult tobacco survey in India[8] revealed that more than one-third (35%) of Indian adults consumed tobacco in some form or the other with smoking contributing to tobacco consumption in 14% adults. Prevalence of smoking among males was 24% whereas the prevalence among females was 3%. An international multicountry survey in 2012 revealed that in India, the prevalence of smoking in adults was 13.3% (males—23% and females—3.2%).[7] The World Health Organization (WHO) in its global report on trends in prevalence of tobacco smoking 2015[9], projects that in 2025, around 8% of the Indian population will be smokers as compared to the 13% of population who smoked in 2010. Estimates show that by 2025, 15% of smokers shall be males and 1% females. The age-specific estimates regarding current tobacco smoking in 2010 and projected figure in 2025 are depicted in table 1.[9] Tobacco smoking in India is dominated by bidi with cigarette being the second most popular form, mainly in urban localities.[8] Bidi consists of finely ground, sun-dried tobacco rolled in a brown broadleaf plant (*Diospyros melanoxylon* or *Diospyros ebenum*) native to India.[10]

It is estimated that, in India, nearly a trillion bidis are consumed every year.[11] The other forms of smoked tobacco in different parts of India include hookah, chuttas, dhumti, chillum, cigars, cheroots, and pipes.[7] Mortality due to smoking-related diseases is caused by several diseases predominantly lung cancer, chronic obstructive pulmonary disease as well as cardiovascular diseases. Although the tobacco epidemic worldwide causes a significant morbidity and mortality and in spite of best efforts, the global community has not been able to curb this dangerous addiction.

TABLE 1	Age-specific rates of current tobacco smoking in India (2010 and as projected in 2025)			
Age (in years)	2010		2025	
	Males	Females	Males	Females
15–24	12.7	0.2	7.7	0.1
25–39	23.1	1.3	14.0	0.4
40–54	32.9	3.2	19.8	0.9
55–69	30.6	6.1	18.2	1.7
70+	24.7	10.2	14.8	2.8

Source: Adapted from World Health Organization. (2015). WHO global report on trends in prevalence of tobacco smoking 2015. [online] Available from: http://apps.who.int/iris/bitstream/10665/156262/1/9789241564922_eng.pdf [Accessed February, 2016].

Tuberculosis (TB) continues to be a global threat, especially in developing countries. The WHO declared this dreaded disease as a global emergency in 1992 when it was estimated that approximately a third of the world's population was latently infected with *Mycobacterium tuberculosis*.[12] In 2013, around 9 million people developed TB while 1.5 million lost their lives to this disease worldwide. India accounts for the highest burden of TB with over one-fifth of the world's cases with a prevalence of 211 per 100,000 population in 2013. Furthermore, it was observed that economically productive age group was the worst affected with 70% of the cases.[2]

As early as 1918, smoking as a risk factor for TB was thought of and investigated.[13] However, it was Lowe[14] in 1956, after the Second World War who highlighted this association between tobacco smoking and TB. He analyzed the death rates from TB for the time period of 1870s to 1940s and concluded that "patients of over 30 years of age with respiratory TB showed a highly significant deficiency of nonsmokers and light smokers and an excess of moderate and heavy smokers when compared with the controls". From India, this association was first studied in 1959.[15] In a cross-sectional study, out of the 439 employees who underwent mass miniature radiography along with physician's consultation, 46 cases of TB were identified.[15] Subsequently, this association was not emphasized for nearly a half a century. In 2002, Maurya et al.,[16] reviewed the available evidence to determine the association of smoking with increased incidence of TB. Since then there have been a slew of studies, reviews,[6,17-19] and meta-analyses[20-22] for the possible linkage between TB and smoking. In 2007, a WHO statement[4] described smoking and TB as "related epidemics". The WHO report states that the prevalence of smoking among people with TB is often well above 20%.[2]

Epidemiological and mathematical modeling of TB cannot be considered complete without taking into account the effects of tobacco smoking. It is now being advocated that tobacco cessation efforts be incorporated along with the TB control programs.[23] This chapter details the association of smoking and TB and describes the many diverse aspects.

SMOKING AND TUBERCULOSIS: A DEVASTATING COMBINATION

In spite of consistent evidence of increased incidence of infection, disease, and death due to TB among smokers, this relationship is yet to receive the attention that it deserves.

Smoking and Tuberculin Reactivity

An independent association exists between smoking and an increased risk of latent TB infection. In a cross-sectional study comprising 2,665 volunteers from elderly homes; it was observed that the smokers were more likely to develop Heaf grade reaction greater than or equal to 3 as compared to nonsmokers [odd ratio (OR), 1.59].[24] In studies among the prison inmates in America and Pakistan, smoking was observed as an independent risk factor for tuberculin reactivity.[25,26] A study from the United States of America highlighted prevalence of latent TB infection among never-smokers, current smokers, and former smokers to be 4.1, 6.6, and 6.2%, respectively.[27]

The effect of smoking and risk of infection was evaluated in a recent study from Spain, where 439/1,079 patients with TB were found to be smokers. The prevalence of latent TB infection among contacts was higher among contacts of smokers (35.3%) as compared to nonsmokers (25.7%). Decrease in smoking did lower the risk of infection.[28]

Smoking and Tuberculous Disease

Pulmonary Tuberculosis

A number of studies including cross-sectional,[29-31] case-control,[18,32-36] and cohort studies[37-39] corroborated the association of tobacco smoking and tuberculous disease and suggested that smoking is an important risk factor for developing TB. In a cross-sectional study from England,[29] over 76,000 people underwent mass miniature radiography and the smoking history along with development of TB was recorded. It was observed that smokers were significantly more affected with TB as compared to nonsmokers (0.42, 2.09 for men and 0.42, 1.55 for women per 1,000). Furthermore, large prospective studies from Hong Kong showed that "current smoking" increased the risk of developing TB by nearly three times in elderly and by nearly two times in patients with silicosis (adjusted hazard ratio = 2.87 and 1.96, respectively).[37]

A study from China[40] observed that 54.6% of patients with TB were smokers while a similar study from South Africa[41] documented that 56% of patients with active TB were current smokers.

A study from Cambodia has shown that the lifetime TB prevalence was higher for manufactured cigarette smokers (1.60) than for nonsmokers (1.02). The estimated number of cases of lifetime TB infection per 10,000 for manufactured cigarette smokers was 102 while for nonsmokers was 106 cases. Thus, manufactured cigarettes contributed to an annual excess of 58 TB cases per 10,000 men.[42] A study to evaluate smoking habits and degree of nicotine addiction among all registered TB patients in Macedonia, observed that 48.2% were smokers and 51.8% were nonsmokers out of which 69.8% were males. The majority of the smokers (53.8%) belonged to the age group 35-54 years, 38.5% were above 54 years, and 7.7% at the age less than 34 years. The percentage of nicotine addiction was low among 30.07% of the smokers, on average level between 38.6% of the smokers and high among 30.7% of them. The majority of smokers (68.9%) smoked more than 20 cigarettes/day.[43] In a study from California, increased risk for pulmonary TB was observed among ever-smokers (OR, 1.35; 95% CI, 1.19-1.53), as well as current (OR, 1.26; 95% CI, 1.08-1.48), and past smokers (OR, 1.43; 95% CI, 1.23-1.67), compared with never-smokers.[44]

A cross-sectional study designed to study the association of smoking and gender differences of active TB in the 22 WHO-designated high-burden countries showed a higher prevalence of active TB among male smokers. It was observed that the amount of cigarette smoking was a significant predictor of the increased TB notification in males, accounting for 33% of the variance in the gender ratio of TB notification.[45] As the TB notification rates in boys and girls are nearly similar, the difference in rates of association of pulmonary TB in male and female smokers has been speculated to the gender-based differences in smoking rates.[46] In a study from South Africa of nearly 2,000 subjects with newly diagnosed TB, cigarette smoking was present in 38% of the males but in only 5% of the females.[47]

Studies from India: A 1:5 nested case-control was carried out from a community-based survey of 60,000 villagers in Tamil Nadu, which revealed that the smokers were at least twice as likely to develop TB as compared to nonsmokers [adjusted OR (aOR), 2.24].[48] In the Bombay Cohort Study[49] from Mumbai, India, 81,443 men were followed for 12 years and a subgroup analysis revealed that "bidi smoker", "other-mainly cigarette smokers" and altogether, the "smoker" were more likely to give a history of "self-reported TB" as compared to never-smokers (aOR, 5.23, 2.24, and 3.77, respectively). The WHO monograph stated that the 19 studies with significant results highlighting that smoking was a risk factor for pulmonary TB, the risk ratios ranged from 1.012 to 6.26.[4]

In a community-based cross-sectional analysis from central India regarding smoking and pulmonary TB, the adjusted prevalence OR for mild, moderate, and heavy tobacco smokers were 2.28, 2.51, and 2.74, respectively as compared to nonsmokers.[50]

Meta-analyses: Three meta-analyses[20-22] were available which used different selection criteria. These meta-analyses refrained from giving an overall pooled summary estimate due to a substantial variation among the studies but stated that there was a significantly increased risk of clinical tuberculous disease among smokers regardless of the outcome definition. In selected studies, the pooled summary estimates for this association are 2.27 and 2.64.[21,22]

Extrapulmonary Tuberculosis

Although tobacco smoking is known to be deleterious to extrapulmonary tissues, larger studies have failed to find an association between smoking and extrapulmonary TB (OR, 0.57). It is possible that only lungs are more prone to TB among smokers due to the direct effects of smoking.[51]

Smoking and Death due to Tuberculosis

Sufficient amount of evidence exists to support the association between smoking and death from TB. A retrospective study of 1 million deaths from China revealed that both male and female smokers were more likely to die of TB than nonsmokers (weighted mean risk ratio, 1.20 and 1.29, respectively).[52] A study from Korea in 657 subjects, diabetes and smoking were seen to independently increase the risk of death in the first 12 months after enrollment. Diabetic patients who smoked greater than or equal to one pack of cigarettes daily had an increased risk of death from TB.[53]

Studies from India: A large case-control study from South India, among 43,000 adult male deaths and 35,000 controls, showed that smoking tobacco was associated with increased risk of tuberculous death (standardized risk ratio, 4.5). In a study of a nationally representative sample of 1.1 million homes, "verbal autopsy" method assessed the cause of death. Both men and women were more likely to die of TB if they were smokers (adjusted relative risks, 2.3 and 3.0, respectively).[48]

Meta-analyses: The risk ratios for TB deaths are quantitatively lower than that for TB disease. Due to much variation in the mortality data, pooled estimate of the risk of death was not available from the meta-analyses (range of OR, 1.03–5.92).[17,20] In summary, for a patient of TB, who was also a smoker, there was approximately twice the risk of dying from the disease.

Tuberculosis mortality attributable to smoking: Using data on total number of deaths from TB and the likelihood (risk ratios) that smoking leads to death from TB, it was possible to calculate the fraction of deaths from TB that could be attributed to smoking. It was estimated that the percentage of deaths from TB attributable to smoking, in India, were 38%[54] to 61%[48] in men and 9%[54] in women, and in Taiwan, it was 37.7%.[55] Smoking bidi can account for up to one-third of deaths from TB in India.[56]

DOSE-RESPONSE RELATIONSHIP

Dose-response relationship means that as the exposure increases, the associated disease increases. For tobacco smoking, the "dose" may be measured as "amount"—the number of cigarettes or bidis/day, as "duration"—the number of years of smoking, or as a composite measure—"pack-years". There is a sufficient body of evidence to suggest a positive dose-response relationship between smoking and TB infection, disease, and death.[52,56]

Tuberculin Reactivity

The chances of developing latent TB infection increase with the amount, duration, or pack-years of smoking. A case-control study from the United States of America showed that the odds of developing latent TB infection were 1.32, 1.75, 1.6, and 2.12 in subjects who smoked 1–20 cigarettes/day, greater than 20 cigarettes/day, for less than 15 years, and greater than 15 years, respectively as compared to nonsmokers.[25]

Tuberculosis Disease

Smoking increases tuberculous disease in a dose dependent manner. Early studies from England have reported higher rates of TB in heavier smokers.[14,29] In a nested case-control study from India, OR for smoking 1–10/day, 11–20/day, and greater than 20/day were 1.75, 3.17, and 3.68, respectively (P for linear trend <0.0001) and for smoking for a duration of less than 10 years, 11–20 years, and greater than 20 years ORs were 1.72, 2.45, and 3.23, respectively (P for linear trend <0.0001).[33]

Cumulative exposure assessed in the form of pack-years has also been associated with increased risk of the disease. In a fairly recent study from Cambodia,[42] it was observed that smoking at least one pack a day was associated with a more than tenfold increase in odds of TB relative to less than 5 cigarettes/day (OR for cigarettes/day, 1.00 for <5; 6.79 for 5 to <10; 6.11 for 10 to <15; 10.07 for 15–25; 11.65 for >25).

In a systemic meta-analysis[57] to evaluate the dose-response relationship between smoking and TB, in 72,684 individuals from 14 high TB-burden countries including India, it was observed that after removal of confounders, smoking amount and duration showed a stronger dose-response relationship in women than in men. However, in patients with body mass index (BMI) less than 18.5 kg/m^2, stronger dose-response relationship was seen in men.

Tuberculosis Death

There is credible evidence for a dose-response relationship between TB mortality and the amount and duration of smoking. In China, the risk ratios for death due to respiratory TB for smoking 1–10, 11–20, and over 20 cigarettes/day were 1.01, 1.23, and 1.57 in rural areas and 1.24, 1.48, and 2.03 in urban areas, respectively.[52] The risk ratios for starting smoking at age less than 20, 20–24, and greater than or equal to 25 years were 1.25, 1.18, and 1.12 in rural and 1.86, 1.42, and 1.22 in urban China, respectively.[52]

EFFECT OF SMOKING CESSATION

If a noxious stimulus is considered as a risk factor for the disease, then one might assume that cessation of exposure should lead to decreased incidence. Quitting smoking decreases the risk of TB infection, disease, and possibly death but the risk never reaches that of a never-smoker.

Latent Tuberculosis Infection

In epidemiological studies, it is impossible to determine with precision, the time of entry of *M. tuberculosis* bacteria into the body. Hence, it is difficult to be certain whether the observed latent TB infection is due to a bacterium that entered the body before stopping smoking or after. However, it is possible to make reasonable inferences regarding the link of smoking cessation and developing latent TB infection by analyzing the available epidemiological data. It has been reported that when compared to nonsmokers, the OR for Heaf test positivity was 1.59 in smokers and 1.2 in former smokers. Hence, it is reasonable to infer that cessation of smoking could possibly decrease the risk of contracting latent TB infection.[24]

Tuberculosis Death

There is evidence that quitting smoking reduces the risk of tuberculous death. In Taiwan, among 486,341 adults, there were 21 tuberculous deaths in "current smoker" and 6 TB deaths in "ex-smoker". The authors reported that with quitting smoking, there was a 65% reduction in death rates from TB.[55]

EFFECT OF CONFOUNDERS

Certain factors can increase the rates of both TB and smoking. Hence, it is possible that in smokers, in the presence of these factors, the observed increase in TB is actually due to these factors only, and is not an independent direct effect of smoking on TB. In epidemiological studies, statistical techniques can account for this "confounding" effect. If an association is independent of such confounding factors, causality in the association is strengthened.[58]

Socioeconomic Conditions

Lower socioeconomic status is associated with TB and smoking. Different studies vary in their measurements of socioeconomic condition. In spite of this limitation, studies have reported the association of smoking and tuberculous infection, disease, and death after statistically adjusting for socioeconomic condition.[4,20,29]

Alcohol Use

Alcohol use has been associated with both smoking and TB. Gajalakshmi and Peto[36] have reported that in 6,962 adults in rural Tamil Nadu, India, smoking and alcohol were independently associated with TB disease (independent adjusted relative risks 2.2, and 1.5, respectively). There is also a presence of other evidence as well that suggests that the effect of smoking on tuberculous infection, disease, and death is independent of alcohol intake.[36]

Human Immunodeficiency Virus

Human immunodeficiency virus (HIV) is the strongest known risk factor for reactivation of TB. Smoking in these patients has been found to be an independent risk factor for TB infection and disease after statistically adjusting for HIV status.[22]

EFFECT ON CASE MANAGEMENT

Smoking influences the case management issues in TB as suggested by the limited but credible evidence. Tobacco smokers are more likely to default from treatment, relapse after getting cured, and are likely to suffer from a more extensive severe disease. In a study from Hong Kong[19] to evaluate the effect of smoking on treatment outcomes in patients with pulmonary TB, it was found that in both current smokers and ex-smokers, sputum smears and culture positivity persisted even beyond 2 months of antituberculous treatment. Both these categories of smokers were significantly less likely to achieve cure or treatment completion within 2 years.

Default from Treatment

A 1:3 case-control study from Hong Kong presented the statistical models for identifying factors that predict default from treatment of TB. It was observed that smokers could be expected to default even at the start of the treatment (OR for default for "current smokers", "ex-smokers", and "those with a history of default from treatment" 3.44, 2.48, and 10.74, respectively).[59] Pinidiyapathirage et al.[60] studied 892 hospitalized patients with TB in Welisara, Sri Lanka. The rates of treatment default were 10.3% for the 770 patients with newly diagnosed TB and 30.3% for the 122 patients on retreatment regimen. Overall, regular smokers were nearly twice as likely to default from treatment (aOR, 1.9) as compared with nonsmokers. Smoking contributed to 16.7% of unsuccessful treatment outcomes with the default seen in current smokers and death in ex-smokers.[60]

Relapse after Treatment

Smokers have a higher relapse rate after a successful treatment of TB. In a study from India, among treatment-naïve, smear-positive patients with pulmonary TB, all doses of the 6-month treatment regimen were administered under direct observation. The patients were actively followed by sputum smear and culture every 6 months. The overall relapse rate for smokers at 18 months after treatment completion was 18.1% (41 of 226) as compared to 7.3% (19 of 260) in those who did not smoke.[61]

In a study from Hong Kong[19] among 16,345 patients with TB, it was seen that in both current smokers and ex-smokers the overall relapse rates were 4.2 and 3.4%, respectively with bacteriologically confirmed relapse rates being 2.4 and 1.8%, respectively.

Severity of Disease

Both smoking and TB are known to cause lung damage. Smokers with TB tend to have more severe disease with increased incidence of pulmonary tissue destruction, cavities, miliary disease, sputum smear-positive status, and hospitalization for longer duration.[34,62] Patients with TB who are smokers have a clinical, radiological, and microbiological evidence of faster and more aggressive lung involvement.[34,62]

Treatment Failure

Smoking has been associated with higher treatment failures as compared to nonsmokers. A study from Morocco[63] that followed 727 patients with newly diagnosed TB between 2004 and 2009 observed that the rates of failure among smokers were higher as compared with nonsmokers (9.1 and 4.5%, respectively; p <0.01). Smoking was independently associated with treatment failure (aOR, 2.25). In another study from Brazil,[64] 53 patients with pulmonary TB who were culture positive after 2 months and 240 patients who became culture negative after 2 months of therapy were enrolled. The 240 patients with a negative culture functioned as controls. Patients who smoked had a threefold greater odds to remain culture positive after 2 months of treatment than nonsmokers. Smoking had a negative impact on culture conversion during antituberculosis treatment. It was also observed that smoking delays the culture conversion in a dose-dependent manner. Current smokers had a higher risk of nonconversion as compared to never- or ex-smokers.

Leung et al.[19] observed that among never-smokers, ex-smokers, and current smokers the rates of nonconversion of sputum smear at the end of 2 months were 5.8, 11.1, and 9.4%, respectively (p <0.001) while the rates for nonconversion of culture were 4.9, 7.2, and 9.4%, respectively (p <0.001).

In a study to evaluate the effect of smoking on the rate of sputum conversion in patients with multidrug-resistant TB (MDR-TB), it was seen that current smoking was a risk factor for lower rates of sputum culture conversion. On removing the confounding factors, smoking was significantly associated with a 20% reduction in the rate of conversion. These patients may also be infectious for a longer time, which could enhance the transmission of MDR-TB.[65]

ENVIRONMENTAL TOBACCO SMOKE

Environmental tobacco smoke (ETS) increases tuberculous infection and disease. However, there were no data available for association of ETS and death from TB. There are several sociodemographic and household factors responsible for those exposed to secondhand smoke and occurrence of pulmonary TB. In the pediatric population, the factors implicated include age, frequency, and closeness of contact with a TB patient in the household, overcrowding, and relationship with the smoker. Among adults, the factors were age, contact with a TB patient in the household, number of smokers in the household, and number of cigarettes smoked by household members.[66]

Tuberculous Infection

There is increasing likelihood of contracting latent TB infection in subjects with exposure to ETS. In India,[67] in a study of 281 children, it was observed that exposure to ETS was an independent risk factor for tuberculin reactivity in children (OR, 2.68), irrespective of the sputum acid-fast bacillus smear status of the infecting adult patient.

In a study to determine the association between exposure to a smoking index case of TB and latent TB infection, Huang et al.[68] observed that in 21 children (age <15 years) who were exposed to smoking TB patients were more likely to be tuberculin skin test positive at baseline [RR, 2.64; 95% confidence interval (CI), 1.78–3.91], by 6 months (RR, 1.91; 95% CI, 1.40–2.60) and by 12 months (RR, 1.48; 95% CI, 1.07–2.06) than those who were not exposed.

Tuberculous Disease

Environmental tobacco smoke can not only lead to higher chances of contracting latent TB infection, but can also lead to increased risk of developing active TB disease in children and adults. In one study, exposure to smoking was documented by history and urinary cotinine levels. Children who were exposed to ETS at home or outside the home within the family had more chances of developing tuberculous disease (OR, 6.3; p <0.00001).[69] In adults in Hong Kong,[70] ETS accounted for 18.7% of cases of "culture confirmed TB". In a meta-analysis of 18 studies regarding risk of TB following passive smoking in adults and children, the authors concluded that children had more than three-fold increased risk of passive smoking associated active TB as to compared the adults exposed to cigarette smoke.[66]

POSSIBLE BIOLOGICAL MECHANISMS

The mechanisms by which smoking increases the risk for TB are diverse. The possible mechanisms have been depicted in figure 1. Exposure to tobacco smoke leads to a decrease in ciliary function, alterations in number of macrophages[71] and their response to tuberculous infection along with decrease in number of CD4 and CD8 cells that produce various immunomodulatory cytokines like interferon-γ (IFN-γ) and tumor necrosis factor-α (TNF-α).[72] There is ample evidence to suggest the role of passive smoking in producing the ill effects on fetal lung development, decreased innate as well as adaptive immune response within the lungs leading to a predisposition for tuberculous infection.[73] Other plausible mechanisms include inflammatory damage to the lower airway epithelium and bronchiolar collapse.[71]

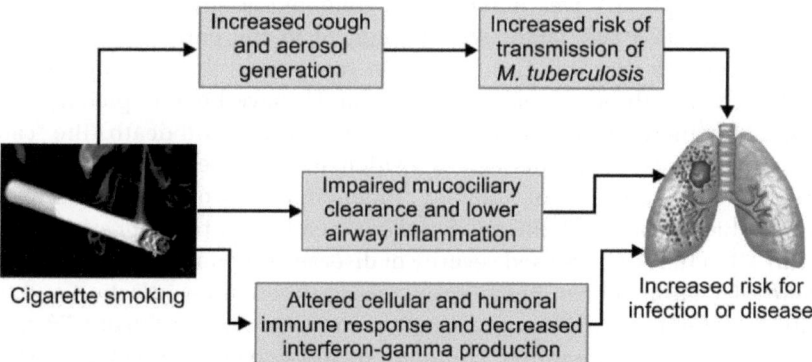

FIG. 1: Cartoon depicting possible mechanisms responsible for the association of smoking and tuberculosis.

There is also clinical data to suggest that smoking increases reactivation of TB as evidenced by more of cavitary and upper zone involvement in smokers.[14,32,62] Smoking alters humoral and cellular immunity and results in increased infections.[74] In mice pulmonary T cells, cigarette smoke decreases the production of IFN-γ, which is known to play a central role in protective immunity against TB.[75] Nicotine can decrease the production of TNF-α in macrophages via a cholinergic anti-inflammatory pathway mediated via vagus nerve.[76]

A study[77] demonstrated that smoking can reduce the effector cytokine responses and further impair mycobacterial containment within infected human macrophages. In a recent study,[78] it was seen that smokers had significantly more alveolar macrophages than nonsmokers or ex-smokers. Furthermore, the ability of macrophages to secrete TNF-α, IFN-γ, and interleukin-1β was impaired in smokers as well as ex-smokers in response to *M. tuberculosis* infection.

TUBERCULOSIS AND TOBACCO CESSATION

When a smoker develops TB, it creates a potent opportunity for tobacco cessation efforts. Among patients with TB who smoke, 54.9–96.4% smokers quit smoking soon after diagnosis of TB but up to 18–50% started smoking again within 6 months of completion of TB treatment.[79,80]

In India, it has been reported that up to half of physicians did not give TB-specific quit smoking advice.[79] In Sudan, in a large study in 24 health centers, tobacco cessation intervention was seen to be feasible and effective within routine TB services.[81] It is now recommended that tobacco cessation efforts be incorporated in TB control program in easily implementable interventions like "ABC (Ask, Brief advice, and Cessation support) for TB".[30] Clinicians and public health programs can exploit this opportunity to help patients with TB quit smoking.

A study from South Africa[47] highlighted that smoking was ubiquitous among male patients with TB in high HIV prevalence population. However, these patients were also highly motivated to quit smoking. The authors suggest that a smoking cessation program should run in conjunction with the TB control program.

CONCLUSION

The association between TB and diabetes is known since antiquity. In the 1980s, the association of TB with HIV was noted and highlighted as "deadly-duo/deadly-duet". Although smoking as a risk factor was thought of in the early 20th century, it was not until this century that this has now been recognized that smoking and TB are definitely linked. The three major risk factors for TB have been depicted in figure 2. Tobacco smoking increases tuberculous infection, disease, and death. The "causality" in this association is strengthened by evidence for dose-response relationship, decreased risk with cessation of smoking, independence from confounding factors, and plausible biological mechanisms. Smoking creates complications in managing a patient with TB in having increased severity of disease and poorer treatment outcomes. Exposure to ETS has also been linked to increased tuberculous infection and disease. A majority of patients with TB are smokers who quit smoking during TB treatment but many start again after treatment completion. Tobacco cessation efforts for patients with TB must be incorporated in the current control programs for better management of patients with TB.

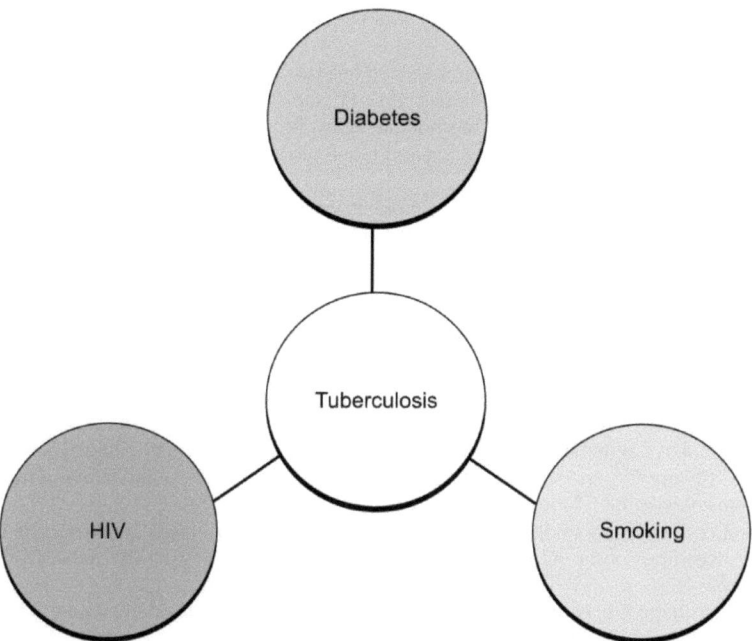

HIV, human immunodeficiency virus.
FIG. 2: The three major risk factors for tuberculosis.

REFERENCES

1. World Health Organization. (2016). The global burden of disease: 2004 update. [online] Available from: http://www.who.int/healthinfo/global_burden_disease/GBD_report_2004update_full.pdf. [Accessed February, 2016].
2. World Health Organization. (2014). Global tuberculosis report 2014. [online] Available from: http://www.who.int/tuberculosis/ publications/global_report/en/. [Accessed February, 2016].
3. World Health Organization. World Health Statistics 2014. Geneva: World Health Organization; 2014.
4. World Health Organization. A WHO/The Union monograph on TB and tobacco control: joining forces to control two related global epidemics. Geneva: World Health Organization; 2007.
5. World Health Organization. (2015). Tobacco. WHO fact sheet no. 339. [online] Available from: http://www.who.int/mediacentre/factsheets/fs339/en/. [Accessed February, 2016].
6. Pai M, Mohan A, Dheda K, et al. Lethal interaction: the colliding epidemics of tobacco and tuberculosis. Expert Rev Anti Infect Ther. 2007;5:385-91.
7. Ng M, Freeman MK, Fleming TD, et al. Smoking prevalence and cigarette consumption in 187 countries, 1980-2012. JAMA. 2014;311:183-92.
8. International Institute for Population Sciences, Ministry of Health and Family Welfare, Government of India. Global Adult Tobacco Survey (GATS), India: 2009-2010.
9. World Health Organization. (2015). WHO global report on trends in prevalence of tobacco smoking 2015. [online] Available from: http://apps.who.int/iris/bitstream/10665/156262/1/9789241564922_eng.pdf. [Accessed February, 2016].
10. Malson JL, Sims K, Murty R, Pickworth WB. Comparison of the nicotine content of tobacco used in bidis and conventional cigarettes. Tob Control. 2001;10:181-3.
11. Lal PG, Wilson NC, Gupta PC. Attributable deaths from smoking in the last 100 years in India. Curr Sci. 2012;103:1085-90.
12. Grange JM, Zumla A. The global emergency of tuberculosis: what is the cause? J R Soc Promot Health. 2002;122:78-81.

13. Webb GB. The effect of the inhalation of cigarette smoke on the lungs. A clinical study. Am Rev Tuberc. 1918;2:25-7.
14. Lowe CR. An association between smoking and respiratory tuberculosis. Br Med J. 1956;2:1081-6.
15. Shah JR, Warawadekar MS, Deshmukh PA, Phutane PN. Institutional survey of pulmonary tuberculosis with special reference to smoking habits. Indian J Med Sci. 1959;13:381-92.
16. Maurya V, Vijayan VK, Shah A. Smoking and tuberculosis: an association overlooked. Int J Tuberc Lung Dis. 2002;6:942-51.
17. Davies PD, Yew WW, Ganguly D, et al. Smoking and tuberculosis: the epidemiological association and immunopathogenesis. Trans R Soc Trop Med Hyg. 2006;100:291-8.
18. Dhamgaye TM. Tobacco smoking and pulmonary tuberculosis: a case-control study. J Indian Med Assoc. 2008;106:216-9.
19. Leung CC, Yew WW, Chan CK, et al. Smoking adversely affects treatment response, outcome and relapse in tuberculosis. Eur Respir J. 2015;45:738-45.
20. Lin HH, Ezzati M, Murray M. Tobacco smoke, indoor air pollution and tuberculosis: a systematic review and meta-analysis. PLoS Med. 2007;4:e20.
21. Bates MN, Khalakdina A, Pai M, Chang L, Lessa F, Smith KR. Risk of tuberculosis from exposure to tobacco smoke: a systematic review and meta-analysis. Arch Intern Med. 2007;167:335-42.
22. Slama K, Chiang CY, Enarson DA, et al. Tobacco and tuberculosis: a qualitative systematic review and meta-analysis. Int J Tuberc Lung Dis. 2007;11:1049-61.
23. Smoking cessation and smoke-free environments for tuberculosis patients: lessons learnt from the field. Proceedings of the 42nd Union World Conference on Lung Health. Lille, France. October 26–30, 2011.
24. Nisar M, Williams CS, Ashby D, Davies PD. Tuberculin testing in residential homes for the elderly. Thorax. 1993;48:1257-60.
25. Anderson RH, Sy FS, Thompson S, Addy C. Cigarette smoking and tuberculin skin test conversion among incarcerated adults. Am J Prev Med. 1997;13:175-81.
26. Hussain H, Akhtar S, Nanan D. Prevalence of and risk factors associated with Mycobacterium tuberculosis infection in prisoners, North West Frontier Province, Pakistan. Int J Epidemiol. 2003;32:794-9.
27. Horne DJ, Campo M, Ortiz JR, et al. Association between smoking and latent tuberculosis in the U.S. population: an analysis of the National Health and Nutrition Examination Survey. PLoS One. 2012;7:e49050.
28. Godoy P, Caylà JA, Carmona G, et al. Smoking in tuberculosis patients increases the risk of infection in their contacts. Int J Tuberc Lung Dis. 2013;17:771-6.
29. Adelstein AM, Rimington J. Smoking and pulmonary tuberculosis: an analysis based on a study of volunteers for mass miniature radiography. Tubercle. 1967;48:219-26.
30. Yu GP, Hsieh CC, Peng J. Risk factors associated with the prevalence of pulmonary tuberculosis among sanitary workers in Shanghai. Tubercle. 1988;69:105-12.
31. Rao VG, Gopi PG, Bhat J, Yadav R, Selvakumar N, Wares DF. Selected risk factors associated with pulmonary tuberculosis among Saharia tribe of Madhya Pradesh, central India. Eur J Public Health. 2012;22:271-3.
32. Brown KE, Campbell AH. Tobacco, alcohol and tuberculosis. Br J Dis Chest. 1961;55:150-8.
33. Kolappan C, Gopi PG. Tobacco smoking and pulmonary tuberculosis. Thorax. 2002;57:964-6.
34. Leung CC, Yew WW, Chan CK, et al. Smoking and tuberculosis in Hong Kong. Int J Tuberc Lung Dis. 2003;7:980-6.
35. Prasad R, Suryakant, Garg R, Singhal S, Dawar R, Agarwal GG. A case-control study of tobacco smoking and tuberculosis in India. Ann Thorac Med. 2009;4:208-10.
36. Gajalakshmi V, Peto R. Smoking, drinking and incident tuberculosis in rural India: population-based case-control study. Int J Epidemiol. 2009;38:1018-25.
37. Leung CC, Li T, Lam TH, et al. Smoking and tuberculosis among the elderly in Hong Kong. Am J Respir Crit Care Med. 2004;170:1027-33.
38. Jee SH, Golub JE, Jo J, Park IS, Ohrr H, Samet JM. Smoking and risk of tuberculosis incidence, mortality, and recurrence in South Korean men and women. Am J Epidemiol. 2009;170:1478-85.
39. Lin HH, Ezzati M, Chang HY, Murray M. Association between tobacco smoking and active tuberculosis in Taiwan: prospective cohort study. Am J Respir Crit Care Med. 2009;180:475-80.

40. Wang J, Shen H. Review of cigarette smoking and tuberculosis in China: intervention is needed for smoking cessation among tuberculosis patients. BMC Public Health. 2009;9:292.
41. Brunet L, Pai M, Davids V, et al. High prevalence of smoking among patients with suspected tuberculosis in South Africa. Eur Respir J. 2011;38:139-46.
42. Singh PN, Yel D, Kheam T, Hurd G, Job JS. Cigarette smoking and tuberculosis in Cambodia: findings from a national sample. Tob Induc Dis. 2013;11:8.
43. Popovska A, Zakoska M. Smoking habits and degree of nicotine addictions among TB patients. Eur Respir J. 2014;44(Suppl 58):334.
44. Smith GS, Van Den Eeden SK, Baxter R, et al. Cigarette smoking and pulmonary tuberculosis in northern California. J Epidemiol Community Health. 2015;69:568-73.
45. Watkins RE, Plant AJ. Does smoking explain sex differences in the global tuberculosis epidemic? Epidemiol Infect. 2006;134:333-9.
46. Diwan VK, Thorson A. Sex, gender, and tuberculosis. Lancet. 1999;353:1000-1.
47. Louwagie GM, Ayo-Yusuf OA. Tobacco use patterns in tuberculosis patients with high rates of human immunodeficiency virus co-infection in South Africa. BMC Public Health. 2013;13:1031.
48. Gajalakshmi V, Peto R, Kanaka TS, Jha P. Smoking and mortality from tuberculosis and other diseases in India: retrospective study of 43,000 adult male deaths and 35,000 controls. Lancet. 2003;362:507-15.
49. Pednekar MS, Gupta PC. Prospective study of smoking and tuberculosis in India. Prev Med. 2007;44:496-8.
50. Rao VG, Bhat J, Yadav R, et al. Tobacco smoking: a major risk factor for pulmonary tuberculosis—evidence from a cross-sectional study in central India. Trans R Soc Trop Med Hyg. 2014;108:474-81.
51. Lin JN, Lai CH, Chen YH, et al. Risk factors for extra-pulmonary tuberculosis compared to pulmonary tuberculosis. Int J Tuberc Lung Dis. 2009;13:620-5.
52. Liu BQ, Peto R, Chen ZM, et al. Emerging tobacco hazards in China: 1. Retrospective proportional mortality study of one million deaths. BMJ. 1998;317:1411-22.
53. Reed GW, Choi H, Lee SY, et al. Impact of diabetes and smoking on mortality in tuberculosis. PLoS One. 2013;8:e58044.
54. Jha P, Jacob B, Gajalakshmi V, et al. A nationally representative case-control study of smoking and death in India. N Engl J Med. 2008;358:1137-47.
55. Wen CP, Chan TC, Chan HT, Tsai MK, Cheng TY, Tsai SP. The reduction of tuberculosis risks by smoking cessation. BMC Infect Dis. 2010;10:156.
56. Gupta PC, Pednekar MS, Parkin DM, Sankaranarayanan R. Tobacco associated mortality in Mumbai (Bombay) India. Results of the Bombay Cohort Study. Int J Epidemiol. 2005;34:1395-402.
57. Patra J, Jha P, Rehm J, Suraweera W. Tobacco smoking, alcohol drinking, diabetes, low body mass index and the risk of self-reported symptoms of active tuberculosis: individual participant data (IPD) meta-analyses of 72,684 individuals in 14 high tuberculosis burden countries. PLoS One. 2014;9:e96433.
58. Hill AB. The environment and disease: association or causation? Proc R Soc Med. 1965;58:295-300.
59. Lam TH, Ho SY, Hedley AJ, Mak KH, Peto R. Mortality and smoking in Hong Kong: case-control study of all adult deaths in 1998. BMJ. 2001;323:361.
60. Pinidiyapathirage J, Senaratne W, Wickremasinghe R. Prevalence and predictors of default with tuberculosis treatment in Sri Lanka. Southeast Asian J Trop Med Public Health. 2008;39:1076-82.
61. Thomas A, Gopi PG, Santha T, et al. Predictors of relapse among pulmonary tuberculosis patients treated in a DOTS programme in South India. Int J Tuberc Lung Dis. 2005;9:556-61.
62. Altet-Gômez MN, Alcaide J, Godoy P, Romero MA, Hernández del Rey I. Clinical and epidemiological aspects of smoking and tuberculosis: a study of 13,038 cases. Int J Tuberc Lung Dis. 2005;9:430-6.
63. Tachfouti N, Nejjari C, Benjelloun MC, et al. Association between smoking status, other factors and tuberculosis treatment failure in Morocco. Int J Tuberc Lung Dis. 2011;15:838-43.
64. Maciel EL, Brioschi AP, Peres RL, et al. Smoking and 2-month culture conversion during anti-tuberculosis treatment. Int J Tuberc Lung Dis. 2013;17:225-8.
65. Magee MJ, Kempker RR, Kipiani M, et al. Diabetes mellitus, smoking status, and rate of sputum culture conversion in patients with multidrug-resistant tuberculosis: a cohort study from the country of Georgia. PLoS One. 2014;9:e94890.

66. Patra J, Bhatia M, Suraweera W, et al. Exposure to second-hand smoke and the risk of tuberculosis in children and adults: a systematic review and meta-analysis of 18 observational studies. PLoS Med. 2015;12:e1001835.
67. Singh M, Mynak ML, Kumar L, Mathew JL, Jindal SK. Prevalence and risk factors for transmission of infection among children in household contact with adults having pulmonary tuberculosis. Arch Dis Child. 2005;90:624-8.
68. Huang CC, Tchetgen ET, Becerra MC, et al. Cigarette smoking among tuberculosis patients increases risk of transmission to child contacts. Int J Tuberc Lung Dis. 2014;18:1285-91.
69. Altet MN, Alcaide J, Plans P, et al. Passive smoking and risk of pulmonary tuberculosis in children immediately following infection. A case-control study. Tuber Lung Dis. 1996;77:537-44.
70. Leung CC, Lam TH, Ho KS, et al. Passive smoking and tuberculosis. Arch Intern Med. 2010;170:287-92.
71. Hodge S, Hodge G, Ahern J, Jersmann H, Holmes M, Reynolds PN. Smoking alters alveolar macrophage recognition and phagocytic ability: implications in chronic obstructive pulmonary disease. Am J Respir Cell Mol Biol. 2007;37:748-55.
72. Shang S, Ordway D, Henao-Tamayo M, et al. Cigarette smoke increases susceptibility to tuberculosis—evidence from in vivo and in vitro models. J Infect Dis. 2011;203:1240-8.
73. Sopori M. Effects of cigarette smoke on the immune system. Nat Rev Immunol. 2002;2:372-7.
74. Arcavi L, Benowitz NL. Cigarette smoking and infection. Arch Intern Med. 2004;164:2206-16.
75. Feng Y, Kong Y, Barnes PF, et al. Exposure to cigarette smoke inhibits the pulmonary T-cell response to influenza virus and Mycobacterium tuberculosis. Infect Immun. 2011;79:229-37.
76. Borovikova LV, Ivanova S, Zhang M, et al. Vagus nerve stimulation attenuates the systemic inflammatory response to endotoxin. Nature. 2000;405:458-62.
77. van Zyl-Smit RN, Binder A, Meldau R, et al. Cigarette smoke impairs cytokine responses and BCG containment in alveolar macrophages. Thorax. 2014;69:363-70.
78. O'Leary SM, Coleman MM, Chew WM, et al. Cigarette smoking impairs human pulmonary immunity to Mycobacterium tuberculosis. Am J Respir Crit Care Med. 2014;190:1430-6.
79. Pradeepkumar AS, Thankappan KR, Nichter M. Smoking among tuberculosis patients in Kerala, India: proactive cessation efforts are urgently needed. Int J Tuberc Lung Dis. 2008;12:1139-45.
80. Ng N, Padmawati RS, Prabandari YS, Nichter M. Smoking behavior among former tuberculosis patients in Indonesia: intervention is needed. Int J Tuberc Lung Dis. 2008;12:567-72.
81. El Sony A, Slama K, Salieh M, et al. Feasibility of brief tobacco cessation advice for tuberculosis patients: a study from Sudan. Int J Tuberc Lung Dis. 2007;11:150-5.

CHAPTER 15
Pulmonary Diseases Caused by Nontuberculous Mycobacterium

Violeta V Mihailovic Vucinic

INTRODUCTION

Nontuberculous mycobacteria (NTM) or atypical mycobacteria—the term that was first coined by Pinner at the beginning of the 20th century, are typically environmental microorganisms residing in soil and water.[1] Up to date genus *Mycobacterium* has grown to more than 140 species.

All NTM have lipid-rich cell walls, confirming the acid-fast staining property which is the main characteristics. Beside two obligate pathogens (*M. tuberculosis* complex and *M. leprae*), there are many of NTM species who live freely in the environment. Out of the whole group of NTM species, some 25 species are associated with NTM manifested diseases while others are truly environmental organisms.[1-3]

Nontuberculous mycobacteria have the ability to cause pulmonary and extra-pulmonary granulomatosis disorders.

Pulmonary infections are most frequent. Because of the similarity of clinical manifestations and the overlap in diagnostic tools to conventional tuberculosis (TB), most of NTM are diagnosed and treated by pulmonologists.[4]

Lung disease represents 65–90% of all clinically manifested NTM comorbidity contributes to NTM infection, i.e., manifested emphysema, diabetes mellitus, leukemia, collagen vascular disease, lung cancer, chronic kidney disease, systemic lupus erythematosus.

Individuals on immune suppressive therapy are on high risk on NTM infection, as well as patients on antitumor necrosis factor-α (TNF-α) therapy, especially in human immunodeficiency virus (HIV) infection; these microbes can cause serious sometimes even deadly infection.[5,6]

In countries with low TB incidence, the incidence of NTM even outnumbers the incidence of TB cases. In the Unites States, the prevalence is 1.4–6.6 per 100,000.[6-11]

Factors that may explain this rising incidence in industrially well-developed countries are raising in the prevalence in HIV infection hematological malignancy, immunological disorders, and patient with immune suppressive therapy.

For these countries, additionally, the financial burden of NTM infection therapy is another serious problem, because the therapy regimes last for almost 2 years (four times longer than the TB treatment and four times expensive than the TB treatment).[7,12,13]

CLINICAL PRESENTATIONS OF NONTUBERCULOUS MYCOBACTERIA LUNG DISEASES

Pulmonary NTM disease is classified into four clinical presentations:
1. Fibrocavitary lung disease
2. Nodular bronchiectatic disease

3. Hypersensitivity-like disease
4. Cystic fibrosis and NTM infection.[1]

Fibrocavitary Lung Disease

In the year 1979, Wolinsky described NTM pulmonary disease "resembling TB with chest radiograph presenting fibrous thin wall cavity in the right upper lobe".[3]

The patient was middle-aged male heavy smoker with underlying chronic obstructive pulmonary disease, pneumoconiosis, and/or previous TB. The patient had history of productive cough and weight loss, and fibrocavitary lung disease caused by *M. avium* complex (MAC) infection. This is the typical presentation of possible MAC infection or *M. kansasii* infection, the two NTM species which are the most often cause of fibrocavitary NTM disease.

This type of lung disease has relatively high mortality because of already preexisting lung disease and possibly present respiratory insufficiency. The potential for progressive cavitary lung destruction requires aggressive therapy in these patients. The sputum from these patients is usually acid-fast bacillus (AFB) positive.[14-17]

In general, MAC is a pathogen commonly found in the environment and with the very low virulence. Since the expanding incidence of HIV infection, MAC has been recognized as the cause of severe pulmonary infection in HIV patients.[18-20]

In patients with already cured TB, old TB lesion may be infected by NTM.

In some patients, disease caused by *M. xenopi* has been superimposed to pulmonary aspergilloma of already cured empty lung cavities. This disease has poor prognosis.

Nodular Bronchiectatic Disease

In the year 1989, Prince and coworkers described patient with progressive noncavitary form of MAC pulmonary disease.[21]

A couple of years later in 1992, Reich and Johnson suggested a term "lady Windermere syndrome" for this form of MAC lung infection.[22]

The term was coined after Oscar Wilde's character from his novel "Lady Windermere's Fan". Lady Windermere was an old aristocrat that willingly suppressed her dry cough so the symptoms such as dry, quiet, discrete, covered cough are predominant symptoms of pulmonary nodular MAC infection in older individuals. Patients are often nonsmoking women with no evidence in previous lung disease except for bronchiectasis.[23]

Unrecognized and uncured infection leads to respiratory insufficiency. Besides MAC, this form of pulmonary disease may be caused by *M. kansasii*, *M. xenopi*, and *M. scrofulaceum*.

Hypersensitivity-like Disease

Mycobacterium avium may be the cause of pulmonary disease called "hot tub lung disease". The cause is the inhalation of mycobacterial antigen through contaminated water in hot tubes. Patients often have acute and subacute onset of dyspnea and cough, they may also have fever and hypoxemia.[24-27]

Histological findings represent nonnecrotizing granulomas or sings of organizing pneumonia or interstitial pneumonia.[26]

Tissue cultures are positive for mycobacteria, thoracic computed tomography (CT) scans resemble infiltrates, nodules, or ground-glass lesions. The differential diagnosis is hypersensitivity pneumonitis or sarcoidosis.[27,28]

Cystic Fibrosis and Nontuberculous Mycobacteria Infection

Patients with cystic fibrosis can often develop NTM infection. The predisposition for NTM infection is very high in these patients due to bronchiectasis.

In the United States study, 13% of patients with cystic fibrosis had NTM lung disease, 72% MAC, and 16% *M. abscessus* while in European cystic fibrosis patients, *M. abscessus* predominates.[29-31]

NONTUBERCULOUS MYCOBACTERIA INFECTION IN THE IMMUNOCOMPROMISED

In the course of HIV infection, NTM infection develops much earlier when the CD4+ cell count is yet significantly higher than 50 cells/mL.

Patients with systemic immune suppression, i.e., hematological malignancy, TNF-α inhibitor therapy, systemic corticosteroid therapy, etc., are at high risk of developing disseminated NTM disease.[12]

Approximately, 30% of HIV patients with NTM infection have manifested lung disease.

Usually, these patients after beginning antiretroviral therapy, develop respiratory and general symptoms like cough 93%, dyspnea 47%, fever 80%, and night sweats 73%. Thoracic CT demonstrates lymphadenopathy, cavitary lesions, nodules, or pericardial effusion.[32]

Nontuberculous mycobacterium pulmonary disease in organ transplant recipients is very rare 0.2–5%.[33-35]

Stem cell transplant recipients often have catheter-related infections and NTM pulmonary disease is the second most common complication.[35]

DIAGNOSIS OF NONTUBERCULOUS MYCOBACTERIA DISEASES

According to the American Thoracic Society and Infectious Disease Society of America, there are clinical, radiological, and microbiological criteria for diagnosis of NTM.[1]

Clinical Criteria

- Pulmonary symptoms including cough, dyspnea, and hemoptysis
- General symptoms like fever and weight loss
- Exclusion of other possible diseases.

Radiological Criteria

- Nodular lesion
- Infiltrations with cavitary opacities on chest X-ray
- High-resolution computed tomography representing multifocal bronchiectasis with multiple small nodules.

Microbiological Criteria

- Positive culture resulting from at least two sputum specimens
- Positive culture resulting from at least one bronchial lavage

- Lung biopsy specimens with typical histological characteristic of either granuloma inflammation or AFB and one (at least) sputum culture positive for NTM
- If NTM are isolated that usually represent in environmental contamination or if NTM isolated are in frequently encountered expert consultation should be obtained
- Patients suspected for NTM disease who do not meet criteria sited above should be followed up until the definite confirmation or exclusion of the diagnosis
- The definite diagnosis of NTM does not obviously mean beginning of therapy; the treatment should be based upon the facts of potential risks and/or benefits of the treatment.

CONSERVATIVE TREATMENT OF NONTUBERCULOUS MYCOBACTERIA DISEASE

Conservative treatment of NTM disease has been shown in table 1.

TABLE 1	Conservative treatment of nontuberculous mycobacteria disease[1]
Nontuberculous mycobacteria disease	**Therapy**
Mycobacterium avium complex (MAC) pulmonary disease	–
Nodular/bronchiectatic disease	Three times-weekly regimen of clarithromycin (1,000 mg) or azithromycin (500 mg), rifampin (600 mg), and ethambutol (25 mg/kg)
Fibrocavitary MAC lung disease or severe nodular/bronchiectatic disease	Daily regimen of clarithromycin (500–1,000 mg) or azithromycin (250 mg), rifampin (600 mg) or rifabutin (150–300 mg), and ethambutol (15 mg/kg) with consideration of three times-weekly amikacin or streptomycin early in therapy. Patients should be treated until culture negative on therapy for 1 year
Disseminated MAC disease	Clarithromycin (1,000 mg/day) or azithromycin (250 mg/day) and ethambutol (15 mg/kg/day) with or without rifabutin (150–350 mg/day). Therapy can be discontinued with resolution of symptoms and recovery of cell-mediated immune function
Treatment of nontuberculous mycobacteria cervical lymphadenitis due to MAC	Primarily by surgical excision, with a greater than 90% cure rate. A macrolide-based regimen should be considered for patients with extensive MAC lymphadenitis or poor response to surgical therapy
Prophylaxis of disseminated Mycobacterium avium complex disease	
Adults with acquired immunodeficiency syndrome with CD4 lymphocyte counts < 50 cells/µL	Azithromycin 1,200 mg/week or clarithromycin 1,000 mg/day has proven efficacy. Rifabutin 300 mg/day is also effective but with reconsidering side effects
M. kansasii pulmonary disease	Daily isoniazid (300 mg/day), rifampin (600 mg/day), and ethambutol (15 mg/kg/day). Treatment until negative culture on therapy for 1 year

Continued

Continued

TABLE 1	Conservative treatment of nontuberculous mycobacteria disease[1]
Nontuberculous mycobacteria disease	**Therapy**
M. abscessus pulmonary disease	Multidrug regimens including clarithromycin 1,000 mg/day may cause improvement of symptoms and disease regression. Surgical resection of localized disease combined with multidrug clarithromycin-based therapy offers the best chance for cure of this disease
Nonpulmonary disease caused by NTM (*M. abscessus, M. chelonae, M. fortuitum*)	Therapy based on *in vitro* susceptibilities. For *M. abscessus* disease, a macrolide-based regimen is frequently used. Surgery may also be an important element of successful therapy

CASE STUDY 1

A 40-year-old patient had pulmonary TB in 1999 when a complete medical treatment in duration of 6 months was performed. About 10 years after the TB treatment was completed, he complained of cough, increased fatigue, loss of body weight. Chest radiography revealed fibrous lesions in the upper lobe of the right lung (Fig. 1). Chest CT showed same lesions of the upper lobe right lung (Fig. 2). Bronchoscopy examination showed signs of inflammation. *Mycobacterium xenopi* was isolated from Lowenstein sputum culture and bronchial aspiration. *Mycobacterium xenopi* was also confirmed by subsequent Mycobacteria Growth Indicator Tube analysis.

The patient responded well to therapy with signs of radiographic regression and clinical improvement with no side effects.

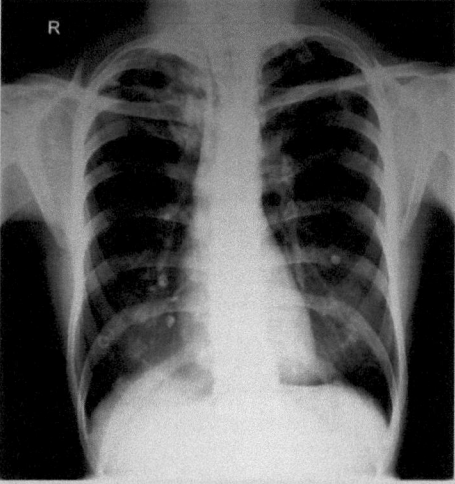

FIG. 1: Chest radiography representing fibrous lesions in the upper lobe of the right lung.

Courtesy: Professor Dr Vesna Skodric-Trifunovic, University Hospital of Pulmonary Diseases, Clinical Center of Serbia, Belgrade, Serbia.

Fibrocavitary lesions that mostly involve the upper lobes and resemble pulmonary TB.

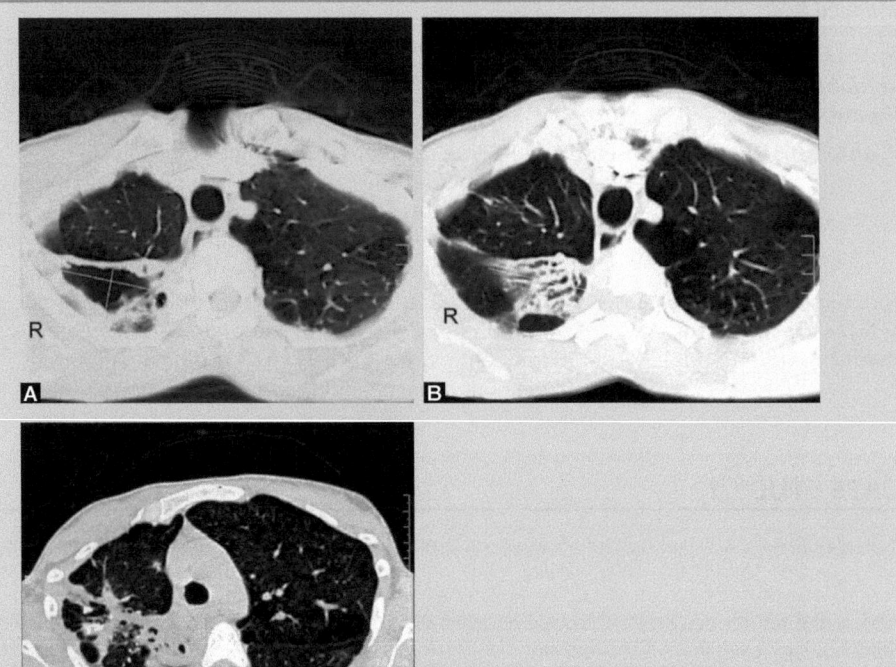

FIG. 2: Composite computed tomography scans case study 1.

Cavitary lesions can sometimes occur in pulmonary malignancy and sarcoidosis as well as in infections by nonmycobacterial pathogens including fungi and *Nocardia* species.[36]

However, some authors suggested that in cavitary disease, caused by NTM, lung lesions are characterized by thin-walled cavities, whereas TB would present with thick-walled cavities; a review of these and later studies has refuted the use of cavity appearance as a diagnostic tool.

Of note that other infectious (e.g., nocardiosis, fungal infection, TB) and noninfectious diseases (e.g., sarcoidosis) that can present with similar clinical and radiographic features have to be properly excluded before a firm diagnosis of NTM lung disease is made. Even in otherwise successful treatment, radiographic abnormalities may persist or even appear to increase in size; only small nodules tend to disappear during successful treatment.[37-39]

CASE STUDY 2

A 54-year-old patient was treated in the University Hospital of Lung Diseases, Clinical Center of Serbia during June and July 2011 when based on clinical findings (cough, sputum production, fever, night sweats), radiographic findings (lesion of the upper and middle lobe right lung) (Fig. 3) and two positive Lowenstein sputum cultures (50 and 30 colonies)—anti-TB treatment was started: isoniazid (H), rifampicin (R), pyrazinamide (Z), and ethambutol (E). Acid-fast bacillus smear negative (three sputum samples).

Chest CT showed excavation located in the upper lobe of the right lung, and bronchiectasis in the middle and lower lobe right lung (Fig. 4). Bronchoscopy examination showed signs of inflammation. Histopathological findings were unrepresentative. In 2011, November, the patient did not improve properly. Subsequently, hybridization of cultures was performed and MAC was identified.

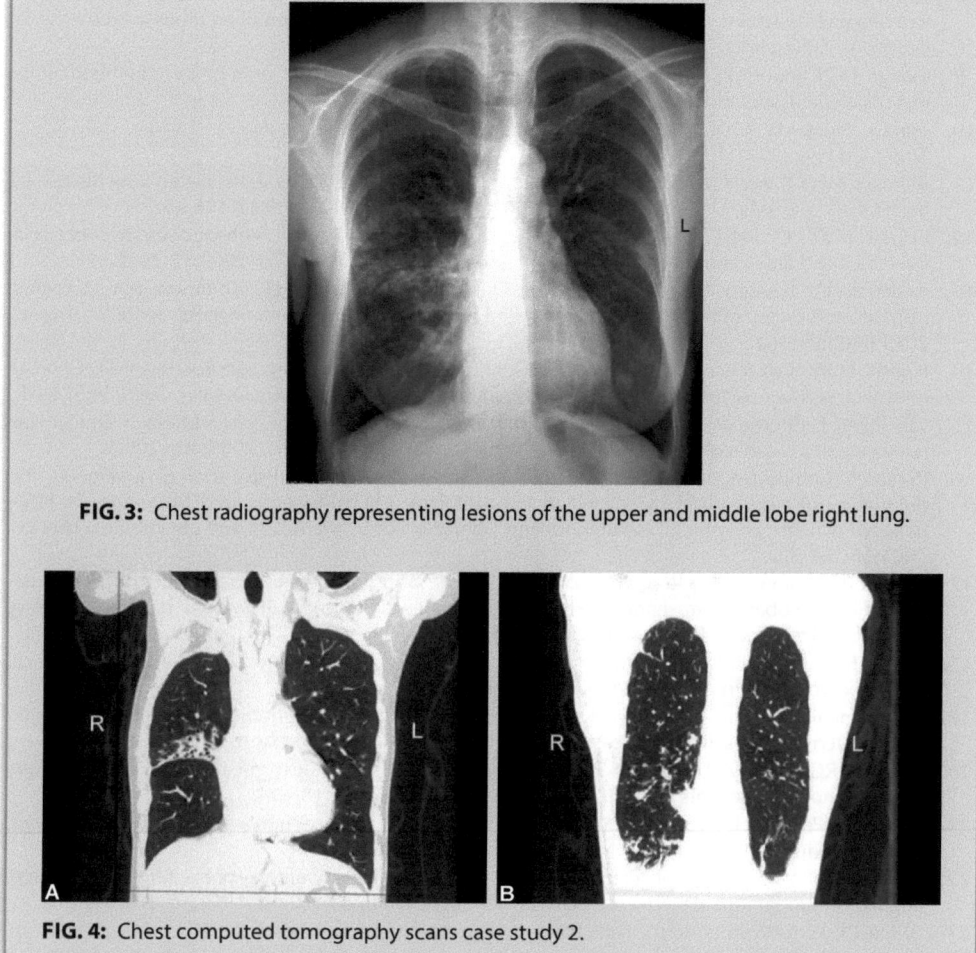

FIG. 3: Chest radiography representing lesions of the upper and middle lobe right lung.

FIG. 4: Chest computed tomography scans case study 2.

REFERENCES

1. Griffith DE, Aksamit T, Brown-Elliott BA, et al. An official ATS/IDSA statement: diagnosis, treatment, and prevention of nontuberculous mycobacterial diseases. Am J Respir Crit Care Med. 2007;175(4):367-416.
2. Falkinham JO. Impact of human activities on the ecology of nontuberculous mycobacteria. Future Microbiol. 2010;5(6):951-60.
3. Wolinsky E. Nontuberculous mycobacteria and associated diseases. Am Rev Respir Dis. 1979;119(1):107-59.
4. O'Connell ML, Birkenkamp KE, Kleiner DE, Folio LR, Holland SM, Olivier KN. Lung manifestations in an autopsy-based series of pulmonary or disseminated nontuberculous mycobacterial disease. Chest. 2012;141(5):1203-9.
5. Wallis RS, Broder MS, Wong JY, Hanson ME, Beenhouwer DO. Granulomatous infectious diseases associated with tumor necrosis factor antagonists. Clin Infect Dis. 2004;38:1261-5.
6. Prevots DR, Shaw PA, Strickland D, et al. Nontuberculous mycobacterial lung disease prevalence at four integrated health care delivery systems. Am J Respir Crit Care Med. 2010;182:970-6.
7. Winthrop KL, McNelley E, Kendall B, et al. Pulmonary nontuberculous mycobacterial disease prevalence and clinical features: an emerging public health disease. Am J Respir Crit Care Med. 2010;182:977-82.

8. Thomson RM; NTM working group at Queensland TB Control Centre and Queensland Mycobacterial Reference Laboratory. Changing epidemiology of pulmonary nontuberculous mycobacteria infections. Emerg Infect Dis. 2010;16:1576-83.
9. Marras TK, Chedore P, Ying AM, Jamieson F. Isolation prevalence of pulmonary non-tuberculous mycobacteria in Ontario, 1997-2003. Thorax. 2007;62:661-6.
10. Tsai CF, Shiau MY, Chang YH, et al. Trends of mycobacterial clinical isolates in Taiwan. Trans R Soc Trop Med Hyg. 2011;105:148-52.
11. Billinger ME, Olivier KN, Viboud C, et al. Nontuberculous mycobacteria-associated lung disease in hospitalized persons, United States, 1998-2005. Emerg Infect Dis. 2009;15:1562-9.
12. Winthrop KL, Chang E, Yamashita S, Iademarco MF, LoBue PA. Nontuberculous mycobacteria infections and anti-tumor necrosis factor-alpha therapy. Emerg Infect Dis. 2009;15:1556-61.
13. Andrejak C, Nielsen RB, Thomsen VØ, Duhaut P, Sørensen HT, Thomsen RW. Chronic respiratory disease, inhaled corticosteroids and risk of non-tuberculous mycobacteriosis. Thorax. 2013;68(3):256-62.
14. Hoefsloot W, van Ingen J, de Lange WC, Dekhuijzen PN, Boeree MJ, van Soolingen D. Clinical relevance of Mycobacterium malmoense isolation in the Netherlands. Eur Respir J. 2009;34:926-31.
15. van Ingen J, Boeree MJ, de Lange WC, de Haas PE, Dekhuijzen PN, van Soolingen D. Clinical relevance of Mycobacterium szulgai in the Netherlands. Clin Infect Dis. 2008;46:1200-5.
16. Research Committee of the British Thoracic Society. First randomised trial of treatments for pulmonary disease caused by M. avium intracellulare, M. malmoense, and M. xenopi in HIV-negative patients: rifampicin, ethambutol and isoniazid versus rifampicin and ethambutol. Thorax. 2001;56:167-72.
17. Jenkins PA, Campbell IA; Research Committee of the British Thoracic Society. Pulmonary disease caused by Mycobacterium xenopi in HIV-negative patients: five year follow-up of patients receiving standardised treatment. Respir Med. 2003;97:439-44.
18. Berger E, Batra P, Ralston J, Sanchez MR, Franks AG Jr. Atypical mycobacteria infection in an immunocompromised patient. Dermatol Online J. 2010;16(11):21.
19. Cattamanchi A, Nahid P, Marras TK, et al. Detailed analysis of the radiographic presentation of Mycobacterium kansasii lung disease in patients with HIV infection. Chest. 2008;133:875-80.
20. Kalayjian RC, Toossi Z, Tomashefski JF Jr, et al. Pulmonary disease due to infection by Mycobacterium avium complex in patients with AIDS. Clin Infect Dis. 1995;20:1186-94.
21. Prince DS, Peterson DD, Steiner RM, et al. Infection with Mycobacterium avium complex in patients without predisposing conditions. N Engl J Med. 1989;321:863-8.
22. Reich JM, Johnson RE. Mycobacterium avium complex pulmonary disease presenting as an isolated lingular or middle lobe pattern. The Lady Windermere syndrome. Chest. 1992;101:1605-9.
23. Wilde O. Lady Windermere's Fan. Plays written or first performed at the St James's Theatre in London; 1892.
24. Hanak V, Kalra S, Aksamit TR, Hartman TE, Tazelaar HD, Ryu JH. Hot tub lung: presenting features and clinical course of 21 patients. Respir Med. 2006;100:610-5.
25. Hanak V, Golbin JM, Ryu JH. Causes and presenting features in 85 consecutive patients with hypersensitivity pneumonitis. Mayo Clin Proc. 2007;82:812-6.
26. Khoor A, Leslie KO, Tazelaar HD, Helmers RA, Colby TV. Diffuse pulmonary disease caused by nontuberculous mycobacteria in immunocompetent people (hot tub lung). Am J Clin Pathol. 2001;115:755-62.
27. Hartman TE, Jensen E, Tazelaar HD, Hanak V, Ryu JH. CT findings of granulomatous pneumonitis secondary to Mycobacterium avium-intracellulare inhalation: "hot tub lung". AJR Am J Roentgenol. 2007;188:1050-3.
28. Martinez S, McAdams HP, Batchu CS. The many faces of pulmonary nontuberculous mycobacterial infection. AJR Am J Roentgenol. 2007;189:177-86.
29. Olivier KN, Weber DJ, Wallace RJ Jr, et al. Nontuberculous mycobacteria. I. multicenter prevalence study in cystic fibrosis. Am J Respir Crit Care Med. 2003;167:828-34.
30. Olivier KN, Weber DJ, Lee JH, et al. Nontuberculous mycobacteria. II. nested-cohort study of impact on cystic fibrosis lung disease. Am J Respir Crit Care Med. 2003;167:835-40.
31. Roux AL, Catherinot E, Ripoll F, et al. Multicenter study of prevalence of nontuberculous mycobacteria in patients with cystic fibrosis in France. J Clin Microbiol. 2009;47:4124-8.

32. Phillips P, Bonner S, Gataric N, et al. Nontuberculous mycobacterial immune reconstitution syndrome in HIV-infected patients: spectrum of disease and long-term follow-up. Clin Infect Dis. 2005;41:1483-97.
33. Doucette K, Fishman JA. Nontuberculous mycobacterial infection in hematopoietic stem cell and solid organ transplant recipients. Clin Infect Dis. 2004;38:1428-39.
34. Daley CL. Nontuberculous mycobacterial disease in transplant recipients: early diagnosis and treatment. Curr Opin Organ Transplant. 2009;14:619-24.
35. Weinstock DM, Feinstein MB, Sepkowitz KA, Jakubowski A. High rates of infection and colonization by nontuberculous mycobacteria after allogeneic hematopoietic stem cell transplantation. Bone Marrow Transplant. 2003;31:1015-21.
36. Kanne JP, Yandow DR, Mohammed TL, Meyer CA. CT findings of pulmonary nocardiosis. AJR Am J Roentgenol. 2011;197(2):W266-72.
37. Albelda SM, Kern JA, Marinelli DL, Miller WT. Expanding spectrum of pulmonary disease caused by nontuberculous mycobacteria. Radiology. 1985;157(2):289-96.
38. Ellis SM. The spectrum of tuberculosis and non-tuberculous mycobacterial infection. Eur Radiol. 2004;14 Suppl 3:E34-42.
39. Fujiuchi S, Matsumoto H, Yamazaki Y, et al. Analysis of chest CT in patients with Mycobacterium avium complex pulmonary disease. Respiration. 2003;70(1):76-81.

CHAPTER 16

Treatment of Tuberculosis

Dragica P Pesut

INTRODUCTION

Before the era of available anti-tuberculosis (TB) drugs, basic principle of TB treatment included bed rest, diet, and hygiene. The first anti-TB drug streptomycin commenced in 1944 followed with para-aminosalicylic acid and, then, with isoniazid and pyrazinamide in 1952, and ethambutol in 1961. Chemical modifications of rifamycins in early 1960s led to synthesis of rifampicin and its therapeutic use in 1968.[1] Its common administration with isoniazid considerably decreased duration of TB treatment (from 18-24 months to 9 months).[2] Together with declaring TB global emergency by the World Health Organization (WHO), the strategy Directly Observed Treatment Short-course (DOTS) was developed in 1990s.[3] The recommended therapy regimen is known as short-course chemotherapy. Pyrazinamide plays a key role in the shortening treatment of TB from 9-12 months to 6 months.[4] The major historical landmarks of TB treatment are presented in table 1.

Successful implementation of DOTS strategy led to a decline in TB incidence and prevalence in some countries such as Peru, Cuba, China, parts of India, and the United States of America[5] while in some other countries in Europe (e.g., Scandinavian, Yugoslavia, the Netherlands, Soviet Union) and in Latin America (Uruguay and Chile), TB declined rapidly from the 1960s to the 1980s. In the majority of the countries, it coincided with implementation of national TB programs, which had the basic DOTS elements in place. Contribution of synchronous social and economic development could not be neglected.

TABLE 1	The major historical landmarks of tuberculosis treatment[1-3]	
Time	*Intervention*	*Therapy duration (months)*
1944	Discovery of effective medication: Streptomycin and para-aminosalicylic acid	>18–24
1952	Administration of "triple therapy" (streptomycin, para-aminosalicylic acid, and isoniazid) assured cure	≈18
1970s	Isoniazid and rifampicin administered together reduced the duration of treatment	9
1980s	Adding of pyrazinamide allowed short-course regimen	6

> **BOX 1** **Drugs with proved action against *Mycobacterium tuberculosis* recommended for treatment of tuberculosis**
> - First line drugs for oral administration: Isoniazid (H), rifampicin (R), pyrazinamide (Z), ethambutol (E)
> - Injectable agents: Streptomycin (S), amikacin, kanamycin, capreomycin
> - Fluoroquinolones: Ciprofloxacin*, ofloxacin*, levofloxacin, moxifloxacin, gatifloxacin
> - Second line oral drugs and reserve drugs: Ethionamide, prothionamide, para-aminosalicylic acid, cycloserine, terizidone, rifabutin, amoxicillin/clavulanic acid, clarithromycin, clofazimine, linezolid, imipenem/cilastatin
> - New drugs: Bedaquiline, delamanid
>
> *Not recommended if newer generation fluoroquinolones are available.

Due to emerging problem of drug-resistant TB, short-course regimen, which contains the first line anti-TB drugs (isoniazid, rifampicin, pyrazinamide, ethamutol, and streptomycin), had to be replaced with the regimens of much longer duration consisting of combinations of the second line anti-TB drugs (listed in the Box 1). Thus, the recommended DOTS strategy was renamed to DOT in 2008 (S stated for short-course).[6]

ANTITUBERCULOSIS DRUGS

Currently, appropriate treatment of TB is chemotherapy consisting of a combination of several anti-TB drugs.[7] Drug combination is important to act against different populations of *Mycobacterium tuberculosis* in human organism (metabolically active mycobacteria under conditions of continuous growth, those in the acid inhibition phase and bacilli in a sporadic multiplication phase), and to prevent or to combat existing drug resistance. Thus, general rules of susccessful TB treatment exclude administration of a single drug alone (drug resistance usually follows and is permanent), and never adding a single drug alone to the existing drug combination in the case of patient's worsening.[8] The list of currently recommended anti-TB drugs is presented in box 1.

A study aimed to explore possible role of fluoroquinolones in treatment of TB showed that gatifloxacin had higher activity against *M. tuberculosis* isolates followed by ofloxacin, levofloxacin, and sparfloxacin whereas ciprofloxacin showed the lowest activity.[9] Gatifloxacin was also found to be the most effective fluoroquinolone against multidrug-resistant isolates both from previously treated and nontreated patients. Thus, except ciprofloxacin, other fluoroquinolones showed potential to be included in the treatment regimens of TB including multidrug-resistant disease. Sparfloxacin, although highly active against mycobacteria, is not in the list of recommended fluoroquinolones in treatment of TB. Its use in clinical practice is restricted by side effects and the contribution to anti-TB therapy is unclear.[9] The prevalence and molecular characterization of fluoroquinolone-resistant *M. tuberculosis* isolates are in focus of current research.[10]

In 2014, a generic policy implementation package was produced by the WHO for the introduction of new anti-TB drugs or combination of drugs.[11] Apart from delivery model design, monitoring and evaluation, it includes pharmacovigilance, financing, procurement, and supply support, as well as private sector engagement, technical assistance, and operational research.

TREATMENT OF NEW TUBERCULOSIS CASE-DRUG SENSITIVE

History taking and careful review of available medical documents are of crucial importance to reveal if the patient has ever been treated for TB or not. This step contributes to proper selection of the patient's category (new case or previously treated patient—relapse of the disease or chronic disease) and proper choice of treatment regimen. Previously treated patients have significantly higher risk of multidrug-resistant TB (MDR-TB) compared with new cases (20.5% vs. 3.5% respectively).[12]

Treatment regimen for newly diagnosed TB cases is also called short-course regimen, which lasts 6 months or longer. It includes use of the first line drugs during 2 months of initial phase (usually combination of at least four drugs) followed by 4 months of continual phase (usually combination of two drugs). The standard short-course anti-TB drug regimen is expressed as 2HRZE (isoniazid, rifampicin, pyrazinamide, ethambutol)/4HR (isoniazid, rifampicin) with numbers 2 and 4 denoting month duration of treatment in the initial and continual phase, respectively. The three drugs, isoniazid, rifampicin, and pyrazinamide, could be enough in initial phase only in the case of known drug susceptibility to isoniazid and rifampicin. Being very active drugs that are responsible for killing and sterilizing *M. tuberculosis*, isoniazid and rifampicin should be retained throughout the entire treatment, if possible. First line anti-TB drugs except streptomycin are used orally 30 minutes before breakfast in a single daily dose. Apart from daily administration, intermittent treatment could be discussed. Based on the good postantibiotic effect of isoniazid and rifampicin, initial phase of treatment may be equally effective if the drugs are administered two or three times a week.[13,14] Currently, daily treatment is recommended during initial therapy phase, while therapy three times a week in the continuation phase may be advocated exceptionally, e.g., when the patients' adherence to treatment is not ideal.[15] Notes on the standard abbreviations of drug names and daily dosage are presented in table 2.

Velayutham et al. demonstrated the sterilizing capacity and potential of five-drug daily regimens which contain moxifloxacin to shorten duration of TB treatment.[16] Compared to the thrice-weekly four-drug regimen [rifampicin, isoniazid, pyrazinamide ethambutol (RHZE)] in patients with newly diagnosed sputum positive pulmonary TB, a five-drug daily regimen with moxifloxacin [isoniazid, rifampicin, pyrazinamide, ethambutol, moxifloxacin (HRZEM)] resulted in significantly higher sputum culture conversion in the first 2 months.

TABLE 2	The first line antituberculosis drugs (abbreviations) and daily dosage	
Drug	*Daily dosage adults*	*Children*
Isoniazid (H)	5–10 mg/kg, max 300 mg orally or IM	5–10 mg/kg
Rifampicin (R)	10 mg/kg, max 600 mg orally	10–20 mg/kg
Pyrazinamide (Z)	25–30 mg/kg, max 2 g orally	40 mg/kg
Streptomycin (S)	15 mg/kg IM; BM < 50 kg: 0.75 g, BM > 50 kg: 1 g	20 mg/kg
Ethambutol (E)	15 mg/kg (up to 25 mg/kg in initial phase) orally	Avoided

IM, intramuscular; BM, body mass.

In some settings, serum drug concentrations are regularly measured, at least in human immunodeficiency virus (HIV)-positive TB patients, those with diabetes mellitus, or at extremes of weight (i.e., extremely under weight or extremely over weight).[17] The measurement is especially useful in the patients who show slow clinical response to treatment. A retrospective study, performed in Northern Alberta, Canada, in a 15-year period, showed that low isoniazid serum concentration, and, to a lesser extent, rifampicin, appeared to be associated with reduced sputum culture conversion after 2 months of treatment.[17]

Special Considerations

In some occasions, treatment of drug-sensitive TB should be fitted. Those special situations include women during pregnancy and lactation and patients with liver and/or renal diseases.[7,18-20] Aged and extremely aged patients require reduced drugs' doses. In HIV-positive patients, special consideration should be given to necessity of antiretroviral therapy and its timing related to anti-TB treatment, having in mind drug-drug reactions. Even more attention is needed in patients under treatment with second line anti-TB drugs.[7]

Tuberculosis in Pregnancy

In the pregnant women with active or recently active TB, there is neither indication for abortion nor for cesarean section due to TB. The recommendation is few decades old.[21] Medical treatment regimen should be applied for the benefit of the both mother and fetus, and protection of the newborn child. All the first line anti-TB drugs can be administered but streptomycin. Delivery under regional anesthesia and techniques to avoid excessive straining during the second stage of labor are advised. Forty years ago, Schaefer et al. found none of followed up 1,588 infants born to the tuberculous mothers had congenital TB and all were of average weight.[21] Pregnancy and TB are actual research topic again.[22]

TREATMENT OF DRUG-RESISTANT TUBERCULOSIS

Drug resistance has become a significant threat to TB control in many parts of the world.[12,23] It is usually a consequence of improper treatment, shortage or intermittent drug supply, and/or poor monitoring of the patients under treatment. Related therapy usually requires second line drugs, which are less effective, more toxic, and more costly.[23-25] Instead of the 6-month short therapy regimen applied for drug-sensitive disease, drug-resistant TB requires longer therapy duration that may exceed 20 months and has a much lower rate of successful outcome. Ideally, all patients would undergo rapid drug-resistance testing, so that an appropriate treatment regimen can be provided. In the settings where the testing is not available, decisions about therapy regimens should be made on an individualized basis. The knowledge on both the local epidemiology and patient-specific factors could be helpful, especially the information about possible source of infection. As previously mentioned, patient's history taking should provide the answer if the patient has ever been treated for TB because the proportion of drug resistance is the highest among people previously treated for tubersulosis.[12] Apart from *M. tuberculosis* resistance to a single drug, resistance may develop to two, three, or more first line or second line drugs.

Multidrug-resistant TB is defined as TB caused by strains of *M. tuberculosis* that are resistant to at least the two most important first line drugs isoniazid and rifampicin. Therapy regimens to treat MDR-TB cases are tailored individually according to drug-susceptibility test (DST) results and information on source of infection if it is available. Following to the WHO recommendations, they contain fluoroquinolones, injectable

TABLE 3	Treatment duration and regimens for multidrug-resistant tuberculosis	
Duration (months)	Preferred regimen	Alternative regimen
8	SL-inj, FQ, Pto/Eto, Cs/Trd, E, Z	SL-inj, FQ, PAS, Cs/Trd, E, Z
12	FQ, Pto/Eto, Cs/Trd, E, Z	FQ, PAS, Cs/Trd, E, Z

Z, pyrazinamide; E, ethambutol; SL-inj, second line injectable; FQ, fluoroquinolone; Pto/Eto, prothionamide/ethionamide; Cs/Trd, cycloserine/terizidone; PAS, para-aminosalicylic acid.

TABLE 4	Treatment of extensively drug-resistant tuberculosis	
Duration (months)	Preferred regimen	Alternative regimen
20	Pto/Eto, Cs/Trd, Lzd, Cfz, Amx-Clv, Mero, E, Z	PAS, Cs/Trd, Lzd, Cfz, Amx-Clv, Mero, E, Z

Z, pyrazinamide; E, ethambutol; Pto/Eto, prothionamide/ethionamide; Cs/Trd, cycloserine/terizidone; PAS, para-aminosalicylic acid; Lzd, linezolid; Cfz, clofazimine; Amx-Clv, amoxicillin-clavulanic acid; Mero, meropenem.

agents, and other second line oral drugs (Table 3). Consultation with TB experts (e.g., *consilium*) is crucial in creating a treatment regimen.

In extensively drug-resistant or extreme drug-resistant TB (XDR-TB) strains are resistant to all the current first line drugs, as well as to any of fluoroquinolones and at least to one of three injectable second line drugs (capreomycin, kanamycin, or amikacin). Extensively drug-resistant-TB, already detected in 100 countries,[12] may progress to total drug-resistant TB if a nonadequate combination of drugs is administered or if patient's adherence to treatment is not achieved.[26] This turns the world back to the times without available anti-TB drugs, making TB an incurable disease again. Treatment duration and regimens for XDR-TB are presented in table 4. In general, duration of individually tailored regimen should not be less than 18 months after culture conversion and injectable agents should be continued for at least first 6 months of therapy.

Apart from MDR-TB and XDR-TB, the other terms exist to denote degree of drug resistance. The term pre-XDRinj denotes MDR-TB with additional resistance to second line injectable drug while pre-XDRfq is related to MDR-TB with additional resistance to fluoroquinolone.[27]

A study on availability, price, and affordability of anti-TB drugs in Europe showed that, compared to capreomycin, kanamycin was markedly cheaper.[27] Additionally, kanamycin-containing regimens showed larger effect on treatment success in MDR-TB.[28] Some other drugs, such as linezolid, previously used in treatment of other infections, especially nontuberculous mycobacterial diseases, found their place in TB drug regimens for those complicated cases of MDR-TB and XDR-TB.[12,29] Linezolid-containing regimens have led to more rapid culture conversion compared to regimens without the drug in treatment of XDR-TB.[30,31] However, use of linezolid carries the high risk of adverse events.[31] Lowering the dose from 1,200 to 600 mg[29] and, especially, from 600 to 300 mg might be beneficial in this terms.[31]

NEW DRUGS AND REGIMENS

The need of new anti-TB agents to address the problem of drug-resistant TB has intensified research and two new medicaments have been developed—delamanid

(OPC-67683) and bedaquiline (TMC207). They emerged over 2013–2014 for use in regimens for drug-resistant TB in cases where other combinations are not effective.[11] Bedaquiline and delamanid seem promising drugs, which demonstrated a protective effect against the emergence of further resistances toward the backbone drugs, in particular, during the development phase.[32]

Bedaquiline

Bedaquiline (TMC207) is a new anti-TB drug with a novel mechanism of action that is available for the first time in over 40 years.[33,34] This diarylquinoline drug works by inhibiting bacterial adenosine triphosphate synthase.[35] Although it has only been through two Phase IIb trials for safety and efficacy, in December 2012, it was granted accelerated approval by the Food and Drug Administration. The WHO issued interim policy guidance for use of bedaquiline.[11] The drug should be used in combination with at least three other anti-TB drugs. The recommended dosage is 400 mg orally once daily for 2 weeks followed by 200 mg orally three times per week for 22 weeks. Bioavailability of the drug is twofold increased if it is taken with food. Bedaquiline is currently registered in several countries and the first results on its effectiveness were published recently: a report on its use in a nontrial setting in Europe—a French cohort[36] and in the first five patients in India,[37] where drug-resistant TB is a major problem. Striking improvement is observed in all the five MDR-TB patients in India. There are still no results on clinical effectiveness of bedaquiline in HIV-coinfected TB patients. Contrary to some other anti-TB drugs, bedaquiline is selective for mycobacterial species, and it is believed that the feature would likely extend its durability by minimizing the emergence of drug resistance.[34]

Delamanid

Delamanid, a dihydro-nitroimidazooxazole derivative, is a mycobacterial cell wall synthesis inhibitor, which received a conditional approval from the European Medicines Agency for the treatment of MDR-TB. Its high potency and better tolerability together with least risk for drug-drug interactions have been demonstrated.[38,39] Delamanid also improved outcomes and reduced mortality in MDR-TB.[40] No significant interactions were observed between delamanid and antiretroviral drugs (tenofovir, lopinavir/ritonavir, and efavirenz) in clinical trials conducted on healthy subjects.[41]

Current Status of Drug Discovery and Development

In the supplement of the Global Tuberculosis Report 2014,[12] the WHO presented current status of discovery and development of potentially new anti-TB drugs as of August 2014 [lead optimization: cyclopeptides, diarylquinolines, DprE inhibitors, InhA inhibitor, indazoles, LeuRS inhibitors, ureas, macrolides, azaindoles, mycobacterial gyrase inhibitors, pyrazinamide analogs, ruthenium (II) complexes, spectinamides, SPR-10199, translocase-1 inhibitors; preclinical development: CPZEN-45, BTZ043, DC-159a, SQ609, SQ641, TBI-166; good laboratory practice toxicity: PBTZ169, TBA-354, Q203; clinical development phase II: AZD5847, bedaquiline (TMC207), linezolid novel regimens b, PA-824, rifapentine, SQ-109, sutezolid (PNU-100480); clinical development phase III: delamanid (OPC-67683), gatifloxacin, moxifloxacin, rifapentine].[12]

The preliminary results of two studies presented recently at the 2014 World Conference on Lung Health appointed to high success rate of shortened MDR-TB regimen, i.e., suggested that 9-month treatment regimen for MDR-TB appeared to be as effective as a 12-month regimen.[42] Further studies should reveal the effect of MDR-TB treatment with oral anti-TB drugs alone.

Thioridazine

In the era of increasing incidence rates of MDR-TB and XDR-TB, it might be worth to mention an old neuroleptic compound, thioridazine, which has been put to clinicians' attention again as possible agent for treatment of drug-resistant TB cases. The Portuguese authors believe that the agent, shown to inhibit efflux pumps of bacteria, will prove to be effective having small risks and great rewards.[43] They suggest that compassionate therapy with thioridazine should be contemplated when available therapy is predictably ineffective and death is inevitable due to poor prognosis.

VITAMIN SUPPLEMENTATION

Pyridoxine (vitamin B6) is not recommended in routine practice in all the patients treated with isoniazid but in patients with malnutrition, chronic alcoholism, and diabetes mellitus together with start of isonazid. For all the other patients, in the majority of guidelines, its use in dose of 50-100 mg daily is recommended only if peripheral neuropathy occurs.[7]

Vitamin C: Tuberculosis is associated with oxidative stress, and is traditionally linked to vitamin C deficiency, which persisted during conventional treatment.[44] Thus, the vitamin has been used as an adjuvant agent in the treatment of TB.[44] The results of recent study on treatment of TB meningitis confirm increased local and systemic oxidative stress, accompanied by impaired redox status, while not total vitamin C deficiency was found.[45] Oxidative stress and vitamin C status in TB patients is in focus of current research. Starting from the point that the vitamin can prevent oxidative damage, including the toxic effects of anti-TB drugs, further studies are needed to reveal whether its supplementation would be beneficial in treatment of TB.

Vitamin D: The key role of the antirachitic substance in calcium and bone homeostasis has been studied since the early 1920s.[46] It has been also recognized that the vitamin is able to modulate a variety of processes involved in regulatory systems such as host defense—inflammation, immunity, and repair. The role and serum level of vitamin D have been studied in many respiratory diseases including upper respiratory tract infections.[47] Thanks to known effects of vitamin D on antimicrobial immunity *in vitro* (suppresses the intracellular growth of *M. tuberculosis*), the vitamin was used in TB treatment in the preantibiotic era.[48,49] As part of TB treatment in sanatoriums, patients have been encouraged to sit in balconies in the sun making lots of vitamin D. The vitamin is known to induce the expression of cathelicidin, which is involved in the first line of defense in TB.[50] Due to conflicting results, a role of vitamin D in treatment of TB is still discussed. It seems that supplementation of the vitamin may be beneficial to those patients with insufficient vitamin D levels.[51,52] One of the latest studies showed that supplementation with 1,000 IU/day vitamin D3 (25-hydroxyvitamin D) did not significantly reduce the incidence or duration of the infections in adults.[47] The other study demonstrated both a role of vitamin D supplementation in accelerating resolution of inflammatory responses during TB therapy, and attenuation of suppressive effect of anti-TB medicaments on antigen-stimulated secretion of interleukin-4 (IL-4), CC chemokine ligand 5, and interferon-α.[53] Vitamin D receptor polymorphisms are associated with susceptibility to *M. tuberculosis* infection.[50] Findings of a multicenter randomized controlled trial showed that adjunctive vitamin D in adult patients with smear-positive pulmonary TB significantly hastened sputum culture conversion in the patients with the tt genotype of the TaqI vitamin D receptor polymorphism and not in all study population.[49] Further research on larger samples is needed to explore a role of vitamin D in treatment of TB.

ADJUNCTIVE THERAPY

Corticosteroids are traditionally contraindicated in TB patients except in those with pericarditis and meningoencephalitis. Recommended dose of methylprednisolone is 0.6 mg/kg during 4 weeks with gradual decrease of daily dose during the next 2 weeks. Short-term clinical benefits in pulmonary TB found did not appear to be maintained in the long term.[54] Corticosteroids are useful in reducing the outpouring of fluid from serous surfaces.[8] There is no proof that adhesions formation in specific pleuritis could be prevented by corticosteroids. Missing adrenocorticotropic hormones should be supplemented in adrenal glands TB.

Surgery has its place not only in treatment of late complications of TB (constrictive pericarditis, hydrocephalus, obstructive uropathy, Pott's disease, massive pleural adhesions with consecutive restrictive ventilation disturbance) but also in some forms of extrapulmonary TB and MDR-TB.[55] The medical treatment of MDR-TB can cure 50–75% of cases.[56] To increase the treatment success rates, some of the patients with medical treatment failure are selected for surgical resection [lobectomy, segmentectomy, cavernoplasty (speleoplasty)].[56] The patients should receive medical anti-TB treatment for at least 1 month, optimally 2 months, preoperatively as well as postoperatively to prevent disseminated disease. Individual drug regimens should include at least five drugs. Some innovative endoscopic methods have been proposed by Russian authors[57] in treatment of MDR-TB and some old almost forgotten methods such as artificial pneumothorax are used again in the combined therapy of destructive pulmonary TB.[58,59]

OTHER TREATMENT MODALITIES

A long time before potent anti-TB drugs appeared, the basic principle of TB treatment included bed rest, diet, and hygiene. The importance of those has never been diminished and, in the era of drug resistance, the actuality arisen. Even in drug-sensitive cases, bed rest is important during the beginning of chemotherapy and especially in severely ill patients. When it comes to diet, some controversies on vitamin D intake are previously mentioned. It is deeply embedded in some populations' beliefs that patients with TB should eat highly caloric and fat food to survive. The food regularly included bacon. It was only in 2003 when a compound with bactericidal effect on *M. tuberculosis* was identified in bacon.[60] Further research on modulating the immune response to shorten treatment duration and/or to overcome drug resistance might be of high importance in the era of drug-resistant disease.

TREATMENT OUTCOME

It is established that TB patients are registered at the time of diagnosis and start of treatment, and disease outcomes are recorded at the end of the therapy course.

Working groups of the WHO and the International Union Against Tuberculosis and Lung Disease recommended mutually exclusive categories of TB treatment outcome (cure, treatment completed, failure, death, treatment interrupted, and transfer out) with possible additional categories (still on treatment, etc.).[61,62] Finally, the WHO defined and standardized treatment outcomes through two important documents: (i) treatment of TB guidelines[7] and (ii) guidelines for the programmatic management of drug-resistant TB.[23] Having in mind duration of TB treatment, the analysis is carried out in the first quarter of the calendar year that follows a full year after the last patient was enrolled. Categories are expressed as a percentage of the total number of cases notified, given separately for newly diagnosed and retreated patients.

Global target of the World Health Assembly to achieve 85% as the rate of treatment success of treated smear-positive cases was reached for the first time in 2007, when the rate of 86% globally exceeded the goal.[63] In that term, coordination of clinical and public health services was crucially important, especially in low-incidence areas.[64] Unfortunately, dramatic increase of MDR-TB cases reported in the Global Tuberculosis Report 2014 of the WHO denoted previous global plan to eradicate TB in the world by 2050 nonreachable.[12] The main reason for the situation is failure of infection control as the most neglected vital intervention of TB prevention and care.[12] Despite new anti-TB agents which appeared in 2013, it seems that fight against TB will proceed to the next 200 years.

Contribution of surgery to disease outcome in TB has been studied in some countries such as Peru, Russia, or Korea, where, apart from standardized treatment regimens, surgery is used to improve treatment success in MDR-TB and XDR-TB cases. In Peru, surgery was used in 14% of the XDR-TB cases,[65] and in 4% of MDR-TB and XDR-TB cases in Korea.[66] Surgical treatment contributed to improved treatment success rate in the patients with MDR-TB (68.3% in surgically treated cases vs. 44.2% in nonsurgically treated).

Many studies focused on treatment outcomes in TB and the prediction of the outcome trying to reveal the factors of treatment failure, especially in drug-resistant TB.[67-69] Studies on default as a problem of treatment failure have shown reasons, timing, and some features of defaulters.[70,71] Thus, factors such as unemployment, alcoholism, homelessness, and being a pensioner were associated with default in Tashkent, Uzbekistan.[70] Default mostly occurred during the intensive phase, while the patients were hospitalized (61%), or just before they were to start the continuation phase (26%). A study from Moldova showed that default risk was the highest in the month following the phase of hospitalized treatment in civilians or, in former prisoners, after leaving prison.[72]

Sputum culture conversion is an important parameter of successful treatment outcome. It denotes achievement of negative sputum culture result in the patient with previously positive ones. Only rarely it happens without treatment in the patients who are able for self-limitation of the process owing to extensive and rapid fibrous tissue reactions. It seems that the carriers of O blood type of the ABO blood type system are more capable for such fibrous reaction leading to favorable disease outcome compared to the others.[73,74] In the majority of the patients, sputum conversion is the result of anti-TB treatment regimen.

The time necessary for conversion of the sputum culture under treatment may vary and depends on sterilizing capacity of anti-TB drugs. It can be achieved in 15 days, requires a month on average in drug-sensitive TB cases. Pyrazinamide is well known for its sputum sterilizing capacity and streptomycin has the proven effective activity inside cavitating lesions. Thus, despite the fact that the latter drug is less present in the newest regimens having ethambutol as alternative, it is recommended in the hospitalized patients with multicavity disease during initial phase of treatment.

ADHERENCE TO TREATMENT, ETHICAL ISSUES, AND PATIENTS' EDUCATION

When patients are offered anti-TB treatment, they should generally be informed and asked for their specific consent, but there is no inherent ethical obligation to do this by using a written form.[75] Treating the patient with a caring and respectful attitude enhances the likelihood that treatment will be completed. Those who refuse to consent to anti-TB treatment should be counseled about the risks to both themselves and the community. Patients rarely persist in refusing treatment when appropriate counseling is provided.

Illness perception assessment by means of the questionnaire, especially its brief version [Brief Illness Perception Questionnaire (BIPQ)], is useful and time-saving method, which may help a physician to understand the reasons the patients are reluctant about treatment and to successfully change their behavior.[76,77] The patients' adherence to treatment can increase the success rate of MDR-TB treatment. Although the patients have the right to refuse care, those with active TB who do not complete the necessary course of therapy, should be informed about the possibility of involuntary isolation or detention as last-resort measures.[75]

Education of the patients and population about TB, its causes, and clinical presentation should be widely offered without linguistic barriers. A new Tuberculosis Network European Trials Group project, ExplainTB, has been developed to meet this purpose worldwide. In the era of intensive electronic communication, the educational material is adapted for internet and iPhone use and offered in many languages.[78]

Tobacco Smoking

In many studies, majority of TB patients were found to be active smokers or exposed to environmental tobacco smoke at the time of diagnosis.[77,79,80] Even more, many of them listed smoking as the main cause of the disease by their own opinion.[77] Tobacco smoking is recognized not only as a major and the most preventable cause of morbidity and mortality in the world but also as an addictive disease.[81] Nicotine is the substance, which is continually necessary to its user.[82] Dependent smokers adjust their smoking behavior to maintain peripheral and central nicotine levels. That is why a high proportion of smokers that failed to quit smoking during the treatment of TB in a cohort was not unexpected.[77] Contents of tobacco smoke has been shown to decrease both humoral and cellular immunity in humans.[79,83-85]

Research on tobacco smoking association with TB demonstrated its influence on the severity and clinical course of the disease, contribution to longer duration of sputum culture conversion, and increased rate of relapses in smokers.[79,80] Thus, education of TB patients on harmful effects of tobacco smoking and its influence in TB is necessary. Due to nicotine dependence, which can be genetically influenced, proper professional help in smoking cessation should be offered to those patients who are not able to quit smoking alone.[81]

SOCIAL SUPPORT

Patients who belong to vulnerable groups of people (migrants, refugees and internally displaced people, homeless people and those dependent on drugs or alcohol, Roma population in slums, elderly in community centers for care, patients in psychiatric asylums, prostitutes, etc.) are in need of special and active approach to TB diagnosis and treatment.[86-88] Early detection of pulmonary TB is crucially important from both clinical and public health view. The prolonged period of infectiousness in undetected cases contributes to further dissemination of the disease in the community.[89-94] Welfare, incentives, and housing services together with other appropriate social support are important part of overall support to the patients which belong to those groups of people.[86] In some settings, lack of access to funds to support vulnerable patients severely compromises treatment access, completion, and cure.[95] In some countries, such as the United Kingdom, guidance on identifying and treating TB in underserved groups is provided.[96] Models of community support for TB patients exist, and a briefing on TB treatment in vulnerable groups was released in 2013.[97]

CONCLUSION

With still 9 million new TB cases and 1.5 million deaths from a curable disease, MDR-TB as a public health crisis in 2013, TB and its treatment remains monumental challenge in the 21st century. Apart from increase of political commitment and financing, successful TB therapy in the future should include high quality treatment of drug-susceptible cases to prevent the development of drug resistance, expanding of rapid testing to detect drug-resistant cases, and provision of immediate access to effective treatment and proper care.

REFERENCES

1. Sensi P. History of the development of rifampin. Rev Infect Dis. 1983;5 Suppl 3:S402-6.
2. Iseman MD. Tuberculosis therapy: past, present and future. Eur Respir J Suppl. 2002;36:87s-94s.
3. The Stop TB Strategy. Building on and enhancing DOTS to meet the TB-related Millennium Development Goals. Geneva, World Health Organization; 2006. [online] Available from: http://whqlibdoc.who.int/hq/2006/WHO_HTM_STB_2006.368_eng.pdf. [Accessed February, 2016].
4. Wade MM, Zhang Y. Effects of weak acids, UV and proton motive force inhibitors on pyrazinamide activity against *Mycobacterium tuberculosis in vitro*. J Antimicrob Chemother. 2006;58:936-41.
5. Lönnroth K, Jaramillo E, Williams BG, Dye C, Raviglione M. Drivers of tuberculosis epidemics: the role of risk factors and social determinants. Soc Sci Med. 2009;68:2240-6.
6. Veen J, Migliori GB, Raviglione M, et al. Harmonisation of TB control in the WHO European region: the history of the Wolfheze Workshops. Eur Respir J. 2011;37(4):950-9.
7. World Health Organization. Treatment of tuberculosis: guidelines. 4th ed. Geneva, Switzerland: WHO; 2009.
8. Crofton J, Horne N, Miller F. Clinical Tuberculosis. 2nd ed. London: Macmillan Educational Ltd; 1999.
9. Singh M, Chauhan DS, Gupta P, Das R, Srivastava RK, Upadhyay P, et al. *In vitro* effect of fluoroquinolones against Mycobacterium tuberculosis isolates from Agra and Kanpur region of north India. Indian J Med Res. 2009;129(5):542-7.
10. Zhang Z, Lu J, Wang Y, Pang Y, Zhao Y. Prevalence and molecular characterization of fluoroquinolone-resistant Mycobacterium tuberculosis isolates in China. Antimicrob Agents Chemother. 2014;58(1):364-9.
11. World Health Organization. The use of bedaquiline in the treatment of multidrug-resistant tuberculosis. Interim policy guidance. [online] Available from: http://www.who.int/tb/challenges/mdr/bedaquiline/en/. [Accessed February, 2016].
12. World Health Organization. (2014). Global tuberculosis report 2014. Geneva: WHO; 2014.
13. Mitchison DA, Dickinson JM. Laboratory aspects of intermittent drug therapy. Postgrad Med J. 1971;47:737-41.

14. Caminero JA, Matteelli A, Lange C. Treatment of TB. In: Migliori GB, Lange C, editors. Tuberculosis. Sheffield: European Respiratory Society; 2012. pp. 154-66.
15. Chang KC, Leung CC, Grosset J, Yew WW. Treatment of tuberculosis and optimal dosing schedules. Thorax. 2011;66:997-1007.
16. Velayutham BV, Allaudeen IS, Sivaramakrishnan GN, et al. Sputum culture conversion with moxifloxacin-containing regimens in the treatment of patients with newly diagnosed sputum-positive pulmonary tuberculosis in South India. Clin Infect Dis. 2014;59(10):e142-9.
17. Mah A, Kharrat H, Ahmed R, et al. Serum drug concentrations of INH and RMP predict 2-month sputum culture results in tuberculosis patients. Int J Tuberc Lung Dis. 2015;19(2):210-5.
18. Milburn HJ. How should we treat tuberculosis in adult patients with chronic kidney disease? Key messages from the British Thoracic Society Guidelines. Pol Arch Med Wewn. 2010;120(10):417-22.
19. Quantrill SJ, Woodhead MA, Bell CE, Hardy CC, Hutchison AJ, Gokal R. Side-effects of antituberculosis drug treatment in patients with chronic renal failure. Eur Respir J. 2002;20:440-3.
20. Unsal A, Ahbap E, Basturk T, et al. Tuberculosis in dialysis patients: a nine-year retrospective analysis. J Infect Dev Ctries. 2013;7(3):208-13.
21. Schaefer G, Zervoudakis IA, Fuchs FF, David S. Pregnancy and pulmonary tuberculosis. Obstet Gynecol. 1975;46(6):706-15.
22. Bothamley GH, TBNET contributors. Tuberculosis and pregnancy. TBNET project 2013. [online] Available from: http://www.tb-net.org/research. [Accessed February, 2016].
23. World Health Organization. Guidelines of the programmatic management of drug-resistant tuberculosis. Geneva, Switzerland: WHO; 2006.
24. Sotgiu G, Ferrara G, Matteelli A, Richardson MD, Centis R, Ruesch-Gerdes S, et al. Epidemiology and clinical management of XDR-TB: a systematic review by TBNET. Eur Respir J. 2009;33(4):871-81.
25. Migliori GB, Lange C, Girardi E, et al. Extensively drug-resistant tuberculosis is worse than multidrug-resistant tuberculosis: different methodology and settings, same results. Clin Infect Dis. 2008;46:958-9.
26. World Health Organization. Extensively drug-resistant tuberculosis (XDR-TB): recommendations for prevention and control. Wkly Epidemiol Rec. 2006;81:430-2.
27. Günther G, Gomez GB, Lange C, Rupert S, van Leth F; TBNET. Availability, price and affordability of anti-tuberculosis drugs in Europe: a TBNET survey. Eur Respir J. 2014;45:1081-8.
28. Ahuja SD, Ashkin D, Avendano M, et al. Multidrug-resistant pulmonary tuberculosis treatment regimens and patient outcomes: an individual patient data meta-analysis of 9,153 patients. PLoS Med. 2012;9:e1001300.
29. Migliori GB, Eker B, Richardson MD, et al. A retrospective TBNET assessment of linezolid safety, tolerability and efficacy in multidrug-resistant tuberculosis. Eur Respir J. 2009;34(2):387-93.
30. Sotgiu G, Centis R, D'Ambrosio L, et al. Efficacy, safety and tolerability of linezolid containing regimens in treating MDR-TB and XDR-TB: systematic review and meta-analysis. Eur Respir J. 2012;40:1430-42.
31. Lee M, Lee J, Carroll MW, et al. Linezolid for treatment of chronic extensively drug-resistant tuberculosis. N Engl J Med. 2012;367:1508-18.
32. Sotgiu G, Migliori GB. Facing multi-drug resistant tuberculosis. Pulm Pharmacol Ther. 2015;32:144-8.
33. Andries K, Verhasselt P, Guillemont J, et al. A diarylquinoline drug active on ATP synthase of Mycobacterium tuberculosis. Science. 2005;307:223-7.
34. Matteelli A, Carvalho AC, Dooley KE, Kritski A. TMC207: the first compound of a new class of potent anti-tuberculosis drugs. Future Microbiol. 2010;5(6):849-58.
35. Worley MV, Estrada SJ. Bedaquiline: a novel antitubercular agent for the treatment of multidrug-resistant tuberculosis. Pharmacotherapy. 2014;34(11):1187-97.
36. Guglielmetti L, Le Dû D, Jachym M, et al. Compassionate use of bedaquiline for the treatment of multidrug-resistant and extensively drug-resistant tuberculosis: interim analysis of a French cohort. Clin Infect Dis. 2015;60(2):188-94.
37. Udwadia ZF, Amale RA, Mullerpattan JB. Initial experience of bedaquiline use in a series of drug-resistant tuberculosis patients from India. Int J Tuberc Lung Dis. 2014;18(11):1315-8.
38. Xavier AS, Lakshmanan M. Delamanid: a new armor in combating drug-resistant tuberculosis. J Pharmacol Pharmacother. 2014;5(3):222-4.
39. Gler MT, Skripconoka V, Sanchez-Garavito E, et al. Delamanid for multidrug-resistant pulmonary tuberculosis. N Engl J Med. 2012;366:2151-60.

40. Skripconoka V, Danilovits M, Pehme L, et al. Delamanid improves outcomes and reduces mortality in multidrug-resistant tuberculosis. Eur Respir J. 2013;41:1393-400.
41. Mallikaarjun S, Wells C, Petersen C, et al. Delamanid Coadministered with Antiretroviral Drugs or Antituberculosis Drugs Shows No Clinically Relevant Drug-Drug Interactions in Healthy Subjects. Antimicrob Agents Chemother. 2016;60(10):5976-85.
42. International Union Against Tuberculosis and Lung Disease—the UNION. The 45th UNION World Conference. [online] Available from: http://www.theunion.org/news-centre/news. [Accessed February, 2016].
43. Amaral L, Martins M, Viveiros M, Molnar J, Kristiansen JE. Promising therapy of XDR-TB/MDR-TB with thioridazine an inhibitor of bacterial efflux pumps. Curr Drug Targets. 2008;9(9):816-9.
44. Pawar BD, Suryakar AN, Khandelwal AS. Effect of micronutrients supplementation on oxidative stress and antioxidants in pulmonary tuberculosis. Biomed Res. 2011;22:455-9.
45. Miric D, Katanic R, Miric B, Kisic B, Popovic-Katanic N, Nestorovic V. Changes in vitamin C and oxidative stress status during the treatment of tuberculous meningitis. Int J Tuberc Lung Dis. 2013;17(11):1495-500.
46. Miragliotta G, Miragliotta L. Vitamin D and infectious diseases. Endocr Metab Immune Disord Drug Targets. 2014;14(4):267-71.
47. Rees JR, Hendricks K, Barry EL, et al. Vitamin D3 supplementation and upper respiratory tract infections in a randomized, controlled trial. Clin Infect Dis. 2013;57(10):1384-92.
48. Rockett KA, Brookes R, Udalova I, Vidal V, Hill AV, Kwiatkowski D. 1,25-dihydroxyvitamin D3 induces nitric oxide synthase and suppresses growth of Mycobacterium tuberculosis in a human macrophage-like cell line. Infect Immun. 1998;66:5314-21.
49. Martineau AR, Timms PM, Bothamley GH, et al. High-dose vitamin D(3) during intensive-phase antimicrobial treatment of pulmonary tuberculosis: a double-blind randomised controlled trial. Lancet. 2011;377(9761):242-50.
50. Luong Kv, Nguyen LT. Impact of vitamin D in the treatment of tuberculosis. Am J Med Sci. 2011;341(6):493-8.
51. Talat N, Perry S, Parsonnet J, Dawood G, Hussain R. Vitamin D deficiency and tuberculosis progression. Emerg Infect Dis. 2010;16(5):853-5.
52. Hasan Z, Salahuddin N, Rao N, et al. Change in serum CXCL10 levels during anti-tuberculosis treatment depends on vitamin D status. Int J Tuberc Lung Dis. 2014;18(4):466-9.
53. Coussens AK, Wilkinson RJ, Hanifa Y, et al. Vitamin D accelerates resolution of inflammatory responses during tuberculosis treatment. Proc Natl Acad Sci U S A. 2012;109(38):15449-54.
54. Critchley JA, Orton LC, Pearson F. Adjunctive steroid therapy for managing pulmonary tuberculosis. Cochrane Database Syst Rev. 2014;11:CD011370.
55. Lesic AR, Pesut DP, Markovic-Denic L, et al. The challenge of osteo-articular tuberculosis in the twenty-first century: a 15-year population-based study. Int J Tuberc Lung Dis. 2010;14(9):1181-6.
56. Man MA, Nicolau D. Surgical treatment to increase the success rate of multidrug-resistant tuberculosis. Eur J Cardiothorac Surg. 2012;42(1):e9-12.
57. Lovacheva OV, Sivokozov IV, Ergeshov AE, Vasil'eva IA, Bagdasarian TR. Use of a valvular bronchoblocker in the treatment of patients with destructive pulmonary tuberculosis. Probl Tuberk Bolezn Legk. 2008;(10):58-61.
58. Andrenko AA, Fedorova MV, Grishchenko NG, Tadzhieva NV. Artificial pneumothorax in the combined therapy of destructive pulmonary tuberculosis. Probl Tuberk. 1995;(1):43-5.
59. Pontali E, Matteelli A, D'Ambrosio L, Centis R, Migliori GB. Rediscovering high technology from the past: thoracic surgery is back on track for multidrug-resistant tuberculosis. Expert Rev Anti Infect Ther. 2012;10(10):1109-15.
60. International Union Against Tuberculosis and Lung Disease. Bactericidal substance isolated from bacon. UNION Newsletter 11, 2003.
61. Veen J, Raviglione M, Rieder HL, et al. Standardized tuberculosis treatment outcome monitoring in Europe. Recommendations of a Working Group of the World Health Organization (WHO) and the European Region of the International Union Against Tuberculosis and Lung Disease (IUATLD) for uniform reporting by cohort analysis of treatment outcome in tuberculosis patients. Eur Respir J. 1998;12:505-10.
62. Laserson KF, Thorpe LE, Leimane V, et al. Speaking the same language: treatment outcome definitions for multidrug-resistant tuberculosis. Int J Tuberc Lung Dis. 2005;9:640-5.

63. Jordan TS, Davies PD. Clinical tuberculosis and treatment outcomes. Int J Tuberc Lung Dis. 2010;14(6):683-8.
64. Veen J. Coordination of clinical and public health services to improve treatment outcome in low-incidence areas: a role for the TB case manager. Int J Tuberc Lung Dis. 2008;12(12):1349.
65. Mitnick CD, Shin SS, Seung KJ, et al. Comprehensive treatment of extensively drug-resistant tuberculosis. N Engl J Med. 2008;359:563-74.
66. Kim DH, Kim HJ, Park SK, et al. Treatment outcomes and long-term survival in patients with extensively drug-resistant tuberculosis. Am J Respir Crit Care Med. 2008;178:1075-82.
67. Baussano I, Pivetta E, Vizzini L, Abbona F, Bugiani M. Predicting tuberculosis treatment outcome in a low-incidence area. Int J Tuberc Lung Dis. 2008;12:1441-8.
68. Kim HR, Hwang SS, Kim HJ, et al. Impact of extensive drug resistance on treatment outcomes in non-HIV-infected patients with multidrug-resistant tuberculosis. Clin Infect Dis. 2007;45:1290-5.
69. Kwon YS, Kim YH, Suh GY, et al. Treatment outcomes for HIV-uninfected patients with multidrug-resistant and extensively drug-resistant tuberculosis. Clin Infect Dis. 2008;47:496-502.
70. Hasker E, Khodjikhanov M, Usarova S, et al. Default from tuberculosis treatment in Tashkent, Uzbekistan; who are these defaulters and why do they default? BMC Infect Dis. 2008;8:97.
71. Vasankari T, Holmstrom P, Ollgren J, Liippo K, Kokki M, Ruutu P. Risk factors for poor tuberculosis treatment outcome in Finland: a cohort study. BMC Public Health. 2007;7:291.
72. Jenkins HE, Ciobanu A, Plesca V, et al. Risk factors and timing of default from treatment for non-multidrug-resistant tuberculosis in Moldova. Int J Tuberc Lung Dis. 2013;17(3):373-80.
73. Volkova KI, Blinetskaia ZS, Fateev IN. Genetic blood markers of the ABO system in patients with pulmonary tuberculosis in relation to ethnic origin. Probl Tuberk. 1991;(10):55-8.
74. Pesut D. Population-genetic approach in studying susceptibility to lung cancer and pulmonary tuberculosis. PhD thesis. University of Belgrade School of Medicine, 1994.
75. World Health Organization. Guidance on ethics of tuberculosis prevention, care and control. 2010.
76. Broadbent E, Petrie KJ, Main J, Weinman J. The brief illness perception questionnaire (BIPQ). J Psychosom Res. 2006;60:631-7.
77. Pesut DP, Bursuc BN, Bulajic MV, et al. Illness perception in tuberculosis by implementation of the Brief Illness Perception Questionnaire—a TBNET study. Springerplus. 2014;3:664.
78. TBNET (Tuberculosis Network European Trials Group) project. ExplainTB. [online] Available from: http://www.explaintb.org. [Accessed February, 2016].
79. Bothamley GH. Smoking and tuberculosis: a chance or causal association? Thorax. 2005;60:527-8.
80. Bates MN, Khalakdina A, Pai M, Chang L, Lessa F, Smith KR. Risk of tuberculosis from exposure to tobacco smoke: a systematic review and meta-analysis. Arch Intern Med. 2007;167(4):335-42.
81. Pesut DP, Bursuc BN, Maat MJ. Nicotiana tabacum—a flower of evil. In: Koskinen CJ, editor. Handbook of Smoking and Health. New York: Nova Biomedical; 2011. pp. 695-721.
82. Pianezza ML, Sellers EM, Tyndale RF. Nicotine metabolism defect reduces smoking. Nature. 1998;393(6687):750.
83. Aoshiba K, Tamaoki J, Nagai A. Acute cigarette smoke exposure induces apoptosis of alveolar macrophages. Am J Physiol Lung Cell Mol Physiol. 2001;281:L1392-401.
84. Sopori M. Effects of cigarette on the immune system. Nat Rev Immunol. 2002;2(5):372-7.
85. Arcavi L, Benowitz NL. Cigarette smoking and infection. Arch Intern Med. 2004;164(20):2206-16.
86. World Health Organization. Tuberculosis control in vulnerable groups. WHO bulletin 2008. [online] Available from: http://www.who.int/bulletin/volumes/86/9/06-038737/en/. [Accessed February, 2016].
87. Pesut D. Active case detection of tuberculosis in risk groups in Serbia. Med Pregl. 2004;57 Suppl 1:75-80.
88. Bothamley GH, Ditiu L, Migliori GB, Lange C; TBNET contributors. Active case finding of tuberculosis in Europe: a Tuberculosis Network European Trials Group (TBNET) survey. Eur Respir J. 2008;32(4):1023-30.
89. Malbasa M, Pesut D. Is there delay in diagnosis of pulmonary tuberculosis in an intermediate-to-low TB incidence setting. Pneumologia. 2011;60(3):138-42.
90. Maciel EL, Golub JE, Peres RL, et al. Delay in diagnosis of pulmonary tuberculosis at a primary health clinic in Vitoria, Brazil. Int J Tuberc Lung Dis. 2010;14(11):1403-10.
91. Mirsaeidi SM, Tabarsi P, Mohajer K, et al. A long delay from the first symptom to definite diagnosis of pulmonary tuberculosis. Arch Iran Med. 2007;10(2):190-3.

92. Sanz B, Blasco T; ATBIM Project. Variables associated with diagnostic delay in immigrant groups with tuberculosis in Madrid. Int J Tuberc Lung Dis. 2007;11(6):639-46.
93. Finnie RK, Khoza LB, van den Borne B, Mabunda T, Abotchie P, Mullen PD. Factors associated with patient and health care system delay in diagnosis and treatment for TB in sub-Saharan African countries with high burdens of TB and HIV. Trop Med Int Health. 2011;16(4):394-411.
94. Andersen RM, Bjørn-Præst SO, Gradel KO, Nielsen C, Nielsen HI. Epidemiology, diagnostic delay and outcome of tuberculosis in North Jutland, Denmark. Dan Med Bull. 2011;58(3):A4256.
95. Hemming S, Windish P, Hall J, Story A, Lipman M. P160 Treating TB patients with no entitlement to social support—welcome to the social jungle. Thorax. 2010;65:A145-6.
96. National Institute for Health and Care Excellence. (2012). Tuberculosis: identification and management in under-served groups. [online] Available from: http://www.nice.org.uk/guidance/ph37. [Accessed February, 2016].
97. National Institute for Health and Care Excellence. (2013). Tuberculosis in vulnerable groups: local government briefing. [online] Available from: http://www.nice.org.uk/advice/lgb11/chapter/about-this-briefing. [Accessed February, 2016].

CHAPTER 17
Management of the Adverse Effects of Antituberculosis Drugs

Dragica P Pesut

INTRODUCTION

Adverse reactions to anti-tuberculosis (TB) drugs have been noticed and reported since the introduction of the drugs.[1,2] The reactions are usually minor, but sometimes can be dramatic necessitating treatment interruption. A major side effect is any adverse reaction that results in temporary or permanent discontinuation of a drug, while a minor side effect requires only dose adjustment and/or addition of concomitant treatment.

Apart from adverse effects of anti-TB drugs alone, drug interactions (among anti-TB drugs or between anti-TB drugs and other drugs) make it sometimes necessary to modify or discontinue therapy. Adverse reactions may develop during therapy with both first line and second line anti-TB drugs.

ADVERSE REACTIONS TO THE FIRST-LINE ANTITUBERCULOSIS DRUGS

First-line anti-TB drugs (isoniazid, rifampicin, pyrazinamide, ethambutol, and streptomycin) are, generally, well tolerated. Among them, adverse events occur most frequently with isoniazid.[3] Apart from polyneuropathy, just like, rifampicin, and pyrazinamide, it may cause liver toxicity. Not only acute but also chronic liver disease may complicate treatment with isoniazid. Increased deaths from liver cirrhosis in those treated with isoniazid were observed in the Massachusetts study.[4] In the same study, an excess of breast cancer cases among the patients who did not receive isoniazid was referred to multiple chest fluoroscopies to monitor pneumothorax.

The need for supplemental vitamin B6 during TB treatment using isoniazid is not clarified and further randomized controlled studies should be conducted. In the past times, wide use of pyridoxine together with isoniazid from the start of treatment is replaced with administration of the vitamin only if the signs of polyneuropathy already exist (patients with diabetes mellitus, chronic alcoholism, and malnutrition) or if they appear during anti-TB treatment.[5]

Apart from allergy, usually reversible renal failure, nausea, skin rash, and neuromuscular blockade, common adverse effect associated with streptomycin use include nonreversible auditory and vestibular nerve damage, which make it necessary to perform auditory examination in the patient before starting the treatment. To protect the fetus from the statoacoustic nerve damage, the agent is never recommended during pregnancy. In children and adults whose initial audiograms are within normal limits, in 98% of the cases, it will continue to be so even after 2-month therapy. Proper dosage (0.75–1.0 g/day; >50 kg: 1.0 g/day; <50 kg: 0.75 g/day; maximum cumulative dose 60 g) decreases the risk of adverse

TABLE 1	The first line antituberculosis drugs' most common adverse reactions
Side effect	Responsible drug
Skin rash	Any agent
Gastrointestinal intolerance	Any agent
Liver toxicity	Isoniazid, rifampicin, and pyrazinamide
Peripheral neuropathy	Isoniazid
Optic neuritis	Ethambutol and, rarely, isoniazid
Uric arthritis (gout)	Pyrazinamide
Statoacoustic nerve damage	Streptomycin

events. If audiometry appoints to already existing auditory disturbance, streptomycin may worsen it irreversibly, and should be avoided. However, its administration then may relay on clinician's estimation of the priorities and eventual vital indications for its use.

A population-based study of adult new smear-positive patients in Kyrgyzstan showed that more than 80% of the reactions to anti-TB drugs occurred during the first month of therapy (most during the first week of treatment), and 2% of the patients had to interrupt treatment for 1 week or more.[6] The most common causative agent was rifampicin while pyrazinamide, followed by rifampicin, most frequently caused serious adverse reactions. Rash, abdominal pain, and jaundice were most commonly observed. Drug reactions studies performed in Canada also appointed to the first line drug reactions leading to modification or discontinuation of a treatment regimen.[7,8] In 6.5% of new TB patients in Argentina, the treatment had to be modified due to adverse anti-TB reactions.[9] The most common adverse reactions to the first line anti-TB drugs and possible responsible drugs are shown in table 1. Due to side effects such as hypersensitivity, gastrointestinal intolerance, vertigo, and hepatitis, thiacetazone should be avoided whenever it is possible and ethambutol used instead.[5,10]

DETECTION OF RESPONSIBLE DRUG

Although, theoretically, any drug can induce an immune response, only 6–10% of adverse drug reactions are immunologically mediated and diagnosis of adverse reaction is mainly based on clinical judgment.[11] It is not always easy to detect the causative agents in patients with adverse anti-TB drug reactions. Detection of responsible drug may not be simple in the patients treated with fixed dose combinations regimens. Attempts have been made to reveal responsible drug by both *in vitro* methods such as the drug lymphocyte stimulation test (DLST), and *in vivo* methods such as a challenge test or skin tests. In a prospective study on adverse drug reactions in human immunodeficiency virus (HIV)-negative TB patients, the events were studied related to skin eruption, hepatitis, or drug fever following their clinical manifestations.[12] The study showed that DLST contributed little to identifying the causative anti-TB drugs.

Gastrointestinal and hematologic toxicity are usually not considered to be immune-mediated side effects. Toxic hepatitis is defined as a liver transaminase value more than three times the upper limit of normal while drug induced fever (usually caused by rifampicin) is recurrence of fever despite microbiological and radiographic improvement by therapy for several weeks. If fever appears due to infection, including TB, drug reaction as a cause can be excluded. Drug related fever spontaneously resolves when drugs are stopped.

TABLE 2	The first line oral antituberculosis drugs, dosages, and common adverse effects[5,13]	
Antituberculosis drug	Recommended daily dosage	Common adverse effect (not exclusive)
Isoniazid	• 5 mg/kg • Should not exceed 300 mg/day • Always consider coadministering vitamin B6	Elevated transaminases; hepatitis; peripheral neuropathy; GI intolerance; CNS toxicity, neutropenia
Rifampicin	• 10 mg/kg • > 50 kg: 600 mg • < 50 kg: 450 mg	Elevation of liver enzymes; hepatitis; hypersensitivity; fever; GI disorders: anorexia, nausea, vomiting, abdominal pain; discoloration (orange or reddish) of urine, tears, and other body fluids; thrombopenia
Pyrazinamide	• 30 mg/kg • Maximum 2.0 g/day	Arthralgia; hyperuricemia; toxic hepatitis; GI discomfort
Ethambutol	• 15–25 mg/kg • Maximum 2.0 g/day	Optic neuritis; hyperuricemia; peripheral neuropathy (rare)

GI, gastrointestinal; CNS, central nervous system.

The most effective management of drug adverse reactions is discontinuation of the medication and their substitution with alternative medications with different chemical structures. However, first line anti-TB drugs, in particular isoniazid and rifampicin, are the most important agents and their continued use should be attempted. Strict administration of recommended daily dosage, shown in table 2, decreases the risk of adverse reactions listed in table 2.

Neutropenia may occur as a rare complication of antituberculous therapy. It is usually due to a single agent, most frequently isoniazid. In a reported case of lymph node TB, neutropenia developed during combination therapy of isoniazid, rifampicin, ethambutol, and streptomycin and was a cause of treatment interruptions.[14] Administration of granulocyte colony stimulating factor twice weekly subcutaneously corrected neutropenia and allowed anti-TB treatment continuation.

Patients with renal disease are found to be at increased risk of toxicity from anti-TB drugs, particularly isoniazid and ethambutol, compared to those with normal renal function.[15-17] These patients need special consideration and treatment monitoring.

ADVERSE REACTIONS TO THE SECOND-LINE ANTITUBERCULOSIS DRUGS

Not only efficacy, but also safety and tolerability profiles of therapeutic regimens based on second line and reserve anti-TB drugs are showed poor.[18] Treatment with second line drugs in multidrug-resistant TB (MDR-TB) and extensively drug-resistant TB (XDR-TB) diseases is frequently influenced by the occurrence of adverse drug events (Tables 3 and 4). Due to higher risk of side effects and lack of reliable indicators to individually guide the duration of treatment, national authorities should identify highly specialized reference centres for treatment of MDR-TB and XDR-TB.[19,20]

TABLE 3	Second line injectable antituberculosis drugs, dosages, and common adverse effects[5,13]	
Drug	**Recommended daily dosage**	**Common adverse effect (not exclusive)**
Amikacin*	• 0.75–1.0 g • >50 kg: 1.0 g/day • <50 kg: 0.75 g/day • Maximum cumulative dose 50 g	• Auditory and vestibular nerve damage (nonreversible); renal failure (usually reversible); allergies; nausea; skin rash; neuromuscular blockade
Capreomycin†	• 0.75–1.0 g • >50 kg: 1.0 g/day • <50 kg: 0.75 g/day • Maximum cumulative dose 50 g	• Auditory and vestibular nerve damage (nonreversible); renal failure (usually reversible); Bartter-like syndrome; allergies; neuromuscular blockade
Kanamycin*	• 375–500 mg/kg • >50 kg: 1.0 g/day • <50 kg: 0.75 g/day • Maximum cumulative dose 50 g	• Auditory and vestibular nerve damage (nonreversible); renal failure (usually reversible); allergies; nausea; skin rash; neuromuscular blockade

*Intravenous administration only.
†Intravenous/intramuscular administration only.

TABLE 4	The second line oral antituberculosis drugs, dosages, and common adverse effects	
Antituberculosis drug	**Recommended daily dosage**	**Common adverse effect (not exclusive)**
Rifabutin	• 150–450 mg • Consider to monitor drug levels	Anemia; gastrointestinal discomfort; discoloration (orange-reddish) of urine and other body fluids; uveitis; elevated liver enzymes
Ethionamide	• 0.75–1.0 g	Severe gastrointestinal intolerance; nausea; vomiting; hepatitis; CNS disorders
Prothionamide	• 0.75–1.0 g	Severe gastrointestinal intolerance; nausea; vomiting; hepatitis; CNS disorders
Cycloserine	• 250 mg TID • Maximum 1,000 mg/day	CNS disorders; anxiety; confusion; dizziness; psychosis; seizures; headache
Terizidone	• 250 mg TID • Maximum 1,000 mg/day	CNS disorders; anxiety; confusion; dizziness; psychosis; seizures; headache
Para-aminosalicylic acid	• 4.0 g TID	Gastrointestinal intolerance; nausea; diarrhea; vomiting; hypersensitivity

CNS, central nervous system; TID, thrice a day.

Fluoroquinolones are found to cause several side effects. Common adverse effects of levofloxacin [recommended dose: 500–1,000 mg four times a day (QD)] and ciprofloxacin (500–750 mg twice a day) are gastrointestinal discomfort, disorders of the central nervous system, rarely—tendon rupture, hypersensitivity, and *Clostridium difficile* colitis.[5,13] Apart from these, moxifloxacin (400 mg) may cause headache, dizziness, hallucinations, increased transaminases level, and QT prolongation on electrocardiography (ECG). Sparfloxacin is highly active against mycobacteria, but the use in clinical practice is restricted by its side effects and the contribution to anti-TB therapy is still unclear. A study showed that it was generally well tolerated. Only mild phototoxic reactions and moderate prolongations of the QT interval were registered in patients without clinical symptoms.[21]

LINEZOLID

Linezolid is one of the drugs used in combinations to treat the most complicated MDR-TB/XDR-TB cases. Its side effects are frequent and often serious, require careful monitoring, particularly when therapy extends beyond 2 months. Previously lacking, clinical data on its safety, tolerability and efficacy in treatment of TB have been studied by the Tuberculosis Network European Trials Group using a sizable cohort of patients with MDR-TB/XDR-TB from Belarus, Germany, Italy, and Switzerland.[22] Based on the retrospective, nonrandomized, unblinded observational study, the results showed that most linezolid side effects occurred after 8 weeks of treatment. In the cohort, linezolid was administered for a mean duration exceeding 32 weeks. The majority of the patients (77%) experienced major side effects while 23% had minor ones. Anemia was the most frequent with about 20% of the cases being severely affected and requiring blood transfusion. The other side effects included thrombocytopenia, nausea/vomiting, and polyneuropathy. In one-third of the patients who experienced major adverse effects, it was possible to successfully reintroduce linezolid while in about 70% of cases the drug was permanently discontinued. Administration of linezolid at 600 mg once daily, versus 1,200 mg (i.e., twice daily) is associated with a lower risk of major side effects as well as a lower risk of any side effects. It is worth to mention that none linezolid-related death has occurred during study period and that the described adverse effects were reversible in all cases when therapy with linezolid was discontinued. However, adverse effects of linezolid therapy are not proven, as they may also be due to other drugs (Table 5).

A recent study in the Netherlands has shown that with well-designed therapy regimens and carefully considered surgical options, the majority of drug-resistant cases of TB could be treated successfully.[27] The development of new drugs, more effective and less toxic, to treat patients with drug resistant TB was urgently needed over years while adherence to internationally agreed standards of care and control practices stayed as imperative. Thus, two new anti-TB drugs (delamanid and bedaquiline) appeared over 2013/2014 to meet the expectations.

TABLE 5	Oral reserve drugs with uncertain antituberculosis activity, dosages, and common adverse effects[5,13,22-26]	
Antituberculosis drug	*Recommended daily dosage*	*Common adverse effect (not exclusive)*
Linezolid	600 mg	Thrombopenia; anemia; neuropathy
Clofazimine	100 mg Optimal dose unknown	Ichthyosis; gastrointestinal discomfort; nausea; vomiting; discoloration of the skin
Amoxicillin-clavulanate	125–875 mg BID or 250–500 mg TID	Gastrointestinal discomfort; diarrhea; rash
Clarithromycin	500 mg BID	Gastrointestinal discomfort

CNS, central nervous system; BID, twice a day; TID, thrice a day.

TABLE 6	New antituberculosis drugs, dosages, and common adverse effects[27-32]	
Antituberculosis drug	Daily dosage	Common adverse effects
Delamanid	200 mg twice daily	QT interval prolongation; mental disorder; increased blood cortisol
Bedaquiline	400 mg orally for 2 weeks followed by 200 mg thrice weekly	Gastrointestinal discomfort; nausea; diarrhea; arthralgia; dizziness; hyperuricemia; eye disorder; headache; increase in QT interval but without pathological prolongation

BEDAQUILINE (TMC207)

Safety and tolerability study showed a low rate of adverse events at a dose of 400 mg daily in the Phase IIa study. The majority of adverse events are of mild or moderate intensity (Table 6). Nausea is significantly more frequently reported by patients treated with TMC207 in the MDR-TB trial. Diarrhea, arthralgia, dizziness, hyperuricemia, and eye disorders are more frequent, but not of statistical significance. TMC207 produces increases in the QT interval, but no pathologically prolonged.[28]

DELAMANID (OPC-67683)

Most adverse events during delamanid therapy were found to be mild to moderate (Table 6). A study showed that QT prolongation was reported significantly more frequently in the groups that received delamanid,[29] and the other study demonstrated that delamanid was well-tolerated, had low rates of discontinuation, and could be effective for treating MDR-TB.[30]

RARE COMPLICATIONS AND OTHER CONSIDERATIONS

Alopecia

Drug-induced alopecia, usually associated with antimitotic drug therapy, although rarely, may be induced by anti-TB drugs. Isoniazid, thiacetazone, and ethionamide have been reported to induce it.[33-38] The effect is reversible after the withdrawal of the offending drug. However, in a complicated case of isoniazid-induced alopecia and generalized lichenoid eruptions in a 32-year-old woman, apart from isoniazid withdrawal, oral prednisolone therapy was administered.[36] In another case of a 30-year-old female with isoniazid-induced alopecia without other side effects, isoniazid withdrawal was the only approach in managing the adverse effect.[37] Regrowth of the hair was observed after 2 months. In some cases, HIV infection has been taken into consideration as possible aggravating factor—3/5 patients with isoniazid-induced alopecia were HIV-positive in a series of 141 TB patients.[33] The newest report is a case of isoniazid-induced alopecia in a 10-year old male child from India.[38]

Hypothyroidism

It seems that hypothyroidism may be more common in MDR-TB patients during treatment than previously recognized.[39] Based on the results from a Lesotho study, where high proportion of cases with hypothyroidism was found (69%), screening of all those patients for hypothyroidism is recommended. This should be performed within 2–3 months of starting MDR-TB treatment in all patients, even in those without symptoms. Prospective studies could offer some new information and proper guidelines in this term.

QT Prolongation

The possibility of QTc prolongation on ECG for patients being treated for MDR-TB with some of the new (bedaquiline, delamanid) and repurposed (moxifloxacin) drugs has been shown to happen.[28,40] Thus, strategies for managing or preventing this condition in the context of treating TB as an infectious disease are in focus of current discussions.[40]

Drug Reaction with Eosinophilia and Systemic Symptoms Syndrome

A severe adverse drug reaction which includes skin eruptions, fever, and hematologic skin abnormalities (eosinophilia or atypical lymphocytes) is known as DRESS (drug reaction with eosinophilia and systemic symptoms) syndrome. It has been reported to develop during anti-TB treatment and included cerebral vasculitis, but the effects have been finally attributed to allopurinol and not to anti-TB drugs.[41] In a case of 71-year old man under anti-TB treatment (isoniazid, rifampicin, pyrazinamide, and ethambutol), skin eruption with eosinophilia and renal and hepatic involvement appeared 4 weeks after start of therapy regimen.[42] The treatments for DRESS syndrome are culprit drug withdrawal and corticosteroids.

PERSPECTIVES

Despite the implementation of MDR-TB treatment strategies, the number of MDR-TB cases has continued to increase.[43] That also means increased number of patients under monitoring for adverse effects of anti-TB drugs. There are no findings to support possible difference in adverse effects between the treatment of XDR-TB compared to MDR-TB that could be important therapy limiting factors.[44-46] Current treatment regimens for these patients are long and complex. In some patients groups, drug toxicity may not be completely profiled.[43,47] Finally, some of these patients will also be treated for other comorbidities, including HIV infection, at the same time.

Patients with Acquired Immunodeficiency Syndrome

Adverse effects of anti-TB drugs are observed more frequently in patients with acquired immunodeficiency syndrome (AIDS). The first reports describing an increased risk of severe cutaneous reactions associated with the use of thiacetazone in persons with AIDS came from Africa in the late 1980s and early 1990s, both in adults and children.[10,48-50] Apart from adverse reactions to anti-TB drugs alone, these patients experience the problems of drug/drug interactions related to antiretroviral treatment.[51] Identifying optimal therapy for them requires special consideration (see Chapter 13).

Inhalation and Fixed Drug Combinations Therapy

Although efficacy of anti-TB fixed dose combinations regimen was noninferior to that of the standardized regimens, hematologic effects were significantly higher in the group of patients treated with fix dose combinations drugs.[52] Possible introduction of inhalation anti-TB therapy, the attempt has been made to apply, might contribute to decreased number of patients with adverse drug reactions to anti-TB drugs.[53]

FORECASTING THE DRUG ADVERSE EFFECTS

Thanks to the attempts to develop forecasting methods for appearance of anti-TB drugs adverse effects, especially in the patients with MDR-TB, clinicians now can easier predict medicinal complications in those patients.[53] In that terms, intolerance to chemical preparations in the past is a risk factor for adverse drug effects during anti-TB drug therapy, and the other risk factors are kidney and liver biochemical disturbances, leukocytosis, existence of associated diseases, and increased erythrocyte sedimentation rate to more than 40 mm/h, in a rank order. Risk factors such as existence of lymphopenia or pernicious habits, changes in electrolyte metabolism, and disease duration from 4 to 5 years are also found to be in positive correlation with appearance of adverse effects.[53] The patients with fibrocaseous pulmonary TB and those aged 30–40 years also are found to be at higher risk for developing medicinal complications during the treatment. Generally, the risk of development of hepatic toxicity following treatment with first line anti-TB treatment increased with the patients' age.[54]

Toward Personalized Treatment of Tuberculosis

High incidence of drug-induced hepatotoxicity and other adverse drug reactions makes anti-TB treatment challenging. Not only environmental factors, but also some genetic factors are recognized to contribute to the adverse effects of anti-TB drugs. Previous reports have shown that some polymorphisms were associated with large interindividual and inter-racial differences in the toxicity and efficacy of isoniazid.[55] Apart from known single nucleotide polymorphisms (SNPs) in drug-metabolizing enzymes, a new research on Western Indian population, demonstrated 18 new SNPs, nuclear receptors, and transporter proteins that contributed to drug-induced hepatptoxicity.[56] The well-known patient's isoniazid acetylation status (rapid acetylator or slow acetylator) has been shown to influence treatment success, based on microbiological sputum conversion, and adverse drug reactions rate.[57] Having in mind that pharmacokinetic variability to a single drug in the regimen was significantly associated with failure of therapy and adverse drug reactions, individualized dosing of anti-TB drugs is expected to be more effective than standardized dosing. Although anti-TB therapy is still not personalized, new technologies might enable this approach (e.g., use of N-acetyltransferase type 2 genotyping). Pharmacogenetic basis of adverse drug reactions stays in focus of current research[58] hopefully to lead to safer and more efficacious treatment of TB in the future.[59]

REFERENCES

1. Girling DJ. Adverse effects of antituberculosis drugs. Drugs. 1982;23:56-74.
2. Rieder HL. Interventions for tuberculosis control and elimination. Paris, France: International Union Against Tuberculosis and Lung Disease, 2002. pp. 15-93.
3. Schaberg T, Rebhan K, Lode H. Risk factors for side effects of isoniazid, rifampin and pyrazinamide in patients hospitalized for pulmonary tuberculosis. Eur Respir J. 1996;9(10):2026-30.
4. Boice JD, Fraumeni JF Jr. Late effects following isoniazid therapy. Am J Public Health. 1980;70(9):987-9.
5. World Health Organization. Treatment of tuberculosis: guidelines. 4th ed. Geneva: World Health Organization, 2010.
6. Hinderaker SG, Ysykeeva J, Veen J, Enarson DA. Serious adverse reactions in a tuberculosis programme setting in Kyrgyzstan. Int J Tuberc Lung Dis. 2009;13(12):1560-2.

7. Yee D, Valiquette C, Pelletier M, Parisien I, Rocher I, Menzies D. Incidence of serious side effects from first-line antituberculosis drugs among patients treated for active tuberculosis. Am J Respir Crit Care Med. 2003;167:1472-7.
8. Marra F, Marra CA, Bruchet N, et al. Adverse drug reactions associated with first-line anti-tuberculosis drug regimens. Int J Tuberc Lung Dis. 2007;11:868-75.
9. Gonzalez Montaner LJ, Dambrosi A, Manassero M, Dambrosi VM. Adverse effects of antituberculosis drugs causing changes in treatment. Tubercle. 1982;63:291-4.
10. Falzon D, Hill G, Pal SN, Suwankesawong W, Jaramillo E. Pharmacovigilance and tuberculosis: applying the lessons of thioacetazone. Bull World Health Organ. 2014;92(12):918-9.
11. Gruchalla RS. 10. Drug allergy. J Allergy Clin Immunol. 2003;111(2 Suppl):S548-59.
12. Suzuki Y, Miwa S, Shirai M, et al. Drug lymphocyte stimulation test in the diagnosis of adverse reactions to antituberculosis drugs. Chest. 2008;134(5):1027-32.
13. Sotgiu G, Lange C, Migliori GB. Pulmonary tuberculosis. In: Palange P, Simonds A, editors. ERS Handbook of Respiratory Medicine. Sheffield, UK: European Respiratory Society; 2010. pp. 200-8.
14. Cormican LJ, Schey S, Milburn HJ. G-CSF enables completion of tuberculosis therapy associated with iatrogenic neutropenia. Eur Respir J. 2004;23:649-50.
15. Quantrill SJ, Woodhead MA, Bell CE, Hardy CC, Hutchison AJ, Gokal R. Side-effects of antituberculosis drug treatment in patients with chronic renal failure. Eur Respir J. 2002;20:440-3.
16. Unsal A, Ahbap E, Basturk T, et al. Tuberculosis in dialysis patients: a nine-year retrospective analysis. J Infect Dev Ctries. 2013;7(3):208-13.
17. Milburn HJ. How should we treat tuberculosis in adult patients with chronic kidney disease? Key messages from the British Thoracic Society Guidelines. Pol Arch Med Wewn. 2010;120(10):417-22.
18. Sotgiu G, Migliori GB. Facing multi-drug resistant tuberculosis. Pulm Pharmacol Ther. 2015;32:144-8.
19. World Health Organization. Guidelines of the programmatic management of drug-resistant tuberculosis. Geneva, Switzerland: WHO, 2006.
20. World Health Organization. Guidelines for the programmatic management of drug-resistant tuberculosis. 2011 update. Geneva: WHO; 2011.
21. Lubasch A, Erbes R, Mauch H, Lode H. Sparfloxacin in the treatment of drug resistant tuberculosis or intolerance of first line therapy. Eur Respir J. 2001;17(4):641-6.
22. Migliori GB, Eker B, Richardson MD, et al. A retrospective TBNET assessment of linezolid safety, tolerability and efficacy in multidrug-resistant tuberculosis. Eur Respir J. 2009;34(2):387-93.
23. Ahuja SD, Ashkin D, Avendano M, et al. Multidrug resistant pulmonary tuberculosis treatment regimens and patient outcomes: an individual patient data meta-analysis of 9,153 patients. PLoS Med. 2012;9:e1001300.
24. Sotgiu G, Centis R, D'Ambrosio L, et al. Efficacy, safety and tolerability of linezolid containing regimens in treating MDR-TB and XDR-TB: systematic review and meta-analysis. Eur Respir J. 2012;40:1430-42.
25. Lee M, Lee J, Carroll MW, et al. Linezolid for treatment of chronic extensively drug-resistant tuberculosis. N Engl J Med. 2012;367:1508-18.
26. Sotgiu G, Ferrara G, Matteelli A, et al. Epidemiology and clinical management of XDR-TB: a systematic review by TBNET. Eur Respir J. 2009;33:871-81.
27. van Altena R, de Vries G, Haar CH, et al. Highly successful treatment outcome of multidrug-resistant tuberculosis in the Netherlands, 2000-2009. Int J Tuberc Lung Dis. 2015;19(4):406-12.
28. World Health Organization. The use of bedaquiline in the treatment of multidrug-resistant tuberculosis. Interim policy guidance. [online] Available from: http://www.who.int/tb/challenges/mdr/bedaquiline/en/. [Accessed February, 2016].
29. Gler MT, Skripconoka V, Sanchez-Garavito E, et al. Delamanid for multidrug-resistant pulmonary tuberculosis. N Engl J Med. 2012;366(23):2151-60.
30. Zhang Q, Liu Y, Tang S, Sha W, Xiao H. Clinical benefit of delamanid (OPC-67683) in the treatment of multidrug-resistant tuberculosis patients in China. Cell Biochem Biophys. 2013;67(3):957-63.
31. Udwadia ZF, Amale RA, Mullerpattan JB. Initial experience of bedaquiline use in a series of drug-resistant tuberculosis patients from India. Int J Tuberc Lung Dis. 2014;18(11):1315-8.
32. Guglielmetti L, Le Dû D, Jachym M, et al. Compassionate use of bedaquiline for the treatment of multidrug-resistant and extensively drug-resistant tuberculosis: interim analysis of a French cohort. Clin Infect Dis. 2015;60(2):188-94.
33. FitzGerald JM, Tuner MT, Dean S, Elwood RK. Alopecia-side effect of antituberculosis drugs. Lancet. 1996;347:472.

34. Gupta DK, Kumar R, Kumar V, Aggarwal AK. Diffuse toxic alopecia due to thiacetazone. Indian J Chest Dis Allied Sci. 1983;25:74-5.
35. Arshad N, Jain RC, Verma K. Ethionamide induced alopecia. Indian J Tub. 1984;31:173-4.
36. Sharma PK, Gautam RK, Bhardwaj M, Kar HK. Isonicotinic acid hydrazide induced anagen effluvium and associated lichenoid eruption. J Dermatol. 2001;28:737-41.
37. Gupta KB, Kumar V, Vishvkarma S, Shandily R. Isoniazid-induced alopecia. Lung India. 2011;28:60-1.
38. Dixit R, Qureshi D, Mathur S. Alopecia caused by isoniazid. J Pharmacol Pharmacother. 2014;5(2):155-7.
39. Satti H, Mafukidze A, Jooste PL, McLaughlin MM, Farmer PE, Seung KJ. High rate of hypothyroidism among patients treated for multidrug-resistant tuberculosis in Lesotho. Int J Tuberc Lung Dis. 2012;16(4):468-72.
40. Harausz E, Cox H, Rich M, Mitnick CD, Zimetbaum P, Furin J. QTc prolongation and treatment of multidrug-resistant tuberculosis. Int J Tuberc Lung Dis. 2015;19(4):385-91.
41. Sola D, Rossi L, Sainaghi PP, Pirisi M. DRESS syndrome with cerebral vasculitis. Intern Med. 2013;52(12):1403-5.
42. Lee JY, Seol YJ, Shin DW, et al. A case of the drug reaction with eosinophilia and systemic symptom (DRESS) following isoniazid treatment. Tuberc Respir Dis (Seoul). 2015;78(1):27-30.
43. World Health Organization. Global tuberculosis report 2014. Geneva: WHO; 2014.
44. Kim HR, Hwang SS, Kim HJ, et al. Impact of extensive drug resistance on treatment outcomes in non-HIV-infected patients with multidrug-resistant tuberculosis. Clin Infect Dis. 2007;45:1290-5.
45. Eker B, Ortmann J, Migliori GB, et al. Multidrug- and extensively drug-resistant tuberculosis, Germany. Emerg Infect Dis. 2008;14:1700-6.
46. Keshavjee S, Gelmanova IY, Farmer PE, et al. Treatment of extensively drug-resistant tuberculosis in Tomsk, Russia: a retrospective cohort study. Lancet. 2008;372:1403-9.
47. Companion handbook to the WHO guidelines for the programmatic management of drug-resistant tuberculosis. Geneva: World Health Organization; 2014. [online] Available from: http://apps.who.int/iris/bitstream/10665/130918/1/9789241548809_eng.pdf. [Accessed February, 2016].
48. Vieira DE, Gomes M. Adverse effects of tuberculosis treatment: experience at an outpatient clinic of a teaching hospital in the city of São Paulo, Brazil. J Bras Pneumol. 2008;34(12):1049-55.
49. Nunn P, Kibuga D, Gathua S, et al. Cutaneous hypersensitivity reactions due to thiacetazone in HIV-1 seropositive patients treated for tuberculosis. Lancet. 1991;337(8742):627-30.
50. Chintu C, Luo C, Bhat G, Raviglione M, DuPont H, Zumla A. Cutaneous hypersensitivity reactions due to thiacetazone in the treatment of tuberculosis in Zambian children infected with HIV-I. Arch Dis Child. 1993;68(5):665-8.
51. Khan FA, Minion J, Pai M, et al. Treatment of active tuberculosis in HIV-coinfected patients: a systematic review and meta-analysis. Clin Infect Dis. 2010;50:1288-99.
52. Hao LH, Guo SC, Liu CC, et al. Comparative bioavailability of rifampicin and isoniazid in fixed-dose combinations and single-drug formulations. Int J Tuberc Lung Dis. 2014;18(12):1505-12.
53. Tashpulatova F. Forecasting the risk of medicinal complications from the chemical therapy in patients with multi-resistant pulmonary tuberculosis. Eur Respir J. 2011;38:4370.
54. Abbasi MA, Ahmed N, Suleman A, et al. Common risk factors for the development of antituberculosis treatment induced hepatotoxicity. J Ayub Med Coll Abbottabad. 2014;26(3):384-8.
55. Matsumoto T, Ohno M, Azuma J. Future of pharmacogenetics-based therapy for tuberculosis. Pharmacogenomics. 2014;15(5):601-7.
56. Singh M, Gupta VH, Amarapurkar DN, et al. Association of genetic variants with anti-tuberculosis drug induced hepatotoxicity: a high resolution melting analysis. Infect Genet Evol. 2014;23:42-8.
57. Pasipanodya JG, Srivastava S, Gumbo T. Meta-analysis of clinical studies supports the pharmacokinetic variability hypothesis for acquired drug resistance and failure of antituberculosis therapy. Clin Infect Dis. 2012;55(2):169-77.
58. Sharma SK, Jha BK, Sharma A, et al. Genetic polymorphisms of CYP2E1 and GSTM1 loci and susceptibility to anti-tuberculosis drug-induced hepatotoxicity. Int J Tuberc Lung Dis. 2014;18(5):588-93.
59. Mouton JP, Mehta U, Parrish AG, et al. Mortality from adverse drug reactions in adult medical inpatients at four hospitals in South Africa: a cross-sectional survey. Br J Clin Pharmacol. 2015;80(4):818-26.

CHAPTER 18

Vitamin D and Tuberculosis

Snežana Jovičić, Zorica Šumarac

INTRODUCTION

The growing evidence from the past decade established vitamin D as essential for life in higher animals. The elements of this endocrine system are present in almost all cell types, thus proving its vital role in many additional biological actions, besides the traditional calcium homeostasis regulation. One of them is the role in proper functioning of the innate and adaptive immune system, indicating its significance in responses to infection. In this chapter we elaborate the role of vitamin D endocrine system in *Mycobacterium tuberculosis* infection through its effect to immune reaction to this infection, as well as the potential of vitamin D treatments of tuberculosis patients.

VITAMIN D—BIOCHEMISTRY AND METABOLISM

The basic chemical structure of vitamin D is cyclopentanoperhydrophenanthrene ring, the fundamental structure of all steroids, but with the broken 9,10 carbon-carbon bond in B ring, which makes it a secosteroid (Fig. 1).[1]

Vitamin D occurs in nature in two main forms:

1. Vitamin D3 (cholecalciferol), produced in the skin from 7-dehydrocholesterol upon exposure to ultraviolet B portion of sunlight
2. Vitamin D2 (ergocalciferol), synthesized in yeasts by irradiation of ergosterol. The differences between the two forms of vitamin D are in the side chain—vitamin D2 has the double bond between carbon 22 and carbon 23 and a methyl group on carbon 24.[2] Vitamin D2 has only one-third of vitamin D3's potency in biological activity.[3]

The sources of vitamin D3, besides synthesis in the skin expressed during summer months, are only few types of food with significant amounts of this ingredient, like cod liver oil, fatty fish (i.e., salmon, mackerel, sardines), and egg yolk.[2] Therefore, limitations of adequate intake and production of vitamin D in the skin might be old age, pigmented skin, sunscreen use, and clothing.[4]

Vitamin D alone has no known biologic action. Either originated from the skin or food intake, it has to be metabolized first in the liver through hydroxylation into 25-hydroxyvitamin D3 [25(OH)D3], the main vitamin D form in circulation, and then into the biologically active metabolite 1,25-dihydroxyvitamin D3 [1,25(OH)$_2$D3] in the kidney.[5] Since vitamin D and its metabolites are fat soluble, they are carried in the circulation by a transport protein—vitamin D-binding protein—produced in the liver.[2] The key enzymes responsible for transformation and metabolic activation of vitamin D are hepatic vitamin D-25-hydroxylase (CYP27A1 and CYP2R1) and highly regulated renal 25-hydroxyvitamin D-1α-hydroxylase (CYP27B1). The metabolic action of vitamin D is carried out through binding of 1,25(OH)$_2$D3 to a nuclear receptor—vitamin D receptor (VDR), which regulates

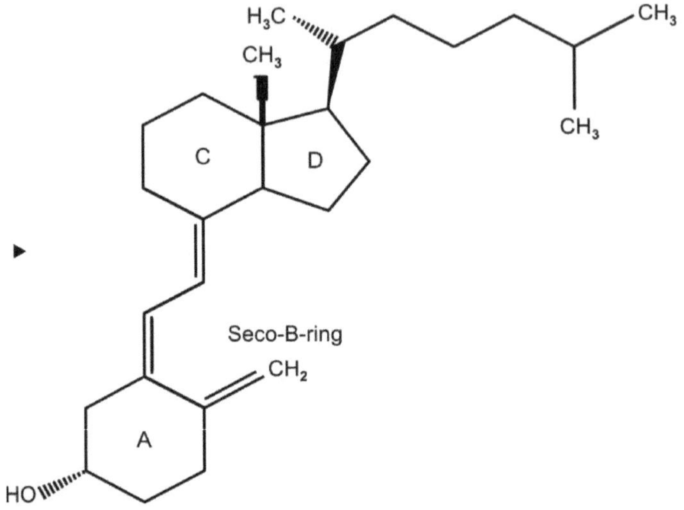

FIG. 1: Chemical structure of vitamin D3.

gene transcription in various vitamin D target cells. Differences in various tissues in whose cells VDR is expressed, in terms of differentiation stage and presence of specific transcription factors, cause wide variability of genes modulated in each tissue at any time.[5]

Namely, VDR represents a transcription factor dependent on 1,25(OH)$_2$D3. Through heterodimer formation with retinoid X receptors and specific association with vitamin D responsive elements (VDREs) in target genes, it controls gene expression. Vitamin D responsive elements are, among others, identified in genes whose transcription 1,25(OH)$_2$D3 activates, including osteocalcin and osteopontin, β_3 integrin, calbindin-D$_{28k}$, and p21.[6]

Besides these effects of 1,25(OH)$_2$D3 on genome upon binding with VDR, which lead to upregulation or downregulation of gene expression that can take hours or days to achieve, it has another, more rapid mechanism of action. Namely, 1,25(OH)$_2$D3 can bind to a receptor located on plasma membrane, thus achieving its biological action through calcium channels in monocytes, vascular smooth muscle, pancreas β-cell and on the intestine, which is mediated with second messengers like MAP kinase or cyclic AMP.[4]

The predominant catabolic pathway for inactivating 1,25(OH)$_2$D3 to calcitroic acid is the inducible 24-hydroxylase pathway. The responsible enzyme is the mitochondrial 25-hydroxyvitamin D-24-hydroxylase (CYP24A1), regulated through negative feedback control with 1,25(OH)$_2$D3 concentrations. It weakens the activity of 1,25(OH)$_2$D3 in order to prevent hypercalcemia.[5]

Vitamin D pathway regulates almost 3% of the mouse and human genome. Together with the presence of all elements of the vitamin D system and VDR in almost all cell types, this indicates that vitamin D endocrine system is essential for life in higher animals.[7] The central role in calcium homeostasis is well established, but it is involved in many additional biological actions in the adaptive as well as in the innate immune system, and functioning of the pancreatic β-cells, heart, brain, and fetal growth and development.[1] Accordingly, growing epidemiological data support the role vitamin D might play in suppression of many chronic illnesses, including cancers, cardiovascular disease, diabetes, the metabolic syndrome, autoimmune disease, myopathy, and infections.[7,8]

IMMUNOMODULATORY EFFECTS OF VITAMIN D

The primary defense against infection is the innate immune system, which includes the complement system, neutrophils, and macrophages, as well as antigen presentation to lymphocytes, part of the adaptive immune system. According to accumulating evidence, vitamin D may be the key player of human responses to infection due to its involvement in regulation of different components of the innate immune system.[9] In monocytes, the results of studies showed specific induction of CYP27B1 and VDR upon binding *Mycobacterium tuberculosis* to monocytic toll-like receptor (TLR) 2/1.[10] Therefore, locally synthesized 1,25(OH)$_2$D3 binds to nuclear VDR and regulate gene expression in monocytes, particularly of the antibiotic protein cathelicidin (LL37).[11]

Except through TLR 2/1-mediated mechanism, the expression of CYP27B1 is also induced by TLR 4 ligands [i.e., lipopolysaccharide (LPS)].[12] The mechanism of enhanced transcription of VDR and CYP27B1 is not fully defined. Studies showed that JAK-STAT, p38 MAP kinase, and nuclear factor-κB (NF-κB) pathways are included in the expression of CYP27B1 in the presence of either LPS or interferon-γ (IFN-γ), for which is long known to enhance the effect of vitamin D on bacterial killing.[13] It is still unclear which pathways are associated with induction of CYP27B1 by TLR ligands, but recent studies have shown that a potential intermediate in promotion of localized activity of CYP27B1 may be interleukin (IL)-15.[14]

Another key determinant of monocyte responses to vitamin D may be CYP24A1. Its activity is promoted by IL-4, and with that IL-4 attenuates intracrine induction of LL37 expression mediated with TLR 2/1. This effect is opposite to IFN-γ which potentiates intracrine vitamin D responses. Since IFN-γ is the product of T-helper 1 (Th1) T-cells and Th2 T-cells synthesize IL-4, this could mean that the two types of adaptive immune responses which are mediated with T-cells have opposite influence on vitamin D metabolism.[15] Through this influence of cytokines on regulation of activation and catabolism of vitamin D, it may represent the connection between innate and adaptive immunity.[16]

The binding of VDR to a VDRE in the proximal promoter of the LL37 gene is followed by the activation of LL37 transcription. Human gene for β-defensin 2 (DEFB4) also contains VDRE in its proximal promoter.[11] The induction of its transcription is mediated via NF-κB response elements.[17] Promotion of NF-κB signaling may involve not only inflammatory cytokines, but also nucleotide-binding oligomerization domain containing 2 (NOD2), an intracellular pathogen recognition receptor for muramyl dipeptide, originated from bacterial cellular membrane. This may also be induced with 1,25(OH)$_2$D3.[18]

Vitamin D also affects innate immunity VDR presence on macrophages or dendritic cells (DCs), which have the antigen presenting role. Antigen presentation and promotion of a tolerogenic T-cell response is diminished through DC maturation inhibition caused by treatment with 1,25(OH)$_2$D3. Also, DCs express CYP27B1, so antigen presentation by DCs may be suppressed.[19,20]

ROLE OF VITAMIN D IN MYCOBACTERIUM TUBERCULOSIS INFECTION

Historically, the treatment of tuberculosis consisted of exposure to sunlight, especially as part of therapy for cutaneous tuberculosis. Since vitamin D3 was isolated from cod liver oil, which was first used to treat tuberculosis, this initiated its common use in treatment and prevention until the introduction of antibiotics in the mid-20th century.[21]

The active metabolite of vitamin D, 1,25(OH)$_2$D3 affects immune reaction to *M. tuberculosis* infection. The active disease is characterized by granulomas which consist of macrophages containing bacteria in the central core and T-cells surrounding them. As it was mentioned before, CYP27A1 expression in macrophages is promoted by binding *M. tuberculosis* antigens with TLR 2/1 receptors.[10] Therefore, 1,25(OH)$_2$D3 is synthesized locally. The Th1 cells secrete IFN-γ, which amplifies this effect by upregulating CYP27A1 and suppressing the inactivating enzyme—CYP27B1.[13,22] Several mechanisms of antimicrobial action of 1,25(OH)$_2$D3 include the induction of a superoxide burst and promotion of phagosome and lysosome fusion in *M. tuberculosis*-infected macrophages.[23,24] These mechanisms are mediated by phosphatidylinositol 3-kinase, implying the initiation from binding to VDRs located on plasma membrane.[25] Another interaction of 1,25(OH)$_2$D3 and the innate immune response to *M. tuberculosis* infection is via nuclear VDR, when it enhances the responses through induction of LL37 synthesis.[10] Besides its direct bactericidal activity, LL37 is also involved in the immune response by monocytes, T-cells, and neutrophils attraction to the infection focus.[26]

Besides the involvement in the phagolysosome fusion process in macrophages, vitamin D is also the mediator of the preceding process of autophagy [encapsulation of organelles or cell aspect of the 1,25(OH)$_2$D3-induced response to *M. tuberculosis* infection], since the autophagy response to the activation of TLR 2/1 receptors is connected with the activation of an intracrine vitamin D system.[27,28]

Together with the paracrine action of locally produced 1,25(OH)$_2$D3 during *M. tuberculosis* infection, it may be released into the systemic circulation and cause hypercalcemia through influence on target organs—kidney, gut, and bone. This may be present in patients with active tuberculosis in the early phases of treatment.[26]

RESPONSE TO VITAMIN D TREATMENT IN TUBERCULOSIS

Vitamin D status is determined with serum 25(OH)D concentration, since it is the main circulating form. The concentration of 25(OH)D less than 50 nmol/L (20 µg/L) is considered vitamin D deficiency.[29] When serum concentration is below 75-100 nmol/L (30-40 µg/L), the elevation of parathyroid hormone occurs.[30] However, intestinal transport of calcium rises for 45-60% when 25(OH)D concentration reaches values from 50 to 80 nmol/L (20-32 µg/L), so the values of 25(OH)D in the range of 52-72 nmol/L (21-29 µg/L) are considered vitamin D insufficient. If the concentration of 25(OH)D is greater than or equal to 75 nmol/L (30 µg/L), the vitamin D status is sufficient.[8] The minimum daily requirement is 400 IU/day for all ages, but treatment doses of 10,000 IU/day, or a single bolus dose of up to 600,000 IU in adults have been safely administered in deficiency state.[31,32]

Several studies have evaluated vitamin D status in patients with tuberculosis in different populations. In the study of Talat et al. in Pakistan, an increased risk for progression of tuberculosis was associated with low vitamin D levels.[33] Sato et al. investigated the connection between 25(OH)D concentration in plasma and the course of treatment of tuberculosis and concluded that low serum levels of vitamin D were good in predicting prolonged clinical course.[34] Martineau et al. used single oral dose of 2.5 mg of vitamin D and it suppressed the growth of *M. tuberculosis* in patients' blood samples.[35] In other studies, results showed that vitamin D supplementation together with the conventional therapy for tuberculosis shortened time needed for conversion of sputum smears from positive to negative bacteria status.[16] In a randomized, placebo-controlled trial of vitamin D supplementation in patients with pulmonary tuberculosis, supplementation with high doses (600,000 IU in two doses, 1 month apart) of vitamin D accelerated patients' recovery, which was confirmed with radiological findings, in all patients with tuberculosis and improved immune system in patients who were vitamin D deficient at baseline.[36]

Vitamin D receptor gene polymorphism is not rare in many populations and the prevalence varies in different groups. They may lead to changes in the protein structure or to defects in gene activation. Although nucleotide changes in 3' end of the VDR gene are considered to be silent (*BsmI, ApaI, TaqI*), with no effect on the protein structure, they may affect regulation of VDR gene expression. It was proposed that mRNA coded with the *TaqI* t allele of the VDR gene is more stable than the one from the T allele. Also, a nonsilent VDR gene polymorphism is the *FokI*, on the exon 2, which is a translation initiation start site. The point mutation found in the F allele produces a VDR protein which is three amino acids shorter than the f variant, and the shorter protein is more active.[37] In the report of Martineau et al. from a double-blind randomized controlled trial in a vitamin D deficient population, results showed no significant improvement of the outcome of standard tuberculosis treatment with vitamin D supplementation (four oral doses of 2.5 mg vitamin D3 administered in 42 days, every 2 weeks), even though it increased serum vitamin 25(OH)D concentrations. However, a significant shortening of the time needed for conversion of sputum culture was noticed in participants with the *tt* genotype of the *TaqI* polymorphism of the *VDR* gene.[38] The genetic influence in the susceptibility to tuberculosis was also reported in a case-control study of the influence of vitamin D deficiency and VDR polymorphisms on tuberculosis among Gujarati Asians.[39] Deficiency of 25(OH)D was associated with active tuberculosis. Also, the association of combination of 25(OH)D deficiency and TT/Tt genotype, as well as of undetectable levels of 25(OH)D and ff genotype, were associated strongly with the disease.

Vitamin D, with its significant impact on the immune system, definitely could play a significant role in susceptibility, progression, and outcome of *M. tuberculosis* infection and tuberculosis. Introduction of vitamin D supplementation for prevention in high-risk populations, as a safe agent that improves innate mechanisms for mycobacterial destruction, would be a major breakthrough. Also, it might improve outcome in drug-resistant cases considering the increasing prevalence of multidrug-resistance in patients with tuberculosis. However, properly designed, randomized controlled trials are needed to assess all aspects of this implementation, including the influence of gene polymorphisms in the vitamin D biologic system.

REFERENCES

1. Norman AW. From vitamin D to hormone D: fundamentals of the vitamin D endocrine system essential for good health. Am J Clin Nutr. 2008;88(2):491S-9S.
2. Endres DB, Rude RK. Mineral and bone metabolism. In: Burtis CA, Ashwood ER, Bruns DE, editors. Tietz Textbook of Clinical Chemistry and Molecular Diagnostics. 4th ed. Philadelphia: WB Saunders; 2006. pp. 1929-6.
3. Armas LA, Hollis BW, Heaney RP. Vitamin D2 is much less effective than vitamin D3 in humans. J Clin Endocrinol Metab. 2004;89:5387-91.
4. Lips P. Vitamin D physiology. Prog Biophys Mol Biol. 2006;92:4-8.
5. Prosser DE, Jones G. Enzymes involved in the activation and inactivation of vitamin D. Trends Biochem Sci. 2004;29(12):664-73.
6. Haussler MR, Whitfield GK, Haussler CA, et al. The nuclear vitamin D receptor: biological and molecular regulatory properties revealed. J Bone Miner Res. 1998;13:325-49.
7. Bouillon R, Bischoff-Ferrari H, Willett W. Vitamin D and health: perspectives from mice to man. J Bone Miner Res. 2008;23(7):974-9.

8. Holick MF. Vitamin D deficiency. N Engl J Med. 2007;357(3):266-81.
9. Hewison M. Vitamin D and the intracrinology of innate immunity. Mol Cell Endocrinol. 2010;321:103-11.
10. Liu PT, Stenger S, Li H, Wenzel L, Tan BH, Krutzik SR, et al. Toll-like receptor triggering of a vitamin D-mediated human antimicrobial response. Science. 2006;311:1770-3.
11. Wang TT, Nestel FP, Bourdeau V, et al. Cutting edge: 1,25-dihydroxyvitamin D3 is a direct inducer of antimicrobial peptide gene expression. J Immunol. 2004;173:2909-12.
12. Adams JS, Ren S, Liu PT, et al. Vitamin D-directed rheostatic regulation of monocyte antibacterial responses. J Immunol. 2009;182:4289-95.
13. Stoffels K, Overbergh L, Giulietti A, Verlinden L, Bouillon R, Mathieu C. Immune regulation of 25-hydroxyvitamin-D3-1alpha-hydroxylase in human monocytes. J Bone Miner Res. 2006;21:37-47.
14. Krutzik SR, Hewison M, Liu PT, et al. IL-15 links TLR2/1-induced macrophage differentiation to the vitamin D-dependent antimicrobial pathway. J Immunol. 2008;181:7115-20.
15. Edfeldt K, Liu PT, Chun R, et al. T-cell cytokines differentially control human monocyte antimicrobial responses by regulating vitamin D metabolism. Proc Natl Acad Sci U S A. 2010;107:22593-8.
16. Lagishetty V, Liu NQ, Hewison M. Vitamin D metabolism and innate immunity. Mol Cell Endocrinol. 2011;347:97-105.
17. Kao CY, Kim C, Huang F, Wu R. Requirements for two proximal NF-kappaB binding sites and IkappaB-zeta in IL-17A-induced human beta-defensin 2 expression by conducting airway epithelium. J Biol Chem. 2008;283:15309-18.
18. Wang TT, Dabbas B, Laperriere D, et al. Direct and indirect induction by 1,25-dihydroxyvitamin D3 of the NOD2/CARD15-beta defensin 2 innate immune pathway defective in Crohn disease. J Biol Chem. 2010;285:2227-31.
19. Adorini L, Penna G, Giarratana N, Uskokovic M. Tolerogenic dendritic cells induced by vitamin D receptor ligands enhance regulatory T cells inhibiting allograft rejection and autoimmune diseases. J Cell Biochem. 2003;88:227-33.
20. Hewison M, Freeman L, Hughes SV, et al. Differential regulation of vitamin D receptor and its ligand in human monocyte-derived dendritic cells. J Immunol. 2003;170:5382-90.
21. Hawthorne GM, Thickett DR. Vitamin D and tuberculosis. J Postgrad Med Inst. 2011;25:185-7.
22. Vidal M, Ramana CV, Dusso AS. Stat1-vitamin D receptor interactions antagonize 1,25-dihydroxyvitamin D transcriptional activity and enhance stat1-mediated transcription. Mol Cell Biol. 2002;22:2777-87.
23. Sly LM, Lopez M, Nauseef WM, Reiner NE. 1alpha,25-dihydroxyvitamin D3-induced monocyte antimycobacterial activity is regulated by phosphatidylinositol 3-kinase and mediated by the NAPDH-dependent phagocyte oxidase. J Biol Chem. 2001;276:35482-93.
24. Hmama Z, Sendide K, Talal A, Garcia R, Dobos K, Reiner NE. Quantitative analysis of phagolysosome fusion in intact cells: inhibition by mycobacterial lipoarabinomannan and rescue by an 1alpha,25-dihydroxyvitamin D3-phosphoinositide 3-kinase pathway. J Cell Sci. 2004;117:2131-40.
25. Norman AW, Mizwicki MT, Norman DP. Steroid-hormone rapid actions, membrane receptors and a conformational ensemble model. Nat Rev Drug Discov. 2004;3:27-41.
26. Martineau AR, Honecker FU, Wilkinson RJ, Griffiths CJ. Vitamin D in the treatment of pulmonary tuberculosis. J Steroid Biochem Mol Biol. 2007;103:793-8.
27. Yuk JM, Shin DM, Lee HM, et al. Vitamin D3 induces autophagy in human monocytes/macrophages via cathelicidin. Cell Host Microbe. 2009;6:231-43.
28. Shin DM, Yuk JM, Lee HM, et al. Mycobacterial lipoprotein activates autophagy via TLR2/1/CD14 and a functional vitamin D receptor signalling. Cell Microbiol. 2010;12:1648-65.
29. Bischoff-Ferrari HA, Giovannucci E, Willett WC, Dietrich T, Dawson-Hughes B. Estimation of optimal serum concentrations of 25-hydroxyvitamin D for multiple health outcomes. Am J Clin Nutr. 2006;84:18-28.
30. Holick MF, Siris ES, Binkley N, et al. Prevalence of vitamin D inadequacy among postmenopausal North American women receiving osteoporosis therapy. J Clin Endocrinol Metab. 2005;90:3215-24.
31. Pearce SH, Cheetham TD. Diagnosis and management of vitamin D deficiency. BMJ. 2010;340:b5664.
32. Wagner CL, Greer FR. Prevention of rickets and vitamin D deficiency in infants, children, and adolescents. Pediatrics. 2008;122:1142-52.

33. Talat N, Perry S, Parsonnet J, Dawood G, Hussain R. Vitamin D deficiency and tuberculosis progression. Emerg Infect Dis. 2010;16:853-5.
34. Martineau AR, Wilkinson RJ, Wilkinson KA, et al. A single dose of vitamin D enhances immunity to mycobacteria. Am J Respir Crit Care Med. 2007;176:208-13.
35. Sato S, Tanino Y, Saito J, et al. The relationship between 25-hydroxyvitamin D levels and treatment course of pulmonary tuberculosis. Respir Investig. 2012;50:40-5.
36. Salahuddin N, Ali F, Hasan Z, Rao N, Aqeel M, Mahmood F. Vitamin D accelerates clinical recovery from tuberculosis: results of the SUCCINCT study (supplementary cholecalciferol in recovery from tuberculosis). A randomized, placebo-controlled, clinical trial of vitamin D supplementation in patients with pulmonary tuberculosis. BMC Infect Dis. 2013;13:22.
37. Chocano-Bedoya P, Ronnenberg AG. Vitamin D and tuberculosis. Nutr Rev. 2009;67:289-93.
38. Martineau AR, Timms PM, Bothamley GH, et al. High-dose vitamin D(3) during intensive-phase antimicrobial treatment of pulmonary tuberculosis: a double-blind randomised controlled trial. Lancet. 2011;377:242-50.
39. Wilkinson RJ, Llewelyn M, Toossi Z, et al. Influence of vitamin D deficiency and vitamin D receptor polymorphisms on tuberculosis among Gujarati Asians in west London: a case-control study. Lancet. 2000;355:618-21.

CHAPTER 19
Surgery for Pulmonary Tuberculosis

Ravindra K Dewan

INTRODUCTION

Most of thoracic surgery developed in late 19th century and early 20th century specifically to deal with the management of tuberculosis (TB) patients.[1,2] Surgical operations for the treatment of TB have a long history, predating the discovery of *Mycobacterium tuberculosis*. For almost two centuries before the introduction of effective anti-TB medicines, surgery was one of the main treatment options for TB. In 1726, the British surgeon E Barry drained a purulent TB lung cavity (pneumotomy). In 1882, Carlo Forlanini introduced collapse therapy into the treatment of pulmonary TB, provoking artificial pneumothorax. However, it was only after the development of radiographic imaging methods and the introduction of the manometer that surgical procedures became safer and more reliable. After the discovery of *M. tuberculosis* by Robert Koch in 1882, surgical intervention remained one of the most common therapeutic options for the treatment of TB patients, although this approach was not always successful. In 1890, Spengler successfully performed thoracoplasty and in 1891, Theodore Tuffier performed a wedge lung resection in a TB patient. In the period 1910–1912, Hans Christian Jacobaeus developed thoracoscopy and an effective operation for closed cauterization of pleural adhesions. In 1938, Vincent Monaldi introduced thoracostomy (drainage) for the treatment of cavitary TB. In 1933, Heidenhain Lilienthal performed the first successful pneumonectomy for TB treatment, and the first lobectomy was reported by Samuel Freedlander in 1935. In 1947, LK Bogush performed the first pneumonectomy in the former Soviet Union for the treatment of a patient with progressive cavitary pulmonary TB.

With the introduction of modern anti-TB chemotherapy in 1952, surgery was largely abandoned and, until the present day, chemotherapy has been the main treatment method for TB, including its drug-resistant forms. In the industrialized countries of Australia, Europe, Japan, and North America, the number of operations fell considerably because the incidence and prevalence of TB declined and medicines were effective. However, the problem of TB continued to exist in developing countries in sizable numbers. For the last five decades, caseloads of thoracic surgeons working in developing countries and recently, emerging economies, have been much higher than those working in Europe, United States of America, and advanced countries. After globalization in 1990s, many case reports from former Soviet states, African countries, Italy, Japan, India, and Pakistan are being published with regular frequency.[3]

The specter of human immunodeficiency virus (HIV)-acquired immunodeficiency syndrome has added new dimensions, challenges, and complexities in the last two decades. However, TB with or without HIV remains the single most important challenge.

Since there are no randomized prospective studies, surgical recommendations for surgery are based primarily on case reports, retrospective studies, experience, and consensus.[1] The management of TB is primarily medical, with surgery being indicated only occasionally.

INDICATIONS OF SURGICAL INTERVENTION

- Diagnostic procedures to confirm TB and to rule out other causes including cancer
- Excision surgery to remove worrisome disease in drug-resistant cases
- Symptom control for conditions like hemoptysis, empyema, or recurrent chest infections.

Some authors have suggested that pulmonary resection combined with anti-TB chemotherapy for multidrug-resistant TB (MDR-TB) has achieved treatment success rates in some settings of up to 88–92% of cases. Despite these favorable results, the role of surgery remains rather controversial in the most recently published MDR-TB treatment guidelines.[4-6] Its indication is limited to the management of complicated forms of TB [including massive hemoptysis, bronchiectasis, bronchial stenosis, bronchopleural fistula (BPF), and aspergilloma] and, mostly, to cases in which medical treatment is failing. Among studies assessing surgery for all forms of TB, several authors have postulated the following absolute indications for surgery in TB treatment:

- A high probability of failure of medical therapy in MDR-TB patients (due to persistent cavitary disease and lung or lobar destruction) and massive hemoptysis or tension pneumothorax
- Persistent positivity of sputum smear or sputum culture despite adequate chemotherapy
- A high risk of relapse based upon the drug-resistance profile and radiological findings
- Localized lesion
- Progression of TB despite adequate chemotherapy
- Repeated hemoptysis or secondary infection
- Multidrug-resistant TB or polyresistant TB
- Absence of any radiological or bacteriological improvement after 4 months of supervised therapy
- Allergic or toxic side effects of drugs
- Issues of gastrointestinal absorption of drugs.

Those patients in which the total cavity diameter was more than 15 cm or the bilateral parenchymal infiltration covered more than 75% of the total lung area are considered to have extended disease. Occasionally, resection is considered for patients with cavitary disease due to the difficulty of antibiotic penetration and the high number of organisms contained within the cavity. Some authors emphasize that surgical treatment is most often used in cases of tuberculoma and fibrotic-cavitary TB, and one of the most important indications for surgery is irreversible morphological changes of the lungs and other respiratory organs due to the development of the fibrotic tissues during the progress of TB over the long term. In cases of tuberculoma of more than 3 cm, early pulmonary resection will prevent progression and shorten the period of treatment. In some cases, surgical treatment avoids errors in differential diagnosis of tuberculoma and lung cancer.

Among studies that specifically consider MDR-TB, while the majority of authors agree on the absolute indication for the surgical treatment of MDR-TB in cases of persistent cavitary disease with treatment failure, some authors consider that even in sputum smear-negative MDR-TB patients, a radiologically persistent fibrous cavitation or destroyed lung (suggesting no clinical improvement) represents an indication for surgery because of the high probability of relapse. Other investigators call to mind that the purpose of surgery is to remove a large, focal burden of bacilli localized in necrotic and nonviable lung tissue. The TB cavity is an ideal growth environment because its wall can restrict drug penetration, and it probably protects *M. tuberculosis* from the host's immune defenses. Many patients who are preoperatively sputum culture-negative have positive cultures from resected lung tissue. Furthermore, cavities might be sites for the development of drug resistance. In a study of resected TB lung tissue, bacillary growth was shown to be most active in macrophages located on the cavity surface, where the majority of new drug-resistance mutations occur. The investigators reported an absence of CD4 and CD8 T-cells at the luminal surface, which might explain active bacillary proliferation. Additionally, after removal of a major TB focus, the immune response to residual infection might be enhanced, similar to paradoxical reactions sometimes noted during TB treatment. The successful treatment of any infectious disease involves a delicate balance of host and pathogen processes. In the human lung, selection of drug-resistance mutations in *M. tuberculosis* occurs predominantly within lung cavities in which high bacterial loads, active mycobacterial replication, and reduced exposure to the host's defense mechanisms can be detected.

Thus, an approach combining chemotherapy and surgery is increasingly being used in many parts of the world to treat patients with MDR-TB/extensively drug-resistant TB (XDR-TB).

Although most surgery for TB is elective, life-threatening conditions that may require emergency surgery are at times found with all forms of TB like profuse lung hemorrhage, spontaneous tension pneumothorax. However, complications and sequelae of the TB process like spontaneous pneumothorax and pyopneumothorax, aspergilloma, pleural empyema with or without BPF, broncholith, pachypleuritis or pericarditis with respiratory and blood circulation insufficiency, post-TB stenosis of trachea and large bronchi, symptomatic and chronic post-TB bronchiectasis, or complications of previous TB surgery form a greater number of surgical interventions performed for intrathoracic TB.

PREOPERATIVE WORKUP OF A PATIENT TO BE TAKEN UP FOR SURGERY

Proper patient selection and the timing of operations are crucial to avoid relapses and to provide a higher chance of cure. Good cooperation between treating physicians and thoracic surgeons, as well as patients' adherence to pre- and postoperative intervention chemotherapy can increase the success rate of MDR-TB treatment.

For patients to be considered as candidates for surgery, three major criteria need to be met:
- The patient must have localized disease amenable to resection and with an adequate respiratory reserve
- The patient must have extensive drug resistance, making the likelihood of treatment failure or relapse very high
- A sufficient quantity of second-line drugs must be available to ensure healing after surgery. In all cases, surgery is only indicated if it is possible to perform surgery (resection of the lung or other type of operation) without significant damage to the patient's lung function.

Surgery is a very serious step for patients with TB, in particular for those with MDR/XDR-TB, given the history of their long and difficult-to-treat disease. For many of these

patients, their disease will be too extensive and characterized by lung destruction and/ or lung function that are too poor, making them unsuitable for surgery. In addition, each operation is rather dangerous and carries certain risks. It is, therefore, crucial to discuss individually with each patient and his/her family all details about the planned surgery and to perform all necessary preoperative examinations and treatments. The following steps are crucial:
- A comprehensive and open discussion should be carried out with patients and their relatives about the nature of their TB and the necessity of surgical intervention, as well as the risks and benefits of surgery, and the short- and long-term prognosis with and without surgical intervention. Possible complications in terms of anesthesia and the operation must be discussed with all patients and their relatives. Consent for surgery must be obtained for all patients who are to undergo surgery
- The following preoperative investigations need to be carried out: full blood analysis, biochemistry tests (liver and kidney, blood sugar, electrolytes and coagulation), HIV testing, sputum smear microscopy, sputum culture testing and drug susceptibility testing (DST), standard chest X-ray
- The patient's cardiorespiratory reserve must be carefully evaluated based on pulmonary function testing: body plethysmography [to evaluate vital capacity, forced expiratory volume in one second and diffusion of the lung(s)], electrocardiogram and echocardiogram (to rule out heart failure and pulmonary hypertension), perfusion lung scintigraphy [in patients with marginal spirometric results and diffusion of the lung(s)], arterial blood gas analysis, and routine cardiological consultation
- Nutritional assessment (body mass index) should be carried out to ensure the patient can tolerate and recover from surgery
- Airways should be sanitized: respiratory exercises, postural drainage, and routine aerosol inhalation should be carried out, or nebulized bronchodilators and antibiotics should be used
- Smoking cessation must be encouraged.

TYPES OF OPERATION

The following are the types of operation currently performed:
- Lung resections like wedge resection, segmentectomy, lobectomy, bilobectomy, combined resection (lobectomy plus minor resection), pneumonectomy or pleuropneumonectomy
- Extrapleural thoracoplasty
- Extrapleural pneumolysis
- Thoracomyoplasty
- Pleurectomy and decortications of the lung
- Operations on the bronchi like occlusion, resection, bronchoplasty, and reamputation of the stump
- Thracocentesis and thoracostomy
- Artificial pneumothorax and pneumoperitoneum.

The principal types of operation to treat TB today are lung resections of different sizes, using posterolateral thoracotomy under general anesthesia with double-lumen endotracheal tube and artificial ventilation of the lung. Mobilization of the lung (or the part of it to be resected) is approached in such a way as to avoid contamination of the pleural space. It should be mentioned, however, that anatomical resections are preferable.

CONTRAINDICATIONS FOR ELECTIVE SURGICAL TREATMENT OF PULMONARY TUBERCULOSIS AND MDR/XDR-TB

In the majority of cases, contraindications for the surgical treatment of TB patients depend on how extensive the process is to be, assessment of the patients' cardiopulmonary function and their general state of heath. The following contraindications can be considered for lung resection:

- Extensive cavitary lesion of the both lungs
- Impaired pulmonary function test, that is forced expiratory volume in 1 second less than 1.5 L in cases of lobectomy and less than 2.0 L where pneumonectomy is planned
- Pulmonary heart failure III–IV (functional classification of the New York Heart Association)
- Body mass index up to 40–50% of the normal range
- Severe comorbidity (decompensation in diabetes, exacerbation of stomach and duodenum ulcers, hepatic or renal impairment)
- Active bronchial TB.

PERSISTENTLY POSITIVE SPUTUM

Surgery plays an important role in the overall management of MDR-TB with acceptable mortality and morbidity.[4,7-12] Surgical interventions, in carefully selected cases, along with second line antitubercular treatment (ATT) appears as the most favorable option since even the best available medical therapy alone only provides bacteriological cure in the order of 44–77% vis-à-vis more than 90% success rate with adjuvant surgery.[10] Operative mortality is no longer a prohibitive issue, with most series reporting fewer than 3% early mortality.[7,13] Though operative mortality has decreased, significant morbidity continues to be a nagging problem, BPF with empyema formation being the most distressing manifestation. In thoracic surgery,[14] poor nutritional status and positive sputum are associated with higher rate of complications. Unequivocal consensus is lacking in the literature regarding the application of perioperative ATT. The rationale behind selecting the exact timing of intervention needs to be logical and scientific, and whereas it appears logical to use surgery after a defined induction phase of chemotherapy, a scientifically defined induction phase has yet to be worked out. Generally accepted timing of surgery is after 3 months of carefully prescribed second line ATT, achieving optimal bacterial suppression at the time of surgery yet avoiding delaying the surgery to a point where the bacillary load is at a perilous high. Continuation of drugs for 18–24 months postoperatively seems reasonable by most authors, though given the economics involved, completion of this task is frankly daunting, if not utopian. Indications of surgery in MDR-TB remain a contentious issue, however, broad consensus is now apparent. Bacteriological cure in many series has been fairly impressive, with well over 90% success achieved with adjuvant surgery. Occasionally, thoracoplasty rather than lung resection surgery is justified in some.

HEMOPTYSIS

Surgery is not immediately required in cases of hemoptysis caused by pulmonary TB. Massive recurrent hemoptysis is the only justified indication in this setting. Conservative measures like positioning the good lung up after localizing the site, antibiotics, rest, and sedation are almost always successful in controlling lung bleeding and surgery can be planned on an elective basis. Very often, post-tubercular cavities

are colonized by *Aspergillus* fungus (aspergilloma) resulting in recurrent hemoptysis. There are interventional measures other than surgery, which have their selected role in appropriate situations:[3]
- Endotracheal intubation to secure airway, suctioning
- Endobronchial tamponade with Fogarty catheter
- Laser photocoagulation [neodymium-doped yttrium-aluminum-garnet (Nd:YAG) or argon]
- Endobronchial hemostatic agents
- Selective bronchial artery embolization.

However, surgical resection of involved portions of the lung is the most definitive and curative modality for treating massive and recurrent hemoptysis.[15] These are challenging surgeries involving careful dissection because of dense and unpredictable adhesions. A properly placed double-lumen endotracheal tube, by which the anesthesiologist can collapse or inflate the lung depending upon the needs of the surgeon, is crucial. Position of this tube is confirmed with pediatric fiberoptic bronchoscope and the time spent here is time well spent. This also protects the other healthy lung and ensures safety during surgery. The dissection of vascular structures at hilum or in the fissure requires precise combination of sharp and blunt dissection. Adhesions are always a major challenge in this surgery. Use of a transfixation suture or double ligature on the proximal side while dividing arteries and veins is crucial to prevent catastrophic postoperative hemorrhage. Bronchus is closed with a bronchial stump stapler or interrupted sutures. Equally good results have been shown by either of these techniques.

EMPYEMA

Empyema is a challenge, and requires a common sense approach, for its management.[3,16] The management depends upon the stage of presentation. Most of the cases can be effectively managed with prolonged and expert intercostal tube management. In the subacute stage, drainage can be assisted by either video-assisted thoracic debridement or instillation of intrapleural antifibrinolytic agents like streptokinase or urokinase. Decortication is indicated in persistent pleural spaces with late fibrinopurulent stage. Thoracoplasty is partial decostalization of the thoracic cage to obliterate persistent pleural space. Whenever lung is unlikely to expand because of extensive disease or multiple BPF, thoracoplasty is an appropriate intervention and is required quite often. Postoperative empyema or persisting space problems almost always require thoracoplasty for ultimate resolution.

POSTOPERATIVE MANAGEMENT

Results in surgery for TB and inflammatory lung disease improve if attention to detail is given in postoperative period. Initial management is ideally done in an intensive care unit. Antibiotics and painkillers are routinely given. Blood is transfused as per requirements. Respiratory exercises should be encouraged and all measures to relieve pain should be taken. Incentive spirometry is a useful tool to achieve these aims. Care of the chest tubes is an essential ingredient of this care and they should be removed only when their output has minimized sufficiently. Persistent air leaks, development of BPF, and residual pleural space are the most important issues to be watched for in the postoperative period and onward. These complications may require various kinds of intervention, including open-window thoracostomy and thoracoplasty.

Recent published series have demonstrated mortality ranging from 0 to 3.1%.[3,4,17-21] Morbidity reported in most series ranges from 3 to 53.7%. Postoperative empyema and BPF are best managed by prolonged tube drainage followed by open-window thoracostomy and thoracoplasty, if required.

CONCLUSION

Surgery for complications and sequel of pulmonary TB still remain an important intervention for alleviation of human misery. It is a high cost and sophisticated intervention, which demands high levels of surgical skill and judgment. There is a continued need to further develop skills and techniques in this area. All these issues require continued commitment from all the stakeholders to improve the results of this highly complicated and complex set of surgical patients.[3]

Uses of newer technologies like surgical staplers, refined blood transfusion technologies, argon beam coagulation, monitoring devices, and safer anesthesia have improved the results of surgery substantially. The number of surgeons engaged in this specific field of pathology has declined tremendously with the advent of ATT. The ravages of TB are on the rise again especially since drug-resistant TB has come to the fore. This calls for a dire need to reinvent the wheel of TB-surgery to adequately address this health hazard. The amalgamation of the older TB surgical techniques with the current developments of surgery in general is needed.

REFERENCES

1. Pezzella AT, Fang W. Surgical aspects of thoracic tuberculosis: a contemporary review—part 1. Curr Probl Surg. 2008;45:675-758.
2. Pezzella AT, Fang W. Surgical aspects of thoracic tuberculosis: a contemporary review—part 2. Curr Probl Surg. 2008;45:771-829.
3. Dewan RK. Surgery for pulmonary tuberculosis: a 15-year experience. Eur J Cardiothorac Surg. 2010;37:473-7.
4. Treasure RL, Seaworth BJ. Current role of surgery in Mycobacterium tuberculosis. Ann Thorac Surg. 1995;59:1405-7; discussion 1408-9.
5. Chiang CY, Yu MC, Bai KJ, Suo J, Lin TP, Lee YC. Pulmonary resection in the treatment of patients with pulmonary multidrug-resistant tuberculosis in Taiwan. Int J Tuberc Lung Dis. 2001;5:272-7.
6. Shiraishi Y, Nakajima Y, Katsuragi N, Kurai M, Takahashi N. Resectional surgery combined with chemotherapy remains the treatment of choice for multidrug-resistant tuberculosis. J Thorac Cardiovasc Surg. 2004;128:523-8.
7. Pomerantz M, Brown JM. Surgery in the treatment of multidrug-resistant tuberculosis. Clin Chest Med. 1997;18:123-30.
8. Sharma SK, Mohan A. Multidrug-resistant tuberculosis. Indian J Med Res. 2004;120:354-76.
9. Dewan RK, Pratap H. Surgical interventions in multi-drug resistant tuberculosis: retrospective analysis of 74 cases treated at a tertiary care level institution. Ind J Thorac Cardiovasc Surg. 2006;22:15-8.
10. Loddenkemper R, Sagebiel D, Brendel A. Strategies against multidrug-resistant tuberculosis. Eur Respir J Suppl. 2002;36:66s-77s.
11. MDR-TB Fact sheet, American Lung Association, March 2005.
12. Iseman MD, Madsen L, Goble M, Pomerantz M. Surgical intervention in the treatment of pulmonary disease caused by drug-resistant Mycobacterium tuberculosis. Am Rev Respir Dis. 1990;141:623-5.
13. Takeda S, Maeda H, Hayakawa M, Sawabata N, Maekura R. Current surgical intervention for pulmonary tuberculosis. Ann Thorac Surg. 2005;79:959-63.
14. Somocursio J, Sotomayor A, Furin J, et al. Identifying a subset of MDR-TB with bilateral pulmonary disease suitable for adjunctive thoracic surgery. Website and personal communication.
15. Corey R, Hla KM. Major and massive hemoptysis: reassessment of conservative management. Am J Med Sci. 1987;294:301-9.

16. Kohli A, Singh G, Vig A, Dubey KR, Singh R. Pleurocutaneous flap: how useful it is in management of chronic empyema. Indian J Chest Dis Allied Sci. 2006;48:257-9.
17. Naidoo R. Active pulmonary tuberculosis: experience with resection in 106 cases. Asian Cardiovasc Thorac Ann. 2007;15:134-8.
18. Souilamas R, Riquet M, Barthes FP, Chehab A, Capuani A, Faure E. Surgical treatment of active and sequelar forms of pulmonary tuberculosis. Ann Thorac Surg. 2001;71:443-7.
19. Furák J, Troján I, Szöke T, et al. Surgical intervention for pulmonary tuberculosis: analysis of indications and perioperative data relating to diagnostic and therapeutic resections. Eur J Cardiothorac Surg. 2001;20:722-7.
20. Olcmen A, Gunluoglu MZ, Demir A, Akin H, Kara HV, Dincer SI. Role and outcome of surgery for pulmonary tuberculosis. Asian Cardiovasc Thorac Ann. 2006;14:363-6.
21. Kim YT, Kim HK, Sung SW, Kim JH. Long-term outcomes and risk factor analysis after pneumonectomy for active and sequela forms of pulmonary tuberculosis. Eur J Cardiothorac Surg. 2003;23:833-9.

CHAPTER 20
Prevention of Tuberculosis in Areas with High Tuberculosis Incidence

Dragana M Jovanovic, Violeta V Mihailovic Vucinic

INTRODUCTION

In settings with poor epidemic control and frequent *Mycobacterium tuberculosis* transmission, reinfection limits the ability to eradicate latent infection and reduces the duration of protection provided by preventive therapy. The standard of care universally accepted is preventive therapy to vulnerable individuals following documented tuberculosis (TB) exposure and/or infection but there are multiple barriers resulting in a pronounced policy-practice gap, with nearly absent implementation in many TB-endemic areas.

Implementation of the directly observed treatment short-course (DOTS) strategy throughout the world over the past 20 years has resulted in decrease of mortality rates by more than 30% with improved epidemiological outcomes in most regions of the world.[1,2] Nevertheless, the impact of DOTS strategy implementation has been limited in the poorest countries and in areas affected by human immunodeficiency virus (HIV) infection, where exclusive focus has been on sputum smear-positive disease essentially excluding children from care. The emergence of drug-resistant TB (DR-TB) is additionally a major threat and requires new measures to enhance early case detection and rapid initiation of treatment.[1,2]

In TB-endemic areas, there is a persistent ongoing transmission due to high numbers of patients and prolonged diagnostic and treatment delay.[3,4]

Annual risk of *M. tuberculosis* infection studies are very limited by the age restriction. There is obvious huge underestimation of the infection pressure experienced by adolescents and adults within the same community, especially among those with high-risk social behavior. It seems impossible to determine the true infection pressure within these high-risk subpopulations in the absence of a tool to measure reinfection which is relevant for the ability to eradicate the pool of latent infection and the duration of benefit resulting from treating latent infection.

Previous *M. tuberculosis* infection is shown to offer some protection against future disease, like a retrospective analysis noted a 79% risk reduction among those with previous infection,[5] indicating uninfected individuals living in areas with a high TB exposure risk as a vulnerable group. Despite the protection provided by previous infection, reinfection disease dominates the epidemic in TB-endemic areas, as suggested by simultaneous infection with multiple strains and the fact that most adult cases harbor currently circulating strains (suggestive of recent infection/reinfection), noting even 77% of TB recurrences attributed to reinfection.[6,7]

Tuberculosis patients previously unable to control *M. tuberculosis* infection are as well at increased risk of TB recurrence.[7]

PREVENTION OF INFECTION

The risk of infection (primary or reinfection) is associated with the proximity and duration of contact, as well as the infectivity of the source case[8] with sputum smear-positive cases as greatest transmission risk.[9]

Higher infection rates reported in child contacts of primary caregivers[10] have particular relevance in HIV-affected communities with sputum smear-negative caregivers posing a significant transmission risk to young and vulnerable children.[11,12]

The most effective means to reduce the TB infection pressure within communities is to improve epidemic control. Early detection and effective treatment end transmission and reduce the high reproductive rate that maintains the TB epidemic. A high proportion of transmission in TB-endemic areas occurs outside of the household, especially among older children and adults[13,14] and within well-recognized "transmission hotspots".

The emergence of DR-TB re-emphasized the importance of classical infection control measures as the World Health Organization (WHO) strategies to reduce *M. tuberculosis* transmission within households, healthcare facilities, and congregate settings.

Studies demonstrated that effective treatment terminates transmission within days of initiation.[15] So, ensuring early and effective treatment of all TB patients is of utmost importance.

For patients not on effective treatment, wearing a simple surgical facemask cuts transmission in half (56% reduction).[16] Careful screening of vulnerable contacts remains important.

Tuberculosis infection/disease in a young child serves as marker of recent transmission and should trigger contact tracing and due to their limited social contact, the source case is usually identified among household members or other caregivers.

PREVENTION OF PROGRESSION TO DISEASE

Given the absence of a fully protective vaccine, preventive therapy defined as any chemotherapeutic intervention that aims to prevent or reduce the risk of TB disease following TB exposure/infection provides additional protection.

Although neonatal Bacille Calmette-Guérin (BCG) vaccination reduces the risk of severe TB disease in infancy, the TB risk is not eliminated and the impact on adults is minimal.[17]

"Treatment of latent infection" implies documented subclinical infection[18] but subclinical lesions may represent recent infection (not yet "latent") or well-controlled asymptomatic ("truly latent") infection. A limited course (either in duration or number of drugs) of treatment is aimed to sterilize existing subclinical lesions and reduces the risk of future disease. "Primary prophylaxis" is therapy during a period of exposure without proof of infection. Post-treatment or "secondary prophylaxis" aims to reduce the risk of TB recurrence after completing a course of TB treatment in immunocompromised HIV-infected patients based on two mechanisms:
1. Improved sterilization of existing lesions
2. Preventing reinfection events from becoming established (analogous to primary prophylaxis).[19]

CANDIDATES FOR PREVENTIVE THERAPY

Different levels of TB control between high-income countries where TB elimination is within reach and TB-endemic countries struggling to control the epidemic have

TABLE 1	Priority groups for preventive therapy in different epidemiological settings		
Preventive therapy target groups	*Most vulnerable groups*	*Other groups to consider*	
High-incidence settings: In order to reduce tuberculosis-related morbidity and mortality	• Young child contacts • HIV-infected patients • Patients with pronounced immune compromise	• Prisoners • People in refugee camps	
Low-incidence settings: In order to reduce tuberculosis-related morbidity and mortality and to eliminate the "pool of latent infection"		• Prisoners • Refugees • Asylum seekers • Additional relevant pockets of infection • Recent immigrants • Old people • Tuberculosis contacts (all ages)	

influenced the implementation of preventive therapy programs. While young children and HIV-infected and other immunocompromised individuals are universally prioritized, low-incidence settings often expand their focus to include recent immigrants, the socially destitute, and the elderly, etc.

Priority groups for preventive therapy in different epidemiological settings have been shown in table 1.

In young and vulnerable children, once infected, the risk of developing TB disease depends on the maturation and integrity of their immune system. Young age at the time of infection is a major risk factor for TB disease development and studies on natural history of disease quantified the risk in different age groups as: 40–50% during infancy; 20–30% during the second year of life; 5% for the 2–5-year age group; and 2% for those 5–10 years of age.[20]

Judging from autopsy studies showing increased mortality of those aged under 5 years in TB-exposed households,[21,22] successful implementation of TB prevention strategies is very important.

HIV-infected individuals have high relative risk of developing TB compared with HIV-uninfected individuals with incidence rate ratios exceeding 20 (20.6).[23]

The CD4 cell count predicts TB risk, which might be greatly reduced by antiretroviral therapy, although the residual risk remains higher (three to five times that of HIV-uninfected).[24,25] Thus, antiretroviral therapy should be initiated in all HIV-infected children within the first month of life to minimize mortality and TB risk.[26]

In adults, the use of isoniazid preventive therapy reduces TB risk but the benefit is restricted to those with a positive tuberculin skin test (TST).[27]

The WHO recommends standard isoniazid preventive therapy for all HIV-infected adults in settings where a TST is not feasible,[28] with prolonged isoniazid preventive therapy courses preferably to TST-positive individuals.[29] The International Union Against Tuberculosis and Lung Disease produced pragmatic guidance for TB/HIV management in resource-limited settings.[30]

Concerning other vulnerable groups, the risk increase is associated with different types of immune compromise and highly variable and dependent on the likelihood of TB exposure/infection. Vulnerable groups include renal dialysis and transplant patients,[24] and those receiving cancer chemotherapy[25] and long-term steroid[31] or tumor necrosis factor-α (TNF-α) treatment.[32] Immunomodulating conditions, such as diabetes mellitus and cigarette smoking, also increase TB risk. Insulin-dependent diabetes in children is associated with a six- to seven-fold risk increase in TB-endemic areas, with a two- to fourfold increase documented among adult patients with lifestyle-related diabetes.[33]

Cigarette smoking doubles the TB risk, while smoking-related lung disease is associated with diagnostic delay and poor treatment outcome.[34] High levels of emotional stress and malnutrition situations combined with a high likelihood of TB exposure, as occur in refugee or detention camps and prisons, also increase TB disease risk,[35] but the impact of preventive strategies is poorly documented.[36] Healthcare workers and TB research assistants experience high rates of annual risk of *M. tuberculosis* infection (11.3% documented in healthcare workers) with increased risk of TB disease.[37,38] Those with a negative TST or any form of immune compromise are particularly vulnerable.[39]

CONTACT SCREENING AND CASE FINDING

Contact screening represents an important opportunity for active case finding while lacking the capacity to perform a TST and/or chest radiograph often serves as a barrier to screening vulnerable contacts. Symptom-based screening is an alternative even in the most resource-limited settings, since safe and effective even in young children and in HIV-infected adults.[40-42]

Flowchart 1 reflects the WHO symptom-based screening approach for child TB contacts;[43] all children with symptoms suggestive of HIV infection and/or TB disease should be tested for HIV, including those with an HIV-infected parent, while HIV-infected individuals should be screened for TB exposure and/or disease at every healthcare contact. Repeated courses of isoniazid preventive therapy may be required in children with multiple exposures.

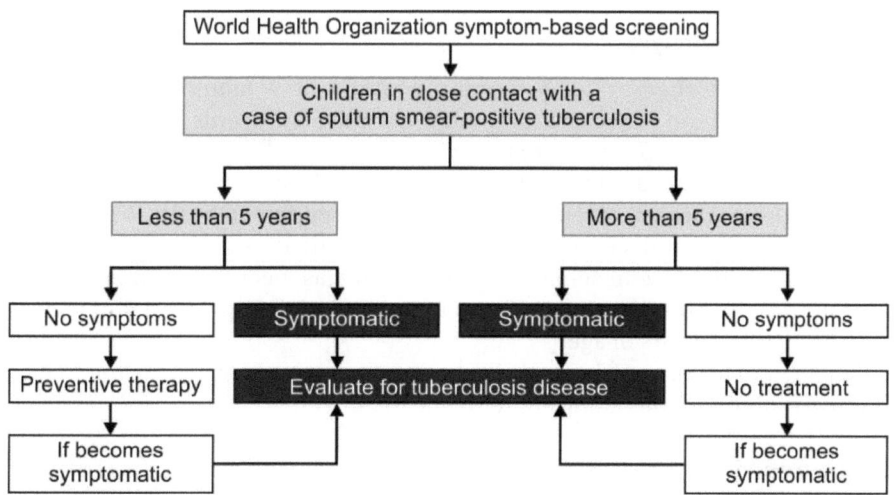

FLOWCHART 1: Guidance for National Tuberculosis Programs on the management of tuberculosis in children.

PREVENTIVE THERAPY OPTIONS

Several regimens have been evaluated, including isoniazid and rifampicin monotherapy, and combination therapy using isoniazid plus rifampicin or rifapentine and/or pyrazinamide, for durations of 2–12 months.

Isoniazid Monotherapy

Isoniazid monotherapy reduced the risk of TB disease by 60%, with no significant difference between 6- and 12-month courses,[44] while combined evidence from the US public health studies suggested a benefit from 9 months compared with 6 months of postexposure isoniazid preventive therapy. The Centers for Disease Control and Prevention (CDC) recommends to use 9 months[45] compared with the 6 months advised by the WHO.[43]

In HIV-infected individuals, a 36% overall reduction in TB disease risk was demonstrated, but the benefit was restricted to those with a positive TST (RR 0.38).[27] Prolonged or repeated isoniazid preventive therapy courses may also protect against reinfection disease.

In HIV-infected children, postexposure prophylaxis and the need for ongoing exposure screening is universally recognized, but the potential value of routine (pre-exposure) isoniazid preventive therapy in the most vulnerable young children remains controversial. Isoniazid alone reduced the risk of TB disease by 78% (RR 0.22), antiretroviral therapy alone by 67% (RR 0.32), and the combination of isoniazid and antiretroviral therapy by 89% (RR 0.11).[46]

In a trial that enrolled infants at a young age (3–4 months), excluding those with any TB exposure and provided early antiretroviral therapy to all HIV-infected infants,[47] no difference in TB disease or mortality was noted, implying that routine isoniazid preventive therapy has little value if HIV-infected infants enter management programs early, with careful TB exposure monitoring and provision of postexposure isoniazid preventive therapy.

Combination Therapy

Isoniazid preventive therapy for 9 months versus 4 or 3 months of isoniazid and rifampicin reported no TB cases and minimal adverse events in children, while adherence was greatly improved with the shorter regimens.[48]

Equivalence between 3 months of isoniazid and rifampicin versus isoniazid alone for 6–12 months was reported,[49] but this has not been endorsed by the WHO.

Strategy using 3 months of weekly long-acting rifapentine and isoniazid (12 doses in total) proved highly efficacious in adults and has been recommended by the CDC,[50] but with the exception of people on antiretroviral therapy, pregnant females, or children less than 12 years of age.

A limitation of all rifampicin- and rifapentine-containing regimens is the interaction with protease inhibitor-containing antiretroviral treatment.

Adverse Events

Severe adverse events are uncommon with the use of preventive therapy[51] and in general, children tolerate TB drugs better than adults, with frequent subclinical transient transaminase elevation, and very rare severe isoniazid-induced hepatitis. Hepatotoxicity is the major concern with the combined use of rifampicin and pyrazinamide being more common in HIV-uninfected adults[52] while children tolerate better standard first-line therapy and no hepatotoxicity was reported from trials that evaluated 2 months of rifampicin and pyrazinamide.[53,54] Increased rates of hypersensitivity reactions were reported with the use of isoniazid and rifapentine.[55]

POLICY-PRACTICE GAP

A massive policy-practice gap exists and contact management is almost nonexistent in areas of high incidence,[56] with just an example of only 12% of HIV-infected patients receiving isoniazid preventive therapy during 2010.[1]

Key implementation barriers include ignorance regarding TB disease burdens in vulnerable individuals, especially young children; concerns about reliable exclusion of TB disease and poor treatment adherence leading to the emergence of DR strains; resource constraints and prioritization; and the absence of effective monitoring and evaluation systems.

Crucial need for basic training and capacity building demands adequate political commitment and resource allocation. Preventive therapy is preventing severe disease in vulnerable individuals, but cost-effective as well from a TB control perspective, if high rates of implementation can be achieved.[57]

DRUG-RESISTANT TUBERCULOSIS

Empirical evidence from clinical experience and available data poses the basis for useful guidance in DR-TB management.

Monoresistance

For isoniazid resistance, often the first step in the development of multidrug-resistant TB (MDR-TB), rifampicin monotherapy for 4 months is advised. Rifampicin monoresistance is less common[58] and following standard isoniazid preventive therapy should be sufficient in such cases. However, rifampicin resistance is usually managed as MDR-TB, since rapid drug-susceptibility testing does not test for isoniazid resistance, which poses problems for the provision of effective preventive therapy.

Multidrug Resistance

Since evidence limited in clinical practice, preventive therapy has been restricted to the most vulnerable contacts, providing two drugs to which the organism is susceptible (or naïve) for at least 6 months with regular follow-up for 1-2 years. Later generation quinolones demonstrate similar potency to rifampicin and 4-6 months of monotherapy should conceivably be adequate, if quinolone resistance is reliably excluded.[59-64]

In conclusion, improved epidemic control through early case finding and treatment initiation remains the crucial point, but different infection control measures should be considered.

Tuberculosis preventive therapy in limited resources and high rates of ongoing transmission is restricted to the most vulnerable, which includes child contacts and HIV-infected.

TUBERCULOSIS PREVENTION IN LOW-INCIDENCE COUNTRIES

Defined by the WHO, the low incidence of TB means a rough notification of less than 200 cases per 100,000 population.[65]

In most countries of the Western Europe and the United States of America, the epidemiological situation in respect to TB infection has shown a favorable 10- to 100-fold decline. For this reason in the developed industrial countries with low TB incidence, TB prevention measures are considered to enable early TB cases detection in high-risk groups and as well to reduce the prevalence of latent TB infection (LTBI) in populations with an increased risk of evolution to active TB disease.[66]

According to the American Thoracic Society/CDC, groups at high risk of emerging active TB should be put on preventive treatment.

Those groups are:
- Individuals in recent contacts with persons with active TB disease
- Children
- HIV-positive
- Immunocompromised individuals (persons undergoing immunosuppressive therapy)
- Patients with kidney failure
- Patients with silicosis
- Homeless
- Intravenous drug users
- Immigrants or crossing borders persons from high-incidence countries.[67]

In a study from the United Kingdom, the rate of active TB among foreign-born population was 21 times higher than the rate of TB among native United Kingdom born.

The immigration of persons from high-prevalence countries into the big cities is the reason why capitals like London have increased rate of active TB cases than other parts of the country.[68,69]

The United States of America procedures require all immigrants to undergo TB screening in their native countries. If persons are with pulmonary infiltrates on the chest X-ray, entering the United States of America is possible only with previous smear testings and negative smear results.[70]

However, the screening programs of TB detection based on chest radiographs and acid-fast smear (AFS) have low capacity to detect individuals with TB infection as these screening tests can miss individuals with AFS-negative active TB.[71]

Methods to Detect Latent Tuberculosis Infection in Countries with Low-incidence Tuberculosis

For LTBI, screening has been performed using TST and recently interferon-gamma release assay (IGRA) tools have been shown to be more helpful.

Tuberculin Skin Test

Historically, the TST or Mantoux test was the only screening tool for LTBI.[72] Although the TST is an inexpensive diagnostic tool without laboratory analysis with clear definitions for interpretation, the intradermal administration and interpretation must be completed by experienced clinicians.[73] The test has low specificity, causing false positives in patients who had a previous history of the BCG vaccination or exposure to nontuberculous mycobacteria (NTM).[74,75]

It has low sensitivity in some populations, causing false negatives in immunocompromised patients with HIV infection, systemic infections, and chronic renal disease; people with prior gastrointestinal surgical procedures; people who had a live vaccination within the previous 2 months; people who are malnourished; or people taking systematic immunosuppressive medications.[67,76]

Interferon-gamma Release Assay Tools in Detecting Latent Tuberculosis Infection in Low-incidence Countries

Interferon-gamma release assays together with chest X-ray considered to be a reliable tool for screening immigrants from countries with high-incidence TB (over 150–200 cases per 100,000 population).[77]

Interferon-gamma release assays are immunological tools used for more than a decade to detect the presence of cellular immune response toward the *M. tuberculosis* specific antigens (ESAT6, CFP10, and TB7.7). The results are not confused by BCG vaccination or NTM infection, because the antigens are absent in most of NTM (with exception of *M. flavescens, M. marinum, M. kansasii,* and *M. szulgai*) and in BCG stains too.[78]

Two IGRA tests are nowadays in use:
1. Quantiferon-Gold (QFT) [enzyme-linked immunosorbent assay on whole blood]
2. T-Spot (enzyme-linked immunospot assay on peripheral blood mononuclear cells).

The overall sensitivity in general population is 75–89% of TST and QFT 75–83% while T-Spot sensitivity in general population is about 90%. The overall specificity of TST in general population is 85–95%, QFT greater than 95%, and T-Spot 88–95%.

In low TB incidence countries where BCG vaccination is not mandatory, specificity and sensitivity of TST is 97%, QFT greater than 95%, and T-Spot 88%. Unfortunately, the specificity of TST in BCG-vaccinated population is only 60%, while QFT 96%, and T-Spot 93%.[77,78]

Besides the difference in sensitivity and specificity, there are several more advantages of IGRAs over TST. Interferon gamma release assay tools are immunological assays done *in vitro*, and the whole procedure is standardized accordingly. This obviously decreases the effects of interpersonal inconsistency in interpreting the results.

Interferon-gamma release assays are quite costly diagnostic (screening) tools, requiring besides laboratory equipment, trained personal, and quality approved procedures, but in low TB incidence countries, economically developed this might not be an obstacle.

Of note, the high specificity of IGRAs decreases the number of false-positive results, especially investigating LTBI, and thus preventing further diagnostic procedures and mistreatment.[73,79,80]

Interferon-gamma release assays permit several advantages over the TST in clinical practice. Because IGRAs have specific antigens that target *M. tuberculosis*, they do not react with common NTM or BCG vaccine strains and do not produce an immunologic "boost".[81-83]

Interferon-gamma release assays follow a standard, objective protocol and provide results within 24 hours, enabling the identification and management of patients with LTBI from hard-to-reach groups.

Interferon-gamma release assays have been recommended as tests in the diagnosis of *M. tuberculosis* infection in several different clinical scenarios: in adults, including BCG-vaccinated individuals or people with immunocompromising conditions; also in situations where the TST has a positive result or in hard-to-reach population groups; in addition, IGRAs may be considered in children greater than 5 years old who have a suspected LTBI, whether from a high-incidence country or with confirmed household contacts.[84-86]

Bacillus Calmette–Guérin vaccination has been widely used since the year 1921. As a part of the WHO Expanded Program for Immunization, BCG vaccination has been used by regulations in countries with high-burden TB, as mandatory on birth or within 1 year of birth (22 countries).[87]

However, the efficiency of BCG vaccination has been shown only in decreasing the risk of severe forms of TB infection in children, like disseminated infection, miliary TB, and TB meningitis.[88,89] So definitely, the BCG vaccination does not prevent TB.

In the United States of America, Canada, Italy, and the Netherlands, BCG vaccination has never been implemented by country regulations. None countries with low-incidence of TB ceased mandatory TB vaccination in all populations.

Germany ceased BCG vaccination as mandatory since 1998. In Germany, the incidence of TB cases is very low, in children and young adults under 15 years, 1.4 cases per 100,000 children population.[90,91]

It is up to national TB programs to consider BCG vaccination as a part of package of TB control depending on the incidence of TB infection.

In low TB incidence countries, BCG vaccination should be considered for specific population groups, i.e., immigrants from high-incidence countries or healthcare workers working with DR-TB patients. However, these groups obviously require better vaccine.

Currently, there are 12 vaccines in an investigation process (into the phase of clinical trials). These vaccines are considered to be potential enough to replace present BCG vaccine or to enhance the immunity developed by BCG.[92]

Tuberculosis Prevention in Human Immunodeficiency Virus-infected Persons in Low Tuberculosis Incidence Countries

The rate of TB infection, reactivation, has decreased in HIV-negative individuals in the last decade of the twentieth century to 0.04–0.058 cases per 100 person-years.[93]

Human immunodeficiency virus infection however accelerates TB reactivation due to the failure of immune response; approximately one-third (30%) of HIV-positive individuals will get active TB.[27]

In general, however, the data on prevalence of the TB/HIV coinfection in low TB incidence countries is insufficient (i.e., in Germany, it is estimated to 3%).

In general, in European countries, TB/HIV coinfection therapy failed in almost 35% of patients.[94,95]

Multidrug-resistant Tuberculosis in Low-incidence Countries

In low TB incidence European countries, the current incidence of MDR-TB ranges up to maximum 6.4%.[96]

In the United States of America, the primary MDR-TB did not increase beyond 1.2% according to the epidemiological data from 2010 among native-born Americans; however, the incidence of MDR-TB among foreign-born persons was significantly higher up to 82% in 2010.[97,98]

The incidence of MDR-TB cases resistant to at least rifampin and isoniazid definitely depends on the efficiency of treatment of previous TB infection. The reason is in hard-to-reach risk groups (homeless, drug abusers). The proper treatment of these populations requires special attention of public health authorities.

Of note, there is an increasing incidence of MDR-TB in high TB burden countries and the boundaries toward low TB incidence countries are not closed.

In low TB incidence countries with developed tools, resistance testing is not a problem as well as the proper treatment. However, the treatment of the particular contact persons is still not sufficient. In Cochrane review up to date, no controlled trial has been published on the efficiency of the possible treatment combinations for LTBI.[99]

The European Centre for Disease Prevention and Control guidelines did not give a clear recommendation for these cases; the suggestion is the follow-up of the identified person from the contact considering to be latently infected with MDR-TB strain.[96]

In low TB burden countries, this suggestion should relay on the well-established public health system. The significant fact is that in low TB incidence countries the targeted groups at high risk for TB and MDR-TB are concentrated in urban areas.

RISK OF TUBERCULOSIS INFECTION AND TUMOR NECROSIS FACTOR-α INHIBITORS

Tumor necrosis factor-α is a significant proinflammatory cytokine. It is also a significant part of the host immunity system necessary to continue TB infection in the latent phase.

Tumor necrosis factor-α inhibitors such as etanercept, infliximab, and adalimumab are nowadays widely used as successful therapeutics in patients with a variety of autoimmune and chronic inflammatory diseases.

Since the introduction of TNF-α inhibitors, a significant increase of TB cases among the treated patients population has been observed. In the United States of America, TB rate increased significantly to 144 per 100,000 in patients treated with infliximab and 35 cases per 100,000 in patients treated with etanercept.[100]

Before starting the treatment with TNF-α inhibitors, patients should be mandatory tested for active TB and the LTBI tests should be performed. Besides obligatory chest X-ray examination the recommendations for which test to use in order to detect LTBI vary depending on the country regulations.

In four low incidence countries (Germany, France, Austria, and Switzerland), TST is recommended only exceptionally and IGRAs are usually performed.

Other low TB incidence countries recommend the use of both TST and IGRAs either at the same time or alternatively, meaning IGRAs if TST is positive (in Spain and Norway) or IGRAs if TST is negative (Canada and Italy).[101]

The global approach of TB prevention in low TB incidence countries depends on control and managing the disease in high-risk groups. It is also of the utmost significance to enable the health system to recognize and diagnose the TB case as early as possible. This requires high awareness of the physicians that TB is possible in any and every patient.

CASE STUDY (FIGS. 1 TO 3)

A 24-year-old patient was treated with infliximab for the serious form of Crohn's disease.
He was also treated with azathioprine at the same time (dose of 125 mg daily).
After 4 months of the therapy, he experienced high temperature, dry cough, weight loss.

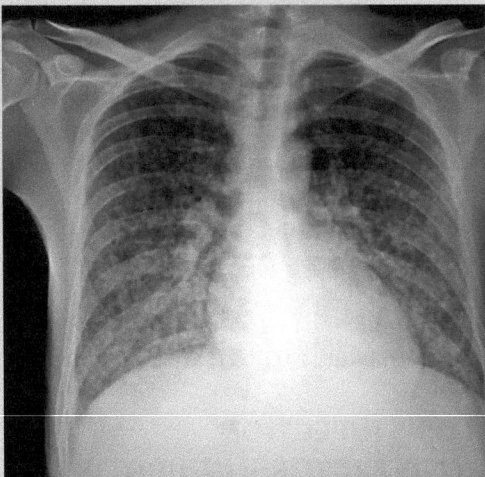

FIG. 1: Chest X-ray lesions resembling miliary tuberculosis infection.

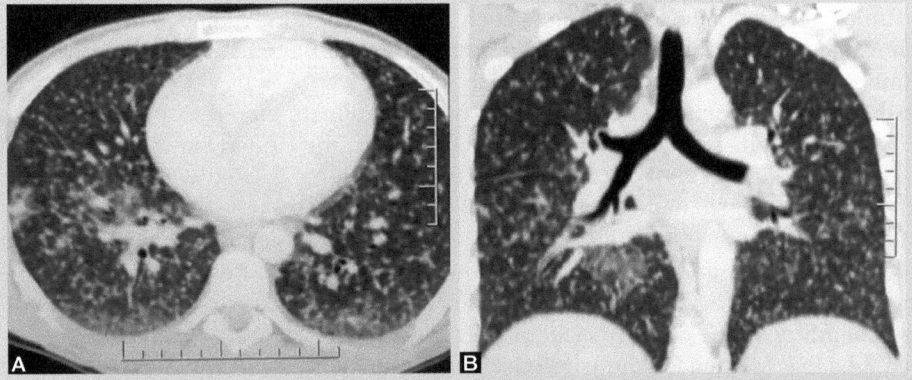

FIG. 2: A and **B,** Thoracic computed tomography presenting typical small nodules and parenchymal lesions resembling miliary tuberculosis.

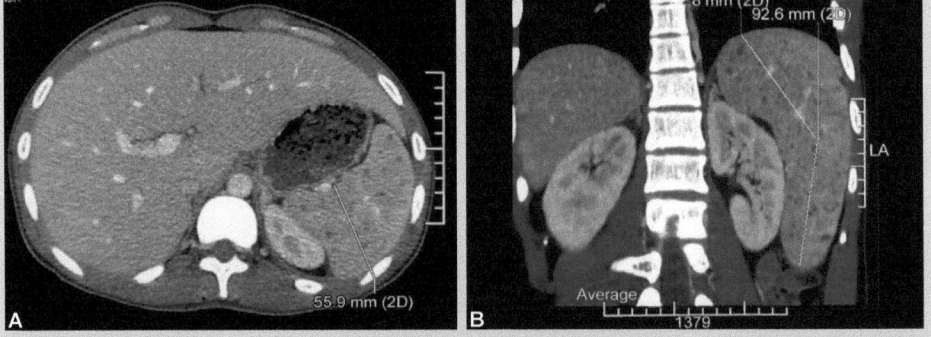

FIG. 3: A, Abdominal scans with enlargement of liver and spleen (spleen with nodular lesions); **B,** The bone marrow biopsy showed necrotic (caseous) granulomas due to tuberculosis infection.

REFERENCES

1. World Health Organization. Global tuberculosis control: WHO report 2011. [online] Available from www.who.int/tb/publications/global_report/en/ index.html. [Accessed February, 2016].
2. Raviglione M, Marais B, Floyd K, et al. Scaling up of interventions to achieve global tuberculosis control: progress and new developments. Lancet. 2012;379:1902-13.
3. Charalambous S, Grant AD, Moloi V, et al. Contribution of reinfection to recurrent tuberculosis in South African gold miners. Int J Tuberc Lung Dis. 2008;12:942-8.
4. Verver S, Warren RM, Beyers N, et al. Rate of reinfection tuberculosis after successful treatment is higher than rate of new tuberculosis. Am J Respir Crit Care Med. 2005;171:1430-5.
5. Andrews JR, Noubary F, Walensky RP, Cerda R, Losina E, Horsburgh CR. Risk of progression to active tuberculosis following reinfection with Mycobacterium tuberculosis. Clin Infect Dis. 2012;54:784-91.
6. Warren RM, Victor TC, Streicher EM, et al. Patients with active tuberculosis often have different strains in the same sputum specimen. Am J Respir Crit Care Med. 2004;169:610-4.
7. den Boon S, van Lill SW, Borgdorff MW, et al. High prevalence of tuberculosis in previously treated patients, Cape Town, South Africa. Emerg Infect Dis. 2007;13:1189-94.
8. Marais BJ, Obihara CC, Warren RW, Schaaf HS, Gie RP, Donald PR. The burden of childhood tuberculosis: a public health perspective. Int J Tuberc Lung Dis. 2005;9:1305-13.
9. Tostmann A, Kik SV, Kalisvaart NA, et al. Tuberculosis transmission by patients with smear-negative pulmonary tuberculosis in a large cohort in the Netherlands. Clin Infect Dis. 2008;47:1135-42.
10. Sinfield RL, Nyirenda M, Hayes S, Molyneux EM, Graham SM. Risk factors for TB infection and disease in young childhood contacts in Malawi. Ann Trop Paediatr. 2006;26:205-13.
11. Kenyon TA, Creek T, Laserson K, et al. Risk factors for transmission of Mycobacterium tuberculosis from HIV-infected tuberculosis patients, Botswana. Int J Tuberc Lung Dis. 2002;6:843-50.
12. Cotton MF, Schaaf HS, Lottering G, et al. Tuberculosis exposure in HIV-exposed infants in a high-prevalence setting. Int J Tuberc Lung Dis. 2008;12:225-7.
13. Schaaf HS, Michaelis IA, Richardson M, et al. Adult-to-child transmission of tuberculosis: household or community contact? Int J Tuberc Lung Dis. 2003;7:426-31.
14. Verver S, Warren RM, Munch Z, et al. Proportion of tuberculosis transmission that takes place in households in a high-incidence area. Lancet. 2004;363:212-4.
15. Riley RL, Mills C, O'Grady F, Sultan LU, Wittstadt F, Shivpuri DN. Infectiousness of air from a tuberculosis ward. Ultraviolet irradiation of infected air: comparative infectiousness of different patients. Am Rev Respir Dis. 1962;85:511-25.
16. Dharmadhikari AS, Mphahlele M, Stolz A, et al. Surgical face masks worn by patients with multi-drug resistant tuberculosis: impact on infectivity of air on a hospital ward. Am J Respir Crit Care Med. 2012;185:1104-9.
17. Trunz BB, Fine P, Dye C. Effect of BCG vaccination on childhood tuberculous meningitis and miliary tuberculosis worldwide: a meta-analysis and assessment of cost-effectiveness. Lancet. 2006;367:1173-80.
18. Mack U, Migliori GB, Sester M, et al. LTBI: latent tuberculosis infection or lasting immune responses to M. tuberculosis? A TBNET consensus statement. Eur Respir J. 2009;33:956-73.
19. Fitzgerald DW, Desvarieux M, Severe P, Joseph P, Johnson WD Jr, Pape JW. Effect of post-treatment isoniazid on prevention of recurrent tuberculosis in HIV-1-infected individuals: a randomised trial. Lancet. 2000;356:1470-4.
20. Marais BJ, Gie RP, Schaaf HS, et al. The natural history of childhood intra-thoracic tuberculosis: a ritical review of literature from the pre-chemotherapy era. Int J Tuberc Lung Dis. 2004;8:392-402.
21. Chintu C, Mudenda V, Lucas S, et al. Lung diseases at necropsy in African children dying from respiratory illnesses: a descriptive necropsy study. Lancet. 2002;360:985-90.
22. Gomez VF, Andersen A, Wejse C, et al. Impact of tuberculosis exposure at home on mortality in children under 5 years of age in Guinea-Bissau. Thorax. 2011;66:163-7.
23. World Health Organization. Global tuberculosis control 2009. Geneva: WHO; 2009.
24. EBPG Expert Group on Renal Transplantation. European best practice guidelines for renal transplantation. Section IV: Long-term management of the transplant recipient. IV.7.2. Late infections. Tuberculosis. Nephrol Dial Transplant. 2002;17 Suppl 4:39-43.
25. Stefan DC, Kruis AL, Schaaf HS, Wessels G. Tuberculosis in oncology patients. Ann Trop Paediatr. 2008;28:111-6.

26. Violari A, Cotton MF, Gibb DM, et al. Early antiretroviral therapy and mortality among HIV-infected infants. N Engl J Med. 2008;359:2233-44.
27. Akolo C, Adetifa I, Shepperd S, Volmink J. Treatment of latent tuberculosis infection in HIV infected persons. Cochrane Database Syst Rev. 2010;(1):CD000171.
28. World Health Organization. (2011). Guidelines for intensified tuberculosis case-finding and isoniazid preventive therapy for people living with HIV in resource-constrained settings. [online] Available from http://whqlibdoc.who.int/publications/2011/9789241500708_eng.pdf. [Accessed February, 2016].
29. Boyles TH, Maartens G. Should tuberculin skin testing be a prerequisite to prolonged IPT for HIV-infected adults? Int J Tuberc Lung Dis. 2012;16:857-9.
30. International Union Against Tuberculosis and Lung Disease. Implementing collaborative TB-HIV activities: a programmatic guide. [online] Available from www.theunion.org/index.php/en/resources/scientific-publications/item/2091-implementing-collaborative-tb-hiv-activities-a-programmatic-guide. [Accessed February, 2016].
31. Chan YC, Yosipovitch G. Suggested guidelines for screening and management of tuberculosis in patients taking oral glucocorticoids: an important but often neglected issue. J Am Acad Dermatol. 2003;49:91-5.
32. Ferrara G, Murray M, Winthrop K, et al. Risk factors associated with pulmonary tuberculosis: smoking, diabetes and anti-TNF-α drugs. Curr Opin Pulm Med. 2012;18:233-40.
33. Webb EA, Hesseling AC, Schaaf HS, et al. High prevalence of Mycobacterium tuberculosis infection and disease in children and adolescents with type 1 diabetes mellitus. Int J Tuberc Lung Dis. 2009;13:868-74.
34. Centers for Disease Control and Prevention, National Center for HIV/AIDS, Viral Hepatitis, STD, and TB Prevention. Prevention and control of tuberculosis in correctional and detention facilities: recommendations from CDC. Endorsed by the Advisory Council for the Elimination of Tuberculosis, the National Commission on Correctional Health Care, and the American Correctional Association. MMWR Recomm Rep. 2006;55:1-44.
35. Al-Darraji HA, Kamarulzaman A, Altice FL. Isoniazid preventive therapy in correctional facilities: a systematic review. Int J Tuberc Lung Dis. 2012;16:871-9.
36. Menzies D, Joshi R, Pai M. Risk of tuberculosis infection and disease associated with work in health care settings. Int J Tuberc Lung Dis. 2007;11:593-605.
37. Claassens MM, Sismanidis C, Lawrence KA, et al. Tuberculosis among community-based health care researchers. Int J Tuberc Lung Dis. 2010;14:1576-81.
38. Bjartveit K. Olaf Scheel and Johannes Heimbeck: their contribution to understanding the pathogenesis and prevention of tuberculosis. Int J Tuberc Lung Dis. 2003;7:306-11.
39. Kruk A, Gie RP, Schaaf HS, Marais BJ. Symptom-based screening of child tuberculosis contacts: improved feasibility in resource-limited settings. Pediatrics. 2008;121:e1646-52.
40. Cain KP, Kimberly D, McCarthy MM, et al. An algorithm for tuberculosis screening and diagnosis in people living with HIV. N Engl J Med. 2010;362:707-16.
41. Getahun H, Kittikraisak W, Heilig CM, et al. Development of a standardized screening rule for tuberculosis in people living with HIV in resource-constrained settings: individual participant data meta-analysis of observational studies. PLoS Med. 2011;8:e1000391.
42. World Health Organization. Guidance for national tuberculosis programmes on the management of tuberculosis in children. [online] Available from http://whqlibdoc.who.int/hq/2006/WHO_HTM_TB_2006.371_eng.pdf. [Accessed February, 2016].
43. World Health Organization. Toward zero deaths. Prevention of childhood TB. Guidance for national tuberculosis programmes on the management of tuberculosis in children. World Health Organization and International Union Against Tuberculosis and Lung Disease.
44. Smieja MJ, Marchetti CA, Cook DJ, Smaill FM. Isoniazid for preventing tuberculosis in non-HIV infected persons. Cochrane Database Syst Rev. 2000;2:CD001363.
45. National Tuberculosis Controllers Association; Centers for Disease Control and Prevention. Guidelines for the investigation of contacts of persons with infectious tuberculosis. MMWR Recomm Rep. 2005;54:1-47.
46. Frigati LJ, Kranzer K, Cotton MF, Schaaf HS, Lombard CJ, Zar HJ. The impact of isoniazid preventive therapy and antiretroviral therapy on tuberculosis in children infected with HIV in a high tuberculosis incidence setting. Thorax. 2011;66:496-501.

47. Madhi SA, Nachman S, Violari A, et al. Primary isoniazid prophylaxis against tuberculosis in HIV-exposed children. N Engl J Med. 2011;365:21-31.
48. Spyridis NP, Spyridis PG, Gelesme A, et al. The effectiveness of a 9-month regimen of isoniazid alone versus 3- and 4-month regimens of isoniazid plus rifampin for treatment of latent tuberculosis infection in children: results of an 11-year randomized study. Clin Infect Dis. 2007;45:715-22.
49. Ena J, Valls V. Short-course therapy with rifampicin plus isoniazid, compared with standard therapy with isoniazid, for latent tuberculosis infection: a meta-analysis. Clin Infect Dis. 2005;40:670-6.
50. Centers for Disease Control and Prevention. Recommendations for use of an isoniazid-rifapentine regimen with direct observation to treat latent Mycobacterium tuberculosis infection. MMWR Morb Mortal Wkly Rep. 2011;60:1650-3.
51. Marais BJ, Ayles H, Graham SM, Godfrey-Faussett P. Screening and preventive therapy for tuberculosis. Chest Clin N Am. 2009;30:827-46.
52. Gao XF, Wang L, Liu GJ, et al. Rifampicin plus pyrazinamide versus isoniazid for treating latent tuberculosis infection: a meta-analysis. Int J Tuberc Lung Dis. 2006;10:1080-90.
53. Magdorf K, Arizzi-Rusche AF, Geiter LJ, O'Brien RJ, Wahn U. Compliance and tolerance of new antitubercular short-term chemopreventive regimens in childhood—a pilot project. Pneumologie. 1994;48:761-4.
54. Priest DH, Vossel LF Jr, Sherfy EA, Hoy DP, Haley CA. Use of intermittent rifampin and pyrazinamide therapy for latent tuberculosis infection in a targeted tuberculin testing program. Clin Infect Dis. 2004;39:1764-71.
55. Sterling TR, Villarino ME, Borisov AS, et al. Three months of rifapentine and isoniazid for latent tuberculosis infection. N Engl J Med. 2011;365:2155-66.
56. Hill PC, Rutherford ME, Audas R, van Crevel R, Graham SM. Closing the policy-practice gap in the management of child contacts of tuberculosis cases in developing countries. PLoS Med. 2011;8:e10001105.
57. Macintyre CR, Plant AJ, Hendrie D. The cost-effectiveness of evidence-based guidelines and practice for screening and prevention of tuberculosis. Health Econ. 2000;9:411-21.
58. Warren RM, Streicher EM, Gey van Pittius NC, et al. The clinical relevance of mycobacterial pharmacogenetics. Tuberculosis. 2009;89:199-202.
59. Mukinda FK, Theron D, van der Spuy GD, et al. Rise in rifampicin-monoresistant tuberculosis in Western Cape, South Africa. Int J Tuberc Lung Dis. 2012;16:196-202.
60. Schaaf HS, Marais BJ. Management of multidrug-resistant tuberculosis in children: a survival guide for paediatricians. Paediatr Respir Rev. 2011;12:31-8.
61. Schaaf HS, Gie RP, Kennedy M, Beyers N, Hesseling PB, Donald PR. Evaluation of young children in contact with adult multidrug-resistant pulmonary tuberculosis: a 30-month follow-up. Pediatrics. 2002;109:765-71.
62. van der Werf MJ, Langendam MW, Sandgren A, Manissero D. Lack of evidence to support policy development for management of contacts of MDR-TB patients: two systematic reviews. Int J Tuberc Lung Dis. 2012;16:288-96.
63. European Center for Disease Prevention and Control. Management of contacts of MDR-TB and XDR-TB patients. [online] Available from http://ecdc.europa.eu/en/publications/Publications/201203-Guidance-MDR-TB-contacts.pdf. [Accessed February, 2016].
64. World Health Organization. Guidelines for the programmatic management of drug-resistant tuberculosis. 2011 update. http://whqlibdoc.who.int/publications/2011/9789241501583_eng.pdf. [Accessed February, 2016]..
65. World Health Organization. Global tuberculosis report 2014. [online] Available from http://www.who.int/tb/publications/global_report/en/. [Accessed February, 2016].
66. Mor Z, Migliori GB, Althomsons SP, Loddenkemper R, Trnka L, Iademarco MF. Comparison of tuberculosis surveillance systems in low-incidence industrialised countries. Eur Respir J. 2008;32:1616-24.
67. Diagnostic Standards and Classification of Tuberculosis in Adults and Children. This official statement of the American Thoracic Society and the Centers for Disease Control and Prevention was adopted by the ATS Board of Directors, July 1999. This statement was endorsed by the Council of the Infectious Disease Society of America, September 1999. Am J Respir Crit Care Med. 2000;161(4 Pt 1):1376-95.
68. Tuberculosis in the UK: Annual report on tuberculosis surveillance in the UK, 2010. London: Health Protection Agency Centre for Infections; 2010.

69. Moore-Gillon J, Davies PD, Ormerod LP. Rethinking TB screening: politics, practicalities and the press. Thorax. 2010;65:663-5.
70. Thorpe LE, Laserson K, Cookson S, et al. Infectious tuberculosis among newly arrived refugees in the United States. N Engl J Med. 2004;350:2105-6.
71. Maloney SA, Fielding KL, Laserson KF, et al. Assessing the performance of overseas tuberculosis screening programs: a study among US-bound immigrants in Vietnam. Arch Intern Med. 2006;166:234-40.
72. Andersen P, Doherty TM, Pai M, Weldingh K. The prognosis of latent tuberculosis: can disease be predicted? Trends Mol Med. 2007;13:175-82.
73. Schluger NW. Advances in the diagnosis of latent tuberculosis infection. Semin Respir Crit Care Med. 2013;34:60-6.
74. Hwang LY, Grimes CZ, Beasley RP, Graviss EA. Latent tuberculosis infections in hard-to-reach drug using population-detection, prevention and control. Tuberculosis (Edinb). 2009;89 Suppl 1:S41-5.
75. Andersen P, Munk ME, Pollock JM, Doherty TM. Specific immune-based diagnosis of tuberculosis. Lancet. 2000;356:1099-104.
76. Hauck FR, Neese BH, Panchal AS, El-Amin W. Identification and management of latent tuberculosis infection. Am Fam Physician. 2009;79:879-86.
77. Hardy AB, Varma R, Collyns T, Moffitt SJ, Mullarkey C, Watson JP. Cost-effectiveness of the NICE guidelines for screening for latent tuberculosis infection: the QuantiFERON-TB Gold IGRA alone is more cost-effective for immigrants from high burden countries. Thorax. 2010;65:178-80.
78. Canadian Tuberculosis Committee. Recommendations on interferon gamma release assays for diagnosis of latent tuberculosis infection. An Advisory Committee Statement (ACS). CCDR. 2010;36(ACS-5):1-22.
79. ECDC. Use of interferon-gamma release assays in support of TB diagnosis. Stockholm: European Centre for Disease Prevention and Control; 2011. [online] Available from http://ecdc.europa.eu/en/publications/Publications/1103_GUI_IGRA.pdf. [Accessed February, 2016].
80. Gordin FM, Masur H. Current approaches to tuberculosis in the United States. JAMA. 2012;308:283-9.
81. Simpson T, Fox J, Crouse K, Field K. Screening for Mycobacterium tuberculosis using an interferon-gamma release assay. J Public Health Manag Pract. 2012;18:E19-25.
82. Pinto LM, Grenier J, Schumacher SG, Denkinger CM, Steingart KR, Pai M. Immunodiagnosis of tuberculosis: state of the art. Med Princ Pract. 2012;21:4-13.
83. Chiappini E, Fossi F, Bonsignori F, Sollai S, Galli L, de Martino M. Utility of interferon-γ release assay results to monitor anti-tubercular treatment in adults and children. Clin Ther. 2012;34:1041-8.
84. Diel R, Goletti D, Ferrara G, et al. Interferon-γ release assays for the diagnosis of latent Mycobacterium tuberculosis infection: a systematic review and meta-analysis. Eur Respir J. 2011;37:88-99.
85. National Collaborating Centre for Chronic Conditions. Tuberculosis: clinical diagnosis and management of tuberculosis, and measures for its prevention and control. Clinical guideline no. 117. London: National Institute for Health and Clinical Excellence (NICE); 2011.
86. Mandalakas AM, Detjen AK, Hesseling AC, Benedetti A, Menzies D. Interferon-gamma release assays and childhood tuberculosis: systematic review and meta-analysis. Int J Tuberc Lung Dis. 2011;15:1018-32.
87. Zwerling A, Behr MA, Verma A, Brewer TF, Menzies D, Pai M. The BCG World Atlas: a database of global BCG vaccination policies and practices. PLoS Med. 2011;8:e1001012.
88. Fine PE. Bacille Calmette-Guérin vaccines: a rough guide. Clin Infect Dis. 1995;20:11-4.
89. Fine PE, Carneiro IA, Milstien J, Clements JC. Issues relating to the use of BCG in immunization programmes: a discussion document. Geneva: World Health Organization; 1999.
90. Manissero D, Lopalco PL, Levy-Bruhl D, Ciofi Degli Atti ML, Giesecke J. Assessing the impact of different BCG vaccination strategies on severe childhood TB in low-intermediate prevalence settings. Vaccine. 2008;26:2253-9.
91. Altes HK, Dijkstra F, Lugnér A, Cobelens F, Wallinga J. Targeted BCG vaccination against severe tuberculosis in low-prevalence settings: epidemiologic and economic assessment. Epidemiology. 2009;20:562-8.
92. Pacific Health Summit. (2011). The challenges of developing new tuberculosis vaccines. [online] Available from http://www.pacifichealthsummit.org/downloads/mdr-tb/The%20Challenges%20of%20Developing%20New%20Tuberculosis%20Vaccines.pdf. [Accessed February, 2016].
93. Horsburgh CR Jr, O'Donnell M, Chamblee S, et al. Revisiting rates of reactivation tuberculosis: a population-based approach. Am J Respir Crit Care Med. 2010;182:420-5.

94. Schaberg T, Bauer T, Castell S, et al. Recommendations for therapy, chemoprevention and chemoprophylaxis of tuberculosis in adults and children. German Central Committee against Tuberculosis (DZK), German Respiratory Society (DGP). Pneumologie. 2012;66:133-71.
95. Migliori GB, Sotgiu G, D'Ambrosio L, et al. TB and MDR/XDR-TB in European Union and European Economic Area countries: managed or mismanaged? Eur Respir J. 2012;39:619-25.
96. European Centre for Disease Prevention and ControlWHO Regional Office for Europe. Tuberculosis surveillance and monitoring in Europe 2012. Stockholm: European Centre for Disease Prevention and Control; 2012.
97. CDC. Reported tuberculosis in the United States, 2010. Atlanta, GA: US Department of Health and Human Services, CDC; 2011.
98. Burman WJ, Reves RR. How much directly observed therapy is enough? Am J Respir Crit Care Med. 2004;170:474-5.
99. Fraser A, Paul M, Attamna A, Leibovici L. Drugs for preventing tuberculosis in people at risk of multiple-drug-resistant pulmonary tuberculosis. Cochrane Database Syst Rev. 2006;(2):CD005435.
100. Wallis RS, Broder MS, Wong JY, Hanson ME, Beenhouwer DO. Granulomatous infectious diseases associated with tumor necrosis factor antagonists. Clin Infect Dis. 2004;38:1261-5.
101. Denkinger CM, Dheda K, Pai M. Guidelines on interferon-γ release assays for tuberculosis infection: concordance, discordance or confusion? Clin Microbiol Infect. 2011;17:806-14.

INDEX

Page numbers followed by *b* refer to box, *f* refer to figure, *fc* refer to flowchart, and *t* refer to table.

A

Abdomen
  computed tomography scan of 140, 181*f*
  ultrasound 72
Abscess formation 63*f*
Acid-fast bacilli 5, 5*f*, 57, 64, 69*f*, 70*f*, 77, 106, 135, 157, 172, 180, 190, 207, 215, 258
  smears, microscopy of 6*t*
Acquired immune deficiency syndrome 77, 170, 105, 128, 226, 287, 298
Acute respiratory distress syndrome 134
Adalimumab 230
Addison's disease 135
Adenopathy
  bilateral hilar 178*f*
  intrathoracic 103*f*
  ipsilateral hilar 98*f*
Adenosine deaminase 90, 158-160, 207
  and lysozyme, estimation of 90
  levels, diagnostic utility of 144
Adrenaline 86
Adverse drug reactions 282
Adynamia 173
Airway
  fistulas 81
    benign 85
      occlusion of 84
  peripheral 54*f*
  stenosis 87
Alcohol use 249
Alcoholism, chronic 281
Alkaline phosphatase levels 132
Alopecia 286
  drug-induced 286
American Thoracic Society 42, 44
Amikacin 16, 200, 284
Amoxicillin 194, 196, 270, 285
Amplified molecular tests 65
Ancillary diagnostic tests 66
Anemia 97, 134
Animacula 128
Anorexia 97, 173, 206, 223
Antigens, mycobacterial 115

Antirejection drugs 35
Antiretroviral therapy 27, 70, 197
Anti-T-cell antibodies 119
Anti-tuberculosis
  chemotherapy 298
  drugs 185, 187, 217, 266, 267, 281, 283, 286
    adverse effects of 281, 287
    causative 282
    common adverse effects 284*t*
    dosages 218*t*, 284*t*
    first line 268*t*, 281, 282*t*, 283*t*
    major side effects 218*t*
    second-line 283
  therapy 136
  treatment 69*f*, 147, 165*f*, 215, 302
Anti-tumor necrosis factor 27, 35, 257
Argon plasma coagulation 81, 85*f*
Artery
  bronchial 86
  pulmonary 131
Arthralgia 286
Arthritis 182*f*
  rheumatoid 231
Asbestosis 171
Aspartate aminotransferase 132
Aspergilloma 107, 299, 303
Aspergillosis 58, 59*f*, 231
  chronic pulmonary 107, 108, 109*f*
Aspergillus fungus 303
Aspirates 172
Aspiration, bronchial 79
Asthma, history of 100*f*
Atrial septostomy catheters 85
Auramine 5, 208
Autoimmune disease 292
Axial contrast enhanced computed
  tomography 69*f*
Azaindoles 271

B

Bacillus calmette-guérin 1, 41, 129
  vaccinated populations 162
  vaccination 66, 307, 314
    role of 149

Bacterial cellular membrane 293
Bacterial infection 107, 109f
  symptoms of 216
Balloon dilatation 81, 83, 83f
Bedaquiline 194, 196, 201, 271, 285-287
Berylliosis 64
Biochemistry tests 301
Biopsy
  bronchial 3, 81
  endobronchial 79-81, 87
  role of 143
  tissue, joint sensitivity of 158
Blood 3
  gas analysis 143
  sugar 301
Body fluid evaluation 212
Body mass index 301
Bone marrow biopsy 316f
Borborygmi 216
Bovine tuberculosis 1
Bowel habits, altered 216
Brain, magnetic resonance imaging of 235f
Breast, abscess of 227
Bronchial brushing 79
Bronchial stenosis 299
  balloon dilatation of 83f
Bronchiectasis 58, 102f, 107, 108, 236f, 238f, 299
Bronchoesophageal fistula 82, 84, 85
  computed tomography image of 86f
Broncholithiasis 97
Bronchopneumonia, caseous 51f
Bronchoscopic methods 80t, 87t
Bronchoscopy 56, 78, 79, 91
  conventional 77, 78
  interventional 77, 81
Brucellosis 64, 132, 160

C

Calmette-guérin strains 10
Cancers 292
Capreomycin 16, 284
Carbon monoxide, diffusion capacity for 142
Cardiovascular disease 110, 292
Cartridge based nucleic acid amplification test 213, 215
Casein hydrolysate 7
Caseous necrosis, small areas of 177f
Cat-scratch lymphadenitis 64
Cavitary formation 53f
Cell
  membrane 5
  types 291

Centers for Disease Control and Prevention 2, 44, 91, 310
Central nervous system 131, 133, 200, 214, 227, 283
  disorders of 284
Centrifugation 4
Centrilobular nodules, reactivation tuberculosis of 101f
Cepheid geneXpert 66
Cerebral
  cortex 214
  edema 214
Cerebrospinal fluid 3, 200, 208
Cervical
  lymph node 63f, 70f
  tuberculosis, complications of 63f
  lymphadenitis, mycobacterial 62
  lymphadenopathy 72
Chemoprophylaxis 223
Chest
  computed tomography 68f, 101, 180f, 236f, 237f, 240f
  scans 263f
  contrast-enhanced computed tomography of 140f
  multislice computed tomography of 178f
  radiograph 68f, 70f, 138f, 180f, 263f
  X-ray 39, 51f, 53f, 178f, 234f, 236f, 237f, 239f, 240f
  lesions 316f
Chlamydia pneumonia 160
Cholecalciferol 291
Choroidal tubercles 145
Chromatography, gas-liquid 11
Chronic obstructive pulmonary disease 110
Cilastatin 196
Clarithromycin 194, 196, 285
Classical miliary pattern 136f
Clavulanate 194, 196, 285
Clavulanic acid 270
Clofazimine 194, 196, 270, 285
Clostridium difficile colitis 284
Coagulation 301
Collapse-consolidation lesions 219
Combination therapy 310
Computed tomography scan 54, 55f, 99f-102f, 157f, 262f
Congenital infection, symptoms of 216
Conjunctiva 62
Connective tissue diseases 231
Consilium 270
Corticosteroids 35, 54, 175, 230
  role of 219

Corynebacterium 6
Cough 98*f*-100*f*, 156*f*, 206, 223
   productive 171
Craniocaudal propagation 236*f*
C-reactive protein 97
Critical drug concentration 189
Cryotherapy 81, 84, 85*f*
Cryptococcosis 231
Cyanoacrylate glue, bronchoscopic injection of 86
Cyclophosphamide 230
Cycloserine 196, 200, 222, 270, 284
Cystic fibrosis 259

D

Dangerous addiction 243
Delamanid 194, 196, 271, 285-287
Deoxyribonucleic acid 1, 5, 65, 78
Diabetes 130, 232, 252, 292
   insulin dependent 309
   mellitus 51, 112, 113, 113*t*, 115, 115*b*, 229, 269, 281
      controlled 96
      higher risk of 112
Diarrhea 286
Diarylquinoline 201
Dihydro-nitroimidazooxazole 271
Diospyros
   ebenum 243
   melanoxylon 243
Directly observed therapy 195
   strategy 22
Directly observed treatment short-course 77, 266, 306
Disease-modifying drugs 27
Disseminated *Mycobacterium avium* complex disease 260
Dithiothreitol plus 4
Dizziness 284, 286
Dragging sensation 133
Drug
   abusers 314
   interactions 281
   lymphocyte stimulation test 282
   reaction 287
   resistant tuberculosis 13, 22, 200, 222, 270, 311
      causes of 187
      emergence of 306
      infection 188
      management of 196, 209
      risk factors of 187
      treatment of 198*t*, 200, 218*t*, 269

sensitive tuberculosis, treatment of 218*t*
susceptibility testing 15, 188, 189, 193, 209, 269
   limitations of 194
   methods 192*t*
Dry bronchiectasis 107
Dry cough 101*f*, 157*f*
Dysphagia 67
Dyspnea 97, 156

E

Electrocautery 81
Electrolyte 301
   disturbances 137
   metabolism 288
Emphysema, subcutaneous 136
Empyema 303
   mixed 107
Endobronchial tuberculosis 83*f*, 87, 88*f*, 105, 106*f*, 206
   types of 87
Endobronchial ultrasound 67, 81, 82
   guided transbronchial needle aspiration 80, 87
Enteritis 132
Enzyme
   drug-metabolizing 288
   linked immunospot assay 313
Eosinophilia 287
Epithelioid cells 176*f*, 177*f*
Epitheloid hystiocytes 238*f*
Ergocalciferol 291
Erythrocytes 179*f*
Estimated tuberculosis
   incidence rates 23*f*
   mortality rates 24*f*
Etanercept 230
Ethambutol 185, 191, 218, 222, 268, 270, 281-283
Ethionamide 16, 196, 200, 222, 270, 284
Extensive pulmonary destruction 56*f*, 58, 107, 108*f*
Extensively drug-resistant tuberculosis 185, 186, 188, 192*t*, 195, 199, 200*b*, 201
   regimen 199
   treatment of 270*t*
Eye disorders 286

F

Fatigue 156*f*
Febrile episodes 157*f*
Fever 52, 100*f*, 165, 173, 223
   mild 206

Fiberoptic bronchoscopy 143
Fibrinogen 86
Fibroblasts 176f
Fibrocavitary
 disease, adult type 211f
 lung disease 258
Fibrotic lesions 42
Fibrotic tissues 299
Fine needle aspiration cytology 64, 70f, 214
Fistula
 bronchopleural 82, 299
 esophagomediastinal 67
 tracheoesophageal 67
Fixed drug combinations
 place of 219
 therapy 287
Flexible bronchoscopy 78
Fluorescent staining 208
Fluorochrome stained smears 5
Fluoroquinolones 191, 201, 269, 270
Fluoroscopy 89
Forced vital capacity 142
Forecasting drug adverse effects 288
Fungal infection 64
 respiratory 171
Fungus 1

G

Gallium scintigraphy 141
Gamma-interferon 161
Gangrene, pulmonary 58
Gastrectomy 35
Gastric
 aspirates 213
 lavage 3, 5, 208
Gastrointestinal discomfort 284
Gastrointestinal intolerance 282
Gatifloxacin 196
Giant multinucleated cells 176f, 177f
Gingiva 62
Glycemic control, worsening of 171
Gram-ghost 5
Gram-neutral bacilli 5
Granulie curable 145
Granulie d'Empis 145
Granuloma 34, 238f
 formation of 231
 necrotic 316f
 tuberculous 179f
Granulomatous disease 1, 132
Granulomatous pathology 82
Granulomatous tissues 85f
Guinea pigs 37

H

Hallucinations 284
Headache 284
Heart 137
Helper T-cell 113
Hematogenous dissemination 133
Hemodialysis 35
Hemoptysis 58, 81, 82, 98f, 99f, 107, 302
 bronchoscopic interventions for 86
 low-grade 107
 massive 109f, 299
 mild 107
Hepatic injury, risk of 42
Hepatitis
 B surface antigen 181
 toxic 111, 282
Hepatosplenomegaly 223
High performance liquid chromatography 11
Highly active antiretroviral therapy 70
Histoplasmosis 132, 231
Hot tub lung disease 258
Human immunodeficiency virus 22, 24f, 27, 28, 35, 41, 51, 63, 67, 77, 96, 102, 103f, 128, 146, 170, 199, 205, 225, 228, 249, 257, 269, 298
 disease, late stage 78
 infection 26, 102, 111, 130, 146, 170, 226, 306
  course of 259
  treatment of 46
 negative 42, 70, 282
 positive 36, 38, 42, 227
 related disease 23
 seronegative 63
 status, positive 67
Hybridization assays, solid phase 13
Hydrocephalus 216, 273
Hypergammaglobulinemia 97
Hyperhemia 88f
Hyperkalemia 135
Hyperparathyroidism 230
Hypersensitivity 258, 284
Hypertension, pulmonary 301
Hyperuricemia 286
Hypoalbuminemia 97
Hypocholesterolemia 149
Hyponatremia 97, 135
Hypotension 135
Hypothyroidism 286
Hypoxia 34

I

Imipenem 194, 196
Immune system 25

Immunity, adaptive 112
Immunochromatographic tests 11
Immunodeficient states, clinical spectrum of 225*fc*
Immunosuppressive agents 129
Immunosuppressive therapy 225
Infarction 214
Infections 292
    prevention of 307
    risk of 307
Infectious agents 108
Infectious disease 22, 160, 170
Infectious Diseases Society of America 67
Inflammation, granulomatous 57
Infliximab 230
Innate immune system 293
Interferon-gamma release assay 16, 33, 37, 39, 41, 66, 90, 102, 162, 212, 312, 313
    role of 142
Interleukin 113
Isoniazid 44, 185, 193, 200, 209, 218, 268, 281-283, 310, 311
    acetylation status 288
    high dose 196
    monotherapy 310
    prophylaxis 232
Isotonic saline lavage 86

J

Jejunal bypass surgery 35

K

Kanamycin 200, 201, 222, 284
Ketoacidosis 229
Ketosis, development of 229
Kidney 134, 177*f*, 288, 301
    abscess of 227
    disease, chronic 35, 230
    insufficiency, chronic 51

L

Lactate dehydrogenase, estimation of 90
Langhans cells 176*f*, 177*f*
Langhans type, giant cells of 238*f*
Laser photoresection 81
Latent tuberculosis 33, 43, 44*t*, 111, 116
    diagnosis of 33, 39*fc*, 142
    infection 26, 33, 39, 102, 142, 247, 248, 312, 313
Lavage
    bronchial 79
    bronchoalveolar 3, 79, 80, 87, 131, 208

Leprosy 64
Leukemia 231
Leukocytosis 97, 288
Levofloxacin 196, 202, 222
    adverse effects of 284
Lidocaine 79
Ligase chain reaction 90
Line-probe assays 191
Linezolid 16, 194, 196, 270, 285
Lipopolysaccharide 293
Listeriosis 231
Liver 132, 301
    abscess of 227
    biochemical disturbances 288
    cirrhosis 281
    disease, chronic 281
    enlargement of 316*f*
    enzymes 148
    toxicity 281, 282
Lobectomy
    first 298
    plus minor resection 301
Low glucose concentration 158
Löwenstein-Jensen medium 9*f*, 209
Lung 179*f*
    abscesses 171
    cancer 105*f*
    decortications of 301
    disease
        chronic 174
        inflammatory 303
        parenchymal 97
    hemorrhage 300
    malignancies 171
    parenchyma 234*f*, 236*f*, 238*f*
    resection of 300
    transplant 118
Lymph node 61, 69*f*, 70*f*
    axillary 227
    biopsy 64
    bronchial 50
    enlargement 51*f*, 181*f*
    intra-abdominal 227
    intrathoracic 89, 227
    left hilar 70*f*
    mediastinal 68*f*, 69*f*
    pulmonary hilar 179*f*
    regional 206
    retroperitoneal 227
    right hilar 69*f*
    suprasternal 69*f*
    tuberculosis 61, 214
        nontuberculous 71

Lymphadenitis 62
  granulomatous 182f
  retroperitoneal 132
Lymphadenopathy 223
  abdominal 216
  mediastinal 178f
  paratracheal 70f, 210f
  tuberculous 89
Lymphocytes 176f, 177f
  atypical 287
Lymphocytopenia, severe 149
Lymphogranuloma venereum 64
Lymphohematogenous dissemination 214
Lymphoma 64, 160, 171

M

Macrolides 271
Macrophages 217
Malaise 165
Malignancy 228
  hematological 35
Malignant diseases, treatment of 225
Malnutrition 230, 281
Mantoux procedure 35
Massive pleural adhesions 273
Measles 205
Mediastinal lymphadenitis, diagnosis of 67
Meningitis, tuberculous 133
Meningoencephalitis 273
Meropenem 194, 196, 270
Metabolic disorders 97, 229
Metabolic syndrome 292
Metallic stents, expandable 84
Methotrexate 230, 231
Microabscesses, multiple 136
Miliary nodules 138f, 140f
Miliary tuberculosis 86, 128-132, 132t, 134,
    135-138, 137t, 139, 144, 146, 148, 207, 210f,
    235f, 316f
  diagnosis of 86, 104
  epidemiology of 129
  infection 316f
  pathogenesis of 130fc, 133
Molecular methods 12, 13, 90
Molecular tests 57, 65
Monoresistance 311
Morphozinamide 185
Moxifloxacin 196, 202, 287
Multidrug-resistant tuberculosis 29, 29f, 43,
    185, 186, 192t, 269, 270t, 299, 314
  development of 311
  diagnosis of 188
  presumptive 194

regimen 196
second-line drugs in 283
treatment 195, 201, 300
Multiple scar formation 63f
Mycobacteria 159, 284
  cell wall 4
  disease, pulmonary nontuberculous 257
  isolation of 64
Mycobacterial stain and culture 159
Mycobacterium 11, 13, 141, 144, 257
  africanum 1, 2, 10
  avium 258
    intracellulare complex 62, 79, 226
  bovis 1, 7
  canetti 2
  caprae 2
  chelonae 10
  complex 228
  drug-resistant 118, 147
  flavescens 313
  kansasii 38, 62, 258, 313
    infection 258
  leprae 1
  marinum 10, 38, 313
  microti 2
  nontuberculous 257
  pinnipedii 2
  riyadhense 38
  scrofulaceum 62, 258
  szulgai 38, 313
  tuberculosis 1, 2, 7, 10, 10f, 13, 15, 17, 33,
      34, 37, 45, 46, 56, 57, 61, 62, 64, 65, 71,
      87, 96, 112, 113, 113t, 115, 129, 130, 157,
      162, 163, 171, 172, 185, 186, 189, 190,
      205, 212, 215, 217, 229, 232, 244, 267,
      267b, 268, 269, 293, 298, 300, 306, 313
    colonies 9f
    complex 1, 189, 257
    culture of 190
    detection of 12, 13, 228
    direct test 12
    identification of 10, 12
    in vitro 226
    infection 66, 91, 252, 291, 293-295, 306,
        313
    microbiology of 1
    replication 50
    specific antigens 33
    test 12
    transmission 307
  xenopi 258
Mycoplasma 160
Myopathy 292

N

N-acetyl-l-cysteine 4
N-acetyltransferase type 2 genotyping 288
National Institute for Clinical Excellence 40, 44
National Tuberculosis Programs on Management of Tuberculosis, guidance for 309*fc*
Nausea 281
Negative predictive value 41
Neodymium-doped yttrium-aluminum-garnet 303
Neuropathy, peripheral 221, 282
Neutropenia 283
New anti-tuberculosis drugs
  common adverse effects 286*t*
  dosages 286*t*
Night fever 98*f*
Night sweats 52, 97, 99*f*, 156
Nocardia 6
Nodular bronchiectatic disease 258
Non-Hodgkin's lymphoma 231
Nonsteroidal anti-inflammatory drugs 221
Nontuberculous mycobacteria 1, 41, 57, 61, 62, 190, 257, 312
  disease 260, 270
    conservative treatment of 260, 260*t*
    diagnosis of 259
  infection 66, 102, 259
  lung diseases 257
Nuclear imaging techniques 141
Nucleic acid amplification 57, 65, 104, 162
  based techniques 12
  tests 11, 112, 162, 207

O

Ofloxacin 16
Optic neuritis 282
Oral anti-tuberculosis drugs, second-line 284*t*
Oral reserve drugs 285*t*
Organ transplantation 233
Oropharyngeal mucosa 62

P

Pain
  abdominal 132
  chest 157*f*
  colicky abdominal 216
Pancreas, posterior of head of 181*f*
Para-aminosalicylate sodium 196
Para-aminosalicylic acid 196, 270, 284
Paradoxical reaction 67
Paradoxical worsening 70*f*, 164
Parenchymal lesions 316*f*
Pediatric tubercular lymphadenopathy, diagnosis of 215*fc*
Pelvis 72
Peptide nucleic acids 6
Perfusion lung scintigraphy 301
Pericarditis, constrictive 273
Pericardium 227
Peripheral blood mononuclear cells 17
Peritonitis 132
Pertussis 205
Phenomena 40
Phototoxic reactions, mild 285
Piringer-Kuchinka lymphadenopathy 64
Pleura 227
Pleural biopsy 163
Pleural effusion 206, 212*f*
  bilateral 138*f*
Pleural fluid
  analysis 157
  characteristics 158
  cultures 159
  elevated 158
Pleurectomy 301
Pleuritic chest pain 53, 165
Pleuropneumonectomy 301
Pneumoconiosis 139
Pneumocystis
  carinii 226
  jirovecii 148
Pneumolysis, extrapleural 301
Pneumomediastinum 136, 137
Pneumonectomy 298, 301
Pneumonia 171
  lower lobe 211*f*
Pneumothorax 58, 107, 108*f*, 136
  artificial 298
  left-sided 136*f*
Pneumotomy 298
Polymerase chain reaction 65, 80, 90
  role of 144
Positive predictive value 41
Posteroanterior chest radiograph 99*f*, 100*f*-103*f*, 109*f*, 108*f*, 157*f*, 165*f*, 166*f*
Pott's disease 273
Pregnancy 135
Preventive therapy
  options 310
  target groups 308
Proinflammatory cytokines 34
Prothionamide 16, 196, 200, 201, 270, 284
Pseudoinfections 91
Psoriasis 231
Puerperium 135

Pulmonary disease 61, 104, 257
Pulmonary function
  development of 232
  tests, role of 142
Pulmonary tuberculosis 52, 53f, 54, 77, 96, 111, 114, 116, 209, 245, 294, 298
  diagnosis of 172, 207, 213fc
  elective surgical treatment of 302
  infection 55f
  postoperative management 303
  sequel of 304
Purified protein derivative 1, 35
Pus 172
Pyrazinamide 185, 198, 200, 217, 218, 222, 266, 268, 270, 274, 281-283, 311
  analogs 271
  testing 194
Pyrexia of unknown origin 134
Pyridoxine 272
  role of 219

Q

Q fever 160

R

Radius, distal parts of 182f
Randomized controlled trials 149
Rapid acetylator 288
Rapid immunochromatographic tests, performance of 10
Rasmussen's aneurysm 97, 107
Real-time polymerase chain reaction assay 14
Renal disease, chronic 174
Renal failure 221
  reversible 281
Renal insufficiency 232
  chronic 229
Respiratory distress mimicking asthma 206
Respiratory failure
  acute 149
  signs of 239
Respiratory infection, upper 171
Respiratory specimens 3
Respiratory symptoms 52
  analysis of 173
Revised National Tuberculosis Control Program 208, 218t
Rhodamine 5
Rhodococcus species 6
Ribonucleic acid 5
Rifabutin 16, 284

Rifampicin 13, 44, 185, 191, 193, 201, 209, 221, 268, 281-283, 310, 311
  monotherapy 311
  resistant tuberculosis 185
Rifampin 162, 217, 218
Rifapentine 311
  long-acting 310
Ruthenium 271

S

Salivary glands 62
Sanatoriums 272
Sarcoidosis 64, 132, 139
Serpentine cord 10f
Serum alkaline phosphatase 227
Serum bilirubin, elevated 132
Shock 221
Short-course chemotherapy 266
Silicosis 35, 171
Single nucleotide polymorphisms 288
Skin 133, 227
  abnormalities 287
  abscess of 227
  induration 36
  lesions 133
  rash 282
  reaction 37
    false-positive 102
  tests 159
Smoking and tuberculosis 243, 244
  disease 245
Sodium hydroxide 4
Soft tissue 227
Solid culture media 7
Solid organ transplant 117, 118
Sparfloxacin 267
Spleen 132, 316f
  enlargement of 316f
Sputum smear
  and culture 172
  microscopy 301
    and culture, role of 142
  negative
    disease 12
    thoracic tuberculosis 80t
  positive disease 306
Sputum test 111
Statoacoustic nerve damage 282
Stenosis
  incomplete 84
  tracheal 84f
Stent placement 81, 83
Steroids, role of 148

Stevens-Johnson syndrome 221
Streptomycin 209, 218, 268, 281, 282
Submandibular nodes 214
Swelling, glandular 61
Syndrome of inappropriate antidiuretic
    hormone secretion 97
Syphilis 64

T

Tendon rupture 284
Terizidone 196, 270, 284
Tetracaine 79
Thioacetazone 194, 196
Thiophene-2-carboxylic acid hydrazide 9
Thioridazine 272
Thoracic computed tomography 316f
Thoracic surgery 298
Thoracic tuberculosis 79, 81, 87t
    complications, management of 82t
Thoracomyoplasty 301
Thoracoplasty, extrapleural 301
Thoracoscopy 163
Thoracostomy 298
Thorax, axial computed tomography 69f
Thrombin 86
Thrombocytopenia 221
Thyroid 135
Tissue
    biopsy 3, 172
    transplantation 232
Tobacco
    cessation 252
    smoke 246, 275
        environmental 250
    usage 243
Tonsils 62
Toxoplasma lymphadenitis 64
Trachea, edematous mucosa of 106f
Tracheobronchial malacia 83
Tracheobronchial stenosis 81, 82
    management of 81
Traction diverticula, development of 85
Transbronchial biopsy 79, 80, 81, 87
Transbronchial needle aspiration 79, 80, 87
Tubercle bacilli 157, 217
Tuberculin reactivity 247
Tuberculin skin test 16, 26, 35, 36, 39, 40t, 41,
    66, 102, 142, 205, 210, 216, 308, 312
    method 36f
    positive 33
Tuberculin units 36
Tuberculoma 55, 55f, 78, 89, 105f, 216
    diagnosis of 89
    pulmonary 105, 109f

Tuberculosis 22, 24f, 28, 39, 52f, 55f, 58, 61,
    77, 84f, 96, 103f, 110, 112, 113, 117, 128,
    155, 170, 174, 185, 205, 213, 215, 219, 225,
    226, 228, 229, 232, 246, 251f, 252, 253f,
    291, 294
  abdominal 216
  active 111, 116
    pulmonary 96, 116
  acute miliary 145
  bacilli 206
  bilateral cavitary pulmonary 109f
  bronchogenic 96, 105
  bronchoscopic biopsy revealed 106f
  care and control, global progress in 22t
  cavity 59f
    large 100f
    typical 99f
  central nervous system 214
  characteristics of 115b
  childhood 205
  chronic bilateral multicavitary 108f
  clinically unrecognized 170
  coinfection 27
  complications of 58, 58t, 82, 273
  congenital 216
  control, different levels of 307
  cutis miliaris acuta generalisata 133
  death 248
  diagnosis 50, 64, 70f, 77b, 171, 227
    methods for 190
  disease 22, 52, 247
    postprimary 52, 53
  drug resistance patterns 186t
  during bronchoscopy, transmission of 91
  effusion 155
  epidemiology of 22
  extrapulmonary 61, 213, 246
  extrathoracic 214
  granulomas 235f
  granulomatous reactions, staining of 104
  immunodiagnostic tests for 16
  immunopathology of 45
  in pregnancy 110, 269
  in solid organ transplant recipients 117
  incidence of 113
  infection 43, 52, 54f, 56, 57, 316f
    clinical manifestations of 50
    healed primary 52f
    less nosocomial 78
    rate of 314
    risk of 315
    symptoms of 54
  infiltrates 97

intrathoracic 86, 206
laboratory 2
  diagnosis of 1
latent 33
lesions 103*f*
lower
  lobe cavitary 100*f*
  lung field 54, 100
low-incidence 312
lung lesion 99*f*
lymph node 61, 62
lymphadenitis 61, 82, 89, 214
  management of 71
management of 298
mortality 247
multicavitary 108*f*
natural history of 112*f*
new cases of 29*f*
osteoarticular 216
pleural 109*f*
presentations, atypical 54
prevalence of 24
prevention 306, 312, 314
primary 50, 51*f*, 96, 97, 210*f*
progressive 56*f*
  primary 211*f*
rapid diagnosis of 90
reactivation 53, 96, 98, 207
relapse, history of 102*f*
related deaths 28
risk factors for 110
self-reported 246
surgery for 303
toward personalized treatment of 288
tracheobronchial 106*f*
treatment 111, 228, 266, 267*b*
  major historical landmarks of 266*t*
worldwide, prevalence of 25
Tuberculostearic acid, estimation of 90
Tuberculous disease 247
Tuberculous infection 249, 252
Tuberculous lymphadenitis 62-64, 70
  development of 62
Tuberculous pleural
  disease 165*f*
    history of 166*f*
  effusions, diagnosis of 157, 164*t*
Tuberculous pleuritis 155, 156, 158
  treatment of 164
Tularemia lymphadenitis 64
Tumor necrosis factor-alpha 309
  inhibitors 315
Tumor-like lesion 105*f*

U

Ulna, distal parts of 182*f*
Upper lobe infiltration 100
Ureas 271
Uric arthritis 282
Urine 3, 172
Uropathy, obstructive 273

V

Vasculitis 214
Visual impairment 221
Vitamin
  B6 272
  C 272
    status 272
  D 272, 273, 291, 295
    biochemistry and metabolism 291
    biologic system 295
    catabolism of 293
    chemical structure of 291, 292*f*
    deficiency 230
    effect of 293
    endocrine system, role of 291
    immunomodulatory effects of 293
    metabolic activation of 291
    receptor 291
    responsive elements 292
    role of 293
    status 294
    supplementation 294
    treatment 294
  D2 291
  D3 272, 291
  supplementation 272
Vomiting 216

W

Watanabe spigots 85
Weakness 156
"Weigert" tubercle 129
Weight loss 101*f*, 156, 156*f*, 206, 223
World Health Organization 44, 110, 307
  Recommended Grouping of Anti-Tuberculosis Drugs 195*t*

Y

Yersinia lymphadenitis 64

Z

Ziehl-Neelsen method 5*f*
Ziehl-Neelsen stain 208

Printed by Libri Plureos GmbH in Hamburg, Germany